Master Techniques in Orthopaedic Surgery

Soft Tissue Surgery

First Edition

Master Techniques in Orthopaedic Surgery

Editor-in-Chief

Bernard F. Morrey, MD

Founding Editor

Roby C. Thompson, Jr., MD

Volume Editors

Surgical Exposures
Bernard F. Morrey, MD
Matthew C. Morrey, MD

The Hand
James Strickland, MD
Thomas Graham, MD

The Wrist
Richard H. Gelberman, MD

The Elbow
Bernard F. Morrey, MD

The Shoulder
Edward V. Craig, MD

The Spine
David S. Bradford, MD
Thomas L. Zdeblick, MD

The Hip
Robert L. Barrack, MD

Reconstructive Knee Surgery
Douglas W. Jackson, MD

Knee Arthroplasty
Paul A. Lotke, MD
Jess H. Lonner, MD

The Foot & Anke
Harold B. Kitaoka, MD

Fractures
Donald A. Wiss, MD

Pediatrics
Vernon T. Tolo, MD
David L. Skaggs, MD

Soft Tissue Surgery
Steven L. Moran, MD
William P. Cooney III, MD

Master Techniques in Orthopaedic Surgery

Soft Tissue Surgery

First Edition

Editors
Steven L. Moran
William P. Cooney III

Wolters Kluwer | Lippincott
Health | Williams & Wilkins

Acquisitions Editor: Robert Hurley
Managing Editor: David Murphy, Jr.
Developmental Editor: Keith Donnellan
Marketing Manager: Sharon Zinner
Project Manager: Paula C. Williams
Designer: Doug Smock
Production Services: Maryland Composition, Inc.

First Edition

Library of Congress Cataloging-in-Publication Data

Soft tissue surgery / editors, Steven L. Moran and William P. Cooney III. — 1st ed.
    p. ; cm. — (Master techniques in orthopaedic surgery)
  Includes bibliographical references.
  ISBN 978-0-7817-6368-4
  1. Soft tissues injuries—Surgery. 2. Extremities (Anatomy)—Surgery. I. Moran, Steven L. II. Cooney, William Patrick, 1943– III. Series: Master techniques in orthopaedic surgery (3rd ed.)
  [DNLM: 1. Soft Tissue Injuries—surgery. 2. Extremities—surgery. 3. Skin Transplantation.
4. Surgical Flaps. 5. Vacuum. WO 700 S6815 2007]
  RD93.S66 2007
  617.4'7--dc22

                                                              2007031773

Care has been taken to confirm the accuracy of the information present and to describe generally accepted practices. However, the authors, editors, and publisher are not responsible for errors or omissions or for any consequences from application of the information in this book and make no warranty, expressed or implied, with respect to the currency, completeness, or accuracy of the contents of the publication. Application of this information in a particular situation remains the professional responsibility of the practitioner; the clinical treatments described and recommended may not be considered absolute and universal recommendations.

The authors, editors, and publisher have exerted every effort to ensure that drug selection and dosage set forth in this text are in accordance with the current recommendations and practice at the time of publication. However, in view of ongoing research, changes in government regulations, and the constant flow of information relating to drug therapy and drug reactions, the reader is urged to check the package insert for each drug for any change in indications and dosage and for added warnings and precautions. This is particularly important when the recommended agent is a new or infrequently employed drug.

Some drugs and medical devices presented in this publication have Food and Drug Administration (FDA) clearance for limited use in restricted research settings. It is the responsibility of the health care provider to ascertain the FDA status of each drug or device planned for use in their clinical practice.

To purchase additional copies of this book, call our customer service department at **(800) 638-3030** or fax orders to **(301) 223-2320**. International customers should call **(301) 223-2300**.

Visit Lippincott Williams & Wilkins on the Internet: http://www.lww.com. Lippincott Williams & Wilkins customer service representatives are available from 8:30 am to 6:00 pm, EST.

To my mother and father, Nancy and Albert Lawrence Moran.
—The journey of a thousand miles begins with the first step.—

Steven Moran, MD

To my wife Mickey and family. They allowed me to take and
shared in taking "the one less traveled by, and that has made all
the difference."

WP Cooney, MD

Contents

Series Preface

Since its inception in 1994, the *Master Techniques in Orthopaedic Surgery* series has become the gold standard for both physicians in training and experienced surgeons. Its exceptional success may be traced to the leadership of the original series editor, Roby Thompson, whose clarity of thought and focused vision sought "to provide direct, detailed access to techniques preferred by orthopaedic surgeons who are recognized by their colleagues as 'masters' in their specialty," as he stated in his series preface. It is personally very rewarding to hear testimonials from both residents and practicing orthopaedic surgeons on the value of these volumes to their training and practice.

A key element of the success of the series is its format. The effectiveness of the format is reflected by the fact that it is now being replicated by others. An essential feature is the standardized presentation of information replete with tips and pearls shared by experts with years of experience. Abundant color photographs and drawings guide the reader through the procedures step by step.

The second key to the success of the *Master Techniques* series rests in the reputation and experience of our volume editors. The editors are truly dedicated "masters" with a commitment to share their rich experience through these texts. We feel a great debt of gratitude to them and a real responsibility to maintain and enhance the reputation of the *Master Techniques* series that has developed over the years. We are proud of the progress made in formulating the third edition volumes and are particularly pleased with the expanded content of this series. Six new volumes will soon be available covering topics that are exciting and relevant to a broad cross-section of our profession. While we are in the process of carefully expanding *Master Techniques* topics and editors, we are committed to the now-classic format.

The first of the new volumes will be *Relevant Surgical Exposures*, which I will edit. The second new volume is *Essential Procedures in Pediatrics.* Subsequent new topics to be introduced are *Soft Tissue Reconstruction, Management of Peripheral Nerve Dysfunction, Advanced Reconstructive Techniques in the Joint,* and finally *Essential Procedures in Sports Medicine.* The full library thus will consist of 16 useful and relevant titles.

I am pleased to have accepted the position of series editor, feeling so strongly about the value of this series to educate the orthopaedic surgeon in the full array of expert surgical procedures. The true worth of this endeavor will continue to be measured by the ever-increasing success and critical acceptance of the series. I remain indebted to Dr. Thompson for his inaugural vision and leadership, as well as to the *Master Techniques* volume editors and numerous contributors who have been true to the series style and vision. As I indicated in the preface to the second edition of *The Hip* volume, the words of William Mayo are especially relevant to characterize the ultimate goal of this endeavor: "The best interest of the patient is the only interest to be considered." We are confident that the information in the expanded *Master Techniques* offers the surgeon an opportunity to realize the patient-centric view of our surgical practice.

Bernard F. Morrey, MD

Preface

Over the past 30 years options for the soft tissue management of traumatic defects have increased with an improved understanding of pedicled flaps, the advent of microsurgery, and the development of negative pressure sponge therapy. Wound complications have decreased due to advances in antibiotic therapy and better debridement techniques. Improved knowledge of surgical anatomy has helped develop surgical incisions which provide better exposure while preserving regional blood supply. Despite these advances, there is still a need for every surgeon to know the techniques of debridement, soft tissue management, and proper incision placement—for these are the foundation of successful surgery.

The educational goal of this text is to demonstrate how to avoid wound problems and how to cover wound problems if they should occur. Chapters illustrate pertinent anatomy, indications and contraindications for specific incisions, and methods for flap coverage in cases of soft tissue loss. Step-by-step accounts of the technical details are provided to carry out these exposures and procedures so that readers will feel they are watching over the shoulder of the contributing author in the operating room. Contributors are experienced in both soft tissue and bony management. Though all surgeons may not feel comfortable with performing all procedures presented in this book, they will at least know what they can expect or request during specialist consultation. This volume of the *Master Techniques in Orthopaedic Surgery* series focuses on the management of the soft tissues as they relate to orthopaedic trauma, but is a text designed for all traumatologists, orthopaedic surgeons, plastic surgeons, and anyone who has had the pleasure (or displeasure) of taking care of a difficult wound.

Steven L. Moran, MD
William P. Cooney III, MD

Acknowledgments

The creation of this text was the result of a tremendous effort of many people. Lippincott, Williams & Wilkins has provided us with incredible resources and a dedicated and knowledgeable staff. We are deeply indebted to the team of Robert Hurley, Executive Editor; Dave Murphy, Managing Editor; Keith Donnellan, Developmental Editor; and Kristen Spina, Editorial Project Manager. We also are deeply indebted to our medical illustrator Wendy Beth Jackelow, who has provided countless hours of work bringing the surgeons' sketches to life. We would also like to thank Dr. Bernard Morrey for giving us the opportunity to write this book. Finally, we are deeply indebted to our coauthors who have provided insightful, organized, and beautifully illustrated chapters explaining the techniques involved in these reconstructive procedures. It is through their hard work that we are able to provide you with this text.

Steven Moran and William P. Cooney

Contributors

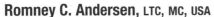

Romney C. Andersen, LTC, MC, USA
Assistant Chief, Orthopaedic Surgery Service
Walter Reed National Military Medical Center
Bethesda, Maryland

Louis C. Argenta, MD
Professor and Chairman Emeritus
Department of Plastic and Reconstructive Surgery
Wake Forest Medical Center
Winston-Salem, North Carolina

Kodi K. Azari, MD, FACS
Chief, Mercy Hospital of Pittsburgh Division of Hand
Surgery
Director, Hand Surgery Fellowship
University of Pittsburgh School of Medicine
Pittsburgh, Pennsylvania

Alessio Baccarani, MD
Fellow, Division of Plastic, Reconstructive, Maxillofacial,
and Oral Surgery
Duke University Medical Center
Durham, North Carolina

Allen T. Bishop, MD
Chair, Division of Hand Surgery
Department of Orthopaedic Surgery
Mayo Clinic
Rochester, Minnesota

William J. Casey III, MD
Mayo Clinic Arizona
Phoenix, Arizona

Kuang-Te Chen, MD
Attending Surgeon
Department of Plastic and Reconstructive Surgery
Chang Gung Memorial Hospital
Taipei, Taiwan

Emilie Cheung
Orthopaedic Surgery
Stanford University
Stanford, California

Kevin C. Chung, MD, MS
Professor, Division of Plastic Surgery
University of Michigan
Ann Arbor, Michigan

Michael P. Clare, MD
Director of Fellowship Education
Foot and Ankle Fellowship
Florida Orthopaedic Institute
Tampa, Florida

Henry D. Clarke, MD
Assistant Professor of Orthopaedic Surgery
Mayo Clinic College of Medicine
Rochester, Minnesota

Damon Cooney, MD
Resident, Department of Plastic Surgery
Southern Illinois University
Springfield, Illinois

William P. Cooney III, MD
Professor Emeritus
Department of Orthopaedic Surgery
Mayo Medical School
Rochester, Minnesota

Anthony DeFranzo, MD
Wake Forest University School of Medicine
North Carolina Baptist Hospital
Winston-Salem, North Carolina

Matthew DeOrio, MD
Foot and Ankle Fellow
Duke University Medical Center
Durham, North Carolina

Seth D. Dodds, MD
Assistant Professor, Hand and Upper Extremity Surgery
Department of Orthopaedics and Rehabilitation
Yale University School of Medicine
New Haven, Connecticut

Scott F. M. Duncan, MD
Assistant Professor
Mayo Medical School
Consultant, Owatonna Clinic
Mayo Health System
Owatonna, Minnesota

Bassem T. Elhassan, MD
Assistant Professor and Consultant of Orthopaedic Surgery
Mayo Clinic
Rochester, Minnesota

David Elliot, MA (Oxon), BM, BCh
Consultant and Plastic Hand Surgeon
St. Andrew's Centre for Plastic Surgery
Broomfield Hospital
Chelmsford, England

Robert Esther, MD
Department of Orthopaedic Surgery
Mayo Clinic
Rochester, Minnesota

Jeffrey B. Friedrich, MD
Assistant Professor of Surgery and Orthopaedics
University of Washington
Children's Hospital and Regional Medical Center
Seattle, Washington

Günter Germann, MD, PhD
Professor of Surgery
Department of Plastic, Hand, and Reconstructive Surgery
University of Heidelberg
Heidelberg, Germany

Goetz A. Gessler, MD
Department of Plastic, Hand, and Reconstructive Surgery
University of Heidelberg
Heidelberg, Germany

Douglas P. Hanel, MD
Professor, Hand and Microvascular Surgery
Department of Orthopaedics and Sports Medicine
University of Washington
Seattle, Washington

Thomas F. Higgins, MD
Assistant Professor, Orthopaedic Trauma
Department of Orthopaedic Surgery
University of Utah School of Medicine
Salt Lake City, Utah

John B. Hijjawi, MD
Froedtert Memorial Lutheran Hospital
Milwaukee, Wisconsin

Nathan A. Hoekzema
Department of Orthopaedic Surgery
Mayo Clinic
Rochester, Minnesota

David J. Jacofsky, MD
Chairman
The Core Institute
Sun City West, Arizona

Amir Jamali, MD
Assistant Professor
University of California—Davis
Department of Orthopaedic Surgery
Sacramento, California

Mark H. Jensen, MD
General Surgery Resident
Mayo Clinic
Rochester, Minnesota

Kenji Kawamura, MD, PhD
Assistant Professor
Department of Emergency and Critical Care
Nara Medical University
Nara, Japan

Thomas Kremer
Department of Plastic, Hand, and Reconstructive Surgery
University of Heidelberg
Heidelberg, Germany

W.P. Andrew Lee, MD, FACS
Professor and Chief, Division of Plastic Surgery
University of Pittsburgh School of Medicine
Pittsburgh, Pennsylvania

Salvatore C. Lettieri, MD
Mayo Graduate School of Medicine
Mayo Clinic
Rochester, Minnesota

L. Scott Levin, MD, FACS
Professor of Surgery
Duke University Medical Center
Durham, North Carolina

Lawrence C. Lin, MD
Plastic Surgery Fellow
Division of Plastic and Reconstructive Surgery
Mayo Clinic
Rochester, Minnesota

Susan E. Mackinnon
Shoenberg Professor and Chief
Division of Plastic and Reconstructive Surgery
Washington University School of Medicine
St. Louis, Missouri

Samir Mardini, MD
Associate Professor of Surgery
Department of Plastic Surgery
Mayo Clinic
Rochester, Minnesota

Patricia L. McKay, CDR, MC, USN
Residency Director
National Capital Consortium
National Naval Medical Center
Walter Reed Army Medical Center
Washington, DC

Bradley Medling
Plastic Surgery Institute
Southern Illinois University School of Medicine
Springfield, Illinois

Steven L. Moran, MD
Associate Professor of Orthopaedics and Plastic Surgery
Department of Plastic Surgery
Mayo Clinic
Rochester, Minnesota

Steven Myerthall, BPE, BSC, MD, FRCSC
The Core Institute
John C. Lincoln Deer Valley Hospital
Sun City West, Arizona

George Nanos, MD
US Navy
Oak Harbor Naval Hospital
Oak Harbor, Washington

Jason Nascone, MD
Assistant Professor
University of Maryland School of Medicine
RA Cowley Shock Trauma Center
Baltimore, Maryland

Michael W. Neumeister, MD
Professor and Chairman
Division of Plastic Surgery
SIU School of Medicine
Springfield, Illinois

Gustavo S. Oderich, MD
Assistant Professor of Surgery
Mayo Clinic College of Medicine
Rochester, Minnesota

Katrim Palm-Bröking, MD
Department of Plastic, Hand, and Reconstructive Surgery
University of Heidelberg
Heidelberg, Germany

Marco Rizzo, MD
Associate Professor of Orthopaedic Surgery
Mayo Clinic
Rochester, Minnesota

Christopher J. Salgado, MD
Assistant Professor of Surgery
Division of Plastic Surgery
Cooper University Hospital
Camden, New Jersey

Roy W. Sanders, MD
Chief, Orthopaedic Trauma Service
Florida Orthopaedic Institute
Tampa, Florida

Michael Sauerbier, MD, PhD
Associate Professor, University of Heidelberg
Department of Plastic, Hand, and Reconstructive Surgery
University of Heidelberg
Heidelberg, Germany

S. Andrew Sems, MD
Department of Orthopaedic Surgery
Mayo Clinic
Rochester, Minnesota

Alex Senchenkov, MD
Clinical Instructor
Department of Otolaryngology—Head and Neck Surgery
University of Cincinnati
Cincinnati, Ohio

Alexander Y. Shin, MD
Professor and Consultant
Division of Hand Surgery
Department of Orthopaedic Surgery
Rochester, Minnesota

Thomas C. Shives
Professor of Orthopaedic Surgery
Mayo Clinic
Rochester, Minnesota

Franklin H. Sim, MD
Professor of Orthopaedics
Mayo Clinic
Rochester, Minnesota

Mark J. Spangehl, MD
Assistant Professor of Orthopaedics
Mayo Clinic College of Medicine
Mayo Clinic Arizona
Phoenix, Arizona

John W. Sperling, MD, MBA
Department of Orthopaedic Surgery
Mayo Clinic
Rochester, Minnesota

Scott Steinmann, MD
Associate Professor
Department of Orthopaedic Surgery
Mayo Clinic
Rochester, Minnesota

Timothy M. Sullivan
Professor of Surgery
Division of Vascular Surgery, Gonda Vascular Center
Mayo Clinic
Rochester, Minnesota

Shian Chao Tay, MD, MS
Assistant Professor of Orthopaedics
Mayo Clinic
Rochester, Minnesota

Lam Chuan Teoh, FRCS
Clinical Associate Professor, Hand Surgery
Singapore General Hospital
Singapore

Huey Y. Tien
Clinical Instructor of Surgery
University of Louisville School of Medicine
Louisville, Kentucky

Tsu-Min Tsai, MD
Clinical Professor of Orthopaedic Surgery
University of Louisville School of Medicine
Louisville, Kentucky

Norman S. Turner, MD
Assistant Professor
Mayo Graduate School of Medicine
Rochester, Minnesota

Nicholas B. Vedder, MD, FACS
Professor of Surgery and Orthopaedics
Chief, Division of Plastic Surgery
University of Washington
Seattle, Washington

Renata V. Weber, MD
Assistant Professor of Plastic and Reconstructive Surgery
Albert Einstein College of Medicine
Montefiore Medical Center
Bronx, New York

Fu-Chan Wei, MD, FACS
Professor, Department of Plastic Surgery
Chang Gung Memorial Hospital
Dean, Medical College
Chang Gung University
Taipei, Taiwan

Bradon J. Wilhelmi, MD
Professor and Chief Program Director
University of Louisville
Louisville, Kentucky

Eduardo A. Zancolli
National Academy of Medicine
Orthopaedics and Traumatology
Buenos Aires, Argentina

PART I
OVERVIEW AND FOUNDATION

1 Why Wounds Fail to Heal

Mark H. Jensen and Steven L. Moran

Surgical wound complications can be a significant problem resulting in prolonged hospital stay, reoperations, and significant morbidity for our patients. Often the surgeon can predict preoperatively which patients will have problems healing wounds or will need additional soft tissue coverage. Surgical planning should not only include the surgical approach but also an assessment of the patient's healing risks. It is our hope that preoperative risk reduction may avoid wound healing complications.

Prevention of wound healing complications starts with an understanding of the healing process. Risk factors can be recognized and modified. Techniques and practices that are proven to prevent wound infections must be employed. This chapter will focus on understanding wound healing and identifying patients at risk for wound complications; we will also attempt to offer means to minimize risk factors for complications through surgical technique and preoperative planning.

PHASES OF WOUND HEALING

Surgically induced wounds heal in several stages. The wound passes through phases of coagulation, inflammation, matrix synthesis and deposition, angiogenesis, fibroplasia, epithelialization, contraction, and remodeling. These processes have been grouped into three main stages: inflammation, fibroplasia, and maturation. Interruption in any one of these stages can lead to wound healing complications.

The inflammatory phase of wound healing involves cellular responses to clear the wound of debris and devitalized tissue. Increased capillary permeability and leukocyte infiltration occur secondary to inflammatory mediators and vasoactive substances. Polymorphonuclear cells (PMNs) are the first cell population in the wound followed by mononuclear leukocytes which mature into wound macrophages. Inflammatory cells clean the wound of harmful bacteria and devitalized tissue. Adequate tissue oxygen tension is necessary for the release of oxygen free radicals by neutrophils. Following the initial introduction of PMNs into the wound, lymphocytes enter the wound in great number, clearing the wound of old neutrophils and secreting important cytokines and chemoattractants for fibroblasts. Fibronectin and hyaluronate deposition from fibroblasts in the first 24 to 48 hours provides scaffolding for further fibroblast migration (1,2).

The fibroblast proliferation phase starts within the initial 2 to 3 days as large populations of fibroblasts migrate to the wound. Secretion of a variety of substances necessary for wound healing and includes large quantities of glycosaminoglycans and collagen. Ground substance formed from the four main glycosaminoglycans (hyaluronic acid, chondroitin-4-sulfate, dermatan sulfate, and heparin sulfate) acts as an amorphous gel that is necessary for collagen aggregation. Collagen levels rise for approximately 3 weeks corresponding to increasing tensile strength. After 3 weeks the rate of degradation equals the rate of deposition. Angiogenesis is an important aspect of the fibroblast proliferation phase as it helps to support new cells in the healing wound.

The maturation phase starts around 3 weeks and lasts up to 2 years. It is characterized by collagen remodeling and wound strengthening. Collagen is the principal building block of connective tissue and is found in at least 13 different types. Types I to IV are the most common in the human body. Each has a distinct feature and is found in different levels in many tissues. For example, type III collagen is high in hydroxyproline and low in hydroxylysine. It is commonly found in skin, arteries, bowel wall, and healing wounds. Type I collagen is found in skin, tendon, and bone; is low in hydroxylysine content; and is the most common collagen type, accounting for more than 90% of body collagen. Early wounds are comprised of a majority of type III collagen. As the wound matures, type III collagen is replaced by type I collagen. Collagen cross-linking improves tensile strength. There is a rapid increase in strength of the wound by 6 weeks as the wound reaches 70% of the strength of normal tissue. The wound then gradually plateaus to 80% of normal strength, but never returns to preinjury levels.

Wound re-epithelialization occurs as adjacent cells migrate through a sequence of mobilization, migration, mitosis, and cellular differentiation of epithelial cells. Wound contraction starts at about 1 week. It is facilitated by the transformation of certain fibroblasts into myofibroblasts containing α–smooth muscle actin. These cells adhere to the wound margins as well as each other and effect contraction of the wound. These stages are imperative for proper wound healing as interruption of these processes results in chronic wound complications (1,3).

RISK FACTORS

The identification of patients at risk for aberrant wound healing allows the surgeon to make appropriate plans for skin closure technique, flap utilization, and postoperative wound management. This will ideally result in modification of risk factors prior to surgery. In cases of chronic diseases or nonmodifiable risk factors, patients must be informed of increased wound healing risks. The following discussion focuses on commonly encountered risk factors with recommendations to ameliorate their effects.

Diabetes

Patients with diabetes are both more likely to undergo surgery and develop perioperative complications than nondiabetic patients. This leads to longer hospital stay with higher health care costs and increased perioperative mortality. Diabetic patients have increased rates of hypertension, cardiac disease, and renal failure. These factors lead to much higher wound healing complications (3). Diabetes inhibits wound healing through many mechanisms. It is a disease affecting small vessels which are critical in supplying nutrients to the healing wound. Elevated glucose levels also affect a myriad of inflammatory systems. Neutrophil adherence, chemotaxis, phagocytosis, and intracellular bactericidal activity are all impaired. Pseuodhypoxia develops as a result of altered redox reactions and vascular permeability secondary to hyperglycemia. Furthermore, glucose is a proinflammatory mediator stimulating cytokine production and inhibiting endothelial nitric oxide levels (4). This translates clinically into higher infectious complications. *Tight control of glucose in the perioperative period mitigates the postoperative complications seen in the diabetic patient*. This has been found in both the intensive care setting as well as routine operative cases (3,5).

Management of patients with diabetes starts in the pre-operative period. There is good evidence to suggest that a preoperative hemoglobin A1C of less than 7% drastically decreases postoperative infectious complications (4). Physicians should aggressively improve glucose management using diet, oral hypoglycemic agents, and insulin as needed. Perioperative management should include sliding scale insulin or continuous insulin infusion to maintain glucose levels below 150 mg per deciliter (3). Evidence suggests that improved outcomes are possible with tighter control of glucose levels between 80 and 110 mg per deciliter in critically ill patients (5). After dismissal from the hospital, the patient should continue their preoperative diabetic regiment.

Obesity

Obese patients have a higher rate of wound infections, dehiscence, hematomas, seromas, and pressure ulcers (6–8). This is felt to be due to multiple factors including difficulty with the operation, altered immune response, increased tension with closure, increased dead space, decreased microperfusion, and decreased mobility post operatively (9,10). Patients should be encouraged to lose weight prior to elective operations. Increased levels of physical activity preoperatively translates to an improved postoperative rehabilitation process. Successful weight loss is difficult to achieve in most patients. This has prompted some surgeons to recommend gastric bypass surgery prior to certain operations such as joint replacement. This has been associated with improved outcomes in hip replacement patients with morbid obesity (11).

Smoking

Numerous studies have consistently found that smokers have significantly higher rates of wound healing complications than nonsmokers. This is related to several causes including the vasoactive effect of cigarette smoke through the sympathetic alpha receptors, increased levels of carboxyhemoglobin with a reduction in oxygen-carrying capacity, increased platelet activation leading to microangiopathic thrombosis, increased levels of fibrinogen with decreased fibrinolytic activity, endothelial injury, and increased hemoglobin levels leading to increased blood viscosity. Regardless of the mechanism the effect is significant. Complication rates of 2.5% to 6% in nonsmokers versus 7.5% to 49% in smokers are reported in the literature.

The increased risk of wound complications in smokers is most pronounced in cases where a large area of tissue is undermined. This is most likely related to failure of the dermal and subdermal plexus supplying the resultant skin flap (Fig. 1-1). Poor outcome in smokers prompts many clinicians to postpone elective procedures until the patient has quit smoking for at least 3 to 4 weeks, particularly if the procedure involves large areas of undermining (12,13). Aggressive use of smoking cessation

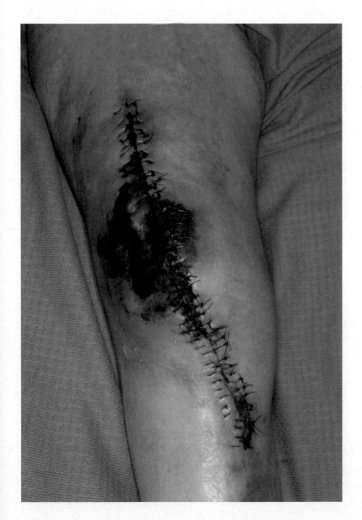

FIGURE 1-1

Following total knee arthroplasty this 76-year-old diabetic smoker developed wound complications necessitating wound debridement and flap coverage.

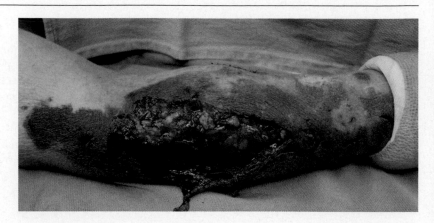

FIGURE 1-2

Chronic steroid use leads to increased skin and vessel fragility. This skin avulsion injury occurred in this 76-year-old steroid dependent man following a fall from a chair.

programs should be implemented. Still, other surgeons feel that this would restrict too many patients from receiving necessary surgery (14,15). We prefer to delay surgery for 4 weeks prior to elective surgical procedures where soft tissue coverage may be an issue and advocate early referral to a nicotine dependence unit. If smoking cessation is not possible, the patient is informed of the likelihood of additional flap coverage for wound closure and a higher likelihood of postoperative wound complications.

Immunosuppressive Medications

Patients with intrinsic or acquired immunodeficiencies are at increased risks for wound healing complications. Patients with MHC class-II deficiency have impaired wound healing because of altered T cell immune function (16). Patient populations at risk for wound healing problems due to altered immune function include patients with hereditary, infectious, and iatrogenic immune deficiencies.

Corticosteroids inhibit wound healing by their anti-inflammatory effect. Decreased numbers of inflammatory cells are noted at the wound site; delays in collagen synthesis, fibroblast proliferation, angiogenesis, wound contracture rates, and epithelial migration are also observed (Fig. 1-2). Vitamin A has been shown to counteract the effects of steroids on wound healing in all areas except wound contraction and infection (17). The exact mechanism is not known, but may be related to the TGF-beta, IGF-I, and hydroxyproline content in the tissue (18). Factors that can help improve wound healing in immunocompromised states include prevention of malnutrition, hypoxia, endocrine disorders, anemia, and other metabolic disorders. Dead tissue, foreign bodies, tissue ischemia, and hematoma should be minimized.

Radiation and Chemotherapy

Radiation and chemotherapy are known to cause delays in wound healing. Operations in irradiated fields are particularly problematic due to dense fibrosis and decreased perfusion caused by small vessel injury (Fig. 1-3). Irradiated fields are more susceptible to infection and delayed healing. Postoperative radiation initiated after the initial 3 to 4 weeks of primary wound healing does not seem to have as marked an effect on wound healing, but can lead to contracture, wound break down, and flap necrosis (21). Neoadjuvant chemotherapy can alter wound healing, especially in cases where chemotherapy has led to neutropenia. Surgery would be ideally delayed until full recovery of platelets and leukocytes. Healing seems to proceed normally in patients who receive their chemotherapy 3 to 4 weeks after surgery, as the wound has been allowed to proceed through the first stages of healing (8,22). Certain chemotherapeutic agents, however, can have a negative effect on wound healing far greater than 4 weeks; for example, Avastin (Bevacizumab), which inhibits vascular endothelial growth factor, has an extremely long half life ranging from day 11 to 50 and has been shown to inhibit wound healing when given in the neoadjuvant setting (23). Surgeons should have a good understanding of specific complications associated with individual chemotherapeutic regiments.

Malnutrition

It has been known for many years that malnutrition has deleterious effects on wound healing. Loss of nutrients alters host immunity through decreased T-cell function, phagocytosis, complement, and antibody levels. Certain patient groups are at particular risk of malnutrition. Severe catabolic states can be induced after multi-system trauma, sepsis, and burns. Significant increases in metabolic rate

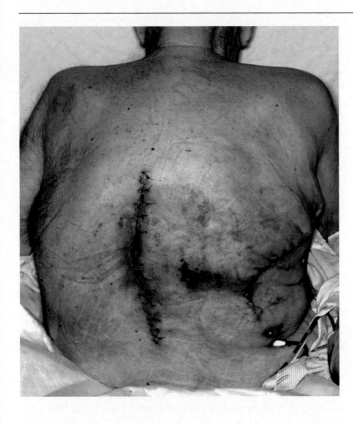

FIGURE 1-3

Signs of trouble in this 80-year-old gentleman who has undergone preoperative radiation with subsequent resection of a spinal tumor and coverage with a latissimus flap. Spinal tumor resection and flap harvest were preformed through separate and parallel incisions. The parallel incision in conjunction with the radiation damage has lead to ischemia within the center portion of skin bridge, which now shows signs of early ischemia with epidermolysis and ulceration.

can also follow uncomplicated abdominal surgery (increase by 10%), uncomplicated injuries such as femoral fracture (20%), peritonitis (40%), and fever (10% for every 1°C above normothermia). This is particularly alarming considering the high portion of trauma patients who are unable to eat for extended periods leading up to and following surgery (24,25).

Assessment of nutritional status becomes an important task for the surgeon. Patients at risk include those with moderate weight loss (10%–20%), severe weight loss (>20%) and serum albumin <3.2 to 2.5 g/dL. Other groups include patients with trauma, burns, gastrointestinal (GI) dysfunction, cancer, fever, and those on chemotherapy. Consideration for preoperative total parenteral nutrition (TPN) should be given to patients who are severely malnourished, however this must be weighted against the risks associated with line infection and liver failure (24). Prealbumin is a laboratory value that can be followed as a surrogate of albumin due to its shorter half life.

Postoperatively patients should be started on a diet as soon as possible. Rapid diet advancement has been shown to decrease postoperative complications and decrease hospital stay (26). In patients who are unable to restart a diet, but have a functioning GI tract, tube feeds should be administered. TPN should be started early on patients who are expected to not tolerate GI feeds. The benefit risk ratio of TPN is equal for patients with normal metabolic demands after 1 week of fasting or inability to take oral intake. Patients with hypermetabolic states can benefit from earlier initiation of TPN (25,26).

Peripheral Vascular Disease

Peripheral artery disease is present in an estimated 0.9% of patients aged 40 to 49 compared with 15% to 29% of patients over the age of 70. Risk factors for the development of PVD include diabetes mellitus, hyperlipidemia, cigarette smoking, and hypertension. Patients at risk for PVD should be screened with blood pressure measurements of the arm and ankle to determine the patient's ankle brachial index; a normal value should produce a ratio >0.9. Symptoms of PVD include claudication, rest pain, atypical leg pain, and ischemic tissue loss. Aggressive lifestyle and risk factor modification is indicated to prevent progression of disease and death from cardiovascular or cerebrovascular events. These patients should undergo cardiac risk evaluation as peri-operative myocardial infarction (MI) and stroke are very common (27).

Wounds in the setting of peripheral vascular disease heal very slowly and can be difficult to manage. Patients with nonhealing wounds in spite of maximal medical management should undergo evaluation for revascularization. Amputation may be considered in the absence of target vessels for revascularization (27). Transcutaneous oxygen measurements in peripheral occlusive disease can be helpful to determine healing potential. TcPO$_2$ levels greater than 30 mm Hg correlate with a high likelihood of healing whereas levels less than 15 mm Hg rarely heal (28,29).

Infection

Surgical site infections are a major impediment to wound healing and contribute to substantial morbidity and mortality. Postoperative infections increase the hospital length of stay by 7 to 10 days and increase charges by $2,000 to $5,000 (30). Rates of surgical infections vary by type of procedure, health of the patient, and skill of the surgeon. Wound classification corresponds with expected rates of infection as follows: clean (1.3%–2.9%), clean-contaminated (2.4%–7.7%), contaminated (6.4%–15.2%), and dirty (5.1%–40%) (6). Other risk factors for the development of postoperative infections include diabetes, obesity, smoking, steroids, malnutrition, colonization with *S. aureus*, preoperative hospitalization, and patient health.

The most important factors which can be used to prevent surgical site infections are timely use of preoperative antibiotics and operative technique. Other practices that are helpful include preoperative showering with antimicrobial soap, scrubbing and draping the patient with sterile drapes, hand washing, gloving, and the use of sterile gowns, masks, and hats by surgical personnel (31). These practices are aimed at reducing the amount of skin associated bacteria. Pathogens are not eliminated because approximately 20% of bacteria reside in the hair follicles and sweat glands where antiseptics do not reach. Although numerous studies have been aimed at identifying the best skin antiseptic, a systematic review failed to show superiority of one antiseptic over another (32).

Preoperative antibiotics administered within 2 hours of incision correlate strongly with the lowest rate of infections. Choices of antibiotics along with common pathogens are listed in Table 1-1. Endocarditis prophylaxis may need to be added in susceptible patients. In spite of clear benefits with the use of preoperative antibiotics, compliance is not perfect. Institutional policies should be constructed to promoting 100% compliance (33).

Hair removal is commonly performed prior to surgical procedures, however most studies have shown that this is not necessary and is associated with an increased risk of surgical site infections (34). If hair removal is preferred, clippers or depilatory creams are safer than shaving and should be used just prior to skin incision. Razors are associated with microtrauma to the skin and should not be used secondary to increased infection rates (35).

TABLE 1-1.   Antimicrobial Prophylaxis for Surgery

Nature of operation	Common pathogens	Recommended Antimicrobials	Adult dosage before surgery[1]
Cardiac	*Staphylococcus aureus, S. epidermis*	cefazolin or cefuroxime OR vancomycin[3]	1–2 g IV[2] 1.5 g IV[2] 1 g IV
Gastrointestinal			
Esophageal, gastroduodenal	Enteric gram-negative bacilli, gram positive cocci	*High risk[4] only:* cefazolin[7]	1–2 g IV
Biliary Tract	Enteric gram-negative bacilli, enterococci, clostridia	*High risk[5] only:* cefazolin[7]	1–2 g IV
Colorectal	Enteric gram-negative bacilli, anaerobes, enterococci	*Oral:* neomycin + erythromycin base[6] OR metronidazole[6] *Parenteral:* cefoxitin[7] OR cefazolin + metronidazole[7] OR ampicillin/sulbactam	1–2 g IV 1–2 g IV 0.5 g IV 3 g IV
Appendectomy, non-perforated[8]	Enteric gram-negative bacilli, anaerobes, enterococci	cefoxitin[7] OR cefazolin + metrodinazole[7] OR ampicillin/sulbactam[7]	1–2 g IV 1–2 g IV 0.5 g IV 3 g IV
Genitourinary	Enteric gram-negative bacilli, enterococci	*High risk only[9]:* ciprofloxacin	500 mg PO or 400 mg IV

(Continued)

TABLE 1-1. Antimicrobial Prophylaxis for Surgery   *Continued*

Nature of operation	Common pathogens	Recommended Antimicrobials	Adult dosage before surgery[1]
Gynecologic and Obstretric			
Vaginal, abdominal or laparoscopic hysterectomy	Enteric gram-negative bacilli, anaerobes, Gp B strep, enterococci	cefoxitin[7] or cefazolin[7] OR ampicillin/sulbactam[7]	1–2 g IV 3 g IV
Cesarean section	same as for hysterectomy	cefazolin[7]	1–2 g IV after cord clamping
Abortion	same as for hysterectomy	*First trimester, high risk[10]:* aqueous penicillin G OR doxycycline *Second Trimester:* cefazolin[7]	2 mill units IV 300 mg PO[11] 1–2 g IV
Head and Neck Surgery			
Incisions through oral or pharyngeal mucosa	Anaerobes, enteric gram-negative bacilli, *S. aureus*	clindamycin + gentamicin OR cefazolin	600-900 mg IV 1.5 mg/kg IV 1–2 g IV
Neurosurgery	*S. aureus, S. epidermis*	cefazolin OR vancomycin[3]	1–2 g IV 1 g IV
Ophthalmic	*S. epidermis, S. aureus,* streptococci, enteric gram-negative bacilli, *Pseudomonas spp.*	gentamicin, tobramycin, ciprofloxacin, gatifloxacin levofloxacin, moxifloxacin, ofloxacin or neomycin-gramicidin-polymyxin B cefazolin	multiple drops topically over 2 to 24 hours 100 mg subconjunctivally
Orthopedic	*S. aureus, S. epidermis*	cefazolin[12] or cefuroxime[12] OR vancomycin[3,12]	1–2 g IV 1.5 g IV 1 g IV
Thoracic (Non-Cardiac)	*S. aureus, S. epidermis,* streptococci, enteric gram-negative bacilli	cefazolin or cefuroxime OR vancomycin[3]	1–2 g IV 1.5 g IV 1 g IV
Vascular			
Arterial surgery involving a prosthesis, the abdominal aorta, or a groin incision	*S. aureus, S. epidermis,* enteric gram-negative bacilli	cefazolin OR vancomycin[3]	1-2 g IV 1 g IV
Lower extremity amputation for ischemia	*S. aureus, S. epidermis,* enteric gram-negative bacilli, clostridia	cefazolin OR vancomycin[3]	1–2 g IV 1 g IV

Reproduced from Antimicrobial prophylaxis for surgery. *Treat Guide Med Lett* 2006;4(52):83–88, with permission.

1. Parenteral prophylactic antimicrobials can be given as a single IV dose begun 60 minutes or less before the operation. For prolonged operations (>4 hours), or those with major blood loss, additional intraoperative doses should be given at intervals 1–2 times the half-life of the drug for the duration of the procedure in patients with normal renal function. If vancomycin or a fluoroquinolone is used, the infusion should be started 60–120 minutes before the initial incision in order to minimize the possibility of an infusion reaction close to the time of induction of anesthesia and to have adequate tissue levels at the time of incision.
2. Some consultants recommend and additional dose when patients are removed from bypass during open-heart surgery.
3. Vancomycin is used in hospitals in which methicillin-resistant S. aureus and S. epidermis are a frequent cause of postoperative wound infection, for patients previously colonized with MRSA, or for those who are allergic to penicillins or cephalosporins. Rapid IV administration may cause hypotension, which could be especially dangerous during induction of anesthesia. Even when the drug is given over 60 minutes, hypotension may occur; treatment with diphenhydramine (Benadryl) and others) and further slowing of the infusion rate may be helpful. Some experts would give 15 mg/kg of vancomycin to patients weighing more than 75 kg, up to a maximum of 1.5 g, with a slower infusion rate (90 minutes for 1.5 g). To provide coverage against gram-negative bacteria, most Medical Letter consultants would also include cefazolin or cefuroxime in the prophylaxis regimen for patients not allergic to cephalosporins; ciprofloxacin, levofloxacin, gentamicin, or aztreonam, each one in combination with vancomycin, can be used in patients who cannot tolerate a cephalosporin.
4. Morbid obesity, esophageal obstruction, decreased gastric acidity or gastrointestinal motility.
5. Age >70 years, acute cholecystisis, non-functioning gall bladder, obstructive jaundice or common duct stones.
6. After appropriate diet and catharsis, 1 g of neomycin plus 1 g of erythromycin at 1 PM, 2 PM and 11 PM or 2 g of neomycin plus 2 g of metronidazole at 7 PM and 11 PM the day before an 8 AM operation.
7. For patients allergic to penicillins and cephalosporins, clindamycin with either gentamicin, ciprofloxacin, levofloxacin or aztreonam is a reasonable alternative.
8. For a ruptured viscus, therapy is often continued for about five days. Ruptured viscus in postoperative setting (dehiscence) requires antibacterials to include coverage of nosocomial pathogens.
9. Urine culture positive or unavailable, preoperative catheter, transrectal prostatic biopsy, placement of prosthetic material.
10. Patients with previous pelvic inflammatory disease, previous gonorrhea or multiple sex partners.
11. Divided into 100 mg one hour before the abortion and 200 mg one half hour later.
12. If a tourniquet is to be used in the procedure, the entire dose of antibiotic must be infused prior to its inflation.

Hypothermia has benefits of decreasing tissue oxygen consumption and is tissue protective in cardiac bypass and organ transplant. However, hypothermia may predispose to infection through cutaneous vasoconstriction. It has been shown that perioperative normothermia is associated with reduced rates of surgical site infections (36).

Several health care improvement initiative studies have shown that surgical site infection surveillance is effective in reducing the infection rates (37). The mechanism is unknown, but many researchers postulate that surveillance is associated with a greater awareness of sterile technique. Operative teams more rapidly recognize problems and find solutions. Surgeons should seek a program at their institution for health care improvement and operative safety. The Institute for Healthcare Improvement (IHI) is a nonprofit organization that leads health care improvement initiatives. They organized the 100,000 Lives Campaign to implement changes in United States hospitals which focused on increased compliance to four areas: appropriate use of antibiotics, removing razors from operative rooms, maintaining glucose control, and ensuring perioperative normothermia (38). Hospitals in compliance with these changes reported a 27% reduction in surgical site infections (7).

SURGICAL TECHNIQUE

Numerous studies aimed at discovering risk factors for complications have identified surgeons as independent risk factors. This could be due to numerous factors including clinical judgment, baseline characteristics of patient populations, procedure type, and surgical technique. There is no doubt that meticulous surgical technique can improve outcomes. This is particularly important when dealing with a patient at risk for complications. Excess intraoperative blood loss has been associated with surgical site infections and poor wound healing (39). Blood loss leading to hypotension with subsequent vasoconstriction and tissue hypoxia is one explanation for increased wound healing complications. Techniques aimed at improving sterility, minimizing tissue destruction, maintaining meticulous hemostasis, improving speed and accuracy, minimizing foreign body placement, and attention to closure are expected to reduce complications.

The choice of suture and method of suture placement can also have an impact on wound healing. There is a wide array of suture types. In general, sutures can be divided by life expectancy (permanent, absorbable, fast absorbable) and consistency (braided vs. monofilament). Permanent suture is indicated in situations where suture absorption is not desired (e.g., vasculature anastomosis). Drawbacks include development of suture abscesses and chronic infection. Stitch abscesses are less problematic with absorbable sutures, but may lose strength prior to tissue healing. Braided sutures are strong, hold well, and are easy to tie. However, they are more prone to infection than monofilament. Braided sutures may also cause tissue tearing as in the case of venous repairs. Monofilament sutures are smooth and resist infection, but are less forgiving and require more knots to resist slippage.

Placement of sutures can also contribute to wound compromise. Simple interrupted sutures and vertical matrass sutures produce less wound edge ischemia than running and horizontal matrass sutures when tissue viability is in question. Horizontal matrass sutures placed under excessive tension can further impede blood supply to wound edges resulting in infection, necrosis, or dehiscence. Care must be taken not to incorporate or impinge vasculature pedicles when placing sutures.

CONCLUSION

Prevention of wound complications starts with the preoperative evaluation where risk factors for wound healing are identified and modified prior to elective procedures. In the traumatic setting and in the established soft tissue deficit, patient factors such as glucose control and nutritional status can be optimized to maximize the patients healing potential. With this chapter as an introduction, the following chapters will address evaluation of traumatic wounds followed by techniques for recruiting or mobilizing surrounding tissue to close large wounds and soft tissue deficits.

REFERENCES

1. Falanga V. Wound healing and its impairment in the diabetic foot. *Lancet.* 2005;66(9498):1736–1743.
2. Stadelmann WK, Digenis AG, Tobin GR. Physiology and healing dynamics of chronic cutaneous wounds. *Am J Surg.* 1998;176:26S–38S.
3. Smiley DD, Umpierrez GE. Perioperative glucose control in the diabetic or nondiabetic patient. *South Med J.* 2006;99(6):580–589.

4. Dronge AS, Perkal MF, Kancir S, et al. Long-term glycemic control and postoperative infectious complications. *Arch Surg.* 2006;141(4):375–380.
5. Van den Berghe G, Wouters P, Weekers F, et al. Intensive insulin therapy in critically ill patients. *N Engl J Med.* 2001;345(19):1359–1367.
6. Culver DH, Horan TC, Gaynes RP, et al. Surgical wound infection rates by wound class, operative procedure, and patient risk index. National Nosocomial Infections Surveillance System. *Am J Med.* 1991;91(3B): 152S–157S.
7. Dellinger EP, Hausmann SM, Bratzler DW, et al. Hospitals collaborate to decrease surgical site infections. *Am J Surg.* 2005;190(1):9–15.
8. Drake DB, Oishi SN. Wound healing considerations in chemotherapy and radiation therapy. *Clin Plast Surg.* 1995;22(1):31–37.
9. Marti A, Marcos A, Martinez JA. Obesity and immune function relationships. *Obes Rev.* 2001;2(2):131–140.
10. Wilson JA, Clark JJ. Obesity: impediment to wound healing. *Crit Care Nurs Q.* 2003;26(2):119–132.
11. Parvizi J, Trousdale RT, Sarr MG. Total joint arthroplasty in patients surgically treated for morbid obesity. *J Arthroplasty.* 2000;15(8):1003–1008.
12. Krueger JK, Rohrich RJ. Clearing the smoke: the scientific rationale for tobacco abstention with plastic surgery. *Plast Reconstr Surg.* 2001;108(4):1063–1073; discussion 1074–1077.
13. Kuri M, Nakagawa M, Tanaka, et al. Determination of the duration of preoperative smoking cessation to improve wound healing after head and neck surgery. *Anesthesiology.* 2005;102(5):892–896.
14. Etter JF, Burri M, Stapleton J. The impact of pharmaceutical company funding on results of randomized trials of nicotine replacement therapy for smoking cessation: a meta-analysis. *Addiction.* 2007;102(5):815–822.
15. Manassa EH, Hertl CH, Olbrisch RR. Wound healing problems in smokers and nonsmokers after 132 abdominoplasties. *Plast Reconstr Surg.* 2003;111(6):2082–2087.
16. Schaffer M, Bongartz M, Hoffman W, et al. MHC-class-II-deficiency impairs wound healing. *J Surg Res.* 2007;138(1):100–105.
17. Anstead GM. Steroids, retinoids, and wound healing. *Adv Wound Care.* 1998;11(6): 277–285.
18. Wicke C, Halliday B, Allen D, et al. Effects of steroids and retinoids on wound healing. *Arch Surg.* 2000;135(11):1265–1270.
19. Gislason H, Søreide O, Viste A. Wound complications after major gastrointestinal operations. *Dig Surg.* 1999;16:512–514.
20. Mehrabi A, Fonouni H, Wente M, et al. Wound complications following kidney and liver transplantation. *Clinic Transplant.* 2006;20(s17):97–110.
21. Tran NV, Evans GR, Kroll SS, et al. Postoperative adjuvant irradiation: effects on transverse rectus abdominis muscle flap breast reconstruction. *Plast Reconstr Surg.* 2000;106(2):313–317; discussion 318–320.
22. Springfield DS. Surgical wound healing. *Cancer Treat Res.* 1993;67:81–98.
23. Thornton AD, Winslet M, Chester K. Angiogenesis inhibition with bevacizumab and the surgical management of colorectal cancer. *Br J Surg.* 2006;93(12):1456 1463.
24. Mainous MR, Deitch ED. Nutrition and infection. *Surg Clin North Am.* 1994;74(3):659–676.
25. Windsor A, Braga M, Martindale R, et al. Fit for surgery: an expert panel review on optmising patients prior to surgery, with a particular focus on nutrition. *Surgeon.* 2004;2(6):315–319.
26. Goonetilleke KS, Siriwardena AK. Systematic review of peri-operative nutritional supplementation in patients undergoing pancreaticoduodenectomy. *JOP.* 2006;7(1):5–13.
27. Norgren L, Hiatt WR, Dormandy JA, et al. Inter-society consensus for the management of peripheral arterial disease (TASC II). *Int Angiol.* 2007;26(2):81–157.
28. Christensen K, Klarke M. Transcutaneous oxygen measurement in peripheral occlusive disease. An indicator of wound healing in leg amputation. *J Bone Joint Surg Br.* 1986;68(3):423–426.
29. Yablon SA, Novick ES, Jain SS, et al. Postoperative transcutaneous oxygen measurement in the prediction of delayed wound healing and prosthetic fitting among amputees during rehabilitation. A pilot study. *Am J Phys Med Rehabil.* 1995;74(3):193–198.
30. Poulsen KB, Bremmelgaard A, Sørenson AI, et al. Estimated costs of postoperative wound infections. A case-control study of marginal hospital and social security costs. *Epidemiol Infect.* 1994;113(2):283–295.
31. Mangram AJ, Horan TC, Pearson ML, et al. Guideline for prevention of surgical site infection, 1999. Centers for Disease Control and Prevention (CDC) Hospital Infection Control Practices Advisory Committee. *Am J Infect Control.* 1999;27(2):97–132; quiz 133–134; discussion 96.
32. Edwards PS, Lipp A, Holmes A. Preoperative skin antiseptics for preventing surgical wound infections after clean surgery. *Cochrane Database Syst Rev.* 2004;3:CD003949.
33. Bratzler DW, Houck PM, Richards C, et al. Use of antimicrobial prophylaxis for major surgery: baseline results from the National Surgical Infection Prevention Project. *Arch Surg.* 2005;140(2):174–182.
34. Mishriki SF, Law DJ, Jeffery PJ. Factors affecting the incidence of postoperative wound infection. *J Hosp Infect.* 1990;16(3):223–230.
35. Cruse PJ, Foord R. The epidemiology of wound infection. A 10-year prospective study of 62,939 wounds. *Surg Clin North Am.* 1980;60(1):27–40.
36. Kurz A, Sessler DI, Lenhardt R. Perioperative normothermia to reduce the incidence of surgical-wound infection and shorten hospitalization. Study of Wound Infection and Temperature Group. *N Engl J Med.* 1996;334(19):1209–1215.
37. Haley RW, Culver DH, White JW, et al. The efficacy of infection surveillance and control programs in preventing nosocomial infections in US hospitals. *Am J Epidemiol.* 1985;121(2):182–205.
38. Bratzler DW. The Surgical Infection Prevention and Surgical Care Improvement Projects: promises and pitfalls. *Am Surg.* 2006;72(11):1010–1016; discussion 1021–1030, 1133–1148.
39. Shapiro M, Munoz A, Tager IB, et al. Risk factors for infection at the operative site after abdominal or vaginal hysterectomy. *N Engl J Med.* 1982;307(27):1661–1666.

2 Initial Evaluation and Management of Complex Traumatic Wounds

Patricia L. McKay and George Nanos

The principles in this chapter are forged from our experience with the treatment of high energy contaminated wounds resulting from recent overseas military conflicts. The soft tissue injuries discussed within this chapter encompass a broad spectrum of clinical presentations, both acute and chronic. These treatment protocols reflect the ever-growing body of scientific knowledge and technological advances contributing to the successful treatment of our patients. In the following illustrations, we hope to point out the common mistakes and potential pitfalls of operative and perioperative wound management and provide surgeons with a framework for successful treatment of all types of wounds.

INITIAL EVALUATION

A thorough initial patient evaluation gives the surgeon the information by which to formulate a treatment plan with the best chance for success. A complete and accurate history must include the circumstances leading to the current wound presentation, the mechanism of injury if associated with trauma, underlying medical conditions, current occupational and socioeconomic status, and patient social habits such as smoking which may have detrimental effects on reconstructive efforts (Table 2-1).

In cases of trauma the energy level, mechanism, location, and the time course from injury to presentation are invaluable in predicting prognosis and planning treatment. Medical comorbidities such as underlying cardiopulmonary or peripheral vascular disease, endocrinopathy, neuropathic disease, immunocompromising conditions, psychiatric illness, nutritional deficits, and allergies can negatively impact the success of treatment if not identified and optimized. Medical consultation and co-management is recommended in these cases. Tetanus status must be addressed in accordance with Centers for Disease Control guidelines.

Failure to fully recognize the scope of the wound and/or injury can have dreadful consequences to the outcome. A detailed physical examination with critical assessment of vital signs, secondary survey, and multi-system examination is required in all cases to evaluate the wound and exclude other medical conditions or associated injury that may take greater priority in treatment.

In multi-system trauma, the Advanced Trauma Life Support (ATLS) approach, beginning with airway, breathing, and circulation (ABC's) is recommended. Traumatologists or critical care specialists should be the principle coordinators of all initial medical care to ensure appropriate global management of the patient.

TABLE 2-1. Wound Treatment Pitfalls	
Inadequate clinical and surgical resources for proper treatment	Failure to recognize and treat infection
Failure to recognize and optimize host factors	Wound closure with excessive tension
Failure to recognize and treat vascular compromise	Prominent bone or hardware
Inadequate debridement	

Critical attention should be directed to vascular status. If capillary refill and/or pulses are abnormal or absent, or if the mechanism introduces suspicion for vascular injury, Doppler testing and/or perfusion studies must be obtained. Revascularization or repair of vessels should be completed prior to, or concurrent with, surgical wound treatment. Special attention should also be paid to the neurological examination, and all deficits clearly documented. In cases of extremity trauma, a high index of suspicion for compartment syndrome is essential. Continued reevaluation is required with adjunctive use of compartment pressure monitoring if the diagnosis is in question, emergent compartment release should be performed if clinically indicated, and prophylactic release should be considered in trauma cases with revascularization procedures.

Ancillary studies aid in full comprehension of the clinical situation. Plain radiographs should be routinely obtained to evaluate for associated fracture, foreign body, exostosis, osteomyelitis, soft tissue emphysema, vascular calcifications such as those associated with Diabetes Mellitus, or other factors contributing to or resulting from the overlying wound. CT scans and MRI may provide additional valuable information. Markers of hematologic and immune status, clotting factors, electrolyte and renal function, and adequacy of resuscitation must all be accounted for based on the clinical situation.

Careful documentation of every aspect of the evaluation and treatment must be made, and generous use of medical photography is helpful not only for documentation, but also for preoperative planning purposes.

PREOPERATIVE PLANNING

Once the evaluation is complete, the surgeon can formulate a treatment plan and determine if surgical intervention is required. The most important question to consider is whether the surgeon and the facility possess the requisite experience, capability, equipment, and consultative and ancillary services to render optimum treatment (Fig. 2-1). The surgeon must have the technical ability and anatomic knowledge for the given location of the injury. The treating hospital and operating room must also be able to furnish the necessary instruments, implants, and wound treatment dressings. When confronted with cases of multi-system trauma, a multidisciplinary team involving traumatologists, intensivists, medical consultants, infectious disease specialists, and wound care support personnel is generally considered to be mandatory. If unable to meet these basic requirements, the clinical situation should be carefully reviewed and the strongest consideration should be given for referral to a higher level of care.

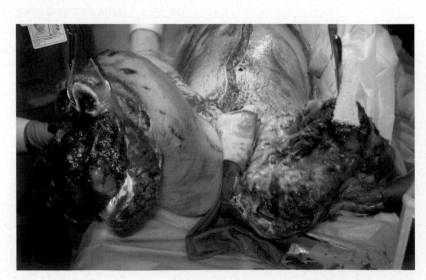

FIGURE 2-1

Injury to multiple extremities and organ systems changes surgical options, increases the risk for systemic problems, and has greater psychological impact. Options for flaps or skin grafts are far more limited. Proper room setup and a hospital team that is prepared to manage comorbidities will facilitate delivery of appropriate care and provide the greatest likelihood of success.

SURGERY

Patient positioning varies depending on the site of the wound in question. General or regional anesthesia may be employed, and consideration for peripheral nerve blocks should be considered for perioperative pain control. A sterile or non-sterile tourniquet is indispensable to ensure optimal visualization for meticulous, thorough debridement and protection of vital structures. Appropriate broad-spectrum antibiotics should be given as scheduled throughout the surgical procedure.

Debridement

Successful surgical treatment of wounds begins with the meticulous and complete removal of foreign material, infection, and devitalized tissue to create a healthy wound bed (Fig. 2-2). In chronic wounds, we attempt to create an acute wound to promote healing. In acute injury, wounds must be extended past the zone of injury to ensure complete treatment, and failure to do so significantly limits the effectiveness of debridement. Judicious use of lavage may help remove foreign matter, but care must be taken not to extend the zone of contamination by forcing debris into the surrounding tissue. Use of a tourniquet early in the case is important to best visualize all contaminants and devitalized tissue and avoid injury to vital structures such as nerves and blood vessels. The tourniquet should be released prior to closure or dressing application to confirm removal of all devascularized tissue and excellent hemostasis.

A systematic approach to wound debridement is required and sharp debridement is the cornerstone of this surgical technique. We prefer the centripetal approach working from superficial tissues to deep, from the margins to the center of the wound. Starting at the skin edges, we meticulously work towards the deeper structures within the wound (Fig. 2-3). In general, we prefer excision of all devitalized tissue to a healthy tissue margin instead of a "wait and see" approach to suspect tissue as we feel this limits persistent contamination and infection. All non-viable or suspect tissue is sharply debrided from the wound until a healthy margin of viable tissue achieved. Every effort to preserve nerves and blood vessels crossing the zone of injury is made, and if they are transected these structures are carefully tagged with dyed monofilament suture and documented in the operative records so that they may be more easily visualized during later wound debridements or reconstructive efforts.

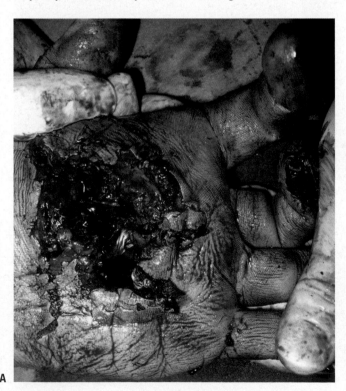
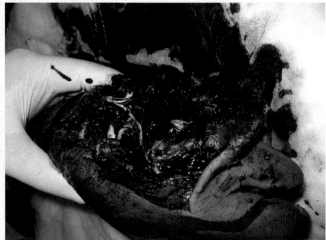

A

B

FIGURE 2-2

Palmar **(A)** and dorsal **(B)** views of an acute hand injury produced by an improvised explosive device. Jagged skin margins, necrotic tissue, foreign material, and hematoma are visible (photos courtesy of Dr. Dana Covey, CAPT, MC, USN).

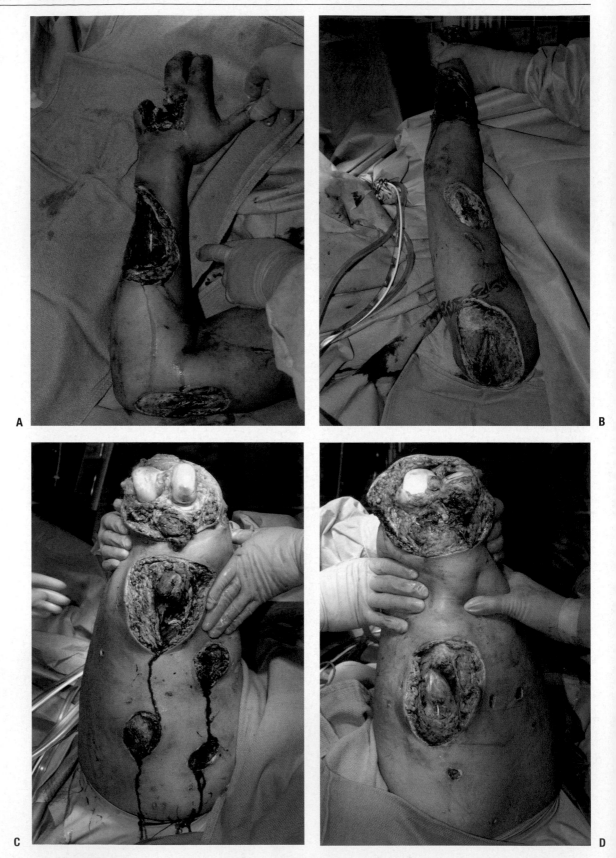

FIGURE 2-3

This patient, injured by an improvised explosive device, sustained left upper **(A,B)** and bilateral lower extremity injuries **(C,D)**. Excellent serial wound debridement results in smooth margins, healthy skin and muscle ready for skeletal stabilization, and delayed primary wound closure for the lower extremities.

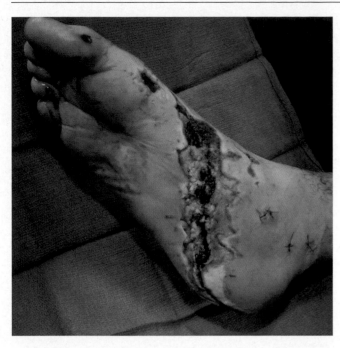

FIGURE 2-4

Plantar wound is not ready for closure or coverage; jagged skin and eschar at the wound edge needs to be sharply debrided. Serial debridements allow the zone of injury to fully declare itself.

Identification of non-viable tissue remains a challenge, and there is no substitute for experience. In general, non-bleeding skin that appears dusky or does not blanch should be excised, creating a smooth wound margin and avoiding the creation of a ragged skin edge that is difficult for subsequent skin grafting or closure. Subcutaneous fat should be soft and yellow; hard, dusky, or gray fat should be excised (Fig. 2-4). It is also important to keep this tissue moist during deeper debridement, as it will easily desiccate. Injured blood vessels or nerves must be carefully assessed for primary or delayed repair or grafting. Smaller sensory nerve branches may not be amenable to salvage, and if so, we like to pull traction on the proximal end, cut sharply, and allow retraction into the soft tissues. If the stump cannot be retracted, we make every effort to bury it in muscle. To the greatest extent possible local soft tissues should be used to cover exposed tendons, nerves, and vessels to prevent desiccation and further injury.

In debridement of muscle, fascia, and tendon, there are several important points to keep in mind. Muscle fascia should be stout, white, and shiny, while non-viable fascia will often appear grey or black, fragile, and stringy. When excising fascia, however, great care should be taken as neurovascular bundles may be in close proximity. Muscle should be red, shiny, of good consistency, contractile, and bleeding (Fig. 2-5). Anything to the contrary should be considered for debridement. Knowledge of anatomy and local blood supply is paramount in this endeavor as overly aggressive

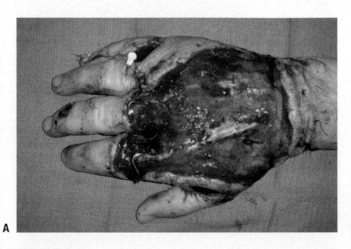
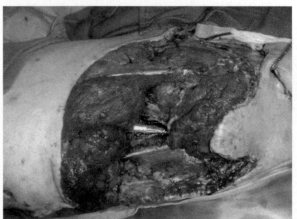

A   B

FIGURE 2-5

A: Right hand and **(B)** left hip open wounds ready for further coverage. Note the healthy, smooth skin margins, clean granulating tissue bed, minimal edema, and skeletal stabilization.

debridement within muscle compartments may devascularize previously viable tissue. Tendon debridement must be carefully considered due to potential loss of function. Tendons are also easily desiccated, especially if overlying paratenon or sheath is missing.

Devascularized bone fragments must be removed from the wound bed, with the exception of substantial articular fragments, which should be retained in an attempt to preserve the articular surface (Fig. 2-6). Curettes, rongeurs, and burs are useful to check for punctated bleeding indicative of healthy bone that should be preserved. Cultures of any contaminated or osteolytic bone will help guide antibiotic selection.

There are many tools available for mechanical debridement. One tool we find useful for very large wounds is the VersaJet™ Hydrosurgery System (Smith and Nephew). This device uses negative pressure from a high-speed stream of water across a small aperture at the tip to remove softer tissue and surface debris by suction. Additional lavage is not required when using this device. However, great care must be used around neurovascular structures to avoid injury.

Strict hemostasis is critical to prevent hematoma and limit further infection and morbidity due to blood loss. Suture ligatures and surgical clips should be used for larger vessels, and bovie or bipolar cautery for smaller vessels. We avoid use of braided suture when possible to avoid harboring bac-

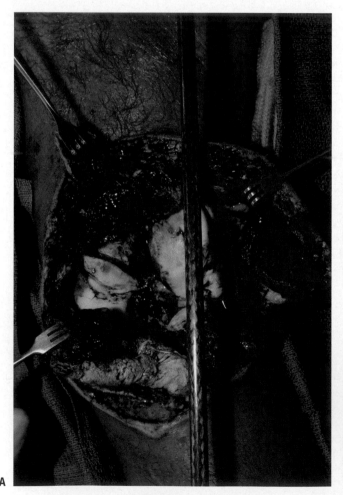

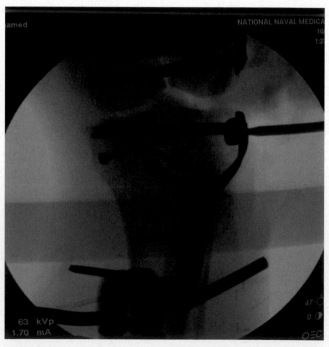

A   B

FIGURE 2-6

During serial debridements every effort is made to preserve substantial articular cartilage fragments. This case also illustrates the value of a team approach, after extensive surgical time to obtain the best possible ORIF of this comminuted intraarticular knee injury **(A,B)**, the plastic surgery service performed a medial gastrocnemius pedicled rotation flap and split thickness skin grafting **(C,D)**. *(Continued)*

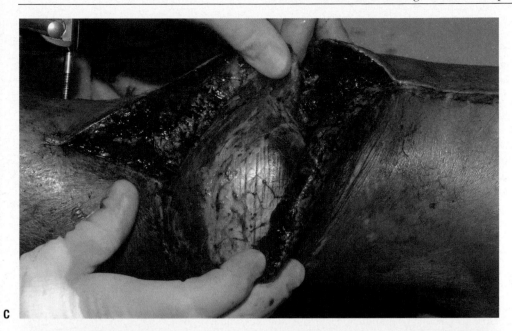

C

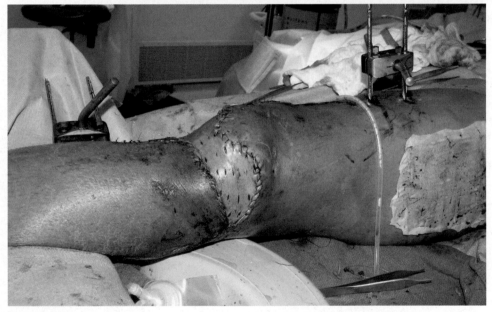

D

FIGURE 2-6   *Continued*

teria. Judicious use of a tourniquet is helpful to identify and control large bleeding vessels and includes release to assess hemostasis prior to closure, grafting, or dressing application. Adjunctive topical hemostatic agents are available and have been used successfully in some of our most severely war injured patients. Lavage is important for removal of foreign debris and lowering bacterial counts. Reflecting prior published research, we use plain saline for lavage without antibiotics. Based on our experience and the literature, we limit use of pulsatile lavage in the forearm and lower leg, and almost never use it in the hand or foot. Pulsatile lavage can further damage delicate tissues, exacerbating the potential for adhesions and functional loss. When pulsatile lavage is used in the hand and foot, it is usually at the half pressure setting. Usually, bulb irrigation is sufficient when combined with careful debridement.

Temporary Coverage and Void Fillers

Negative pressure dressings are a great advance in the treatment of wounds not amenable to primary closure (Fig. 2-7). The wound VAC® (Vacuum Assisted Closure) dressing is commonly employed at our institution. It continues to debride wounds while reducing edema and local bacterial counts and it promotes growth of healthy granulation tissue. It also eliminates the need for multiple daily dressing changes, thereby reducing the patient's discomfort and nursing staff workload. We use portable suction devices supplied by the manufacturer set at the recommended 125 mm Hg intermittent suction. Wall suction can be used if a portable unit is not available, but care must be made to ensure the unit is calibrated to provide a true measurement of suction. We prefer to use less suction in the upper extremity due to the more delicate nature of the soft tissues and have found this to be effective. In the hand, use of the wound VAC® is limited to avoid desiccation and injury to vital nerves, blood vessels, and tendons. It can be of benefit when the underlying tissue is robust such as the thenar or hypothenar eminence, or when the more delicate tissues are absent due to the injury and debridements (Fig. 2-8). When neurovascular structures are exposed we employ standard wet to dry dressings. In general, we try to limit exposure of blood vessels, nerves, or tendons to the wound VAC® and try to rotate available local tissue to provide coverage prior to placement of the wound VAC®. Multiple wounds can be treated with the same suction tube using a foam bridging technique. However, care must be taken to cover the skin with the supplied biofilm or ioban to prevent local skin breakdown.

Adequately eliminating contamination and infection is essential to successful wound treatment. In addition to appropriate broad-spectrum antibiotic use, there are many different options available to provide local infection control that can be tailored to the clinical or surgical situation. Antibiotic bead pouches or fracture spacers have been used effectively to provide local infection control in cases of wounds with associated high-energy fracture patterns. With comminution and bone loss soft tissue space can be maintained for future reconstruction and enhanced mechanical stability provided (Fig. 2-9). In highly resistant bacterial infection, silver impregnated films, colloidal materials, and wound VAC® sponges are additional options for the surgeon and have been utilized with great frequency at our institution. We presently reserve the use of silver for refractory cases due to concerns of resistance and the current high cost of this modality. For extremely large wounds with highly resistant bacterial colonization or infection that are not amenable to wound VAC® treatment, Sulfamylon (mafenide acetate) or Dakin's soaked wet-to-dry dressings have proven effective and resulted in successful wound closure. Infectious disease specialty assistance is recommended in such cases.

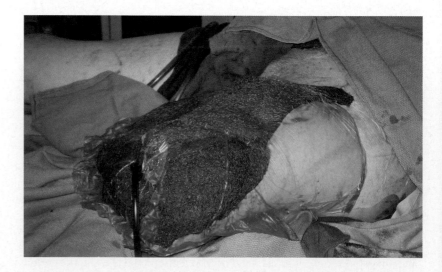

FIGURE 2-7

Use of serial debridements and negative pressure dressings prepare the wound for subsequent flap coverage.

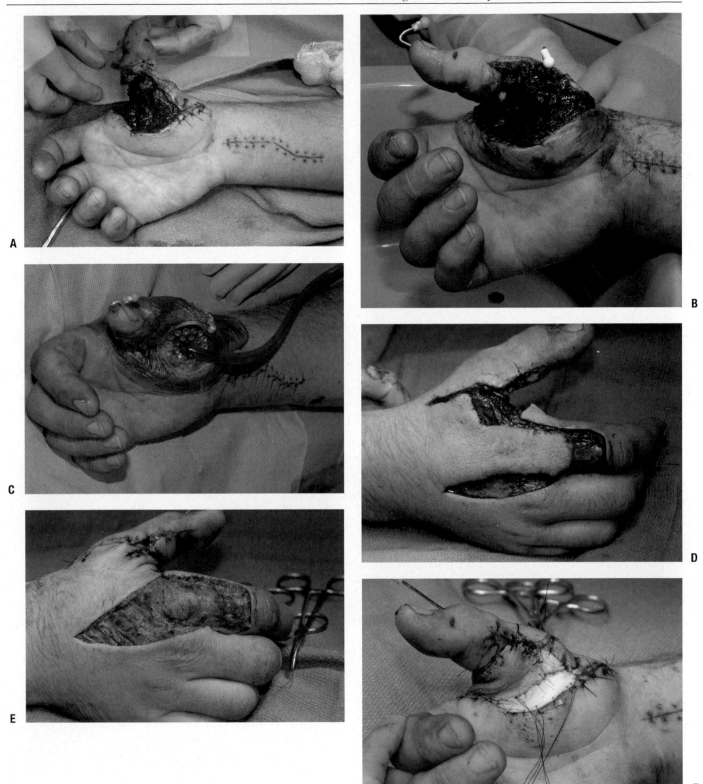

FIGURE 2-8

This case, of a patient who sustained an isolated injury to the thumb from an AK-47 rifle round, illustrates several principles of wound management: thorough debridement preserving vital structures **(A)** and provisional skeletal fixation with K-wires **(B)**; **C:** the use of negative pressure dressings to prepare the wound for coverage. **D-H;** attainment of a closed healthy soft tissue envelope prior to reconstruction, in this case a local rotation flap and full-thickness skin graft were selected. *(Continued)*

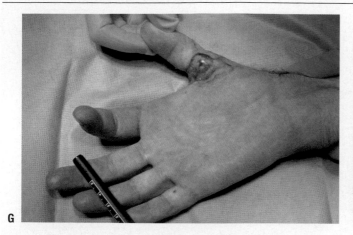

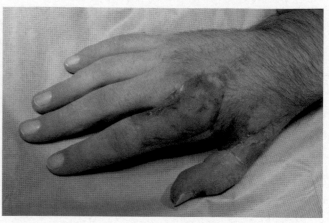

FIGURE 2-8 *Continued*

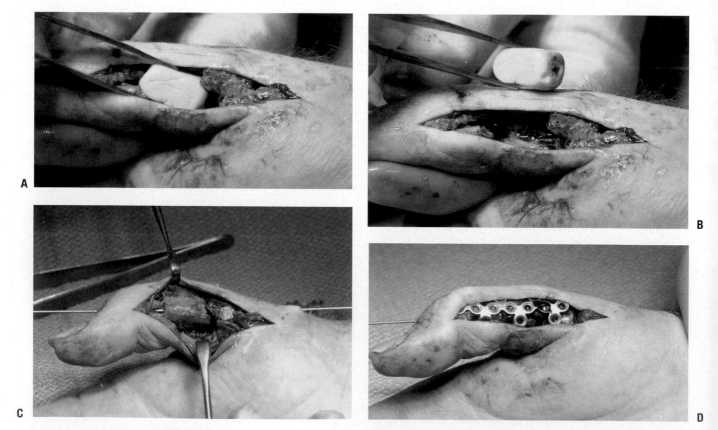

FIGURE 2-9

A,B: In cases of contaminated segmental bone loss (case from Fig. 2-8),an antibiotic impregnated cement spacer can be used to decrease infection risk and maintain space and alignment until the wound is clean enough for soft tissue reconstruction with bone grafting **(C,D)**. *(Continued)*

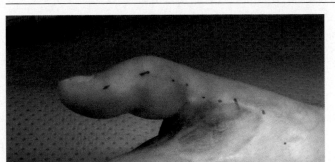
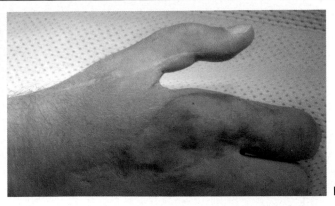

E

F

FIGURE 2-9

Continued **E,F:** A well healed soft tissue envelope, demonstrated here, is necessary prior to performing nerve and tendon grafting.

Choice of Fixation

When wounds are associated with fractures in the acute setting, provisional stabilization should be attempted to maintain soft tissue space, prevent mechanical agitation of the surrounding tissues, and optimize pain control (Fig. 2-10). In general, external fixators are preferred acutely with conversion to definitive fixation as indicated by the injury. In the setting of blast injuries, large amounts of debris are forced into the wounds with tremendous energy and the level of contamination is typically higher than that seen in most blunt open trauma. Our experience has shown the significant potential for widespread osteomyelitis when intramedullary fixation is selected for blast injured patients and we now prefer definitive treatment with an external fixation device in many cases. For the distal extremity, as well as periarticular fractures, Kirschner wires are indispensable for temporary and sometimes definitive fixation. Definitive fixation that requires significant soft tissue stripping may only compound the injury and should be entertained with extreme caution as the clinical situation dictates.

For highly contaminated wounds, or when there is concern for viability in critical areas or structures, repeat operative debridement should be planned every 24 to 36 hours until a healthy, vascularized soft tissue bed is achieved.

Timing of Final Closure

When is the wound ready to close? There are several elements that must be present to ensure success of wound closure. Certainly, all non-viable or necrotic tissue must be absent from the wound. It cannot be overemphasized that good vascular flow must be present for healing of tissues. In addition, a tension free closure must be achieved or blood flow will be compromised at the wound margins leading to wound breakdown and dehiscence. Acute limb shortening can be considered when significant bone and soft tissue defects are present (Fig. 2-11). Soft tissue expanders can also be a valuable tool in the reconstructive phase (Fig. 2-12) One significant marker of excessive tension is blanching at the wound margins. Suture type, configuration, and binding tightness of the suture must all be considered. Mattress sutures can be tension relieving and provide nice eversion of wound edges, but one must also recognize that inappropriate orientation or overtightening of these sutures, especially in horizontal mattress fashion, can create ischemia at the wound edges. In wounds prone to tension in the closure, we typically choose nylon suture sized appropriately to the wound in vertical mattress fashion to distribute tension evenly. At times, we will also utilize "trauma retention" type sutures using heavier gauge nylon to improve local tension. When excessive tension remains, it is better to leave the wound open and return to the operating room later when tension free closure can be obtained. In these cases, we prefer a "Jacob's ladder" type closure with staples and vessel loops, usually over or under a wound VAC® sponge or gauze dressings to create gentle traction at the wound edges and promote future closure attempts. While commercial skin traction devices are available (Fig. 2-13), we have not found them to be more effective, and they are certainly more costly.

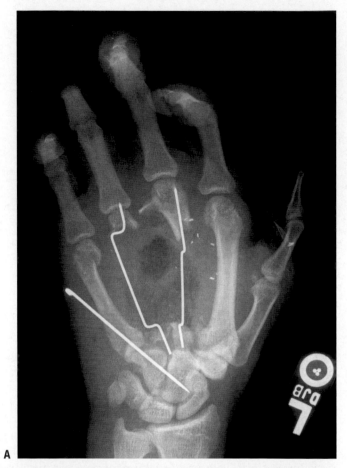

A

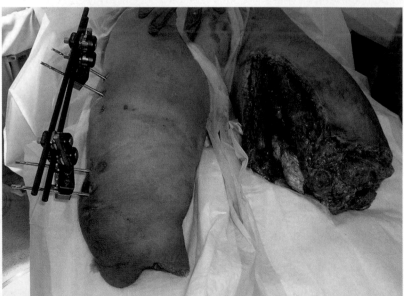

B

FIGURE 2-10

A,B: Fracture stabilization is required to assist in soft tissue management and to maintain structural relationships for subsequent reconstruction. K-wires and external fixation are especially useful in traumatic, highly contaminated wounds.

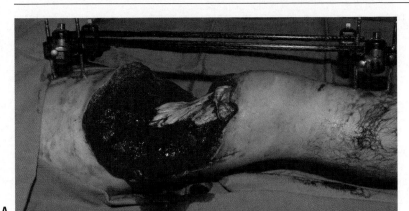

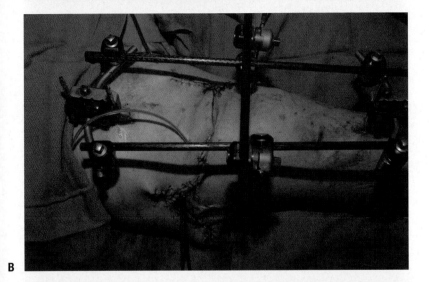

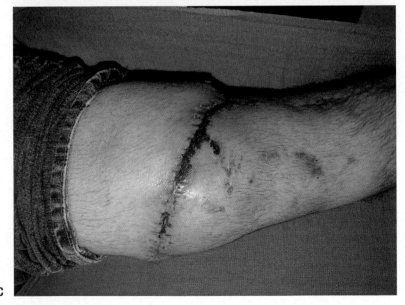

FIGURE 2-11

A-C: Large wound with a segmental femoral defect and associated loss of the anterior thigh soft tissue was managed with acute femoral shortening. Following soft tissue stabilization the femur was subsequently lengthened.

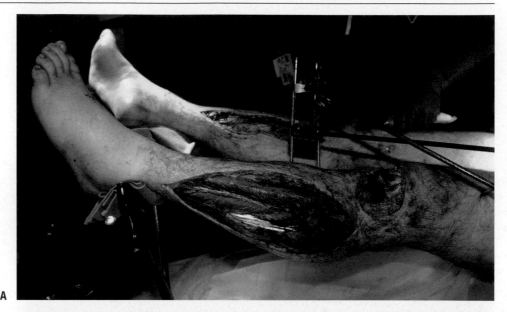

A

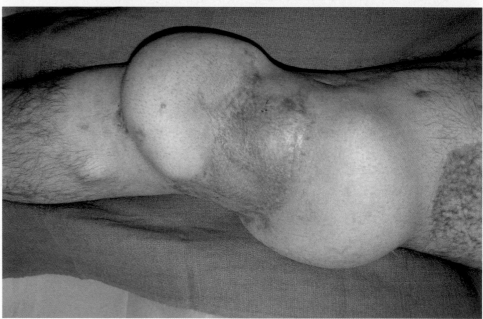

B

FIGURE 2-12

A,B: This patient required extensor mechanism reconstruction after an open knee injury. Soft tissue expanders were used after the initial fracture care, flap, and skin grafting, in order to create adequate skin for reconstruction and knee motion. It is important to remember that soft tissue scarring as well as split thickness skin grafting limit skin excursion and pliability. Subsequent surgery may require release of scar or replacement of damaged skin to obtain motion in affected joints.

Absence of infection is also critical to wound closure. We routinely culture infected or suspicious wounds to help guide antibiotic therapy. Previous literature suggests a culture threshold of less than 10^5 bacteria per gram of tissue is required to allow successful wound closure. However, the utility of cultures is highly dependent on laboratory technician experience, and they have not proven to be clinically helpful at our institution. Clinical and laboratory indicators of infection such as fever, elevated white blood cell count, and elevated inflammatory markers such as C- reactive protein and erythrocyte sedimentation rate can help guide decision making. Examination of the wound may provide obvious clues like purulent material, unhealthy appearing sheen to the tissues, and foul smell. However, even in the most experienced hands, this determination can be exceedingly difficult; surgeons must rely on the clinical appearance and laboratory markers (Fig. 2-14). Current research into

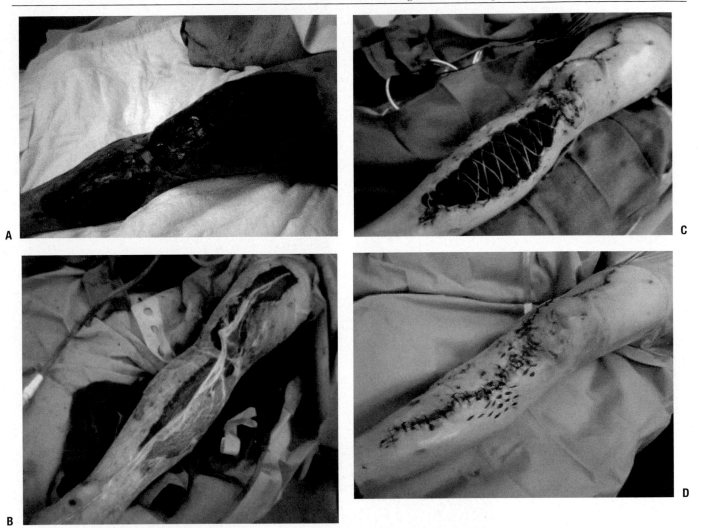

FIGURE 2-13

In some cases tension relieving devices can be used alone or in conjunction with negative pressure dressings to facilitate closure, as in this patient **(A)** with a large wound involving the anterior aspect of the lower extremity. **B,C:** Serial debridements and use of a Jacob's ladder with a negative pressure dressing allowed eventual primary wound closure. **D:** Tension relieving slits in the skin of the lower leg were also used in this case.

other markers or mediators of inflammation and infection is ongoing, but until these efforts bear fruit, this assessment continues to be a significant challenge to the surgeon.

POSTOPERATIVE MANAGEMENT

Postoperative wound care focuses on protecting the healing wound and optimizing medical care to ensure success. Initially, after wound closure or flap coverage, complete soft tissue rest of the involved extremity by splinting or external fixation should be considered (Figs. 2-15 and 2-16). Care should be taken when splinting to ensure functional positions are maintained; the intrinsic plus position for the hand, full extension at the knee, and a plantigrade position for the ankle can facilitate return to function and reduce the need for secondary procedures. Provisional fracture fixation constructs must be checked to ensure integrity of the construct with modifications made as needed to control motion at the fracture site, and ongoing tissue injury.

Elevation of the extremity is critical to reduce local swelling and edema formation. When an external fixation device is present it can be tied to balanced suspension supported by an overhead trapeze. We avoid the use of slings on the lower extremity due to the potential for pressure necrosis.

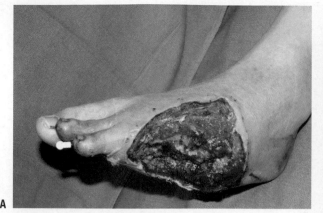

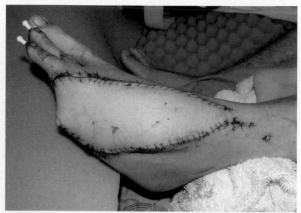

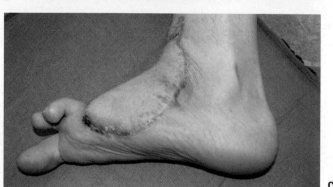

FIGURE 2-14

A–C: In contrast to Figure 2-4, this foot wound was ready for a lateral thigh free flap as evidenced by the healthy wound bed and margins, minimal residual limb edema, and excellent flap healing.

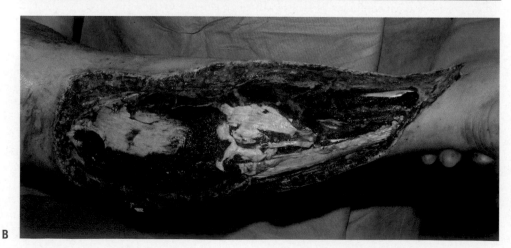

FIGURE 2-15

Patient presented with bilateral lower extremity wounds. His right below knee amputation lacked adequate soft tissue for closure and prosthetic wear **(A)**; his left lower extremity had a large soft tissue wound **(B)**. *(Continued)*

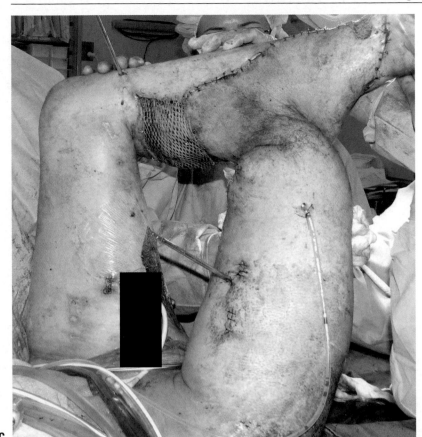

C

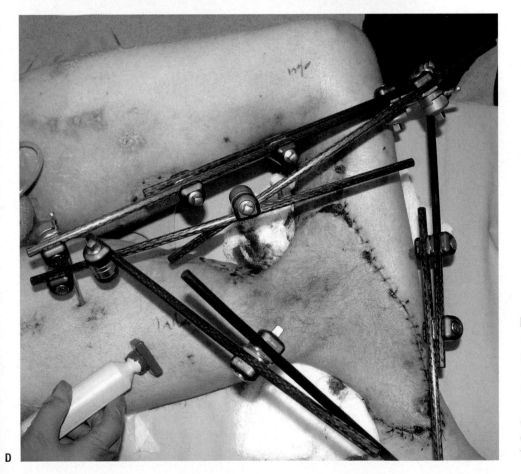

D

FIGURE 2-15

Continued The tissue that would have been discarded in a revision amputation to an above knee level was used in a "cross-leg" flap **(C,D)** with an excellent clinical result **(E)**. Note the external fixator used to protect the flap after inset **(D)**.

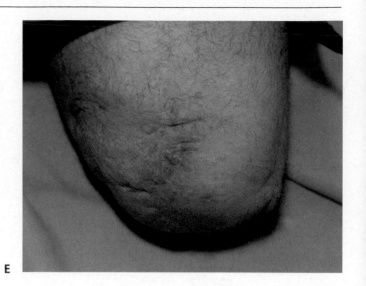

FIGURE 2-15
Continued   **E**

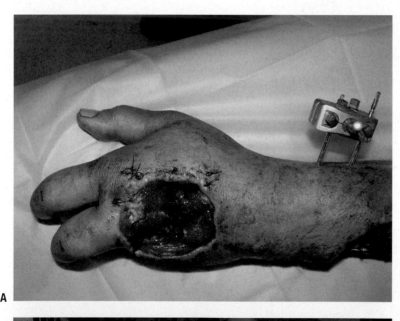

A

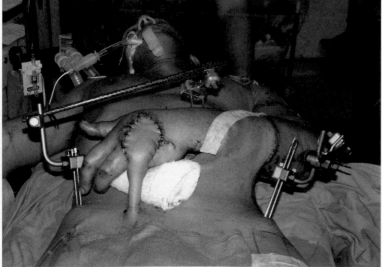

B

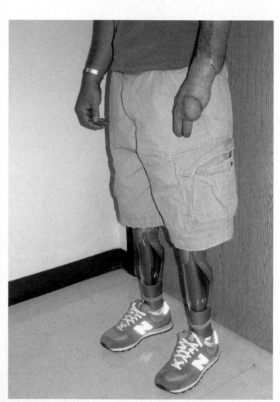

C

FIGURE 2-16

A: After continued treatment with VAC dressings and ORIF, the left upper extremity wounds from Figure 2-3A,B are ready for definitive coverage. In this case flap selection is limited by the injuries. **B:** Bilateral groin flaps were used to obtain coverage of both the hand and forearm wounds. To minimize tension on the pedicles, external fixators were used to stabilize the forearm to the pelvis. **C:** Healed wounds with durable, healthy coverage.

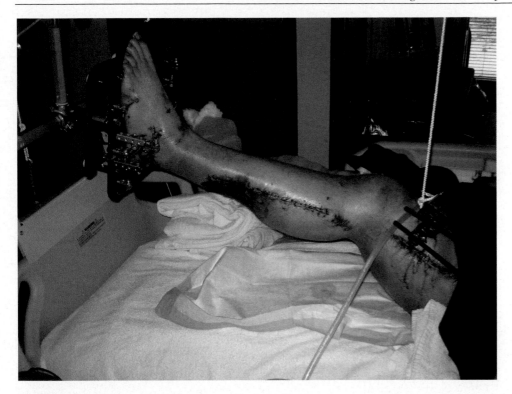

FIGURE 2-17

Elevation is a valuable tool for managing edema. Care must be taken when applying elevation, particularly in the ICU and poly-trauma setting, where patients are often sedated and less mobile. This patient, with multiple bilateral lower extremity fractures eventually received a below knee amputation after development of a full thickness posterior pressure ulcer. The leg was initially elevated by a sheepskin sling tied directly to the overhead bed frame resulting in significant pressure over the posterior calf. Use of a balanced suspension device secured to an external ankle fixator, as demonstrated in the photo, may have prevented this complication.

If an external fixator is not present and a sling is used under the calf, it should always be tied to balanced suspension, not the overhead frame, in this manner. As the patient moves, the pressure on the calf remains constant due to the hanging weights. The skin must be assessed periodically throughout each day (Fig. 2-17).

Mobilization and edema control of the digits should begin as early as possible. Once or twice daily motion begun within seven days of injury can significantly reduce edema and long term stiffness. Burn injuries can be particularly challenging due to pain, contracture, and poor durability of the grafted skin (Fig. 2-18). While consultation with physical and occupational therapists aids in maximizing return of function, a balance between early motion and soft tissue rest must be achieved to ensure proper wound healing. Effective communication with these vital specialists will ultimately benefit both the surgeon and patient.

Patient physiologic factors and comorbidities must continually be reevaluated and optimized in the postoperative period (Figs. 2-19 and 2-20). Markers for infection, hemodynamic status, systemic function, and nutritional status should be reassessed in accordance with the clinical picture. Wound cultures are checked and antibiotic choices are reevaluated in consultation with infectious disease specialists. When using the wound VAC™ system, special attention must be made to the pressure settings and quality of suction. Nursing and ancillary staff education is invaluable. Prominent bone or hardware, especially when combined with inadequate or marginal soft tissue coverage, can lead to wound breakdown and the need for additional surgery (Figs. 2-21 and 2-22).

Pain management is not only humane, but we believe greatly contributes to the success of treatment, especially in cases requiring frequent bedside dressing changes. Reuben et al have shown a reduced incidence of CRPS with aggressive pain management. In many cases, especially trauma, our anesthesia colleagues on the pain service oversee medical management of pain, and provide regional

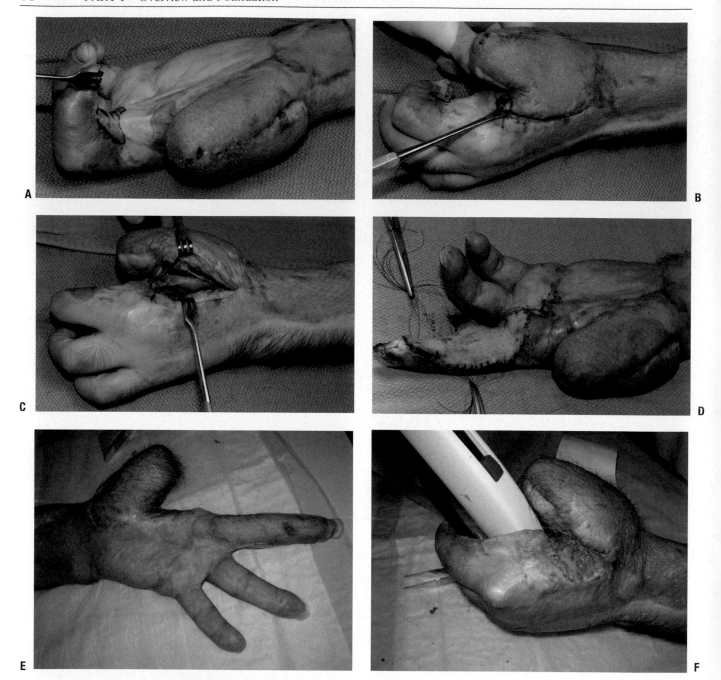

FIGURE 2-18

This patient received severe burns to the upper extremity and chest requiring groin flap to the thumb, and multiple skin grafting procedures complicated by recurrent infections with MRSA. Upon presentation to us he had severe contracture of the long finger **(A)**, erosion of the skin over the residual index metacarpal **(B)**, and essentially no use of the thumb or long finger. Staged reconstruction included thumb metacarpal lengthening, completion of the index ray amputation **(C)**, full thickness skin grafting to the long finger **(D)**, first web-space deepening, thumb carpometacarpal joint arthroplasty, and tendon transfer to the thumb metacarpal for abduction and opposition. The result: a supple, durable soft tissue envelope and functional hand **(E,F)**. Attention to detail through all phases of care can reduce the need for additional procedures.

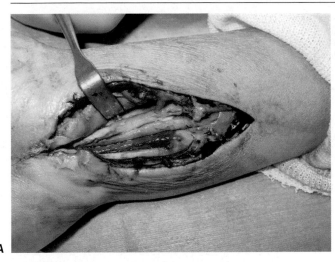
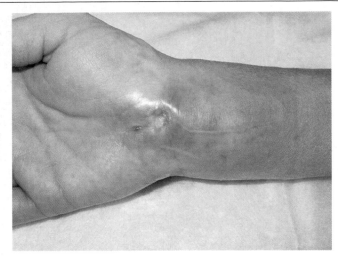

FIGURE 2-19

Underlying medical conditions where immunosuppression is present can lead to wound healing problems even after elective surgery. This rheumatoid arthritis patient underwent routine open carpal tunnel release with subsequent persistent wound drainage. Ultimately, she was diagnosed with Mycobacterium avium. The initial debridement and culture **(A)** failed to heal fully **(B)**. The gelatinous appearing tenosynovium and indolent course are typical of mycobacterial infections. Successful wound healing followed appropriate antibiotic therapy and delayed primary closure.

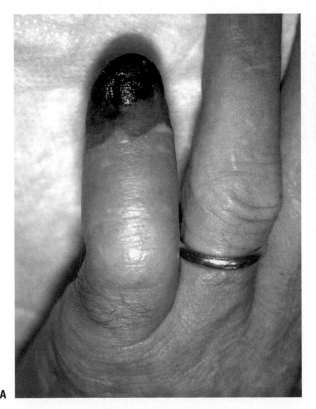
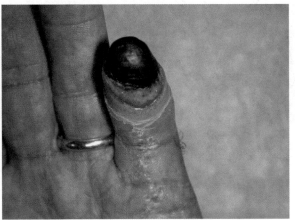

FIGURE 2-20

A,B: Patient had compromised sensation and vascularity following multiple surgeries to the small finger for Dupuytren's disease. The patient sustained a burn to the distal phalanx on the moist heat pads used before therapy. The initial blister and mild erythema were followed by progressive distal tip necrosis; ultimately, the patient requested an amputation of the digit.

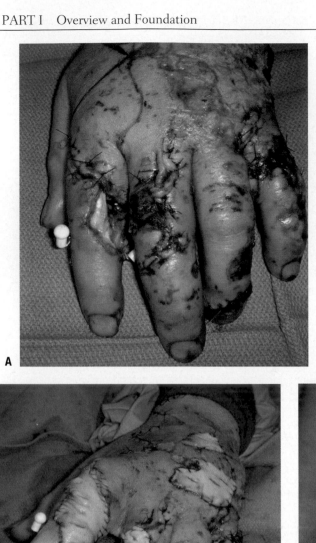

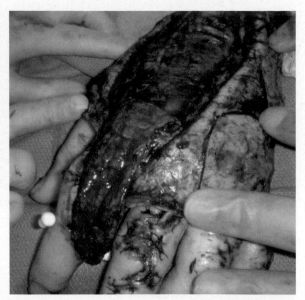

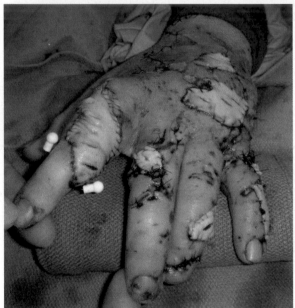

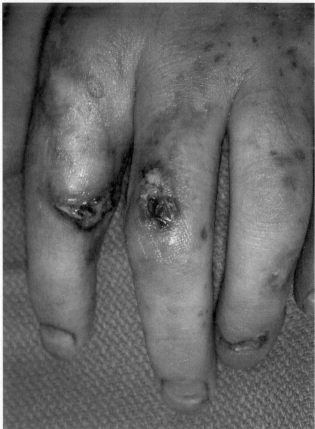

FIGURE 2-21

In this series, the patient's initial wounds were closed primarily but there was inadequate coverage of the PIPJs dorsally **(A)**. A delayed adipofacial flap **(B)** and overlying full thickness skin grafts taken from his amputated lower extremity **(C)** were not robust enough coverage over the dorsally applied plates **(D)**. Removal of the dorsal plates and primary closure lead to successful wound healing **(E)**.

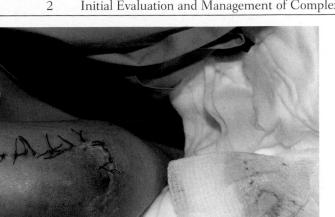

A

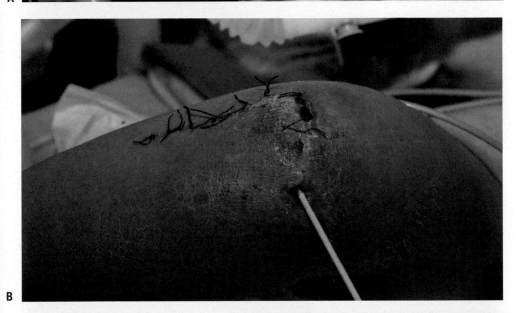

B

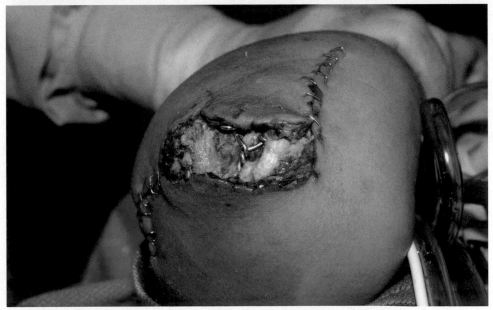

C

FIGURE 2-22

Patient presented with an innocuous appearing wound and persistent serous drainage 3 weeks after ORIF of an open olecranon fracture overseas **(A)**. Careful inspection showed that the wound communicated with the prominent underlying hardware **(B)**. Irrigation, debridement and IV antibiotics combined with removal of the prominent wire knots **(C)** and primary closure resulted in uneventful healing of the wound and fracture.

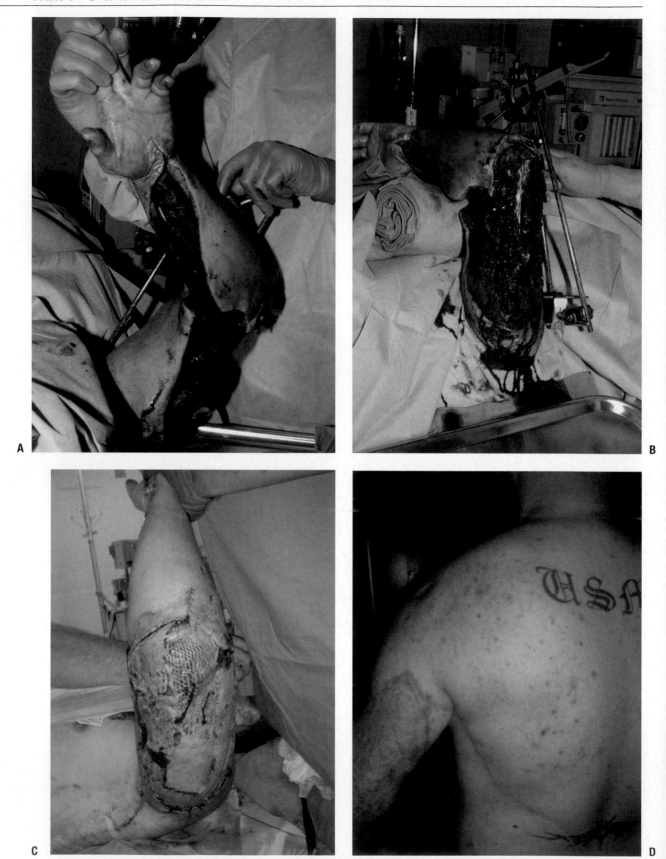

FIGURE 2-23

A-D: Patient suffered a blast injury resulting in an open fracture of the elbow, in addition to severe soft tissue injury and a forearm fasciotomy. He was initially managed with a spanning external fixation device and serial debridements followed by ORIF. (ORIF; pedicled Latissimus Dorsi flap and split thickness skin grafting.)

nerve blocks when appropriate. The mental health of the patient must also never be forgotten, especially in cases of traumatic injury, and appropriate consultation with psychiatric specialists and/or a chaplain should be considered to assist in the patient's overall well-being and ability to participate fully in their own recovery and rehabilitation.

CONCLUSION

Treatment of wounds can be a challenging enterprise, consuming considerable time, energy, and resources. By combining the basic principles of evaluation and treatment set forth in this chapter, and with meticulous attention to detail, the surgeon will have an excellent starting point for the treatment of complicated soft tissue trauma (Fig. 2-23).

Disclaimer. The views expressed in this chapter are those of the authors and do not necessarily reflect the official policy or position of the Department of the Navy, Department of Defense, or the U.S. Government.

RECOMMENDED READING

Anglen JO. Wound irrigation in musculoskeletal injury. *J Am Acad Orthop Surg.* 2001;9:219–226.

Argenta LC, Morykwas MJ. Vacuum-assisted closure: a new method for wound control treatment: clinical experience. *Ann Plast Surg.* 1997;38(6):563–576.

Attinger CE, Janis JE, Steinberg J, et al. Clinical approach to wounds: debridement and wound bed preparation including the use of dressings and wound-healing adjuvants. *Plast Reconstr Surg.* 2006;117(Suppl.): 72–109S.

CDC. Preventing tetanus, diphtheria, and pertussis among adults: use of tetanus toxoid, reduced diphtheria toxoid and acellular pertussis vaccines. Recommendations of the Advisory Committee on Immunization Practices (ACIP) and Recommendation of ACIP, supported by the Healthcare Infection Control Practices Advisory Committee (HICPAC), for Use of Tdap Among Health-Care Personnel. *MMWR.* 2006;55(No. RR-17):1–33.

Klein MB, Hunter S, Heimbach DM, et al. The Versajet water dissector: a new tool for tangential excision. *J Burn Care Rehab.* 2005;26(6):483–487.

Morykwas MJ, Argenta LC, Shelton-Brown EI, et al. Vacuum-assisted closure: a new method for wound control and treatment: animal studies and basic foundation. *Ann Plast Surg.* 1997;38(6): 553–562.

Reuben SS. Buvanendran: preventing the development of chronic pain after orthopaedic surgery with multimodal analgesic techniques. *J Bone Joint Surg Am.* 2007;89:1343–1358.

Reuben SS. Preventing the development of complex regional pain syndrome after surgery. *Anesthesiology.* 2007;101:1215–1224.

Robson MC, Stenberg BD, and Heggers JP. Wound healing alterations caused by infection. *Clin Plast Surg.* 1990;17:485.

3 Management of Simple Wounds: Local Flaps, Z-Plasty, and Skin Grafts

John B. Hijjawi and Allen T. Bishop

Skin grafting and local flap coverage have remained a common means of covering traumatic wounds. Skin grafts, local flaps, and random flaps are not as simple as direct wound closure nor are they are as "elegant" as procedures that are found higher on the reconstructive ladder such as pedicled flaps or free tissue transfer (Fig. 3-1). However, the procedures described in this chapter remain straightforward, reliable, and time-tested and should be an essential component of any surgeon's reconstructive armamentarium.

SKIN GRAFTS

Skin grafts are classified by source and thickness. By far the most common, durable, and successful skin grafts are autografts harvested from the patient's own skin. There are no immunologic issues, since the tissue comes from the patient's own body. Concerns over disease transmission are eliminated and expense is minimal. The only disadvantage is the creation and care of a donor site.

Skin grafts are also available as cadaveric allografts, xenografts (typically porcine skin), and most recently, cultured epithelial grafts. These materials are lifesaving sources of temporary wound coverage in the context of massive burns. Allografts and xenografts do have the disadvantage of immunogenicity and thus impermanence since they are bound to be rejected. However, if the quality of a wound bed is questionable, preserved porcine xenografts may be an excellent option for temporary wound coverage.

Currently available cultured epithelial grafts are expensive, require time to culture, and are not as durable as autografts. Additionally, studies have shown that they are significantly more susceptible to infection than standard autografts.

Skin grafts are also classified based on thickness. The skin is composed of an outer epidermis and a deeper dermis, which is further subdivided into the reticular and papillary dermis (Fig. 3-2). All skin grafts consist of the entire epidermis and a variable amount of dermis. Split-thickness skin grafts contain only a portion of the dermis, whereas full-thickness skin grafts contain the entire dermis and dermal appendages. As a result, full-thickness skin grafts continue to support hair growth following transfer. This needs to be carefully considered when selecting donor sites in situations when a full-thickness skin graft is to be transferred to a conspicuous, previously hairless area.

Since full-thickness skin grafts include all dermal appendages, skin at the donor site will not spontaneously regenerate following harvest; therefore, these donor sites need to be closed primarily or with a split-thickness skin graft. Split-thickness donor sites retain the ability to generate epithelium and will be largely healed within several weeks if cared for properly.

Split-thickness and full-thickness skin grafts have quite different contractile characteristics on harvesting (primary contraction) and after they heal (secondary contraction). Primary contraction is

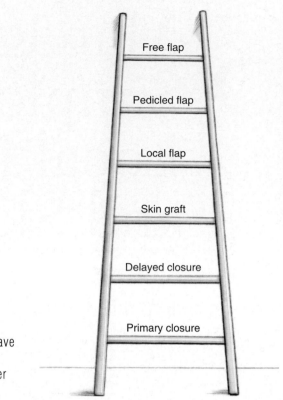

FIGURE 3-1

Reconstructive ladder. Historically, surgeons have closed wounds with the simple procedure first, moving up the rungs of the reconstructive ladder as wounds become larger and more complex.

the initial contraction of a graft when it is harvested. Due to the greater proportion of elastic fibers in a full-thickness skin graft (the dermis is the location of all elastic fibers in the skin), it will undergo more primary contraction than a split-thickness skin graft when harvested. Similarly, a thicker split-thickness skin graft (e.g., 0.018 in) will undergo more primary contraction than a thin split-thickness skin graft. Most skin grafts can be stretched under minimal tension at inset to overcome this contraction, restoring their original size.

Conversely, split-thickness skin grafts undergo more secondary contraction than full-thickness grafts. This can be exploited to provide gradual contraction of a wound over the course of several months. An example is a fasciotomy wound that is under too much tension to close primarily within the days following compartment release. A very thin split-thickness skin graft applied to the wound will undergo significantly more secondary contraction than would a full-thickness skin graft, resulting in contraction of the wound itself. After several months, this may result in a wound that is small enough to allow serial excision of the skin graft and primary closure under minimal tension. In com-

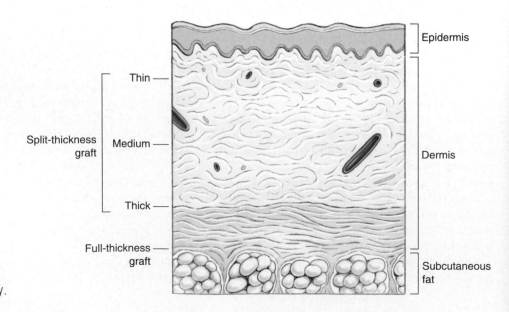

FIGURE 3-2

Skin anatomy.

parison, full-thickness skin grafts can be relied on to undergo virtually no secondary contraction in situations where this is not desirable, such as across a joint surface or in a web space.

Initial adhesion of a skin graft is the result of fibrin present between the graft and the recipient bed. Initial survival of a skin graft relies on plasmatic imbibition, which is the process of nutrient diffusion from the recipient site into the skin graft. Later, vascular channels within the graft line up with vascular channels in the recipient bed through the process of inosculation. Finally, long-term graft survival relies on neovascularization, or the process of new blood vessel growth into the skin graft from the recipient bed. Because skin grafts, both split thickness and full thickness, are completely reliant on the recipient bed for survival, the wound bed must be well-vascularized and free of infection to support skin graft take. Split-thickness skin grafts have lower metabolic demands than do full-thickness grafts, and so they don't require recipient beds with as rich a blood supply. Along the same lines, full-thickness grafts take longer, from 7 to 10 days, to heal. Split-thickness grafts are generally considered healed by 5 days and should be left immobilized and dressed at least that long postoperatively. The time of healing in specific situations depends most on the quality of the recipient wound's blood supply.

Indications/Contraindications

Indications   Skin grafting may be indicated for any defect that cannot be closed primarily and that has a wound bed that can support skin graft take (Table 3-1). Skin grafts survive for the first several days through a process called imbibition. During this stage of skin graft healing, the graft obtains nutrients from the underlying wound bed through a process of diffusion. Wound beds devoid of blood flow, or with little vascularized tissue, will make for poor recipient sites. Exposed structures that will accept a graft include subcutaneous tissue, paratenon, and muscle. Other tissues, such as exposed bone, joint, tendon, and nerve, may be covered temporarily by graft used as a biologic dressing but will not support a graft for permanent coverage. Beds containing tissues of questionable viability, chronic granulation tissue, or frank infection can accept a skin graft but require thorough debridement prior to graft placement. Wounds that contain fewer than 10^5 bacteria per gram of tissue or that allow xenograft adherence within 24 hours allow successful skin grafting.

Contraindications   Skin grafts are contraindicated in areas that are exposed to repetitive trauma or that lie over osseous prominences. Bone, cartilage, and tendons denuded of periosteum, perichondrium, or paratenon cannot be covered with skin grafts as there is inadequate vascular supply to support healing of the skin graft. Controversy exists over whether skin grafts should be placed over bone, cartilage, or tendons with healthy periosteum, perichondrium, or paratenon. It is certainly possible to get skin-graft healing over such structures. However, skin grafts in these situations are rarely optimal for long-term durable coverage. In addition, skin grafting should be avoided in areas that may require secondary surgery for bone or nerve grafting, as adherence to underlying muscle, nerve, and tendon may complicate secondary surgery. All split thickness grafts will undergo some component of contracture over time; thus, if these grafts are placed over large areas of the antecubital fossa, popliteal fossa, or olecranon, there is a risk of limitation in joint motion.

Preoperative Planning

The wound must be debrided and clean prior to attempts at skin grafting. Infection is one of the leading causes of skin graft failure. Since skin grafts are completely dependent on the wound bed they are transplanted to for nutrition, they possess no intrinsic ability to resolve infection. Quantitative wound cultures have been used for many years in some centers to determine the adequacy of a wound's microenvironment for closure. A quantitative culture revealing less than 10^5 bacteria per gram of tissue has been traditionally regarded as an acceptable level of colonization below which a

TABLE 3-1.   Wound Analysis
Is there too much tension across the wound for primary closure?
Is there adequate perfusion of the wound bed?
Are vital structures exposed at the base of the wound?
Is the wound infected or contaminated?
Is the wound geometry favorable for closure?

wound can be closed by skin graft or local flap. However, such cultures are highly dependent on the experience of the technician performing them. A careful clinical evaluation and serial sharp debridement of clinically infected or contaminated wounds are advised.

Donor site selection must also be decided before surgery. Considerations when choosing a donor site for split thickness skin grafts include cosmesis, the thickness of skin in the donor site region, and ease of care of the donor site after graft harvest. The most common split thickness skin donor sites include the buttocks, lateral and anterior thighs, and lower abdomen. These sites are relatively easy to conceal, have thick skin resulting in less pigmentation once healed, and are readily accessible in even a bed-bound patient, easing postoperative care.

Full thickness skin grafts are most commonly harvested from the groin, antecubital fossa, volar wrist crease, medial arm, postauricular sulcus, or lower abdomen. These donor sites all exist in areas where closure can be performed within pre-existing skin creases, thus resulting in relatively inconspicuous donor sites. The hypothenar skin or plantar instep offers the unique quality of glabrous skin if needed for graft material. Always keep in mind that any amputated "spare parts" can provide a good source of viable skin graft with no added morbidity to the patient.

Surgery

Patient Positioning   The patient's position will depend on the location of the graft to be harvested. Most frequently we harvest split thickness grafts from the upper thigh area, where they may easily be concealed under clothing A supine position with a roll underneath one hip is ideal. The majority of full-thickness grafts are harvested from the hairless skin of the groin crease, though the inner upper arm may be used as well. The patient is positioned supine for such harvests. For glaborous skin grafts, the instep of the foot may be positioned so as to allow ease of harvest. For wounds on the posterior aspect of the lower extremity or trunk, a lateral decubitus position readily exposes both the wound and a lateral thigh donor site. With careful planning it is almost never necessary to reposition a patient after harvesting the skin graft.

Split Thickness Grafts   Power dermatomes are the most common method of harvesting split thickness skin grafts, although for very small split thickness grafts hand-driven Weck blades may be more convenient.

Measure the recipient wound and choose a dermatome guard based on that measurement (Fig. 3-3).

- Set and check the dermatome thickness (usually 0.010 to 0.015 in) with a No. 15 scalpel blade. The thin, beveled edge of the knife is about 0.010 in, whereas the thickest portion of the blade is 0.015 in thick (Fig. 3-4).
- Mark the donor site with a ruler so that you will know where the dermatome needs to "touch down" and "lift off." Relying on your memory or estimating how far you will have to drive the dermatome can lead to harvesting too little graft and having to reharvest, creating an unnecessary seam in the graft. In cases of overharvesting, the extra graft can be replaced onto the donor site, but this complicates the donor site dressing.

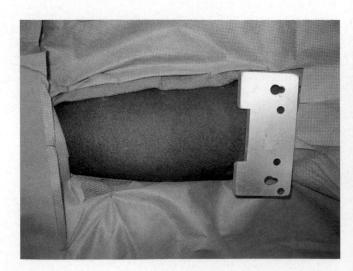

FIGURE 3-3

A dermatome guard of appropriate width is chosen.

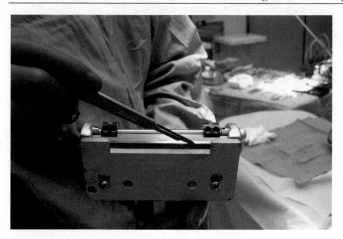

FIGURE 3-4

The thickness setting is double checked.

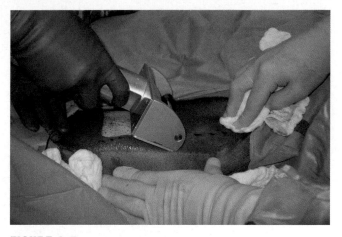

FIGURE 3-5

Countertraction is applied to avoid "skipping" along the skin.

- Clean the donor site to remove any sticky material that will cause the dermatome to stick and apply copious amounts of mineral oil to the donor skin and the dermatome.
- Apply countertraction to the skin in front of and behind the dermatome blade. Dermatomes, particularly when fitted with larger guards, function much more effectively on flat surfaces (Fig. 3-5).
- Activate the dermatome before "touching down" on the skin and plan to keep it activated until after "lifting off" of the skin. Touch down at 45 degrees to the skin, then slightly flatten the angle between the dermatome and skin, maintaining constant firm pressure on the head of the dermatome.
- Realize that if you need to reset a hand for countertraction, you can stop the blade without lifting off of the skin and reset countertraction. The harvest can then be continued without interrupting the continuous sheet of skin graft.
- Transfer the harvested graft onto a dermal carrier with the dermis side up. This side is shinier, and has less friction when rubbed than the epidermis side. If you become confused as to which side is the dermis side, realize that the skin graft edges will always roll toward the dermis side.
- Either make several small slits in the skin graft with a scalpel ("pie crusting") to allow for drainage of accumulated fluid from the wound bed, or run the graft and dermal carrier through a skin graft mesher (Fig. 3-6). Most typically, grafts are meshed at a 1:1.5 ratio. This is done to allow drainage through the graft, to make grafts more conformable to the underlying wound bed, and to increase the area a graft can cover. It is not necessary, however, and many surgeons avoid it since the meshed appearance will be permanently obvious and will significantly compromise the final cosmesis.
- Fix the graft dermis side down to the wound bed with either staples or absorbable sutures such as 5-0 chromic. Traditional bolster or "tie-over" dressings employ silk suture placed circumferentially around the skin graft and left long. They are then tied over mineral oil soaked cotton wrapped in a non-adherent dressing and placed firmly onto the skin graft (Figs. 3-7 through 3-9). A very convenient bolster dressing can be fashioned by placing a non-adherent Nterface dressing (Delasco, Council Bluffs, IA) over the skin graft, followed by mineral oil soaked cotton pushed firmly into the wound bed to compress the skin graft. Finally, a Reston (3M, St. Paul, MN) sponge can be cut to conform to the wound, placed adhesive side up, and stapled to the skin surrounding the wound. This is a very stable bolster construct that resists shearing forces and provides firm compression. For skin grafts placed on an extremity, an Ace wrap can be used to protect this entire dressing.
- Appropriate splints should be applied to immobilize the recipient site until the skin graft is totally healed.

Full Thickness Grafts   Full thickness grafts are harvested after drawing an ellipse, which includes the necessary amount of skin based on the wound measurements. Closure without dogears is best achieved when the length of the ellipse is about four times the width of the ellipse. A scalpel is

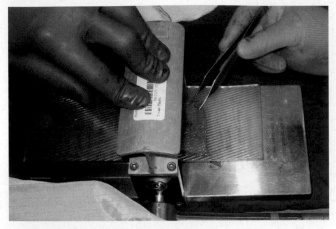

FIGURE 3-6

Meshing the skin graft dermis side up facilitates placement onto the wound.

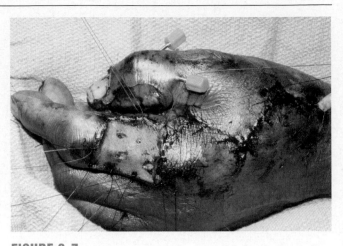

FIGURE 3-7

The bolster or "tie-over" dressing begins with placement of long sutures along the edge of the skin graft.

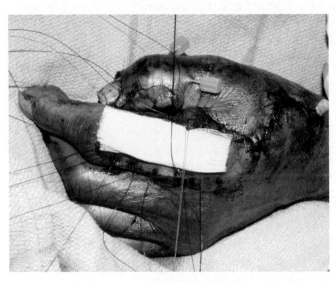

FIGURE 3-8

Cotton balls are wrapped in a non-adherent dressing and compressed onto the skin graft.

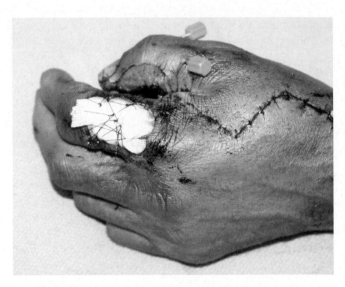

FIGURE 3-9

The completed tie-over.

used to incise the skin just through the dermis. One end of the ellipse is then lifted firmly with a single skin hook or toothed forceps and a fresh scalpel is used to elevate the skin graft just deep to the dermis, taking as little fat as possible with the skin graft. Once harvested, the full-thickness graft can be rolled over a finger or shot glass with the dermis side up, and a curved iris scissors used to remove every bit of residual fat from the dermis.

Full thickness grafts are not typically meshed. Otherwise, they are fixed into position as described for split thickness grafts. They should be left undisturbed for 7 to 10 days. Donor sites are best treated with primary closure after moderate undermining of the wound edge.

Postoperative Management

Split thickness skin grafts should not be disturbed for a minimum of 5 days. The dressing can then be carefully removed to not disturb the healing skin graft, and once daily dressings are begun with an antibacterial ointment and a non-adherent dressing such as Adaptic (Johnson and Johnson, New Brunswick, NJ). Full thickness grafts should remain covered for 7 to 10 days before removing the split or bolster.

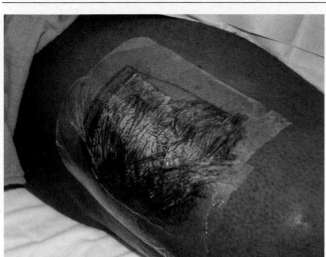

FIGURE 3-10
Donor site dressing.

Donor sites up to 100 cm^2 can be covered with Tegaderm (3M, St. Paul, MN) as long as care is taken to carefully dry the skin surrounding the donor site before applying the dressing. Serum will collect under the Tegaderm after several days, and can be left alone. If the Tegaderm leaks, a patch can be placed over the hole. The benefit of Tegaderm is a completely isolated, moist environment that is virtually painless for the patient (Fig. 3-10). The donor site is typically re-epithelialized by 2 weeks at which point the Tegaderm can be removed and replaced with once daily application of a moisturizing cream and non-adherent dressing. Alternatively, the donor site can be covered with a Xeroform (Sherwood Medical Industries Ltd., Markham, Ontario, Canada), which will dry into an eschar when exposed to air. Once dry this will be painless but is extremely sensitive until the eschar develops.

Rehabilitation   Rehabilitation of the affected extremity can begin once the surgeon is assured of stable graft take. Grafts placed over joints may benefit from 7 to 10 days of immobilization before initiating motion across the joint. For grafts placed away from a joint, normal motion can begin almost immediately if the graft has been securely bolstered to its wound bed.

Complications

Skin graft necrosis or failure is the most common complication following split thickness skin grafting. The formation of fluid under a skin graft, whether hematoma or seroma, is the most common cause of skin graft loss. As noted, the graft is completely reliant on the recipient bed for nutrition and so needs to be in complete contact with the recipient bed to survive. Therefore, precise hemostasis of the wound bed is critical before skin graft application as is firm compression of the graft onto the recipient bed through the use of bolster dressings.

Infection is the next most common cause of skin graft loss. This is best avoided by careful debridement before placement of the graft. Shearing forces can interrupt the formation of vascular connections between the graft and the recipient bed. This will ultimately lead to loss of a graft since healing relies on the formation of genuine vascular connections and is not possible through plasmatic imbibition alone. Therefore, firm immobilization of all skin grafts is critical to their healing.

Finally, an inadequately perfused recipient bed will certainly lead to skin graft loss. Common situations include patients with peripheral vascular disease, previously radiated tissues, and tendon or bone denuded of paratenon or periosteum.

RANDOM FLAPS

Random flaps, by definition, have no named or defined blood supply. They are raised in a subdermal plane and so rely on the subdermal vascular plexus of skin for circulation. To ensure adequate circulation, random flaps should be limited to a length no greater than 2.5 times the width of their base, which is the uncut border of the flap. This ratio may be even more limited in poorly perfused extremities.

Indications/Contraindications

Indications   The elasticity and slight redundancy of local tissue are critical to the success of most random flaps. They are based on local tissue so are typically contraindicated for wounds with significant surrounding soft tissue damage such as radiation wounds. The advantage of random flaps in comparison to skin grafts is that they can provide well-vascularized, full-thickness tissue for wound coverage. Far more durable to friction and repeated stress than skin grafts, local flaps are preferred for closure over vital structures such as tendons, nerves, and blood vessels. An added benefit is that they can be used to close wounds over vital structures denuded of paratenon, periosteum, or perineurium, since a well-vascularized wound bed is not required as it is for skin graft survival. Finally, despite the new scars made to raise random flaps, they are ideal in terms of color match, since they come from local skin.

Contraindications   Gross contamination or frank infection is an absolute contraindication to wound closure with local flaps. In fact, while free flaps and pedicled flaps have been shown to introduce enough independent new blood supply to overcome infectious processes like osteomyelitis, local flaps need to be placed over a clean, uncontaminated wound bed. Finally, local flaps are limited to small wounds usually less than 15 to 20 cm^2; wounds exceeding these dimensions should be covered with another method of soft tissue coverage.

Preoperative Planning

As mentioned previously, adequate surgical debridement is a must before any attempt at closure. Tissue culture is a useful adjunct, particularly in cases of significant blunt trauma with devitalized tissue or cases of gross contamination. Often, serial wound debridement every other day for several days is necessary to obtain negative cultures.

It may not be possible to completely resolve a patient's systemic medical issues, but they should be as optimized as much as possible. Tight control of blood glucose levels in patients with diabetes, management of extremity edema, and nutritional status can all be significantly improved in many patients with several days of focused inpatient care.

Surgery

Z-Plasty   Probably the most familiar random flap to any surgeon, the Z-plasty is not actually indicated for the treatment of open wounds. Rather, the main indications for a Z-plasty include lengthening scars, interrupting linear scars with the transposition of unscarred tissue, and disrupting circumferential or constricting scars (Table 3-2). A common indication in hand surgery is to employ a Z-plasty in contracted web spaces in an effort to introduce healthy adjacent tissue relieving web contractures.

Z-plasties rely on limbs of equal length to facilitate closure. The most common Z-plasty design employs 60-degree angles, which theoretically results in a 75% increase in the length of the central limb of the Z-plasty (Fig. 3-11). Although clinically not feasible, a Z-plasty with angles of 90 degrees would result in the greatest theoretical gain of central limb length, approximately 120%.

Executing an effective Z-plasty is not simply a matter of elevating the triangular flaps and transposing them. Mobility and a tension-free closure are greatly facilitated when the tissue at the bases of the triangular flaps is also elevated.

Four Flap Z-Plasty   Most commonly used for first web space contractures, the four flap Z-plasty results in a 150% gain in length of the original central limb, or scar contracture. Essentially, a 120-degree standard Z-plasty is drawn. Each triangular flap is then bisected, resulting in four equivalent 60-degree triangles that are raised and interdigitated as shown (Fig. 3-12).

TABLE 3-2.   Z-Plasty Indications
Lengthening scars
Interrupting linear scars
Disrupting circumferential or constricting scars

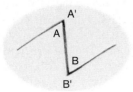
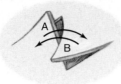
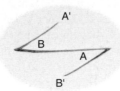

FIGURE 3-11
A basic Z-plasty.

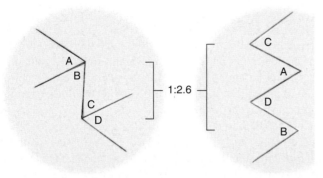

FIGURE 3-12
Four-flap Z-plasty.

Rhomboid Flap   Executing a rhomboid flap begins with converting the defect (even if it is circular) into a rhomboid to better visualize the flap design. A line equivalent in length to the limbs of the rhomboid is then drawn perpendicular to the short axis of the rhomboid (Fig. 3-13). Next, a line (B-C) is drawn at 60 degrees to the A-B line. It will be parallel to one of the limbs of the original rhomboid.

The flap is then elevated. It is also critical to elevate the skin around the base of the flap very liberally to facilitate transposition of the flap and closure of the wound. The flap should not be closed under tension; rather, further undermining of the base of the flap should be executed until the flap closes without tension.

Banner Flap   The banner flap is a type of transposition flap. A pendant or banner of skin is designed with one edge of the banner (near the base of the flap) running tangentially to the wound edge. The flap is elevated and transposed after which any redundant flap can be trimmed. It is important that the original design of the flap places the banner in an area of redundant skin. Since the banner can be designed along any border of the defect, it is helpful for eventual cosmesis if the original banner is designed within a relaxed skin tension line.

Rotational Flap   Rotational flaps are frequently employed on the dorsum of the hand, fingers, and in the scalp to close triangular defects. They are deceptively simple, and poor planning can lead to a large incision with an inadequate flap.

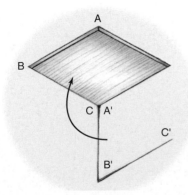
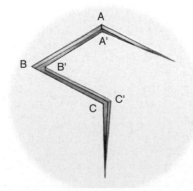

FIGURE 3-13
Rhomboid flap.

Unfortunately, relatively little advancement of the flap edge is possible without making a flap that is approximately four times greater in length than the defect length. Even with an adequately designed flap, tension can develop at a point opposite the pivot point in the base of the flap. This can be overcome by backcutting the base of the flap or excising a Burow's triangle. The pitfall here is the risk of cutting into the base of the flap, which can reduce the circulation of the flap. This added tension in the flap can lead to tip necrosis.

One simple solution for a rotation flap that seems to be under excessive tension is to simply advance the leading edge of the flap into the defect, which results in a new defect at the opposite end of the flap. Since this donor defect should be well vascularized (the flap should be taken from an area of healthy tissue), the donor site can be skin-grafted rather than closed primarily. This strategy, while not elegant, is mush less likely to result in excessive tension on the closure.

V-Y Advancement Flap   V-Y advancement flaps are extremely useful, but their execution differs greatly from transposition flaps. V-Y advancement flaps are not elevated completely, but rather must remain connected to the subcutaneous tissue underlying the flap to maintain their viability. This is because they are incised along all skin borders and so have no connected "base" through which a dermal or subdermal blood supply can provide circulation.

A V-shaped flap is designed immediately adjacent to the defect with the widest portion of the V equivalent in width to the width of the defect (Fig. 3-14). The two limbs of the V are then gradually tapered so that their length is at least 1.5 times the length of the desired advancement. The distance the edge of the flap can be advanced is somewhat determined by the laxity of the local skin.

Following advancement of the flap edge into the defect, the base of the V is closed in a linear fashion, resulting in a "Y."

Postoperative Management

On completion of the operation, a bulky non-compressive dressing is applied to the wound, which may be supported with a plaster splint if immobilization is required. A small window can be left to monitor the flap for signs of ischemia or congestion. Sutures remain for an average of 10 to 14 days, depending on the status and tension of the surrounding tissue. Ideally, flaps are inset under minimal tension, allowing the patient to begin gentle range of motion exercises immediately following surgery. Once sutures are removed, the wounds may be kept moist with a petroleum-based product, which will prevent itching during the early postoperative period.

Complications

The most feared postoperative complication following local flap reconstruction is necrosis or partial necrosis of the transferred tissue. This complication occurs because of inadequate blood supply to the flap. Flap ischemia may result from flap closure under excessive tension, hematoma, or infec-

FIGURE 3-14

The Atasoy-Kleinert V-Y advancement flap. Note that the subcutaneous tissue has remained undisturbed to maintain blood supply. (Redrawn after Louis DS, Jebson PLJ, Graham TJ. Amputations. In: Green DP, Hotchkiss RN, Pederson WC, eds. *Operative hand surgery.* New York: Churchill Livingstone; 1999:48-94.)

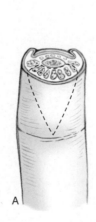
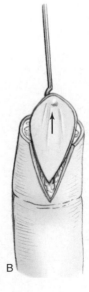
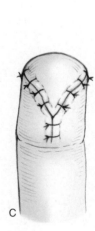

A   B   C

tion. If total flap loss develops, the wound will require closure by another means, either pedicled flap or skin graft. If partial necrosis has occurred, one can debride the necrotic portion of the flap and begin dressing changes to the underlying wound bed. Once the underlying tissues are clean of any infection and necrotic debris, the surgeon can consider allowing the wound to heal through secondary intention or attempt wound closure with an alternative reconstructive method.

PEARLS AND PITFALLS

Pearls

- Use a VAC or Reston bolster to immobilize and compress skin grafts quickly.
- Do not mesh pie-crust skin grafts on hands.
- Exploit secondary contraction of thin split-thickness grafts (0.010–0.012) to induce contraction of fasciotomy wounds.
- Employ Tegaderm for small donor sites (100 cm^2) to decrease pain and provide a moist wound-healing environment.
- Splint extremities to immobilize skin grafts.
- Salvage improperly planned local flaps by skin grafting the local flap donor site.

Pitfalls

- Hematoma
- Seroma
- Inadequate immobilization of grafts or flaps while healing
- Meshing grafts on the hand
- Inadequate initial wound debridement

RECOMMENDED READING

Ablove RH, Howell RM. The physiology and technique of skin grafting. *Hand Clin.* 1997;13:163–173.

Chao JD, Huang JM, Weidrich TA. Local hand flaps. *J Amer Soc Surg Hand.* 2001;1:25–44.

Lin SJ, Hijjawi JB. Skin grafting. In: Lin SJ, Hijjawi JB, eds. *Plastic and reconstructive surgery pearls of wisdom.* New York: McGraw Hill; 2006:435–436.

Louis DS, Jebson PLJ, Graham TJ. Amputations. In: Green DP, Hotchkiss RN, Pederson WC, eds. *Operative hand surgery.* New York: Churchill Livingstone; 1999:48–94.

Tschoi M, Hoy EA, Granick MS. Skin flaps. *Clin Plast Surg.* 2005;32:261–273.

4 Vacuum-Assisted Closure in Extremity Trauma

Anthony J. DeFranzo and Louis C. Argenta

INDICATIONS/CONTRAINDICATIONS

Wounds of the upper and lower extremities provide a constant challenge for orthopaedic and plastic surgeons. Complex severe injuries involving bone and soft tissue demand major reconstructive procedures. Less severe injuries exposing tendon, bone, and joints also demand innovative surgical approaches. Many patients with injured extremities have been the victim of multiple traumas and may have major associated injuries involving head, chest, and abdomen. Major blood loss, disseminated intravascular coagulopathy (DIC), high intracranial pressure, acute respiratory distress syndrome (ARDS), septicemia, and renal failure frequently complicate the treatment of these patients. Vacuum-assisted closure (VAC) has provided a way to effectively manage these wounds until definitive reconstruction can be performed. Vacuum-assisted closure has also greatly simplified reconstruction in many of these patients. Skin grafts are performed in many cases that would have otherwise required major rotational flaps or free flaps prior to the advent of VAC therapy.

The mechanics of the VAC system are straightforward. The system consists of an open cell polyurethane ether foam sponge sealed by an adhesive drape. All pores in the sponge communicate so that negative pressure applied to the sponge is applied equally and completely to the entire wound surface. The effects of the VAC on the wound are multiple. The application of negative pressure causes the sponge to collapse toward its center. Traction forces are thus applied to the wound perimeter pulling the wound edges together progressively making the wound smaller. The VAC sponge should be cut to fit inside the wound to maximize traction forces on the wound edges. The sponge should not overlap intact skin, as skin maceration may occur. In addition, the VAC removes wound edema, appears to increase circulation and decrease bacterial counts, and significantly increases the rate of granulation tissue formation (1,6).

All wounds are thoroughly debrided prior to VAC placement. No clinical infection, purulence, or suspected osteomyelitis should be present prior to VAC placement. Grossly contaminated wounds are a contraindication for VAC placement. The VAC sponge should not be applied directly over major exposed blood vessels in the extremity status posttrauma, especially if the vessel wall has been damaged or a vessel repair has been performed. A protective interface such as Adaptic® may be used. Exposed, repaired, or damaged major vessels should be covered with flaps such as muscle flaps or fasciocutaneous flaps. The VAC may be applied over intact nerves if muscle flap or adequate soft tissue coverage is not possible. A layer of Adaptic may help prevent pain caused by VAC traction especially when VAC sponges are changed. Nerve repairs should also be protected by an interface layer such as Adaptic placed under the VAC sponge. Adequate soft tissue or flap coverage of major peripheral nerves is preferred for final long-term management. The VAC may frequently allow secondary closure of wounds over major peripheral vessels or nerves by pulling together adequate soft tissue as edema is removed. Split-thickness skin grafts placed directly over major exposed vessels or nerves is possible with VAC therapy after granulation tissue occurs, but not preferred.

The VAC sponge may be placed directly on bone if the bone surface bleeds following sharp debridement by an osteotome or low-speed power burr. Occasionally, desiccation of bone may occur with the VAC. If desiccation occurs, further debridement to punctuate bone surface bleeding with the immediate placement of Integra® Dermal Regeneration Template and then VAC placement directly over Integra may be tried. This technique has provided Integra take over bone allowing subsequent skin graft coverage. The Integra must be meshed or holes cut in the outer silicone layer before VAC sponge placement. Relatively small areas of bone have been successfully treated in this manner. Large areas of exposed bone are better treated with pedicle muscle flaps, pedicle fasciocutaneous flaps, or free flaps. The VAC should not be placed over desiccated bone with questionable viability without punctuate bone surface bleeding.

PREOPERATIVE PLANNING

Wounds should be thoroughly debrided before VAC application. Once the wounds are clean, VAC therapy may be initiated. VAC sponges can initially be applied in the operating room following definitive debridement.

SURGERY

To illustrate the application of the VAC device to wounds of the extremities, case studies will be shown to illustrate degloving injuries, gunshot wounds, and a variety of avulsion injuries with exposed tendons, bones, and joints. VAC treatment of traumatic wound complications such as infection and hematoma is also illustrated.

Degloving Injuries

Several degloving injuries to the hand have been treated by the VAC with varying results from 0% to 95% take of replaced degloved skin. The degree of take depends on the condition of the degloved skin and the viability of underlying tissue. The degloved skin is frequently crushed and lacerated. It may be difficult to clinically assess the viability of the degloved avascular skin. Also, roller injuries which frequently cause degloving injuries of the hand may crush as well as deglove the hand. Contusion to the hand intrinsic muscle and crush injury of blood vessels in the hand may also be difficult to evaluate. Progressive loss of viability may occur.

In all hand degloving injuries (N = 6) treated to date at Wake Forest University School of Medicine, fingers were not viable significantly beyond the proximal interphalangeal (PIP) joints and amputations were made at or just distal to that level (4). The thumb has been salvaged at full length in one case. In degloving injuries, most extensor and flexor tendons remain on the hand. If the distal phalanx is avulsed with the skin envelope the flexor digitorum profundus tendon(s) may also be avulsed from the hand and even from the forearm. Extensor peritenon and flexor tendon sheaths are frequently intact, providing vascularized coverage to the tendon.

The clinical approach has been to assess viability of the degloved skin and hand after meticulous debridement and completing the amputations at the appropriate level. The skin is thoroughly defatted, pie-crusted, and placed back on the hand with a few staples and/or sutures. The VAC is then immediately applied. The sponge is cut to fit over the grafted, degloved skin, using one or multiple contiguous pieces of sponge. A "hand VAC" kit is also commercially available. Controlled suction of 125 mm Hg pressure is applied (Fig. 4-1). This procedure takes very little operative time. If successful, the patient is spared a great deal of overall treatment time and morbidity compared to more complicated methods of reconstruction. Therefore, with a degloving injury, our treatment algorithm is as follows: (a) skin defatting and debridement, (b) wound debrideded, (c) skin applied to wound, (d) VAC applied to wound. The VAC is left in place for 4 to 6 days. If there are areas which have not revascularized, the VAC may be replaced for 2 more days for a total of 6 days. After day 6, further take with VAC therapy does not seem to occur and we have not used the VAC longer than 6 days.

If VAC therapy is totally unsuccessful, no more than 6 days are lost with the attempt at degloved skin replacement before other methods of reconstruction are initiated. The best case to date of VAC replacement of degloved skin achieved a 95% take of avulsed skin with preservation of fingers at or just distal to the PIP joints and preservation of the thumb at full length. Excellent range of motion of the metacarpal phalangeal joints was achieved. Further surgery involved outpatient revision of the amputations of the four amputated fingertips and deepening of the first web space (Fig. 4-2).

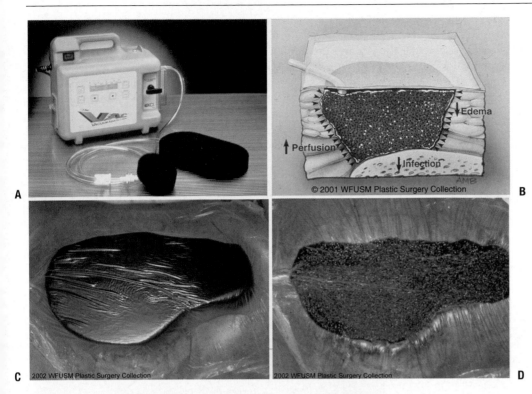

FIGURE 4-1

Mechanics of the VAC system. **A:** Open cell polyurethane ether foam dressing. **B:** A 400–600 micron pore diameter. **C:** Foam dressing cut to fit the wound. **D:** Wound sealed with adhesive drape. There is 50–125 mm Hg controlled suction applied continuously.

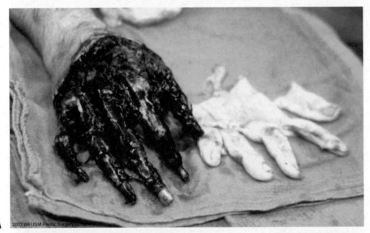
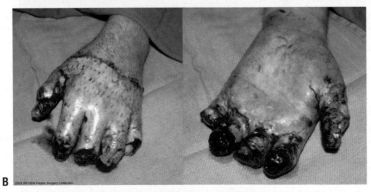
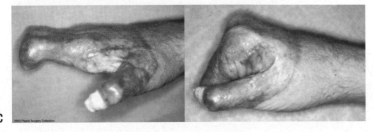

FIGURE 4-2

Degloving injury to the hand. **A:** Entire dorsum and all fingers avulsed to distal palm. Neurovascular bundles present to or just beyond proximal interphalangeal joints. Extensor paratenon intact; flexor tendon sheaths intact. **B:** Fingers surgically amputated at or just distal to PIP joints. Skin defatted, pie-crusted, and reapplied. VAC change day 4 with 95% take of reapplied degloved full-thickness skin. **C:** Final result with good range of motion at metacarpal phalangeal joints.

One degloving injury of the foot has been treated with the VAC. The toes were amputated with the degloved skin at the time of the injury. Metatarsals were shortened surgically so that they were covered by viable soft tissue. The skin was thoroughly defatted, pie-crusted, and returned to the foot. A few staples were used to secure the skin, and the VAC was applied for 4 days. Skin viability was 95%. No revisional surgery has been required. A small area of breakdown on the plantar surface of the heel occurred with ambulation, but healed with simple dressing changes and has not been a recurring problem with proper footwear (Fig. 4-3).

Crush Avulsion Injuries with Exposed Bone, Joints, and/or Tendons

Crush/avulsion injuries are commonly seen after industrial accidents or accidents at home with lawnmowers and farm machinery. Crush/avulsion injuries are also frequently seen with motor vehicle accidents and may be associated with other major critical injuries. Expedient closure of wounds without major reconstructive procedures with long anesthesia times may be beneficial to overall pa-

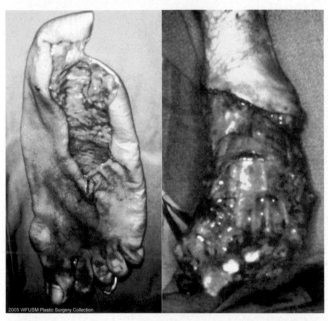

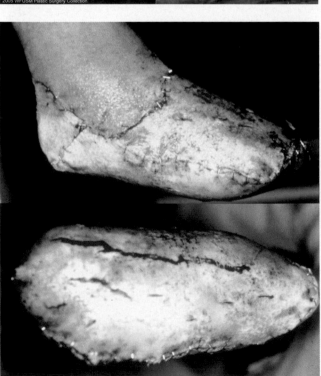

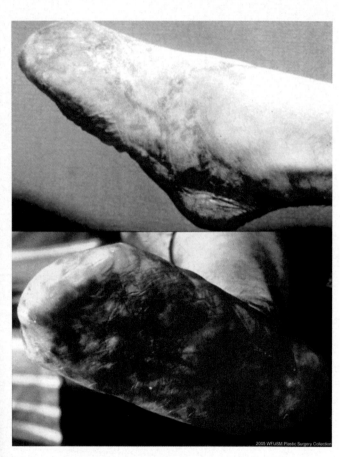

FIGURE 4-3

Degloving injury to the foot. **A:** Entire dorsum, plantar surface, and skin of posterior heel avulsed. All toes traumatically amputated at metatarsal phalangeal joints. **B:** Amputations revised at metatarsal phalangeal joints. Avulsed skin defatted, pie-crusted, and replaced. The VAC is removed on day 4 with 95% of replaced skin viable. **C:** Final result with durable cover with proper footwear at 2 years.

tient care in the critically injured patient. Injuries to the upper extremity and lower extremity from the knee to the ankle result in exposure of tendons, bones, and joints. The VAC has been used on such patients only after one or more thorough operative debridements of all nonviable tissue. In some of these cases, coverage of tendon, bones, and joints has been facilitated by the use of Integra®.

Integra Dermal Regeneration Template is a clear bilayer membrane designed originally for skin replacement in burn patients. It consists of an epidermal layer comprised of a clear thin sheet of silicone (polysiloxane) and a dermal layer comprised of a porous matrix of bovine collagen fibers cross linked with chondroctin-6-sulfate from shark cartilage. The silicone sheet is removed after take of the Integra, and a split-thickness skin graft typically 8 to 12 thousandth of an inch is applied. With VAC therapy over pie-crusted or meshed Integra (noncrushing mesher), take occurs in as little as 6 days. Our practice is to maintain VAC therapy for 6 days undisturbed over Integra. Clinically, the Integra assumes a salmon-pink color when take occurs; but with 6 days of VAC therapy, a more robust red color may be achieved. We now routinely plan to perform split-thickness skin grafts 6 days after VAC placement over Integra.

Integra and split-thickness skin graft provide a pliable durable bilaminar skin reconstruction ideal to cover joint surfaces (3). With VAC therapy, Integra has taken well over a vascularized wound bed, at 6 days in most patients. In addition to simple Integra take, however, viable tendons, bones, and open joints without cover have been bridged for a distance of 1 to 2 cm. At day 6, if structures have not been "bridged" sufficiently, VAC therapy may be continued for a total of 10 to 12 days. Red vascular tissue can be seen spreading transversely through the Integra that is bridging a bone, joint, or tendon.

Tendons and bones can granulate in the abscence of Integra to allow split-thickness skin graft take (2). However, the use of Integra appears to provide a more durable skin cover over bone and over tendon allows tendon glide with appropriate early occupational therapy. Split-thickness skin graft applied over Integra is followed by VAC therapy for another 6 days to achieve take of the split-thickness skin graft to complete the reconstruction. The VAC has been useful in maximizing the take of split-thickness skin grafts over irregular surfaces in many of our cases involving the extremities (7). Whenever

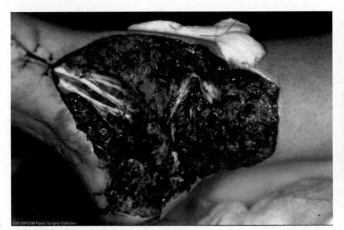

A

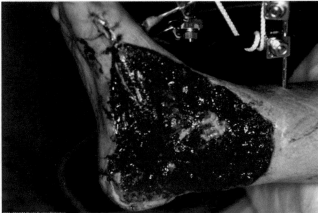

B

FIGURE 4-4

A 68-year-old status post lawnmower avulsion injury. Smoker with atherosclerosis. **A:** Exposed medial malleolus, ankle joint, and tendon. **B:** VAC therapy for 2 weeks with granulation tissue covering exposed tendons and joint. No use of Integra®. **C:** Split-thickness skin graft stable for 4 years with normal footwear.

C

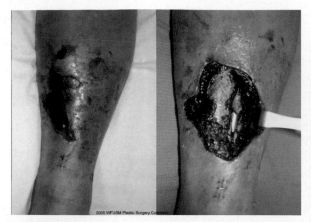

A

FIGURE 4-5

A 67-year-old status post motor vehicle accident with crush of lower extremity and fracture of underlying tibia treated with an intramedullary rod. **A:** Exposure of rod post status debridement. **B:** VAC therapy allowed soft tissue to cover bone by both a decrease in wound size and the formation of granulation tissue. Final skin closure was obtained with a split thickness skin graft. Wound stable at 1 year.

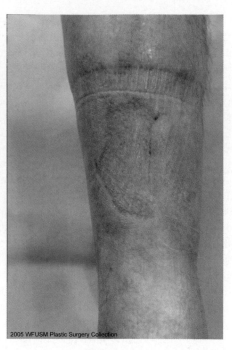

B

FIGURE 4-6

A 17-year-old with skin avulsion of the left arm status post motor vehicle accident. **A:** Exposed ulna is debrided to bleeding bone. **B:** VAC applied for 6 days with formation of granulation tissue. Integra® was then applied and VAC continued for 7 days. Finally split-thickness skin graft was applied. **C:** Stable cover after 3 years for definitive wound closure.

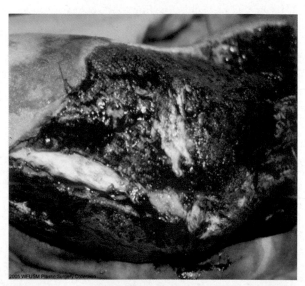

A

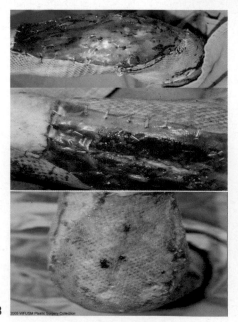

B

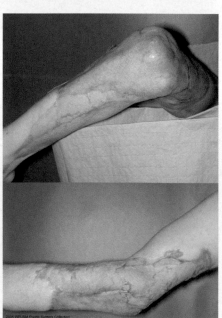

C

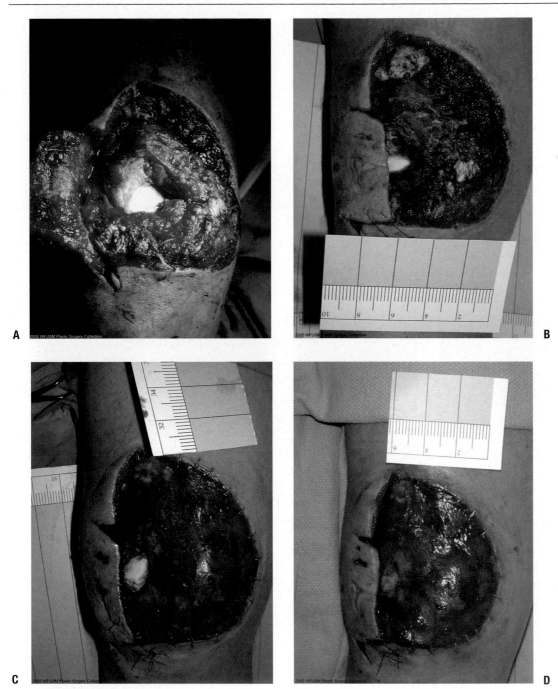

FIGURE 4-7

A 24-year-old male status post motorcycle accident with right brachial plexus injury, right clavicle and right scapula fracture, right occluded axillary artery, right pneumothorax, right open comminuted patella fracture with avulsion of patellar bone and soft tissue with an anterior open knee joint. **A:** Open knee joint post status debridement of nonviable patella and soft tissue. **B:** Soft tissue deficit following ligament reconstruction and VAC placement. **C:** Integra® was placed over the open knee joint. **D:** Granulation bridging knee joint through Integra. *(Continued)*

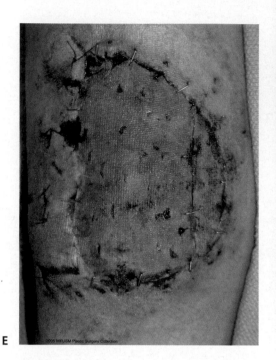

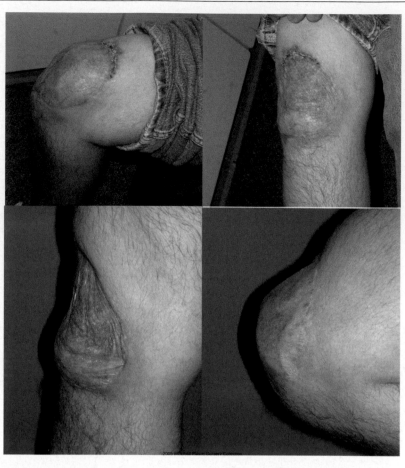

FIGURE 4-7

Continued **E:** A split-thickness skin graft was applied over the Integra® after the Integra showed signs of levascularization. **F:** Excellent range of motion achieved at 3 months with stable cover at 2.5 years.

possible, range of motion of joints and tendons is begun early at 1 to 2 weeks after successful skin graft take (Figs. 4-4 through 4-7).

Gunshot Wounds

Gunshot wounds are associated with blast effect which causes major damage to bone and surrounding soft tissue. Massive wound edema develops. Reconstruction can become exceedingly difficult. When applied immediately after proper debridement, VAC therapy can remove a large amount of edemic fluid from the wound. Multiple operative debridements may be required to ensure that all nonviable bone and muscle have been removed. As much as 2 L of edema fluid have been removed from wounds of the lower extremity over a 24 hour period (5). Application of VAC can also pull retracted wound edges together and promoted the remaining wound to fill with granulation tissue covering exposed bone, tendon, and hardware (Figs. 4-8 and 4-9).

Vacuum-Assisted Closure Therapy for Posttraumatic Wound Complications

Posttraumatic wounds are subject to higher hematoma and infection rates due to tissue devascularization and tissue contamination. If a wound dehisces, rapid edema may make wound reclosure impossible. Bone, tendon, and/or plates become exposed and their coverage is essential to a successful outcome. Vacuum-assisted closure therapy has been useful in regaining closure of posttraumatic open wound complications (Fig. 4-10).

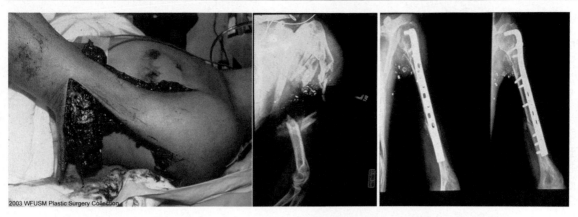

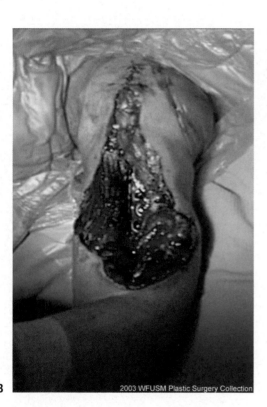

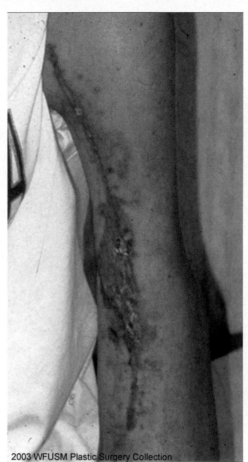

FIGURE 4-8

A 25-year-old with a self inflected gunshot wound to the left arm. **A:** Debridement and plate fixation of the humerus. **B:** Exposed plate status post debridement with decreased wound size and granulation tissue covering plate fixation. **C:** VAC Therapy for 7 days with decreased wound size and granulation tissue beginning to cover plate fixation.

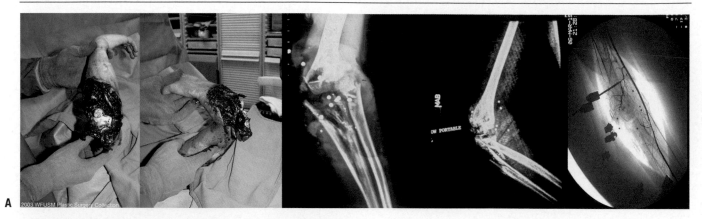

A

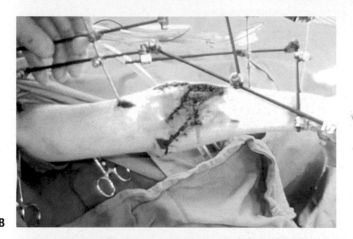

B

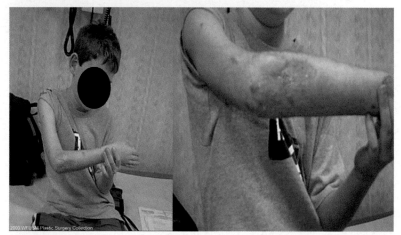

C

FIGURE 4-9

A: A 10-year-old boy with a gunshot wound to the right elbow, forearm, and hand extremity well vascularized. VAC placed on day 4 status post debridement of all nonviable tissue. Three operative debridements were required prior to VAC placement. **B:** Early post-operative course showing a small amount of exposed bone. The soft tissue defect was advanced to closure by VAC therapy. **C:** Split-thickness skin graft placed 10 days status post injury after granulation tissue covers all exposed bone. **D:** Wound stable 2 years. Excellent bone healing and range of motion.

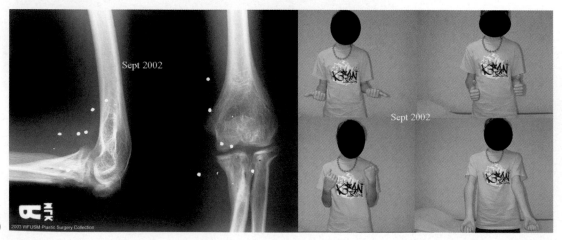

D

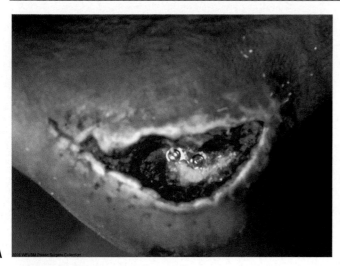
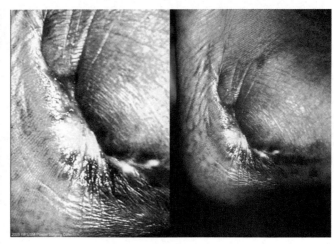

FIGURE 4-10

A 32-year-old status post fractured calcaneus treated by open reduction and plate fixation. **A:** A postoperative hematoma resulted in wound dehiscence and exposed the plate. **B:** Four weeks of VAC therapy were used to obtain wound closure (3.5 weeks as an outpatient). No surgical procedure to achieve skin closure was required. Wounds stable for 3 years with normal foot wear.

POSTOPERATIVE MANAGEMENT

We believe that the VAC sponge ideally should not be left longer than 2 days between changes to maintain proper seal and to avoid infection. Small, clean outpatient wounds may be changed three times a week (Monday, Wednesday, Friday schedule), by visiting home nurses with a 2–3 day change interval.

Oral or intravenous narcotics are usually sufficient for VAC changes in adults. Infusion of Xylocaine into the sponge discontinued from suction 15 minutes before VAC change has been beneficial for local analgesia prior to VAC change. Care must be taken to administer doses of Xylocaine usually well below safe standard dose guidelines. A dose of 10 to 20 cc of 1% Xylocaine with epinephrine for a small to medium size sponge would be sufficient. Much larger wounds may not benefit from Xylocaine infusion. Children granulate more quickly than adults and may require a smaller pore size sponge (white sponge) than the standard black sponge. Granulation tissue may grow into the black sponge and cause increased pain or bleeding with the VAC sponge change in children. Every-24-hour VAC changes may occasionally be required with a standard black sponge in children. However, with granulation tissue development, split-thickness skin grafting is possible even sooner in children, and the uncomfortable course of VAC sponge changes is soon over. Children may require a brief general anesthetic or Ketamine for each VAC change in a dressing room setting staffed by an anesthesiologist.

COMPLICATIONS

Complications are experienced occasionally due to mechanical failure of the machine with loss of suction and unfortunate wound deterioration. The wound may become a sealed abscess cavity if suction is not properly maintained. All new machines have alarms that should signal loss of suction. Every-2-day VAC sponge changes ensures that proper machine function and seal are provided. Technical errors such as an improper seal have occurred with inexperienced personnel. In-service training is mandatory for all nursing and physician staff. Sponge overlap of the skin will cause skin maceration. Bleeding may occur with VAC change, especially in children. Bleeding can usually be controlled with pressure. Generalized bleeding from the wound usually means that sufficient granulation has occurred to allow skin grafting.

Osteomyelitis has occurred infrequently if insufficient bone debridement was performed prior to VAC therapy. Granulation tissue unfortunately may quickly cover a bony sequestrum with VAC therapy. Significant drainage from such wounds soon occurs and points to the need for further debridement of the nonviable bony sequestrum. All questionable bone should be aggressively debrided prior to VAC placement so that all remaining bone bleeds well.

A small number of plates have become infected after VAC coverage with granulation tissue. Plate infection jeopardizes bony union and delays skin closure or skin grafting. Loose plates and screws or plates that do not conform tightly to underlying bone are likely to become infected. Relatively small plate exposures have been successfully treated with the VAC. Major plate exposure should not be treated with the VAC. Clinical judgment should dictate that a major plate exposure, especially with poor-quality surrounding tissue, must be treated with some form of flap.

RESULTS

Vacuum-assisted closure has decreased the requirements for complex wound closure in the extremities. Fewer major pedicle flaps and fewer free tissue transfers are required. With vacuum-assisted closure of traumatic extremity wounds, the number of free tissue transfers now required at our institution is approximately 33% when compared to the number prior to VAC therapy. Long operative and anesthesia times are avoided, which is especially beneficial for critically severely injured patients.

REFERENCES

1. Argenta LC, Morykwas MJ. Vacuum-assisted closure: A new method for wound control and treatment: Clinical experience. *Ann Plast Surg.* 1997;38(6):563–577.
2. David L, DeFranzo A, Argenta L, et al. The use of vacuum-assisted closure therapy for the treatment of lower extremity wounds with exposed bone. *Plast Reconstr Surg.* 2001;108(5):1184–1191.
3. DeFranzo AJ, Argenta LC, David LR, et al. Treatment of traumatic hand/upper extremity wounds with the VAC wound healing device. *Plast Surg Forum.* 2002;264–265.
4. DeFranzo AJ, Marks MW, Argenta LC, et al. Vacuum-assisted closure of treatment of degloving injuries. *Plast and Reconstr Surg.* 1999;104(7):2145–2148.
5. DeFranzo AJ. Vacuum-assisted closure for the treatment of gunshot wounds. *Perspect Plast Surg.* 2001;15(1):91–109.
6. Morykwas MJ, Argenta LC, Shelton-Brown, EI, et al. Vacuum-assisted closure: A new method for wound control and treatment: Animal studies and basic foundation. *Ann Plast Surg.* 1997;38(6):553–562.
7. Schneider AM, Morykwas MJ, Argenta LC. A new and reliable method of securing skin grafts to the difficult recipient bed. *Plast Reconstr Surg.* 1998;102:1195–1198.

PART II
MANAGEMENT OF SOFT TISSUES WITHIN THE UPPER EXTREMITY

5 Evaluation and Management of Nerve Injuries Following Soft Tissue and Bony Trauma

Susan E. Mackinnon and Renata V. Weber

Nerve injuries associated with orthopaedic trauma are usually due to avulsion, crush, or direct laceration of the affected nerve. The extent of the injury can vary from focal lacerations to diffuse nerve root avulsions. In general, the greater the local soft tissue destruction, the more complex the nerve injury and the less likely for return of normal function.

TABLE 5-1.	Typical Nerve Injury Patterns	
Type	**May be Injured**	**Significance**
Stretch/Avulsion Injury		
Avulsion	Nerve roots Nerves exiting Foramen, Bony fx	Unable to be repaired primarily Indication for nerve transfer
Stretch	Any nerve	Mixed nerve injury (Degree VI)
Crush and Compression Injury		
Complex Crush	Skin, Subcutaneous Tissue, Muscle, Nerve, +/- Bone	Varying degree of depth, loss of function is related to amount of tissue destruction
Chronic Compression	Nerve	Slow onset, reversible
Acute Compression	Nerve +/- Muscle	Quick onset, reversible muscle ischemia, variable recovery of both muscle and nerve
Compartment less syndrome	Nerve + Muscle	Quick onset, reversible muscle ischemia if than 6 hrs; variable recovery of muscle and nerve if released after 6 hrs.
Penetrating injury		
Sharp	Skin, Subcutaneous Tissue, Muscle Nerve, +/- Bone All levels	Needs surgical exploration because of high probability for nerve severance
Blunt	Variable	Injury may extend further then expected
Blast	Variable	Injury pattern depends on ballistic makeup and velocity
Electrical	Variable	Neuropathy is from damage to myelin sheath and ranges from neuropathy to causalgia

CLASSIFICATION OF NERVE INJURIES

Nerve injuries can occur with varying degree of soft tissue injury and may be isolated to the nerve(s) or associated with fractures, dislocations, or fracture-dislocations. From an evaluation and treatment perspective, nerve injuries can be grouped as (a) stretch and avulsion injuries, (b) crush and compression injuries, and (c) penetrating injuries. Table 5-1 lists the typical nerve injury patterns and their significance with respect to assessment and treatment.

Originally, peripheral nerve injuries were described by Sir Herbert Seddon in 1943 as neurapraxia, axonotmesis, and neurotmesis (1). The classification was later expanded by Sunderland and further defined by Mackinnon to include six degrees of injuries (Table 5-2) (2). First degree (neurapraxia) and second degree (axonotmesis) injuries recover spontaneously, the latter at the classic rate of 1 in/month or 1 to 1.5 mm/day (3). Third degree injuries must regenerate through some amount of scar tissue, thus recovery is variable and less than normal depending on the amount of scar tissue around the nerve. In fourth degree injuries, also known as a neuroma-in-continuity, regeneration is blocked by scar tissue within the fascicles and recovery is usually very poor or does

TABLE 5-2.		Classification of nerve injury		
Seddon	**Sunderland**	**Mackinnon**	**Injury**	**Recovery**
neurapraxia	Degree I		conduction block resolves spontaneously	fast/excellent
axonotmesis	Degree II		axonal rupture without interruption of the basal lamina tubes	slow/excellent
	Degree III		rupture of both axons and basal lamina tubes, some scar	slow/incomplete
	Degree IV	(neuroma- in-continuity)	complete scar block	none
neurotmesis	Degree V		complete transection	none
	Degree VI		combination of I-V +/- normal fascicles	mixed

not occur. A fifth degree nerve injury (neurotmesis) is a transection of the nerve, which always will require surgical repair, while the sixth degree nerve injury encompasses a variety of nerve injuries within a single nerve. The difficulty with surgical correction of a sixth degree injury is limiting the repair to the fascicles affected by fourth and fifth degree damage and not damaging the fascicles with the potential for spontaneous recovery (Fig. 5-1).

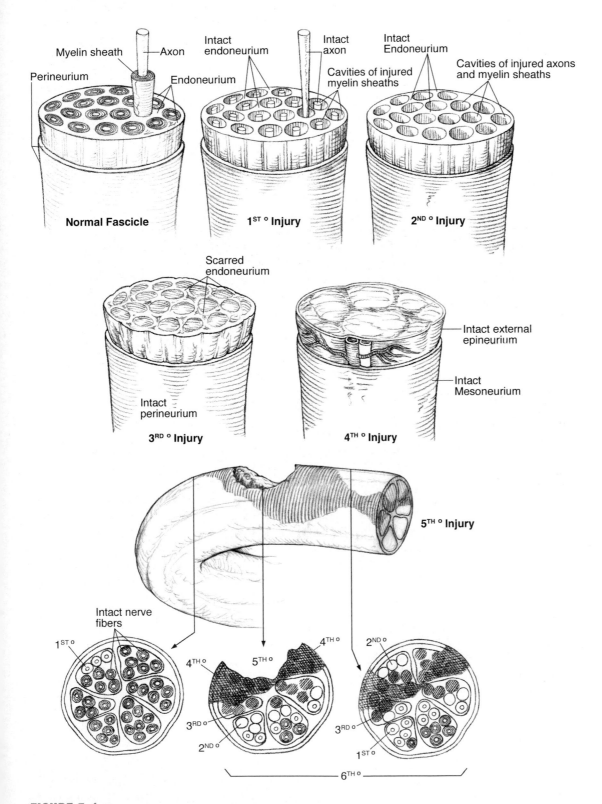

FIGURE 5-1

Schematic depiction of nerve injuries from first through sixth degree. (By permission of Mayo Foundation for Medical Education and Research. All rights reserved.)

Stretch and Nerve Avulsion Injuries

Traction on a nerve can result in a mild stretch injury to the axon with preservation of the basal lamina. The Schwann cells around both myelinated and unmyelinated fibers may be locally injured and, until the cells are replaced from surrounding Schwann cells, will cause a conduction block. Such injuries are classified as first degree injuries and recover completely. As the pulling forces increase across the nerve, the basal lamina, the endoneurium, and perineurium become injured. As the nerve heals, internal scaring of the nerve may occur in some of the fascicles, leading to incomplete recovery. Grossly, the nerve will appear intact as the epineurium is usually not violated. Occasionally, neurolysis or even an internal neurolysis of the injured nerve may improve recovery as long as there is evidence that the nerve recovery is being hindered by scar surrounding the nerve, rather than internal scar to the fascicles.

Nerves that are stretched beyond the breaking point will avulse, resulting in gross disruption of the epineurium, perineurium, and endoneurium. A neuroma will typically form at the proximal end, and these injuries are treated with excision of the neuroma and primary repair when possible. Often, if the time from injury is greater than 2 weeks, even excessive mobilization of the nerve ends will not be enough to overcome the resulting gap that occurs when the unhealthy neuroma tissue at both ends is resected. A nerve graft is then needed to repair the gap.

In extreme cases, nerves can be avulsed from their insertion into the spinal cord. In the past, these injuries were treated conservatively. Once no further nerve recovery was noted, tendon transfers were used to restore the residual functional deficits (4). More recently, the introduction of nerve transfers allows for rewiring of nonfunctioning nerves by using local uninjured nerves to restore electrical continuity to the deinnervated muscles (5). Tendon transfers may be used to augment the nerve transfers once maximum recovery is achieved (6).

Nerves avulsed at the neuromuscular junction present a different problem. Nerves that are injured just prior to entering the muscle, or shortly thereafter, may still be repaired or grafted in most cases as long as a large enough nerve stump is found. Motor nerves that are avulsed from the muscle bellies are treated by implanting proximal nerve, when available, directly into the muscle with the hope that some of the fibers will find a neuromuscular junction and reinnervate at least part of the muscle. Some studies (7) show as good as M4 motor recovery 1 to 2 years after direct nerve to muscle neurotization; however, experimental studies do not support these findings. Rather, recovery is much less than a nerve coaptation would produce (8).

Crush Injuries

Crush injuries comprise the most common peripheral nerve injury to the extremity. External compression may be complicated by increased internal pressure from hematomas, fractures, and local tissue edema. When minor, this may cause a temporary neurapraxia, but with greater compression the likelihood of permanent injury increases. The most severe consequence of a crush injury is the progression to compartment syndrome. Often an early sign of impending compartment syndrome is a decrease in vibration sensibility (9). Compartment syndrome of the upper extremity and lower extremity are surgical emergencies and are reviewed separately within this text.

Nerve compression injuries may also develop distal to the actual soft tissue trauma. Local edema and inflammation after injury can exacerbate a preexisting condition, such as a mild carpal tunnel turning into an acute event after a distal radius fracture. Occasionally, on a case by case basis, surgical decompression is necessary, even though the majority will resolve spontaneously. Likewise, an anterior cruciate ligament tear of the knee requiring reconstruction or repair may precipitate an acute foot drop postoperatively despite the deep peroneal nerve being usually uninjured. Some surgeons postulated that intraoperative positioning of the limb may be a factor in the late development of palsy (10); however, we believe that local tissue inflammation probably exacerbates a preexisting condition that manifests itself as a postoperative foot drop. When conservative nonoperative measures do not lead to sufficient improvement in nerve function after 2 to 3 months, decompression of the peroneal nerve should be considered (11). Figure 5-2 shows an algorithm for treatment of closed nerve injuries.

Penetrating Injuries

Blunt penetrating trauma is usually more locally destructive than a sharp injury. Often nearby structures such as blood vessels and tendons are injured in addition to the nerve. However, the size of a sharp laceration, such as with glass or a knife, can mislead the surgeon into underestimating the extent of injury. A seemingly small skin laceration may in fact extend under the surface and result in

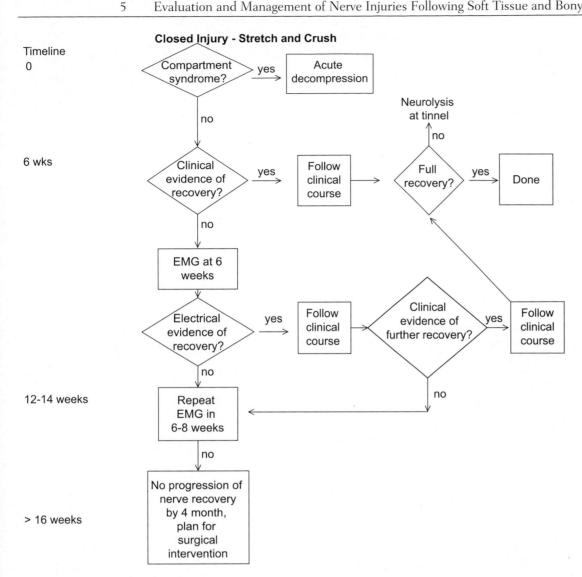

FIGURE 5-2

Algorithm for closed peripheral nerve injuries such as stretch and crush injuries.

a bigger injury than would be expected from the external size of the wound. Exploration is imperative if a nerve palsy is present, as the likelihood that the nerve is partially or completely transected is high. It is recommended to explore these injuries semi-electively within the first 2 weeks. The further from the time of injury, the more likely a nerve graft will be needed to overcome the resulting nerve gap. In the event of a penetrating trauma with an associated vascular injury, immediate exploration is warranted. Often the nerve injury is overlooked and not identified in the face of a more urgent vascular injury. In such cases the functional deficit may be first noticed postoperatively, when it is unclear if the nerve injury is from the inciting event, iatrogenic during the repair of the vascular injury, or secondary to edema or hematoma. While a CT scan or MRI may be helpful to evaluate for the latter, internal scarring of the nerve may not always be seen.

Blunt penetrating injuries are initially treated conservatively, similar to closed crush and stretch injuries, because they are may recover spontaneously. The local tissue edema often causes a neurapraxia that resolves; however, those that do not recover after 3 months should be evaluated by electrodiagnostic studies and treated as a traction injury. Figure 5-3 shows an algorithm for managing nerve injuries and the timing of additional studies.

Two specific blunt penetrating injuries deserve special mention: gun shot wounds and electrical injuries. Gun shot injuries present a unique problem since the trajectory of the bullet is unpredictable. The type, caliber, and velocity of the bullet each play a role in tissue destruction (12). The belief that the higher velocity bullet causes more tissue destruction can lead to early massive debridement; however, current recommendations are for judicious debridement and staged explo-

Penetrating Injuries

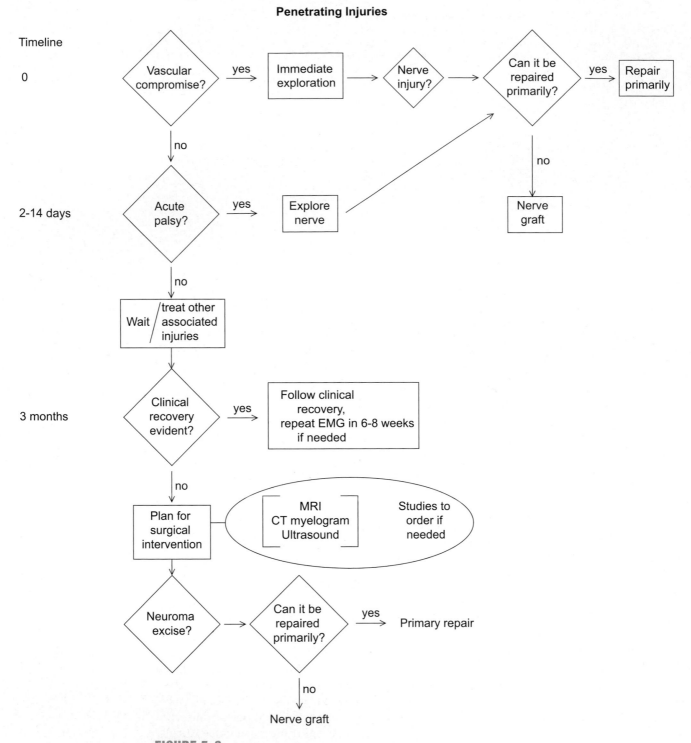

FIGURE 5-3

Algorithm for penetrating injuries.

ration, as in crush injuries (13). In fact, a low velocity bullet like a slug that fragments and stays in the soft tissue will more likely lead to infection and local tissue destruction than an Army issue missile that passes through the tissue with relative ease (14).

Electrical injuries that are not severe enough to cause death from heart arrhythmia and respiratory paralysis cause vigorous nerve stimulation which leads to paralysis and vasospasm. Massive muscle contractions due to nerve stimulation or the direct triggering of striated muscles can cause muscle rupture, ligamentous tears, fractures, and joint dislocations (15). In addition, electric current damages tissue from direct thermal heating; the coagulation necrosis is similar to a burn and is managed in the same manner (16).

One long term sequelae of gun shot wounds to the peripheral nervous system known as causalgia (complex regional pain syndrome I) was first described during the Civil War by Silas Weir Mitchell. The patients present with burning pain, paresthesias, skin atrophy, and temperature changes typical of the syndrome. This condition is also seen in electrical injury patients who survive the electrical contact. Axonal injury is usually from the direct thermal injury. Myelin injury is from direct thermal contact as well as from the electrical destruction of the myofibrils in the muscle. Post-neurological symptoms to the peripheral nervous system can vary from neuropathy to reflex sympathetic dystrophy (complex regional pain syndrome II) (17).

Paresthesias are thought to be due from perineurial fibrosis resulting in symptoms of a compressive peripheral neuropathy (18); surgical decompression can sometimes ameliorate the symptoms. Sympathectomy has been used to provide relief in those patients that respond to sympathetic blocks (19). In general nerve injuries associated with gun shot and electrical injuries are treated as closed nerve injuries.

NERVE INJURY ASSOCIATED WITH SOFT TISSUE AVULSION INJURY

Not to be confused with an avulsion of the nerve itself, a soft tissue avulsion or degloving injury presents a unique problem of coverage. Nerves that are exposed will need coverage to prevent desiccation. The type of soft tissue coverage will depend on the location of the injury and is addressed elsewhere in this book. The coverage can be as simple as replacing missing skin with a skin graft to something more extensive that requires fascia or muscle with skin graft, and ultimately a musculocutaneous or fasciocutaneous flap. If the soft tissue is missing directly over the nerve repair, a flap is needed to cover the nerve repair; this can be either local or a free tissue transfer. The use of vacuum assisted closure dressings has changed our management of complex open fractures and may be used to cover a wound with exposed nerves as well. If the nerves are exposed but uninjured, a protective dressing that keeps the nerves from desiccation may be used, such as a layer of AlloDerm® with or without a wound vacuum assisted closure dressing, or one of the various hydrogels on the market that provides enzymatic debridement at the same time as it absorbs excess fluid from the wound. If the nerves are injured and need to be repaired, primarily or with a nerve graft, the definitive repair should be staged so that it is done at the time of the soft tissue.

NERVE INJURY ASSOCIATED WITH BONY INJURY

Nerve injuries resulting from isolated closed fractures are most often due to compression from surrounding tissue edema or are due to, though less frequently, nerve laceration from the fracture ends. Iatrogenic nerve injury may also occur in the course of fracture fixation (20,21).

The anatomic positions of the radial, median, and ulnar nerves and their major branches make them vulnerable at several sites as they course the upper extremity, which explains the typical relationship seen between particular nerve injuries and fracture patterns (22). The more common nerve injuries with associated fracture patterns are listed in Table 5-3 and include the distal humeral shaft fractures and radial nerve palsy (23), posterior interosseous nerve injury with Monteggia fracture-dislocations (24), and median nerve and/or radial nerve injuries with supracondylar and medial epicondyle fractures in children (25). The time frame to intervention remains controversial; however, dysfunction lasting more than 3 to 4 months necessitates investigation and possible surgical exploration with neurolysis, transposition, repair, and/or reconstruction with nerve grafts or nerve transfers.

TABLE 5-3.   Typical nerve injury associated with fractures

Injury Pattern	Nerve(s) Injured	Treatment
Fracture		
Humerus (mid/distal)	Radial n.	Non-operative if suspect compression
		Exploration if suspect laceration
Supracondylar	PIN	Neurolysis, possible grafting if no
Med epicondylar		recovery after 3 months
Radius (prox)	Median n	Neurolysis, possible grafting if no
Radial n.	recovery after 3 months	
Radius (mid/distal)	Median n.	Carpal tunnel release for neuropathy
Tibia (prox)	Peroneal n.	Peroneal n. release at fibular head for foot drop
Tibia (distal)	Tibial n.	Tarsal tunnel release for neuropathy

TABLE 5-4.	Typical nerve injury associated with dislocations	
Joint affected	**Nerve(s) Injured**	**Treatment if conservative treatment fails**
Shoulder	Axillary Musculocutaneous	Nerve reconstruction with grafts or nerve transfer of Ax or MC
Elbow	Ulnar n. AIN	Ulnar nerve transposition, neurolysis of AIN, reconstruction with nerve grafts or transfers
Hip	Sciatic n. Tibial n. Peroneal n.	Neurolysis, possible graft repair, lower extremity nerve transfers
Knee	Peroneal n. Tibial n.	Peroneal n release at fibular head, tarsal tunnel release, possible graft repair or nerve transfer

For patients with chronic nerve injuries extending beyond 2 years, options for primary repair can be limited. Muscle fibrosis and motor end plate degeneration make attempts at primary muscle reinnervation unsuccessful. Instead, in these situations, tendon transfers can provide improvement in function. In comparison, nerve grafting for sensory nerve recovery is not time dependant and can be performed at any time following trauma.

Dislocations and their associated nerve injuries are listed in Table 5-4. Ulnar nerve injury at the cubital tunnel and/or anterior interosseous nerve injuries are common in elbow dislocations (26,27). Shoulder dislocations have been implicated in upper plexus nerve injuries with the axillary nerve being the most vulnerable to injury (28). In our experience with brachial plexus injuries, a second separate injury at the level of the quadrangular space is also often noted; this "double crush phenomenon" (two separate nerve injuries occurring along the length of a major peripheral nerve) may account for the poor recovery that is cited in the literature with regard to axillary nerve recovery in these injury patterns (29). The double crush syndrome was originally described in the upper extremity to explain nerve problems resulting from a combination of distal nerve compression at the wrist or elbow in conjunction with proximal cervical root or thoracic outlet pathology (30). Nerves that are traumatized proximally may also become more susceptible to compression at distal sites (31).

In the lower extremity, between 10% and 25% of cases of acetabular fracture and traumatic posterior hip dislocation are associated with sciatic nerve injuries (32,33). Tethering of the sciatic nerve at the sciatic notch may exaggerate the traction effect on the nerve in the buttock, thus causing a stretch injury proximally and then a distal compression at the fibular head where the nerve is again tethered. The common peroneal portion of the sciatic nerve is more vulnerable because of its anatomical position and internal architecture (34).

Nerves that are not tethered, but which reside in tight fibro-osseous tunnels (such as the ulnar nerve in the cubital tunnel, the median nerve in the carpal tunnel, and the posterior tibial nerve in the tarsal tunnel), may be affected by a more proximal injury due to tissue edema. For example, the incidence of acute transient median nerve compression syndrome after distal radius fracture is estimated between 12% and 17%, and it occurs regardless of fracture type, the amount of initial displacement, the adequacy of reduction, or the method of operative treatment (35,36). In the majority of cases, the neuropathy resolve spontaneously; however, it certain cases, the symptoms persist after the fracture has healed. This leads to the recommendation of performing prophylactic carpal tunnel decompression whenever there is a distal radius fracture. More recently, the consensus has reversed as there is no advantage to the prophylaxis; in fact, evidence suggests there is increased morbidity to acutely decompress the carpal tunnel in the face of mild median nerve compression (37,38). In contrast, acute severe carpal tunnel with progressive symptoms despite preliminary fracture reduction *is* an indication for surgical release at time of distal radius fixation. Similar conditions are seen in the lower extremity, such as acute foot drop after knee reconstruction for ligament injury or tarsal tunnel with distal tibia or maleolar fractures (39). In general, if a patient has loss of median nerve sensation following forearm fracture or injury, a carpal tunnel release is universally recommended. By contrast, a patient with foot drop following a knee injury is treated expectantly often for several months. We believe there should be *no* distinction between the upper and lower extremities and recommend peroneal nerve release at the fibular head in the case of acute foot drop, just as we would perform a carpal tunnel release for acute compression of the median nerve at the wrist.

PREOPERATIVE ASSESSMENT

Emergency evaluation of a nerve injury should include a thorough motor and sensory exam. Grossly, the muscle function of the nerve in question needs to be evaluated. For the hand, two point static and moving discrimination can be performed to determine the decrease of sensation. Alternatively, the quick and easy "ten test" sensory exam uses the patient's own subjective perception to moving light touch in order to elicit differences in sensation (40). For example, to test for a median nerve injury, both the injured and uninjured index fingers of the patient are touched at the same time over corresponding areas of each finger and the patient is asked if the subjective sensation is the same or different. This technique is particularly useful in children, is extremely sensitive, and requires no instrumentation.

In patients who present with acute motor deficits or palsy, determining if the nerve will recover spontaneously can often be confusing. The mechanism of the injury can often assist in the initial evaluation. Any sharp penetrating injury with no clinical evidence of recovery should be explored. Optimal timing is between 2 to 14 days, as long as the patient is surgically stable. Occasionally, an MRI or CT scan may be useful if there is evidence of a neuroma or neural disruption; however, any injury where there is a high index of suspicion of nerve transection should be explored and repaired. The advantage of repair within the first 2 weeks of injury is that the nerve ends have not retracted and primary repair is often possible.

Closed traction injuries and closed fractures with palsy are the most difficult to assess. Waiting 3 to 4 months for evidence of spontaneous recovery is the gold standard. EMGs at 4 months are advised when no clinical recovery is evident. If there is no evidence of reinnervation occurring (MUPs), surgical exploration and reconstruction will be necessary. Figure 5-2 shows the algorithm for sequence of evaluation and repair. If an initial EMG shows some recovery, a follow up EMG is done 4 to 6 weeks later and correlated with clinical evidence of recovery. Once nerve recovery stops progressing as expected, surgical intervention can be planned based on the EMG results and the clinical exam without further delay.

We always prefer to be involved with the care of the patient early and follow the clinical exam and any additional testing, such as electrodiagnostic testing, ultrasound, MRI, and CT scan in order to minimize delay in recognizing a nerve deficit that will not resolve spontaneously. It is important to be aware that the injury may not be limited to only the site of the trauma, but may affect distal functioning muscle groups and may be impinged at distal sites or proximal sites. The more complex injuries will usually require a team approach, both for the operative reconstruction and for the postoperative management. A pain specialist is paramount to manage the associated chronic pain these patients often have for the more complex injuries. Physical therapy and occupational therapy during the rehabilitative period is essential to prevent joint contracture, to fabricate and adjust protective splints, and to assist in motor and sensory re-education as the recovery process is underway.

OPERATIVE MANAGEMENT

For acutely transected nerves primary repair remains the gold standard. Adequate resection of the nerve ends beyond the zone of nerve injury is essential to ensure healing with or without limited intraneural scaring. Large associated soft tissue wounds with varying levels of tissue destruction, like degloving injuries and crush injuries, with comminuted bony fractures will need serial debridement prior to ultimate reconstruction. In such cases primary nerve repair should be delayed until one can adequately assess the complete nerve defect. If the nerve cannot be approximated after debridement, a graft will be necessary. Nerve grafts may be used as long as the wound is clean. If the wound is significantly contaminated it is preferable to tag the ends of the nerves and return to graft when all devitalized tissue has been debrided. We do not recommend acutely repairing or grafting nerve injuries in contaminated wound beds or in crush injuries, where multiple debridements will be required, as postoperative infection, ongoing tissue necrosis, and progressive soft tissue ischemia will all contribute to poor return of function following nerve repair.

Formal intraoperative nerve stimulation is helpful in complex closed traction injuries, especially of the brachial plexus. Proximal injuries of mixed nerves result in complete or partial deficits to several nerves, as opposed to the discrete single nerve injury pattern of distal peripheral nerve injuries. In most cases, an injury distal to the shoulder level will result in one or two discrete nerve injuries and intraoperative electrical stimulation is not necessary. In the case where several segments along the same nerve are injured, or the brachial plexus is injured, electrical stimulation is useful in guiding intra-operative decision making. Electrical stimulation allows the surgeon to determine which fascicles within the nerve are functional and which ones are not. We limit use of formal intraoperative electrical stimulation to three major situations: (a) in cases where the preoperative EMG results were equivocal; (b) in cases where additional recovery may have occurred between the time of the previous study and the operation; and (c) in situations where the intraoperative mapping of the nerve function can affect the surgical plan. An example of a situation where the intraoperative plan may change is in the case of an incomplete neuroma of the median nerve at the wrist. If the median motor fascicle is intact, the surgeon may try to preserve those fibers and graft the sensory fibers that are injured. Alternatively, if the neuroma is nearly circumferential and the motor fibers poorly conduct to the thenar muscles, the surgeon may opt to completely resect the neuroma and primarily repair or graft the nerve defect.

A handheld 2 mA nerve stimulator will not provide as much information about nerve function as a formal intraoperative electrical stimulation, but is useful in many situations. In the first 72 hours after an acute transaction, the distal half of a motor nerve will contract when stimulated, facilitating the matching of nerves when several are cut, or when the nerve is cut close to the muscle and has begun to branch. The small motor fibers would be otherwise difficult to identify because of their small diameter, which can sometimes be as small as 0.5 to 2 mm in diameter. We find the handheld device a useful aid when performing nerve transfers; it allows us to pick out grossly motor nerve fibers that were uninjured, which will be spliced into nonfunctioning motor nerves to restore animation. For a nerve injury that develops a partial neuroma (as in a 6th degree nerve injury), a nerve stimulator can help determine which nerve fascicles to preserve while resecting the damaged tissue, as long as the fascicles in question are mixed nerves. For injuries to purely or mostly sensory fibers, a handheld nerve stimulator is not useful and formal intraoperative nerve stimulation is the only means to evaluate sensory conduction.

COMMON CLINICAL EXAMPLES

Primary Repair for Nerve Transection

A common soft tissue injury that orthopaedic surgeons may encounter and easily repair is the laceration of a major and minor peripheral nerve as a result of a sharp penetrating injury. In the mid to distal forearm and wrist, the median nerve is fairly superficial, and thus easily injured from a deep laceration with glass or metal. The median nerve can be found deep to the palmaris tendon in patients that have a palmaris longus tendon, and just ulnar to the flexor carpi radialis tendon. Knowledge of the anatomy as well as the topography of the nerve is important in order to align the motor branches when repairing the nerve. Primary repair is the procedure of choice whenever possible and usually can be performed within the first 2 weeks after injury. Repairs performed later than this often need a nerve graft as the nerve retracts with time. The repair should be performed with as little tension as possible at the repair site in order to minimize scarring that occurs within the nerve. A small amount of tension at the repair site is acceptable and has been shown in some animal studies to stimulate neurotropic growth factors and improve healing (41). A useful tool in determining excessive tension is to bring in proximity the two ends of a nerve with a single 8-0 nylon suture. If the freshened nerve ends reach without the suture pulling through the epineurium, the tension is not excessive.

Mobilizing the nerve is crucial. Often sufficient mobilization of the nerve will eliminate the need for a graft. Because of the inherent springiness of nerve tissue, when a nerve is transected it will recoil, leaving a gap. A nerve can stretch 10% to 15% without compromising its inherent blood supply (42). If, when bringing the nerve ends together, there is still a 5 mm gap between the nerve ends, mobilizing 5 cm of nerve (usually 2.5 cm on either side, but not always) will allow the ends to come together. If a 1 cm nerve gap is present when the two freshened ends of nerve are laid in proximity, 10 cm of total nerve needs to be mobilized in order to bring the two halves together with "minimal" tension. This does not mean that any gap should be closed primarily at all costs. If after reasonable mobilization there is a persistent gap, a nerve graft is preferable to forcing a primary repair. It is important to note that if a nerve graft is necessary, the nerve ends should be trimmed generously so that the repair will be outside the zone of injury. When a nerve graft is needed, there is no reason to limit the debridement of the remaining nerve.

External markers such as the native vessel of the nerve on the surface is used along with the different fascicular size and grouping to align the nerve (Fig. 5-4). In the past, it was believed that a

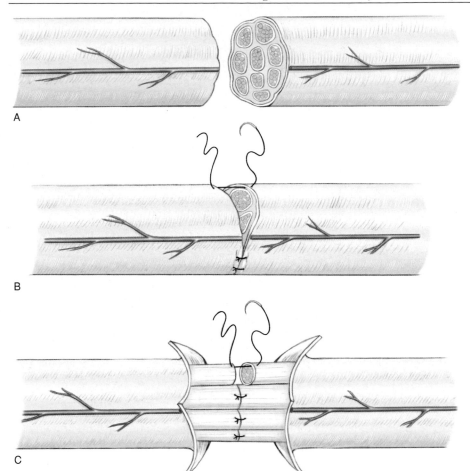

A

B

C

FIGURE 5-4
The two nerve ends are aligned using external markers such as the artery and the grouped fascicle pattern **(A)**, an epineural **(B)** or perineural **(C)** repair may be used, although we prefer the former.

perineural repair of grouped fascicles was better than an epineural repair; however, recent studies show that either technique is equally effective (43). We prefer to use a circumferential epineural repair with 9-0 nylon interrupted sutures to minimize the fibrosis seen with perineural repairs (Fig. 5-4B). Care is taken to prevent overlap (Fig. 5-5); we prefer to have the fascicle slightly retracted with respect to the epineurium, rather than bulging out the side or overlapping internally. At the conclusion of the repair, the area under question is put through the full range of movement to verify that the repair will hold up under gentile protected motion postoperatively. Any repair that withstands gentle range of motion is considered a "tension-free" repair, although in fact it may be still under some mild yet acceptable tension. In larger nerves, such as the sciatic and femoral nerves, or in nerves with significant inflammation in the epineurium, we use 8-0 nylon sutures. In contrast, for cutaneous nerves and digital nerves, 10-0 nylon works best. The least number of epineural sutures to approximate and keep the repair intact through a full range of motion is used. After neurorrhaphy, the area is immobilized for 1 to 2 weeks; however, protected active range of motion is allowed and should be initiated immediately. One exception is in flexor tendon lacerations with associated digital nerve injuries. Both are repaired and the patient begins early protected range of motion under the direction of an occupational therapist. While sensibility is somewhat decreased when compared to patients who are immobilized for 3 to 4 weeks, there is no statistical difference of sensibility at 1 year, and the advantages of early range of motion for the rehabilitation of the tendon injury outweighs the negligible delay in sensory return (44).

Repair of Nerve Gap with Nerve Graft

While a primary repair is preferred, two neurorrhaphy sites under favorable conditions are better than a single neurorrhaphy under unfavorable conditions (45). In contaminated wounds, such as crush injuries from motor vehicle accidents, the wound bed needs to be cleaned before any reconstruction of the resulting deformities can be performed. If a large defect to both the nerve and the soft tissue is present, nerve repair with grafts in addition to soft tissue coverage will be needed. In

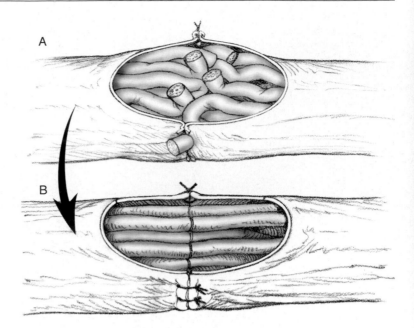

FIGURE 5-5

When aligning the nerve, make sure to trim back the fascicles so that there is no overlap when the epineurium is sutured closed **(B)**. It is preferable to have a small gap internally than to have fibers overlap and potentially "escape" from the edge or "fail to find" the distal half **(A)**. (By permission of Mayo Foundation for Medical Education and Research. All rights reserved.)

areas where local muscle is unavailable, a free tissue transfer may be necessary to cover both bone and nerve repair.

A common situation which may require a nerve graft can be seen in cases of severe knee dislocation with damage to the tibial-peroneal nerve trunk. The stretch injury, if severe enough, will cause internal damage of the nerve. While EMG studies may confirm the suspicion of a third or fourth degree injury, the history and clinical findings are usually enough to warrant surgical exploration with the plan to release the nerve at the very least from the surrounding scar tissue and compression points, and most likely excise the neuroma and graft the resulting nerve defect. If the neuroma is small, a primary repair may be possible; however, the resultant gap following neuroma excision is often not amenable to primary repair as mobilization of the sciatic nerve proximally and the tibial and peroneal nerves distally are limited by nerve branches to the underlying muscles. The resultant 2 to 3 cm gap will need to be repaired with a nerve graft. A sural nerve is the most often used donor nerve. In the case of a tibial-peroneal nerve injury described above, the nerve would be cut in half or thirds and cabled. Once again, 9-0 nylon interrupted sutures are used to repair both sites. The native artery location on the external portion of the nerve as well as the relative size of the fascicles is used to help line up the fascicles. We still prefer to do an epineural repair of the nerve to nerve graft, rather than a perineural repair of the actual fascicles.

Nerve grafts less than 10 cm long work well in vascularized wound beds. The longer the graft, the less optimal the recovery. Some people have suggested using vascularized nerve grafts when the distance is greater than 20 cm (46). However, in general, small caliber nerve grafts, such as sural and medial antibrachial cutaneous nerves, do not need to be vascularized. Large caliber nerves, such as ulnar, do need to be vascularized or the central portion will necrose and then scar, limiting its effectiveness as a graft.

Obtaining a Nerve Graft

The nerve graft serves as a guide for the proximal axon as it regrows toward the distal stump. The sural nerve is by far the most commonly used donor nerve, although other suitable donor nerves include the lateral and medial antibrachial cutaneous nerve (47,48) and the terminal portion of the anterior interosseous nerve (AIN) that innervates the pronator quadratus (49). The sural nerve is often chosen as a nerve donor because of its size, length, and relatively minimal donor site and minimal morbidity. Typically, harvest of the sural nerve will result in numbness over the posterior aspect of the leg and the lateral aspect of the foot and malleolus.

With the patient either prone or supine with the leg frog-legged, the sural nerve is identified lateral to the Achilles tendon. The easiest method for harvest of the sural nerve is to use a posterior midline incision. The closure is slightly lengthier and the resulting scar may be cosmetically undesirable. The alternative is to use a stepwise technique, which requires between 4 and 6 separate horizontal incisions along the back of the calf, each approximately 1 cm in length. The resulting scar is cosmetically more favorable and the technique adds little operative time. An endoscopic or a nerve harvester may be used to limit scars. The trick with using the nerve harvester is that contributions from the lateral and anterior sural nerves, which are cutaneous branches from the peroneal and tibial nerves, may be difficult to incorporate into the sural nerve proper and shorten the overall length that is harvested. Approximately 25 to 30 cm of graft may be harvested from a typical adult patient. The next most often used graft is the medial anti-brachial nerve. It is easily found coursing along side the bacillic vein in the upper arm. Up to 25 cm of nerve graft may be obtained.

While nerve grafts are the gold standard for motor nerve gap repairs, the disadvantage is the limited number of donor nerves available. This has led to the development of new techniques for bridging nerve gaps. For nerve gaps less than or equal to 3 cm on small caliber sensory nerves (50), the nerve may be repaired with a conduit, which may be autologous, such as a vein, or synthetic, such as one of the commercially available nerve tubes (Fig. 5-6A). The end of each nerve is trimmed until healthy fascicles are seen. The end of the nerve is inserted into the tube for approximately 2 to 4 mm and the epineurium is sutured to the end of the conduit with 9-0 nylon using a simple suture technique, a horizontal matrass suture technique, or a half buried matrass suture technique. Clinically, for nerve defects longer than 3 cm, in mixed nerves, and in pure motor nerves the recommendation is still a nerve graft. Alternatively, we have used nerve conduits as a covering over nerve repairs that required several cabled grafts into one larger nerve to serve as a temporary protective covering instead of wrapping a spatulated strip of vein (Fig. 5-6B–D).

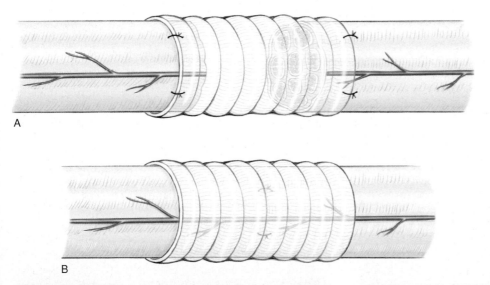

A

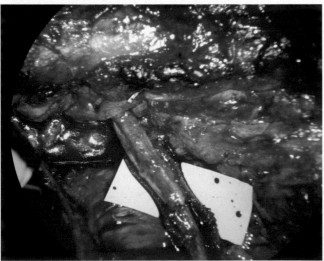

B

C

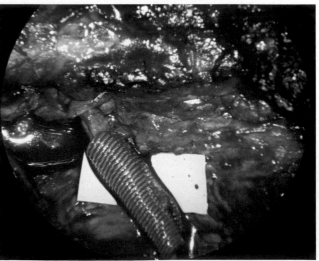

D

FIGURE 5-6

Neural tube may be used to bridge a gap or as a protective covering after nerve repair. When used to bridge a nerve gap **(A)**, the epineurium is sutured to the edge of the neural tube. **B–D:** When used to cover a neurorrhaphy site, the tube may be cut longitudinally and wrapped around the neurorrhaphy site. A suture is placed around the outside of the conduit to help keep it in place.

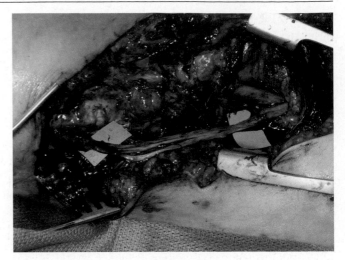

FIGURE 5-7

Three cabled sural nerves, each 2 mm in diameter, were used to bridge the defect in the radial nerve. The diameter of the radial nerve is approximately 6 mm in this location.

Neuroma of Radial Nerve with Humeral Fracture

Considerable controversy remains as to the need for early exploration in closed fracture dislocation injuries with acute nerve palsy. In a recent meta-analysis review of the literature over the last 40 years regarding radial nerve palsy after fracture of the shaft of the humerus, the prevalence of fracture associated nerve palsy was about 12% (51). Over 70% of these compressions resolve spontaneously, therefore the current recommendation is for conservative therapy with closed fractures. If after 3 months there is no clinical recovery, using high-resolution ultrasound to evaluate the injured nerve is less invasive than electrodiagnostic testing and has been used in this specific situation for effectively detecting a neuroma in the presence of a fracture (26,52). However, at 3 to 4 months, if spontaneous recovery is to be anticipated, there should be clinical evidence of reinnervation or electrical evidence of regeneration (motor unit potentials). If radial nerve regeneration stops at the level of the Arcade of Frohse, then decompression of the posterior interosseous nerve is indicated. In addition, open fractures, oblique fractures, and fractures that can compress or transect the radial nerve between the fracture fragments should be explored early (53).

If instead of recovery, all preoperative studies indicate a neuroma of the radial nerve in the distal arm, the nerve should be explored with the plan to resect and graft the defect. Rarely can the nerve be mobilized enough to be repaired primarily. Because the nerve and scar surrounding it are usually densely adherent and are similar in color, entering the scarred area directly is not advised. The uninjured proximal and distal ends of the nerve are exposed first. In the case of a partial palsy or radial nerve weakness, a sixth degree nerve injury is most likely. A handheld nerve stimulator can be used to stimulate fibers proximal to the injury. Those fascicles that result in movement of muscles distal to the injury are intact and these intact fibers are marked and protected from further dissection. The injured fibers are resected until normal fascicles are noted from each end. A nerve graft is used similar to before. If more than one third of the radial nerve has been resected, two or more cabled sural nerve grafts may be needed to bridge the gap (Fig. 5-7). The larger sized fascicles should be lined up and grafted directly whenever possible. 9-0 or 8-0 nylon interrupted sutures are used to repair both sites with an epineural or perineurial repair.

POSTOPERATIVE MANAGEMENT

After any typical nerve repair, whether it is done primarily, with a nerve graft or a synthetic tube, or a primary neurorrhaphy using a nerve transfer, the affected area is splinted or placed in a sling for 2 weeks to minimize movement. The only exception is in digital nerve repairs in conjunction with a tendon repair as noted before. We begin early passive range of motion to prevent tendon adhesion and leave the patient in a dorsal blocking splint to prevent hyperextension and additional strain to the repair site.

In both motor and sensory nerve repairs, an advancing Tinel sign or "tingling" sign seen during the regeneration phase is followed until the patient has restoration of function or sensation. Even before there is clinical evidence of recovery, we begin desensitization of the affected area to assist in sensory reeducation and to prevent hypersensitivity. Formal objective testing, such as Simien-Weinstein testing, and sensory grading is useful for objective data collection, but is not necessarily useful in clinical practice. Motor reeducation begins as soon as the patient has some clinical evidence of muscle contraction.

Occasionally, EMGs are used postoperatively to follow functional recovery. This is useful in cases where a primary repair may not show clinical evidence of recovery and a second stage reconstruction may be planned. In those cases, EMGs are invaluable in answering the question of whether to wait longer in the case of recovery that may not manifest in actual clinical movement yet, versus proceeding with the next phase of reconstruction, if no evidence of recovery is present.

CONCLUSION

Nerve injuries alone are fairly complex and when the soft tissue and bony structures in the vicinity are injured as well, the complexity increases. Bony trauma with or without soft tissue injury indicates a greater force was expended to cause the injury, thus the associated nerve injuries can be severe and at multiple levels. Avulsion and stretch injuries, crush injuries, and penetrating injuries can occur in combination or alone. The mechanism of injury varies greatly, thus no single solution to all nerve injuries exists. The deficits are often not readily apparent because of concomitant injuries or because the patient can not reliably participate in the examination. The reconstruction of both the nerves and the soft tissue will ultimately be tailored to the specific situation. Any study that can aid in the decision process, such as radiology exams and electrical diagnostic testing, should be ordered in a timely fashion. Additional assistance from the following may be needed: (a) a plastic or orthopaedic surgeon knowledgeable about peripheral nerve surgery and soft tissue coverage if the defect is more complex than initially anticipated or if extensive wound coverage issues are beyond the scope of the treating physician; (b) a pain specialist for management of chronic narcotic and non-narcotic pain medication and nonoperative therapies such as nerve blocks and nerve stimulators for chronic pain; (c) a psychiatrist or psychologist for depression if warranted in the complex peripheral nerve injuries; and (d) occupational and physical therapists for motor and sensory reeducation, splinting, and joint mobility maintenance.

REFERENCES

1. Seddon HJ. Three types of nerve injury. *Brain.* 1943;66:237.
2. Mackinnon SE. New directions in peripheral nerve surgery. *Ann Surg.* 1989;22:257–273.
3. Seddon HJ, Medawar PB, Smith H. Rate of regeneration of peripheral nerves in man. *J Physiol.* 1943;102;191–201.
4. Ruhmann O, Schmolke S, Gosse F, et al. Transposition of local muscles to restore elbow flexion in brachial plexus palsy. *Injury.* 2002;33(7):597–609.
5. Weber RV, Mackinnon SE. Nerve transfers in the upper extremity. *J Am Soc Surg Hand.* 2004;4:200–213.
6. Rostoucher P, Alnot JY, Touam C, et al. Tendon transfers to restore elbow flexion after traumatic paralysis of the brachial plexus in adults. *Int Orthop.* 1998;22(4):255–262.
7. Becker M, Lassner F, Fansa H, et al. Refinements in nerve to muscle neurotization. *Muscle Nerve.* 2002;26(3):362–366.
8. Bielecki M, Skowronski R, Skowronski J. A comparative morphological study of direct nerve implantation and neuromuscular pedicle methods in cross reinnervation of the rat skeletal muscle. *Rocz Akad Med Bialymst.* 2004;49:10–17.
9. Phillips JH, Mackinnon SE, Beatty SE, et al. Vibratory sensory testing in acute compartment syndromes: a clinical and experimental study. *Plast Reconstr Surg.* 1987;79(5):796–801.
10. Idusuyi OB, Morrey BF. Peroneal nerve palsy after total knee arthroplasty. Assessment of predisposing and prognostic factors. *J Bone Joint Surg Am.* 1996;78(2):177–184.
11. Krackow KA, Maar DC, Mont MA, et al. Surgical decompression for peroneal nerve palsy after total knee arthroplasty. *Clin Orthop Relat Res.* 1993;(292):223–228.
12. Yoganandan N, Pintar FA. Biomechanics of penetrating trauma. *Crit Rev Biomed Eng.* 1997;25(6):485–501.
13. Santucci RA, Chang YJ. Ballistics for physicians: myths about wound ballistics and gunshot injuries. *J Urol.* 2004;171(4):1408–1414.
14. Davis CA, Cogbill TH, Lambert PJ. Shotgun wound management: a comparison of slug and pellet injuries. *WMJ.* 1998;97(10):40–43.
15. Ten Duis HJ. Acute electrical burns. *Semin Neurol.* 1995;15(4):381–386.
16. Tropea BI, Lee RC. Thermal injury kinetics in electrical trauma. *J Biomech Eng.* 1992;114(2):241–250.
17. Cohen JA. Autonomic nervous system disorders and reflex sympathetic dystrophy in lightning and electrical injuries. *Semin Neurol.* 1995;15:387–390.
18. Smith MA, Muehlberger T, Dellon AL. Peripheral nerve compression associated with low-voltage electrical injury without associated significant cutaneous burn. *Plast Reconstr Surg.* 2002;109(1):137–144.
19. Hassantash SA, Maier RV. Sympathectomy for causalgia: experience with military injuries. *J Trauma.* 2000;49(2):266–271.
20. Yam A, Tan TC, Lim BH. Intraoperative interfragmentary radial nerve compression in a medially plated humeral shaft fracture: a case report. *J Orthop Trauma.* 2005;19(7):491–493.
21. Ozcelik A, Tekcan A, Omeroglu H. Correlation between iatrogenic ulnar nerve injury and angular insertion of the medial pin in supracondylar humerus fractures. *J Pediatr Orthop B.* 2006;15(1):58–61.

22. Hoppenfeld S, de Boer P. *Surgical Exposures in Orthopaedics: The Anatomic Approach,* 2nd ed. Philadelphia: JB Lippincott; 1994:62–66, 107–115.
23. Bodner G, Huber B, Schwabegger A, et al. Sonographic detection of radial nerve entrapment within a humerus fracture. *J Ultrasound Med.* 1999;18:703–706.
24. Ristic S, Strauch RJ, Rosenwasser MP. The assessment and treatment of nerve dysfunction after trauma around the elbow. *Clin Orthop Relat Res.* 2000;370:138–153.
25. Culp RW, Osterman AL, Davidson RS, et al. Neural injuries associated with supracondylar fractures of the humerus in children. *J Bone Joint Surg Am.* 1990;72:1211–1215.
26. Beverly MC, Fearn CB. Anterior interosseous nerve palsy and dislocation of the elbow. *Injury.* 1984;16:126–128.
27. Galbraith KA, McCullough CJ. Acute nerve injury as a complication of closed fractures or dislocations of the elbow. *Injury.* 1979;11:159–164.
28. McIlveen SJ, Duralde XA, D'Alessandro DF, et al. Isolated nerve injuries about the shoulder. *Clin Orthop Relat Res.* 1994;306:54–63.
29. Berry H, Bril V. Axillary nerve palsy following blunt trauma to the shoulder region: a clinical and electrophysiological review. *J Neurol Neurosurg Psychiatry.* 1982;45(11):1027–1032.
30. Upton AR, McComas AJ. The double crush in nerve entrapment syndromes. *Lancet.* 1973;2:359–362.
31. Dellon AL, Mackinnon SE. Chronic nerve compression model for the double crush hypothesis. *Ann Plast Surg.* 1991;26(3):259–264.
32. Fassler PR, Swiontkowski MF, Kilroy AW, et al. Injury of the sciatic nerve associated with acetabular fracture. *J Bone Joint Surg Am.* 1993;75:1157–1166.
33. Jacob JR, Rao JP, Ciccarelli C. Traumatic dislocation and fracture dislocation of the hip: a long-term follow-up study. *Clin Orthop.* 1987;214:249–263.
34. Sunderland S. The relative susceptibility to injury of the medial and lateral popliteal divisions of the sciatic nerve. *Br J Surg.* 1953;41:300–302.
35. Stewart HD, Innes AR, Burke FD. The hand complications of Colles' fractures. *J Hand Surg Br.* 1985;10(1):103–106.
36. Bienek T, Kusz D, Cielinski L. Peripheral nerve compression neuropathy after fractures of the distal radius. *J Hand Surg Br.* 2005;31(3):256–260.
37. Fuller DA, Barrett M, Marburger RK, et al. Carpal canal pressures after volar plating of distal radius fractures. *J Hand Surg Br.* 2006;31(2):236–239.
38. Odumala O, Ayekoloye C, Packer G. Prophylactic carpal tunnel decompression during buttress plating of the distal radius—is it justified? *Injury.* 2001;32(7):577–579.
39. Augustijn P, Vanneste J. The tarsal tunnel syndrome after a proximal lesion. *J Neurol Neurosurg Psychiatry.* 1992;55(1):65–67.
40. Strauch B, Lang A, Ferder M, et al. The ten test. *Plast Reconstr Surg.* 1997;99(4):1074–1078.
41. Sunderland IR, Brenner MJ, Singham J, et al. Effect of tension on nerve regeneration in rat sciatic nerve transection model. *Ann Plast Surg.* 2004;53(4):382–387.
42. Trumble TE, Archibald S, Allan CH. Bioengineering for nerve repair in the future. *J Am Soc Surg Hand.* 2004;4(3):134–142.
43. Cabaud HE, Rodkey WG, McCarroll HR Jr, et al. Epineurial and perineurial fascicular nerve repairs: a critical comparison. *J Hand Surg Am.* 1976;1(2):131–137.
44. Yu RS, Catalano LW 3rd, Barron OA, et al. Limited, protected postsurgical motion does not affect the results of digital nerve repair. *J Hand Surg Am.* 2004;29(2):302–306.
45. Millesi H. Microsurgery of the peripheral nerves. *Hand.* 1973;5:157–160.
46. Doi K, Kuwata N, Kawakami F, et al. The free vascularized sural nerve graft. *Microsurgery.* 1984;5(4):175–184.
47. Dvali L, Mackinnon S. Nerve repair, grafting, and nerve transfers. *Clin Plast Surg.* 2003;30(2):203–221.
48. Myckatyn TM, Mackinnon SE. Surgical techniques of nerve grafting (standard/vascularized/allograft). *Oper Tech Orthop.* 2004;14:171–178.
49. Novak CB, Mackinnon SE. Distal anterior interosseous nerve transfer to the deep motor branch of the ulnar nerve for reconstruction of high ulnar nerve injuries. *J Reconstr Microsurg.* 2002;18(6):459–464.
50. Chiu DT, Strauch B. A prospective clinical evaluation of autogenous vein grafts used as a nerve conduit for distal sensory nerve defects of 3 cm or less. *Plast Reconstr Surg.* 1990;6(5):928–934.
51. Shao YC, Harwood P, Grotz MR, et al. Radial nerve palsy associated with fractures of the shaft of the humerus: a systematic review. *J Bone Joint Surg Br.* 2005;87(12):1647–1652.
52. Bodner G, Buchberger W, Schocke M, et al. Radial nerve palsy associated with humeral shaft fracture: evaluation with US-initial experience. *Radiology.* 2001;219:811–816.
53. Bostman O, Bakalim G, Vainionpaa S, et al. Immediate radial nerve palsy complicating fracture of the shaft of the humerus: when is early exploration justified? *Injury.* 1985;16(7):499–502.

6 Management of Vascular Injuries Following Soft Tissue and Bony Trauma

Gustavo S. Oderich and Timothy M. Sullivan

A ccidental injuries affect 2.6 million people in the United States each year. Mechanisms of injury include penetrating, blunt, and iatrogenic trauma. It is estimated that vascular trauma affects 0.2% to 4% of all injured patients. Therefore, approximately 20 to 100,000 patients will sustain a vascular injury. Over 80% of these vascular injuries will be located in extremities. Ninety percent of all vascular injuries are associated with penetrating trauma, of which 70% are due to gunshot injuries, 20% are due to stab wounds, and 10% are due to blunt trauma. Combined vascular and orthopaedic trauma is relatively uncommon, accounting for less than 1% of all cases of traumatic injuries. Vascular injuries can occur because of the superficial location of vessels, their proximity to bones, and their relatively fixed position across joints. Patients sustaining combined injuries are exposed to substantially increased risk of amputation and limb dysfunction. This chapter focuses on the indications, contraindications, preoperative planning, operative approach, and results of repair of the most common combined vascular and orthopaedic injuries.

INDICATIONS/CONTRAINDICATIONS

Primary repair of arterial and venous injuries is indicated to control bleeding and/or to relieve limb or organ ischemia. Life-threatening injuries should be recognized early during the resuscitation phase and prioritized before proceeding with vascular and orthopaedic repair. Arterial injuries affecting only one of the tibioperoneal or forearm arteries may be treated conservatively provided that there is no evidence of distal ischemia. Nonocclusive arterial injuries (e.g., small intimal flaps or dissections) incidentally found on imaging studies can be safely observed. The benign natural history of these injuries is well documented in several large series; operative repair is required in less than 1% of patients.

Extremity trauma with complex soft tissue, vascular, and skeletal injuries poses one of the most difficult management problems. Patients should be evaluated by a multidisciplinary team. Coordinated interaction of various specialists including a vascular, orthopaedic, and plastic surgeon is of paramount importance to optimize outcome. Injuries of the head, chest, and abdomen may require additional neurosurgical and general trauma consultation. Every effort is made to balance the potential success of an arterial reconstruction and correction of the orthopaedic injury with the overall clinical status of the patient and the potential for complete functional recovery. In general, once life-threatening injuries are stabilized, treatment priorities are as follows:

- Control of bleeding and restoration of arterial inflow.
- Fracture reduction and stabilization.
- Soft tissue coverage.

Vascular repair should be prioritized over definitive orthopaedic repair. Any delay in vascular reconstruction is a gamble and may risk the only opportunity for limb salvage. Patients with stable fractures or dislocations in which minimal manipulation and length discrepancy is anticipated should be treated with immediate definitive arterial revascularization. However, patients with severely comminuted fractures and dislocations, segmental bone loss causing limb discrepancy, or severe soft tissue disruption and contamination should be treated initially with temporary intra-arterial shunts. In these cases, it is wise to delay the definitive vascular reconstruction until wide debridement and initial skeletal repair are accomplished.

Contra-indications for vascular repair include presence of other life-threatening injuries requiring immediate attention or causing hemodynamic instability. Several predictive factors should be taken into consideration when deciding to perform revascularization versus primary amputation (Table 6-1). Overall, approximately 10% to 20% of patients with complex extremity injuries have nonsalvageable limbs and require primary amputation. Assessment of these patients should be individualized. Several factors should be taken into consideration, including the overall clinical status, severity of the arterial, neurologic, and orthopaedic trauma, and expected functional recovery. A primary amputation is considered in cases of dysvascular extremity with complex fractures and extensive soft tissue and nerve damage. Patients with major nerve transections (e.g., tibial nerve transection) and open comminuted tibiofibular fractures with arterial injuries (Gustilo III-C) have very poor functional outcome and high amputation rates; these patients are generally treated with primary amputation. Major nerve transections should be confirmed by direct visualization. Other indication for amputation is prolonged ischemia time (>12 hours) with evidence of a cadaveric extremity (e.g., mottled with absence of motor function, arterial, or venous Doppler signals).

PREOPERATIVE PLANNING

Prolonged ischemia time is the most important factor associated with limb dysfunction or amputation. A high index of suspicion coupled with accurate neurovascular examination is necessary for prompt diagnosis of a vascular injury. Accurate diagnosis of vascular injuries is an essential aspect in the preoperative evaluation of patients with complex extremity trauma. Prompt restoration of arterial blood flow within 6 hours from the time of initial extremity injury is the most critical factor that determines limb salvage and function.

Complete history including the mechanism of trauma, associated injuries, medical history, medications, and allergies should be recorded. Extremity vascular trauma is immediately apparent because of external bleeding, hematoma, or obvious limb ischemia. Physical examination includes inspection of the injured limb for open wounds, obvious deformities, and signs of ischemia. Distal ischemia is manifested by the five Ps: pallor, paresthesia, paralysis, pain, pulselessness, and poikilothermia. A thorough sensory and motor examination and pulse examination should be noted. The presence of hematoma, pulsatile or not, bruit, and thrill must be documented. If distal pulses are diminished or absent, the ankle-brachial index should be determined using a hand-held Doppler device.

Signs of arterial injury have been traditionally classified into "hard" and "soft" signs (Table 6-2). These correlate with the presence of a hemodynamically significant arterial lesion. "Hard" signs in-

---

TABLE 6-1. Factors Associated with Poor Functional Recovery or Need for Primary Amputation After Combined Vascular and Orthopaedic Extremity Trauma

Transected sciatic or tibial nerve	Multiple comminuted fractures
Transection of two of the three upper extremity nerves	Extensive soft tissue loss
Gustillo III-C orthopaedic injury	Crush injury
Below-knee arterial injury with two of the three arteries injured	Severe contamination
Prolonged limb ischemia greater than 12 hours	Elderly patients or multiple medical comorbidities
Cadaveric limb	Shock or other life-threatening injuries

TABLE 6-2. Clinical Signs of Vascular Injury	
Hard Signs	**Soft Signs**
Absent distal pulses	Diminished distal pulses or ABI <0.90
Active pulsatile bleeding	Unexplained hypotension or large blood loss at the scene
Expanding hematoma	Small or moderate nonexpanding hematoma
Bruit	Injury in proximity to a major vessel
Thrill	Neurologic injury in proximity to vessel

ABI, ankle-brachial index.

clude absence of distal pulses, pulsatile bleeding, expanding hematoma, palpable thrill, and audible bruit. "Soft" signs include proximity to the vessel, peripheral nerve deficit, history of moderate hemorrhage, and *diminished* distal pulses.

The general recommendation is that patients with hard signs associated with uncomplicated penetrating trauma should undergo immediate operative exploration, without need for arteriography or duplex ultrasound. The indications for arteriography are summarized in Table 6-3. Patients with multiple penetrating injuries should be evaluated with arteriography to determine the exact location and extent of arterial lesions. Arteriography is also advised in patients with combined arterial and orthopaedic trauma, even in the presence of hard signs. While the presence of hard signs predicts major vascular injury in nearly 100% of patients with uncomplicated penetrating trauma, less than 15% of patients with complex blunt injuries will require vascular repair. The inaccuracy of hard signs in this subgroup is explained by a combination of multiple other factors that ultimately lead to diminished pulses, including fractures, soft tissue disruption, compartment syndrome, and extrinsic arterial compression. Therefore, we generally recommend arteriography in all patients with complex skeletal trauma and hard signs of vascular injury.

We generally prefer a one-shot intraoperative arteriography technique. This avoids the 1 to 3 hour time delay required to obtain a formal arteriography in the angiography suite. An antegrade or retrograde approach in the affected limb is used for most cases. The availability of a portable C-arm and fluoroscopy permits localization of bony landmarks, selective catheterization of arterial branches, and endovascular treatment of arterial lesions. However, because fluoroscopy is usually not readily available in the emergency setting, we usually use ultrasound guidance and a micropuncture set for arterial access. The target artery (e.g., common femoral artery or brachial artery) is accessed with a micropuncture needle (18 gauge) in an antegrade or retrograde fashion. A 0.018 inch guidewire is advanced to allow placement of a sheath. The sheath can be used for contrast injection. Alternatively, the 0.018 inch wire is exchanged into a 0.035 inch wire and a 4 French sheath is advanced. The arterial inflow proximal to the access site should be manually compressed during contrast injection using digital pressure or a tourniquet. A single hand injection of 30 mL of diluted (50:50) iso-osmolar contrast allows adequate visualization of the area of concern and distal runoff vessels.

Other noninvasive imaging modalities are duplex ultrasound, computed tomography angiography (CTA), and magnetic resonance angiography (MRA). Computed tomography angiography is now available in most centers, is quite expeditious, and permits excellent image of the arterial circulation, soft tissue, and bone. This is particularly useful for planning operative approach in patients with centrally located lesions (e.g, aorta, subclavian, or iliac arteries). However, limitations are the relatively large contrast load (150 mL) in a patient who may potentially require additional angiography.

We recommend duplex arterial ultrasound in patients with "soft" signs of vascular injury, including those with an ankle-brachial index of less than 0.90. Arterial imaging is not required in patients

TABLE 6-3. Indications for Preoperative or Intraoperative Diagnostic Arteriography in Patients with Combined Extremity Trauma	
Multiple penetrating injuries	Trajectory parallel to artery
Unclear location or extent of arterial injuries	Underlying peripheral arterial disease
Extensive soft tissue injury	
Fracture or dislocations with hard signs of vascular injury	

with normal pulses and no other sign of arterial injury. Physical examination excludes significant arterial injuries as reliably as arteriography or surgical exploration. This is also true for patients with posterior knee dislocations, in whom arteriography used to be obtained routinely in the 1980s. Results of contemporary series show that in the absence of hard signs, less than 5% of patients had abnormalities on the arteriography but none required operative treatment or had amputation. On the other hand, the incidence of significant vascular injuries is 70% in the presence of hard signs. In patients with normal pulse examination, nonocclusive lesions include small intimal flaps, dissections, contusions, or small pseudoaneurysms; these lesions should be treated with antiplatelet therapy only.

SURGERY

Patient Positioning and General Approach

All vascular injuries can be accessed using the supine anatomic position (Fig. 6-1). Although prone position and a posterior approach may be used for isolated popliteal artery injuries which do not extend into the superficial femoral or tibioperoneal arteries, this approach limits access to the great saphenous vein if harvesting is necessary and may require excessive manipulation of the fractured limb. A generous sterile field should be prepared and draped to allow adequate exposure, proximal and distal control, and options of extra-anatomic reconstruction if indicated. The wise surgeon should always consider the "worst case scenario" (e.g., axillofemoral graft). A noninjured lower extremity should be prepped circumferentially for possible vein harvesting. The ideal conduit is an autologous great or small saphenous vein. Preoperative intravenous antibiotics (e.g., a first-generation cephalosporin) should be administered.

Technique

Repair of vascular injuries can be one of the most challenging aspects of trauma management. Some basic principles of vascular repair are applicable to all vascular injuries (Table 6-4). The operative sequence consists of access, exposure, control, and repair. Initial control of external hemorrhage is usually obtained with simple digital or manual pressure. Use of surgical instruments such as hemostats is not only ineffective but risks iatrogenic injury of adjacent nerves or veins. Manual compression is maintained by a member of the surgical team until definitive proximal and distal control of the injured vessel is obtained. The hematoma should not be entered without first obtaining proxi-

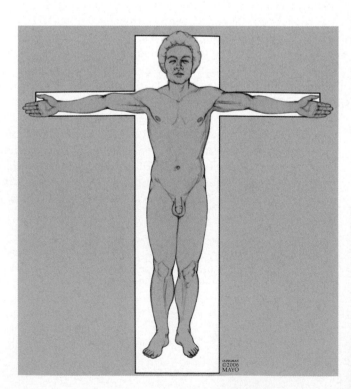

FIGURE 6-1

Patients should be positioned supine with one or both upper extremities abducted. At least one unaffected lower extremity should be circumferentially prepped for vein harvesting if indicated.

TABLE 6-4. Basic Principles of Repair of Vascular Injuries

Manual pressure for vascular control
Access using standard vascular exposure
Ensure proximal and distal control prior to entering a hematoma
Carefully enter the hematoma, avoiding injury to adjacent structures
Assess the extent of injury and presence of concomitant venous injury
Use systemic heparinization whenever possible
Determine type of vascular repair
Debridement of vessel edges
Proximal and distal Fogarty catheter thromboembolectomy

Instill regional heparin after two "clean" passes
Perform vascular anastomosis in a tensionless fashion
Allow prograde and retrograde bleeding prior to completing the anastomosis
Complete suture line, remove distal and proximal clamp sequentially
Assess distal circulation with pulse examination and hand-held Doppler
Obtain completion arteriography
Consider need for fasciotomy
Ensure adequate soft tissue coverage of vascular reconstruction

---

mal and distal control away from the site of injury. Access is gained using the standard exposure techniques described in the following discussion. Vascular clamps should not be applied forcefully and blindly; instead, the artery should be completely dissected, looped with a silastic vessel loop, and clamped under direct vision. One important adjunct is the use of balloon occlusion catheters. This facilitates control in areas of difficult access and avoids excessive dissection. In addition, pressure cuff tourniquets may be used in the extremities to achieve prompt vascular control. Once control is gained, the hematoma is explored with careful attention to avoid injury to adjacent structures. The extent of vascular injury is assessed and clamps are moved closer to the vascular wound. The injured vessel should be debrided and cleaned using tenotomy scissors. The extent of debridement should take into consideration the mechanism of injury, with more extensive debridements for high-velocity gunshot wounds, and blast or crush injuries. One should avoid excising the adventitia of the vessel while dissecting or debriding the artery. Distal and proximal thrombectomy using a Fogarty balloon thromboembolectomy catheter should be performed even in the presence of relatively good prograde or retrograde bleeding. The size of the catheter is generally a 4 or 5 for the iliacs, 4 for the superficial femoral, 3 or 4 for the deep femoral, 2 or 3 for the tibials, and 2 for the pedal and smaller arteries of the forearm. Passage of thromboembolectomy catheters into the deep femoral, tibials, and smaller arteries should be done gently because of risk of arterial rupture, dissection, or intimal injury due to excessive balloon inflation. At least two "clean" passes should be made before considering the artery free of thrombus. Preoperative and intraoperative systemic heparinization (80 mg/kg bolus) should be used unless there is a contraindication (e.g., head injury). An activated clotting time (ACT) above 250 seconds is considered optimal. Liberal regional heparinization should be used with flushes of heparinized saline proximally and distally to prevent propagation of any thrombus.

Restoration of extremity perfusion does not always require definitive arterial reconstruction. Another important adjunct is a temporary arterial shunt placed in the proximal and distal arterial ends. This promptly controls hemorrhage and re-establishes inflow. Our preference is to use either a short or long Sundt intraluminal arterial shunt (Fig. 6-2). The shunt is secured to the artery using silk suture or a Rummel tourniquet. Although systemic heparinization is preferred, this is not an absolute requirement for shunt placement. The main advantage of temporary shunts is the avoidance of damage to a fresh arterial repair during subsequent orthopaedic manipulations in cases of comminuted, unstable skeletal injuries.

The injured vessels are "set up" for the reconstruction using stay sutures and clean white towels. The anastomosis should be performed without any tension using optic magnification and small monofilament suture (e.g., Prolene). In general, a 4 or 5-0 monofilament suture is used for the femoral arteries, and 6 or 7-0 for the popliteal, tibials, and smaller arteries. The type of reconstruction varies and should be tailored to both the patient condition and extent of injury (Fig. 6-3). Simple repair entails a lateral arteriorrhaphy or venorrhaphy. One should avoid excessive narrowing of the lumen and use patch angioplasty if there is any question. A segment of saphenous vein or bovine pericardium can be used for vascular patches. Vessels with injuries involving less than 1.5 cm in length can usually be re-approximated using end-to-end anastomosis. Mobilization of the artery or vein may require ligation of multiple side branches to gain enough length to allow a tensionless anastomosis. The vessel ends should be spatulated to prevent anastomotic narrowing. A running anasto-

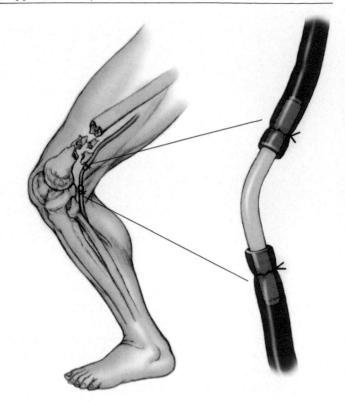

FIGURE 6-2

Intra-arterial Sundt shunt for temporary control and restoration of blood flow.

mosis is used most cases, but interrupted sutures may be required in smaller vessels or pediatric cases. Before completion of the anastomosis, the proximal and distal clamps are temporarily removed to ensure adequate prograde and retrograde bleeding. Absence of back bleeding indicates thrombus formation or a technical defect and warrants further catheter embolectomy or revision. Approximately 80% of all vascular extremity injuries that occur in association with orthopaedic trauma

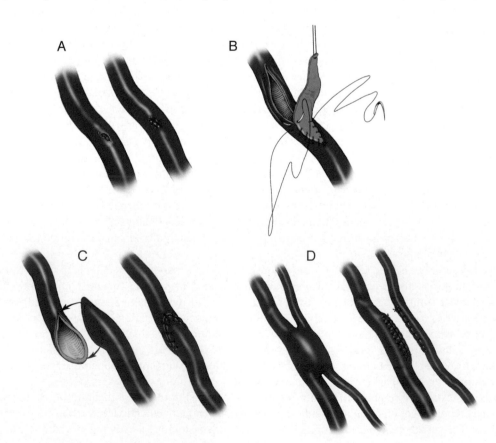

FIGURE 6-3

Types of vascular injuries and repair: simple laceration treated with arteriorrhaphy **(A)**; use of patch angioplasty for longer lesions **(B)**; end-to-end anastomosis **(C)** and lateral arteriorrhaphy **(D)**.

can be repaired using one of these three techniques: simple closure, end-to-end anastomosis, or patch angioplasty.

Insertion of an interposition or bypass graft is required in approximately 20% of cases. Vessels with more extensive injuries of greater than 1.5 cm in length cannot be re-approximated without tension. The preferred conduit in these cases is the great saphenous vein harvested from the contralateral noninjured extremity. The ipsilateral saphenous vein should be avoided due to a high incidence of concomitant deep venous injuries (50%) and postoperative deep venous thrombosis. The great saphenous vein is ideal for vessels 6 mm or smaller. Some size mismatch is acceptable. However, for injuries of larger vessels, a larger conduit should be selected. Spiral or panel vein grafts, or femoral vein grafts, are acceptable options. For arterial injuries of the aorta and major branches, polytetrafluoroethylene (PTFE) or dacron grafts have been used extensively with excellent results. Obviously, contamination of the surgical field represents a limiting factor in these cases. Every attempt should be made to repair both the arterial and venous injury. Although venous repair has limited patency, improved outflow decreases edema and may affect patency of the arterial repair. The traditional recommendation is that all venous injuries involving the popliteal, common femoral, axillary, and portal veins should be repaired because of poor collateral flow. This recommendation has now been extended to all major named veins.

After the vascular reconstruction is complete, the surgeon should assess the adequacy of the repair for any residual stenosis or kinks. The limb should be examined and distal perfusion documented with pulse and hand-held Doppler examination. The goal in a patient without pre-existing vascular disease is to obtain normal distal pulses at the end of the operation. Completion arteriography is important to detect any technical abnormalities that may cause early thrombosis of the repair, as well as to assess the patency of the distal run-off vessels. Finally, the vascular reconstruction should be covered with viable soft tissue. Occasionally, flaps are required to bring vascularized tissue over the reconstruction.

Specific Injuries: Anatomy and Surgical Exposure

Penetrating injuries can affect any arterial segment. Specific patterns of blunt orthopaedic and arterial trauma are well recognized (Table 6-5). The surgical anatomy and exposure of the most common arterial injuries are outlined in the following paragraphs.

Upper Extremity Injuries

SUBCLAVIAN ARTERY   The right subclavian artery originates from the innominate artery, and the left subclavian from the aorta (Fig. 6-4). The subclavian artery is divided into three parts in relation to the anterior scalene muscle: proximal, middle, and distal. The proximal subclavian artery gives off the vertebral, internal thoracic, and thyrocervical trunk. The middle subclavian artery contains the costocervical trunk and the dorsal scapular artery. The distal subclavian artery has no branches. A supraclavicular incision one fingerbreadth above the clavicle allows excellent exposure of the middle and distal subclavian artery (Fig. 6-5). For exposure of the proximal subclavian artery, median sternotomy is required for right-sided injuries and left anterolateral thoracotomy for left-sided injuries.

Subclavian artery injuries are uncommon and represent less than 5% of all vascular injuries. Blunt injuries may occur in association with clavicular or first rib fracture. Over 50% of patients present with massive bleeding. Subclavian artery occlusion is well tolerated in 85% of patients because of a rich collateral system. Amputation is rarely required. Arterial repair usually requires end-to-end

TABLE 6-5. Patterns of Combined Orthopaedic and Vascular Trauma	
Orthopaedic Injury	**Arterial Injury Location**
Supracondylar humeral fracture	Brachial artery
Clavicular fracture	Subclavian and axillary artery
Shoulder dislocation	Axillary artery
First rib fracture	Subclavian artery and aorta
Femoral shaft fracture	Superficial femoral artery and above-knee popliteal artery
Posterior knee dislocation	Popliteal artery
Proximal tibiofibular fracture	Popliteal and tibioperoneal arteries

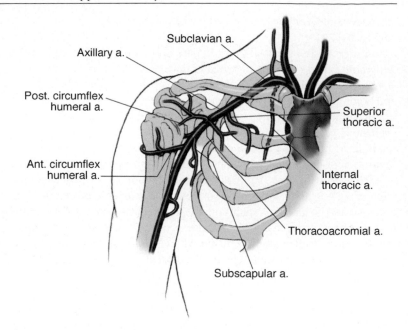

FIGURE 6-4

Surgical anatomy of the subclavian and axillary arteries.

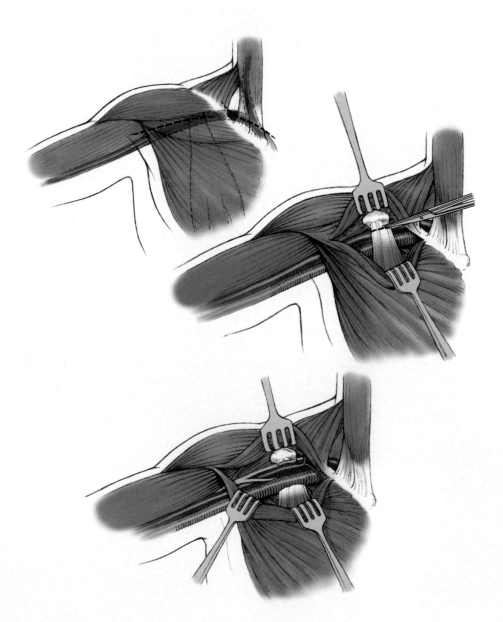

FIGURE 6-5

Preferred surgical approaches for exposure of the subclavian (supracalvicular) and axillary (infraclavicular) arteries.

anastomosis or a small interposition graft using autologous vein. Overall, the mortality rate for subclavian artery injuries is 16%.

AXILLARY ARTERY   The axillary artery extends from the lateral border of the first rib to the lateral border of the teres major muscle (see Fig. 6-4). The artery is divided into three parts in relation to the pectoralis minor muscle: proximal, middle (beneath), and distal. The first part gives of one branch (supreme thoracic), the second two branches (thoracoacromial and lateral thoracic), and the third three branches (subscapular, anterior and posterior humeral circumflex). The artery lies in close proximity to the axillary vein and to the brachial plexus.

Axillary artery injuries represent 5% to 10% of all arterial injuries. The vast majority (95%) are due to penetrating trauma. Although blunt injuries are rare, these occur in 1% of the patients presenting with either a fracture of the proximal humerus or anterior dislocation of the shoulder. In addition, patients who chronically use crutches may develop stenosis or occlusion from repetitive trauma. Patients with axillary artery injuries often sustain associated nerve trauma.

Exposure of the axillary artery is best achieved using an infraclavicular incision one fingerbreadth bellow the clavicle (see Fig. 6-5). Most injuries can be repaired with end-to-end anastomosis or a small interposition graft. The mortality and amputation rates are exceedingly low for axillary injuries. However, two-thirds of the patients have significant neurologic dysfunction or persistent neuralgia from associated trauma to the brachial plexus.

BRACHIAL ARTERY   The brachial artery is a continuation of the axillary artery (Fig. 6-6). It starts at the lower edge of the teres major muscle and terminates approximately 2 cm below the antecubital crease, where it bifurcates into the radial and ulnar arteries. A high bifurcation of the brachial artery above the antecubital crease is found in 20% of the population. In the upper and mid-arm, the brachial artery is accompanied by the median nerve laterally and by the ulnar and radial nerves medially. The median nerve crosses anterior to the artery and is located medially at the level of the elbow joint. The brachial artery has three important branches: deep brachial artery, and superior and inferior ulnar collateral artcrics.

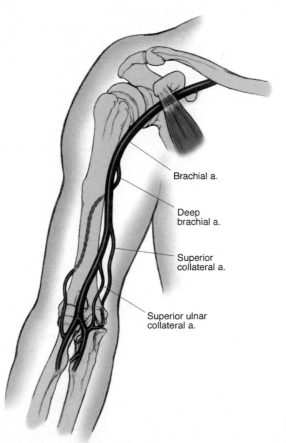

Brachial a.

Deep brachial a.

Superior collateral a.

Superior ulnar collateral a.

FIGURE 6-6

Surgical anatomy of the brachial artery.

The brachial artery is the most commonly injured artery of the upper extremity, accounting for 15% to 30% of all peripheral vascular injuries. Patients typically present with hand ischemia. Patients with supracondylar humeral fractures or elbow dislocations and hard signs of vascular injury should be further evaluated with arteriography to rule out brachial artery injury. The brachial artery is best exposed using a longitudinal incision along the course of the artery medial to the biceps muscle or an S-shaped incision across the antecubital fossa (Fig. 6-7). Most injuries are repaired with either end-to-end anastomosis or interposition vein graft. Clinical outcome after repair is better than for injuries of the axillary or subclavian artery because the incidence of nerve injury is significantly less. Amputation or death is rare.

RADIAL AND ULNAR ARTERIES   The ulnar artery is the larger branch of the brachial artery and gives off the ulnar recurrent arteries and the common interosseus artery (Fig. 6-8). The ulnar artery terminates in the superficial palmar arch. The radial artery gives off the radial recurrent artery, which anastomoses to the deep brachial artery. Distally, the brachial artery gives off a small branch to the superficial palmar arch and terminates in the deep palmar arch.

Injuries to the radial and ulnar artery are also common, but most often result from penetrating trauma. Complete occlusion or transection of either the radial or ulnar artery will often have no adverse effect on the circulation of the hand because of rich collateral circulation. However, patients with marked hematoma in the forearm may develop compartment syndrome requiring fasciotomy. Distal thrombectomy catheters should be handled gently because these arteries are prone to rupture or intimal injury. Repair often requires simple closure, end-to-end anastomosis, or small interposition grafts. Amputation is rare.

Lower Extremity Injuries

COMMON, PROFUNDA, AND SUPERFICIAL FEMORAL ARTERIES   The common femoral artery originates at the level of the inguinal ligament as a continuation of the external iliac artery (Fig. 6-9). The common femoral artery is located adjacent to the femoral nerve (laterally) and common femoral vein (medially). The first branch of the common femoral artery is the superficial circumflex iliac artery, which marks the transition from external iliac to common femoral artery just below the inguinal ligament. The second branch is the superficial epigastric artery. Approximately 5 cm distal to the inguinal ligament the common femoral artery bifurcates into the superficial and deep femoral arteries. The deep (profunda) femoral artery is located in a posterolateral position. This artery gives off the medial and lateral femoral circumflex arteries and four to five perforator branches in the thigh. The superficial femoral artery follows its course underneath the sartorius muscle (Hunter

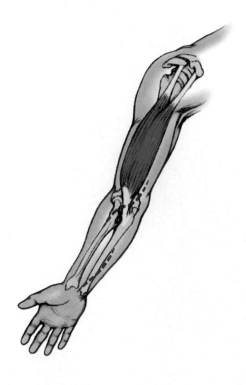

FIGURE 6-7

Preferred surgical approaches for exposure of the distal brachial artery and forearm vessels.

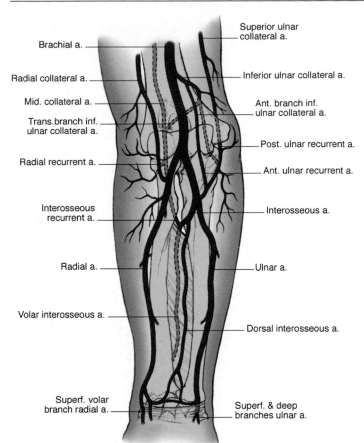

Brachial a.

Superior ulnar collateral a.

Radial collateral a.

Inferior ulnar collateral a.

Mid. collateral a.

Ant. branch inf. ulnar collateral a.

Trans.branch inf. ulnar collateral a.

Post. ulnar recurrent a.

Radial recurrent a.

Ant. ulnar recurrent a.

Interosseous recurrent a.

Interosseous a.

Radial a.

Ulnar a.

Volar interosseous a.

Dorsal interosseous a.

Superf. volar branch radial a.

Superf. & deep branches ulnar a.

FIGURE 6-8

Surgical anatomy of the forearm arteries.

canal) and terminates in the popliteal artery at the level of the adductor hiatus. The artery is adjacent to the saphenous nerve and femoral vein.

Injury to the femoral vessels accounts for one-third of all peripheral vascular injuries in civilian and military series. The most common mechanism of injury is penetrating trauma. Anterior dislocation of the femoral head is a rare cause of blunt injury. The superficial femoral artery is injured in 5% of the patients presenting with femoral shaft fracture. Bleeding is the most common presentation in cases of penetrating trauma, whereas distal limb ischemia predominates in patients with blunt injury.

Exposure of the common femoral artery and femoral bifurcation is best obtained using a longitudinal incision two fingerbreadths lateral to the pubic tubercle (see Fig. 6-9). The incision extends from the level of the inguinal as far distally as necessary, depending on how extensive the injury is to the proximal deep and superficial femoral arteries. Rarely, a suprainguinal curvilinear incision is required for retroperitoneal exposure of the external iliac artery to achieve proximal control. Exposure of the superficial femoral artery can be achieved through a longitudinal incision along the course of the sartorius muscle. Patients with small, clean injuries of the femoral arteries may be treated with primary closure, end-to-end anastomosis, or patch angioplasty. Longer lesions require an interposition graft using autologous saphenous vein from the contralateral thigh. Long-term patency rates approach 100% for interposition grafts. Lower extremity function is predominantly determined by the extent of skeletal and neurologic injury.

POPLITEAL AND TIBIOPERONEAL ARTERIES   The popliteal artery is the continuation of the superficial femoral artery and originates at the adductor magnus hiatus (Fig. 6-10). The popliteal artery gives off multiple genicular collateral branches at the above- and below-knee level. The artery bifurcates in 90% of individuals and gives off the anterior tibial artery and the tibioperoneal trunk. The tibioperoneal trunk gives off the posterior tibial artery and the peroneal artery. The anterior tibial artery follows an anterior and lateral course, perforates the interosseous membrane, and is located in the anterior compartment of the leg along with the deep peroneal nerve. The peroneal artery is the middle branch of the three, follows its course in the deep posterior compartment, and bifurcates into the perforating branch to the anterior artery and communicating artery to the posterior tibial artery.

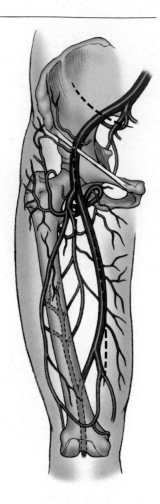

FIGURE 6-9

Surgical anatomy and preferred surgical approaches for exposure of the common, superficial, and deep femoral arteries.

The posterior tibial artery is the most medial branch of the three tibioperoneal arteries and terminates as the common plantar artery below the ankle joint.

Popliteal artery injuries often result from blunt trauma. Fracture or posterior dislocation of the knee is a known mechanism of injury. Most patients with popliteal artery injury present with distal ischemia because the genicular collaterals are not effective in maintaining adequate distal perfusion. Occlusion of a single tibioperoneal artery is well tolerated and does not require repair.

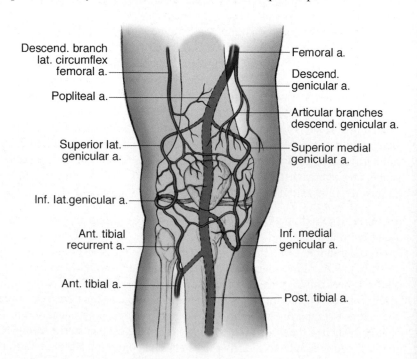

FIGURE 6-10

Surgical anatomy of the popliteal artery.

Most popliteal and tibioperoneal artery injuries can be exposed using a generous medial approach above and/or below the knee level depending on the extent of injury (Fig. 6-11). The great saphenous vein should be identified and protected. Division of the semimembranous and semitendinous muscles is often required for adequate exposure. The posterior tibial and peroneal arteries are also exposed using a medial incision along the posterior margin of the tibia. The soleus muscle is incised longitudinally allowing exposure of the mid- and distal portions of the posterior tibial and peroneal arteries. Although the origin of the anterior tibial artery can be exposed through a medial incision, an incision in the anterior compartment two fingerbreadths lateral to the tibia is required for exposure of the anterior tibial artery.

Injury to the popliteal and tibioperoneal arteries is associated with significant morbidity. Clinical outcome is affected by the extent of skeletal and neurologic trauma, time of ischemia, and adequacy of runoff through the tibial and peroneal arteries.

Venous Injuries   The management of venous injuries is essentially identical to that for any arterial injury. Although venous repair does not yield the same satisfactory results of arterial repair and there is a higher incidence of early thrombosis, current recommendations are to attempt venous repair of any named major vein whenever possible. Large veins such as the inferior vena cava and iliac veins pose a problem in terms of conduit size mismatch. Options in these cases are use of spiral or paneled vein grafts or externally supported PTFE grafts. Injuries affecting minor veins or patients with other life-threatening injuries should be managed with primary ligation. Major veins can be exposed using the same incisions as for their arterial counterpart. Direct pressure using sponge sticks or pressure cuff tourniquets are excellent means of obtaining control in cases of bleeding. Techniques for repair should be the same as for arterial injuries with the caveat that catheter embolectomy often cannot be used because of competent valves.

Mangled Extremity   One should use clinical judgment in cases of severe trauma with complex soft tissue, skeletal, and vascular injuries. Although there are scoring systems to quantify the degree of injury, cases should be individualized. The mangled extremity severity score (MESS) grades skeletal/soft tissue damage, limb ischemia, shock, and age. However, this scoring system is inaccurate in identifying the irretrievable limb requiring primary amputation. Factors associated with need for amputation after below-knee fractures are injury of greater than three muscle compartments, occlusion of greater than two tibial arteries, and presence of cadaveric changes at initial presentation. When more than two of these predictive factors are present, none of the extremities were salvageable. Primary amputation should be considered early in patients with a dysvascular extremity and extensive soft tissue loss, as the chance of functional recovery is minimal.

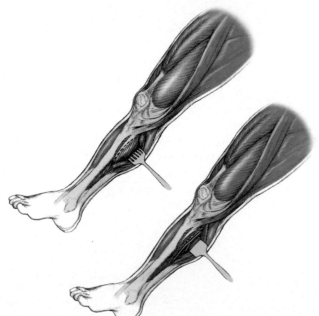

FIGURE 6-11

Preferred medial knee approach for exposure of the below-knee popliteal artery and proximal tibioperoneal vessels.

POSTOPERATIVE MANAGEMENT

Patients should be continuously evaluated for bleeding, distal limb perfusion, and development of compartment syndrome. Following massive bleeding and coagulopathy, one should aggressively resuscitate the patient and monitor laboratory results every 4 hours (complete blood count, platelets, prothrombin and partial thromboplastin times, and fibrinogen levels). We recommend that laboratory levels are kept within normal limits during the first 48 hours. Parameters include hemoglobin above 10 g/dL, platelet count above 100,000, international normalized ratio of less than 1.2, and partial thromboplastin time of less than 40 seconds. Mild abnormalities contribute to postoperative "oozing," large hematoma, and initiate a cascade of coagulopathy that ultimately may lead to bleeding requiring re-exploration. Assessment of vascular pulses should be done routinely with serial examination and hand-held Doppler interrogation. This is repeated every 2 hours for the first 24 hours and every 4 hours thereafter.

The injured extremity should be checked for any signs of infection. Early wound infection, particularly if associated with soft tissue necrosis, is one of the most important determinants of delayed amputation. Aggressive perioperative antibiotic therapy is recommended.

Compartment syndrome is a common occurrence in patients with combined vascular and orthopaedic trauma. Patients with ischemic limbs for more than 4 hours can be expected to have some degree of compartment syndrome. Presentation can be delayed up to 12 to 24 hours after reperfusion of the ischemic limb. Early or prophylactic fasciotomy in this setting may be associated with improved outcome. If fasciotomy is deferred at the time of arterial reconstruction, physical examination and compartment pressure measurements should be repeated frequently. Compartment pressures of higher than 30 cm H^2O strongly indicate fasciotomy.

COMPLICATIONS

The most common complications after vascular reconstructions are bleeding, infection, early thrombosis and development of compartment syndrome. Medical complications involving cardiac, pulmonary, renal, and neurologic systems are also common. Amputation can result because of early technical failure, venous outflow problems, infection, and fracture instability. Deep venous thrombosis is a common occurrence after combined vascular and orthopaedic trauma. Aggressive prophylaxis should be instituted in the early postoperative period. Postoperative duplex ultrasound is indicated for any sign of worsening limb edema or pain. Patients need to be followed regularly because of the potential for late complications. Arterial stenosis or thrombosis, aneurysmal degeneration of vein grafts, and chronic venous insufficiency after primary venous ligation or thrombosis of venous repair can be identified using duplex ultrasound surveillance. We generally re-evaluate patients with combined injuries 6 months after dismissal or earlier if the patient develops symptoms of chronic limb ischemia (e.g., claudication).

RESULTS

The three most important factors affecting clinical outcome in patients with combined vascular and orthopaedic trauma are the mechanism of injury, the time interval from injury to restoration of arterial inflow, and the extent of damage to soft tissue, bone, and nerves. Whereas military trauma is almost universally associated with high-velocity penetrating injuries, the majority of civilian injuries are due to blunt mechanisms. In general, penetrating injuries are associated with better outcome. Blunt injuries with complex fractures, dislocations, and extensive soft tissue damage are associated with much worse results. The results of contemporary clinical series of combined vascular and orthopaedic extremity trauma are summarized in Table 6-6. Overall, the amputation rate in combined series was 6% for penetrating injuries and 31% for blunt trauma.

TABLE 6-6.   Results of Contemporary Series of Combined Orthopaedic and Vascular Trauma

Author	Year	n	n (%) Amputation
Penetrating Trauma			
Bishara et al.	1986	29	0
Swetnam et al.	1986	24	8 (33)
Bongard et al.	1989	11	2 (18)
Russell et al.	1991	35	1 (2.8)
Norman et al.	1995	30	0
Attebery et al.	1996	29	0
Granchi et al.	2000	13	1 (10)
McHenry et al.	2002	27	0
Total		198	12 (6)
Blunt Trauma			
Lange et al.	1985	20	12 (60)
Swetnam et al.	1986	10	8 (80)
Bishara et al.	1986	22	1 (4.5)
Howe et al.	1987	16	6 (37.5)
McNutt et al.*	1989	17	6 (35)
Drost et al.	1989	14	4 (28.5)
Bongard et al.	1989	26	3 (11.5)
Johansen et al.	1990	26	12 (46)
Odland et al.	1990	28	11 (39)
Russell et al.	1991	35	18 (51)
Alexander et al.	1991	29	9 (31)
Schlickewei et al.	1992	113	50 (45)
Attebery et al.	1996	12	3 (25)
Rozycki ct al.	2002	59	11 (18.5)
Hossny[†]	2004	17	4 (23.5)
Menakuru et al.	2005	90	7 (12.8)
Total		534	165 (31)

* All patients had tibial fracture.
[†] All patients had knee dislocation with associated popliteal artery injury.

RECOMMENDED READING

Alexander JJ, Piotrowski JJ, Graham D, et al. Outcome of complex orthopedic and vascular injuries of the lower extremity. *Am J Surg.* 1991;162:111.

Attebery LR, Dennis JW, Russo-Alesi F, et al. Changing patterns of arterial injuries associated with fractures and dislocations. *J Am Coll Surg.* 1996;183:377.

Bongard FS, White GH, Klein SR. Management strategy of complex extremity injuries. *Am J Surg.* 1989;158:151.

Bishara FS, Pasch AR, Lim LT, et al. Improved results in the treatment of civilian vascular injuries associated with fractures and dislocations. *J Vasc Surg.* 1986;3:707.

Drost TF, Rosemurgy AS, Proctor D, et al. Outcome of treatment of combined orthopedic and arterial trauma to the lower extremity. *J Trauma.* 1989;29:1331.

Howe HR, Poole GV, Hansen KJ, et al. Salvage of lower extremities following combined orthopedic and vacular trauma: a predictive salvage index. *Am Surg.* 1987;53:205.

Johansen K, Daines, Howey T, et al. Objective criteria accurately predict amputation following lower extremity trauma. *J Trauma.* 1990;30:568.

Bandyk DF. Vascular injury associated with extremity trauma. *Clin Orthop Relat Res.* 1995;Sep(318):117–124.

McNutt R, Seabrook GR, Schmitt DD, Aprahamian C, Bandyk DF, Towne JB. Blunt tibial artery trauma: predicting the irretrievable extremity. *J Trauma.* 1989;Dec. 29(12):1624–1627.

Lange RH, Bach AW, Hansen ST, et al. Open tibial fractures with associated vascular injuries: prognosis for limb salvage. *J Trauma.* 1985;25:203.

Lin C-H, Weif-C, Levin LS, et al. The functional outcome of lower extremity fractures with vascular injury. *J Trauma.* 1997;43;480.

McCready RA, Logan NM, Dangherty ME, et al. Long-term results with autogenous tissue repair of traumatic extremity vascular injuries. *Ann Surg.* 1997;206:804.

Miranda FE, Dennis JW, Veldenz HC, et al. Confirmation of the safety and accuracy of physical examination in the evaluation of knee dislocation for injury of the popliteal artery: a prospective study. *J Trauma.* 2002;52(2):247–251.

Norman J, Gahtan V Franz M, et al. Occult vascular injuries following gunshot wounds resulting in long bone fractures of the extremities. *Am Surg*. 1995;61:146.

Odland MD, Gisbert VL, Gustilo RB, et al. Combined orthopedic and vascular injury in the lower extremities: indications for amputation. *Surgery*. 1990;108:660.

Palazzo JC, Ristow AB, Cury JM, et al. Traumatic vascular lesions associated with fractures and dislocations. *J Cardiovasc Surg*. 1986;121:607.

Schlickewei W, Kuner EH, Mullaji AB, et al. Upper and lower limb fractures with concomitant arterial injury. *J Bone Joint Surg*. 1992;74:181.

Swetnam JA, Hardin WD, Kerstein MD, et al. Successful management of trifurcation injuries. *Am Surg*. 1986;52:585.

Treiman GS, Yellin AE, Weaver FA, et al. Examination of the patient with a knee dislocation: the case for selective angiography. *Arch Surg*. 1992;127:1056.

Van Wijngaarden M, Omert L, Rodriguez A, et al. Management of blunt vascular trauma to the extremities. *Surg Gynecol Obstet*. 1993;177:41.

7 Management of the Soft Tissue with Shoulder Trauma

Scott F. M. Duncan and John W. Sperling

INDICATIONS/CONTRAINDICATIONS

Shoulder trauma can result in significant soft tissue loss over some of the bony prominences of the shoulder such as the acromion and clavicle. Areas of the scapula can be exposed as well from trauma about the shoulder. Fortunately, the glenohumeral joint itself is covered with a multilayer muscle configuration. If there are concomitant fractures, nerve injuries, or vessel injuries, one must keep in mind not only the pre-existing soft tissue trauma and how to protect the healing of that, but also how to obtain the best exposure to facilitate fixing the concomitant injuries. Open fractures and neurovascular injuries require emergent intervention, or otherwise the extremity may be compromised. In such circumstances, the rescue of the threatened limb takes priority. However, again, one must keep in mind the potential need for soft tissue coverage in these patients. Fortunately, numerous flap options exist about the shoulder for soft tissue coverage (see Chapter 8).

The addition of locking plates, which are fixed angle devices for fixing proximal humerus fractures, has greatly augmented our armamentarium for treating these fractures. In significant injuries, it is not unreasonable to perform a delayed intervention once the soft tissues have been covered or stabilized. Concomitant injuries such as rotator cuff tears can be addressed months down the line, if needed, once the other injuries and soft tissue envelope have finished healing. When the wound bed is grossly purulent, coverage and otherwise operative repair should be delayed until a clean wound can be established. This being said, it is obviously preferable to have all structures fixed prior to any type of soft tissue coverage to minimize injury to the soft tissue flap upon re-operation or re-exploration of the wound.

PREOPERATIVE PLANNING

A thorough examination of the shoulder and the involved extremity as well as a radiographic study of the shoulder are mandatory to recognize soft tissue and bony injuries. Neurovascular injuries may be easily missed if the more distal aspects of the extremity are not examined. Furthermore, radiographic examination must include axillary lateral views to rule out a glenohumeral dislocation. Active flexion, abduction, internal and external rotation should be tested about the shoulder when possible. Active flexion and extension about the elbow, wrist, and fingers will also help delineate more proximal neurovascular compromise. Sensation and motor function of the extremity should be documented. Radial pulses as well as ulnar pulses need to be documented as well as the time for capillary refill.

From a radiographic standpoint in the emergent setting, a computed tomography scan sometimes is required to further delineate the characteristics of bony trauma. Occasionally, an arteriogram may be needed to investigate vascular injuries. The most commonly injured nerve about the shoulder is the axillary nerve, and an examination of deltoid function and shoulder sensation should be performed. When planning the surgical exposure or exposures, one must appreciate what other injuries need to be addressed, if any, and how the incision and exposure will jeopardize any pre-existing skin or muscle trauma. Incisions should be selected that will not compromise the viability of the soft tissue envelope and that once they have healed will not create a tethering-type scar, resulting in loss of shoulder range of motion.

SURGERY

Patient Positioning

We prefer to perform surgery about the shoulder with the patient in a beach-chair position. Depending on the injuries to be addressed, supine and lateral decubitus may be used as well. However, in our experience, the beach-chair position has the advantages of allowing manipulation of the arm as needed to facilitate reduction or retraction as well as providing access to both the anterior and posterior aspects of the shoulder. These surgeries are usually done under general anesthesia, but postoperative pain management can be enhanced by the administration of interscalene blocks by the anesthesiologist. The patient is brought into the regular operating room where preparation and draping are carried out in the usual sterile fashion and manner. As with any surgery, atraumatic technique should be adhered to in an effort to lessen skin, muscle, and other soft tissue necrosis. Poorly executed shoulder surgery can result in greater functional loss than would have otherwise occurred had no surgical intervention been attempted. However, as with any surgery, risks are involved and nerve and vessel injury can occur. Excessive scarring and postoperative joint contractures may result despite the best surgical techniques.

The beach-chair position facilitates the use of fluoroscopy during the course of the procedure (Fig. 7-1). This flexibility is sometimes needed when attempting to image complex injuries. Sometimes it is necessary to extend the wound of the injury both proximally and distally to provide visibility to the area of trauma. However, most important is that an adequate view of the surgical field be created to avoid the need to perform surgical repairs in a challenged manner through a small wound. In general, we try to avoid "T" extensions of transverse lacerations, but occasionally this may need to be done to gain access to neurovascular structures. Again, the type of shoulder injury will necessitate the surgical approach.

Technique

For proximal humerus fractures, there are two basic approaches. The first is a superior deltoid approach in which a skin incision is made in Langer's lines just lateral to the anterior lateral aspect of the acromion. This approach allows the deltoid to be split from the edge of the acromion distally for approximately 4 to 5 cm. Again, care must be taken to protect the axillary nerve. Of note is that the deltoid origin is not removed, but there is still exposure of the superior aspect of the proximal humerus. This type of exposure is quite useful for a fixation of greater tuberosity fractures as well as the insertion of intramedullary nailing. In the beach-chair position rotation, flexion, and extension

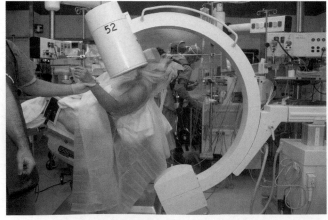
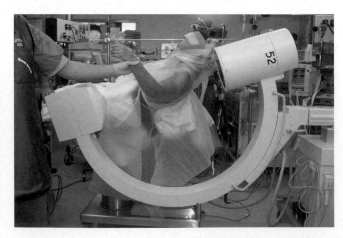

FIGURE 7-1

A,B: The beach-chair position helps facilitate use of intraoperative fluoroscopy.

of the humerus can enhance the exposure of the underlying structures as well as reduction of the fragments.

The second approach is a long deltopectoral approach in which both the deltoid origin and insertion are preserved (Fig. 7-2). The skin incision begins just inferior to the clavicle and extends across the coracoid process and down into the area of insertion of the deltoid on the humerus. The cephalic vein should be preserved and retracted either laterally or medially depending on which is easiest for the surgeon. The cephalic vein is less likely to be injured when taken medially, given that over-vigorous retraction on the cephalic vein and deltoids can result in vein injury. If the vein is accidentally transected or significantly injured, either from the trauma or the surgical approach, ligation can be considered. In the deltopectoral approach, if more exposure is needed to gain access to the proximal aspect of the humerus, the superior part of the pectoralis major tendon insertion can be divided. This may need to be done for multipart fractures. In significant trauma injuries, the pectoralis major tendon may be found to be disrupted and should be repaired when possible using nonabsorbable suture and/or suture anchors.

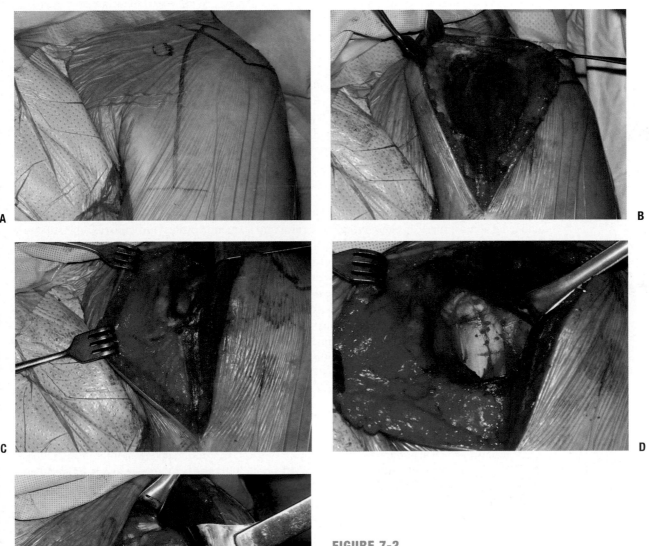

FIGURE 7-2

A: The landmarks of the shoulder are outlined and the incision is marked. **B:** A triangle of fat is usually present at the proximal interval between the pectoralis and deltoid. **C:** Typically, the cephalic vein is left within its bed medially. **D:** One continues the deltopectoral interval distally. **E:** One places a retractor medially beneath the conjoint group and one laterally to retract the deltoid.

We do not advocate procedures that split or remove part of the acromion given the significant risk of complications. Methods of internal fixation of proximal humerus fractures go beyond the scope of what this chapter is intended to provide. However, a brief mention of various options will be discussed. As mentioned earlier in the chapter, there is an improved role for open reduction internal fixation of these fractures given the new fixed angled locking plates that have been developed. However, there still remains a role for intramedullary nailing, tension band techniques, and percutaneous pinning of proximal humerus fractures. Most important, though, is that a majority of proximal humerus fractures in our practices are still treated nonoperatively. Shoulder arthroplasty is still used in those cases where there is significant comminution and adequate fixation cannot be achieved by other means. Successful treatment of shoulder injuries requires understanding of their specific biologic and mechanical challenges. This should also encompass knowledge about the natural history and potential complications from the various treatment options.

With the beach-chair position, we take care to secure the head with use of towels to the head supporting apparatus. This can be done with prefabricated devices such as the Skytron attachment. Care needs to be taken to make sure the neck angle is appropriate. Also, when securing the head, care needs to be taken that there are no pressure points on the eyes. With regard to the anterior approach, the exposure of the shoulder joint is useful for drainage of sepsis, open reduction internal fixation of fractures, hemiarthroplasty, and reconstruction of dislocation trauma. Landmarks for this approach are the coracoid process and the deltoid insertion. The incision starts at about the level of the clavicle and goes over the coracoid process through the area where the deltopectoral groove can be palpated down to the anterior aspect of the shoulder. An alternative to this incision is an axillary incision. The shoulder must be abducted and externally rotated to make this type of approach. The downside of this in the trauma setting is that the skin flaps must be undermined extensively to visualize the area of the deltopectoral groove. However, this approach does have a cosmetic advantage. This approach is also difficult in extremely muscular patients.

The deep surgical dissection involves identifying the short head of the biceps and coracobrachialis; these are retracted medially. The overlying fascia must be carefully incised. The long head of the biceps can be used to identify the division between the lesser and greater tuberosities. This can also be a good marker for where to begin subscapularis dissection. The arm should be kept adducted at most times, because bringing the arm into abduction brings the neurovascular structures closer to the operative field. This is especially true if any work is being done around the coracoid. Care must be taken when retracting the coracoid and coracobrachialis, as over-vigorous retraction can cause musculocutaneous paralysis. Care should be taken with the axillary nerve as well. External rotation of the shoulder increases the distance between the subscapularis and the axillary nerve. A leash of vessels on the inferior border of the subscapularis frequently requires cauterization to maintain good visualization in the surgical field.

The anterolateral approach in the trauma setting is most useful for repair stabilization of the long head of the biceps tendon as well as fixation of greater tuberosity fractures. A transverse or longitudinal incision can be used beginning at the anterolateral corner of the acromion and extending lateral to the coracoid process or going over the anterolateral aspect of the shoulder. The superficial dissection involves subcutaneous fat and deltoid fascia. This is incised in line with the skin incision. The split should not extend more than 5 cm down from the acromion as axillary nerve injury is possible. In the case of rotator cuff tears, one may consider taking the deltoid off the anterior aspect of the acromion, which also improves visualization (Fig. 7-3). Avoid inadvertent inferior retraction as well, which can also injure the axillary nerve. Bleeding will obstruct the view and is frequently encountered during this dissection. Try to obtain good hemostasis and cautery of the acromial branch of the coracoacromial artery; it usually must be electrocauterized. Also avoid excessive stripping and detachment of the deltoid. Deep dissection will reveal the rotator cuff under surface of the acromion and greater tuberosity. A stay suture in the fascia of the deltoid can be useful to prevent excessive splitting and injury to the axillary nerve.

The lateral approach provides limited access in a similar fashion to the anterolateral approach. Again, it can be useful for open reduction internal fixation of greater tuberosity fractures, as well as for open reduction internal fixation of neck fractures using a tension band technique. The rotator cuff is easily accessible through this approach. This is a common approach for insertion of intramedullary rods into the humerus. An incision approximately 5 cm long is made from just above the acromion down the lateral aspect of the arm. Deltoid muscle is split in line with its fibers down to a level no more than 5 cm. Most surgeons insert a suture at the inferior aspect of the split to help prevent it from extending any further and potentially injuring the axillary nerve. Deep surgical dissection is contin-

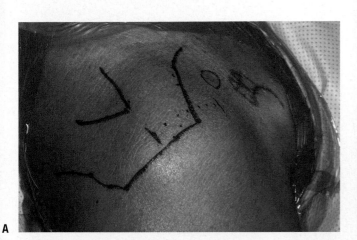
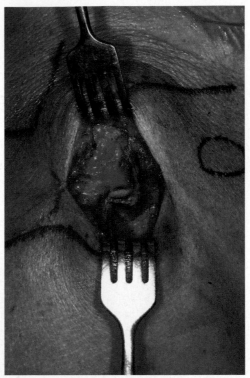
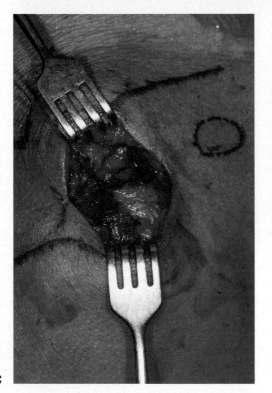
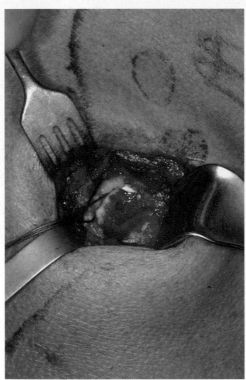

FIGURE 7-3

A: An incision is marked out parallel to the lateral border of the acromion. **B:** The deltoid is taken off of the acromion as outlined. **C:** A stitch is placed in the corner of the deltoid to assist in later repair and ensure proper alignment deltoid repair. **D:** The rotator cuff tear is identified and retention stitches are placed. *(Continued)*

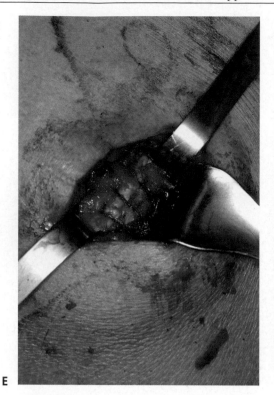
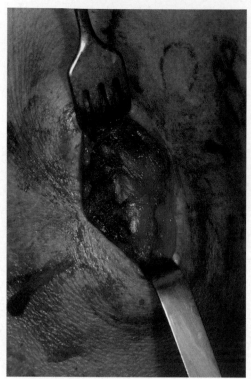

E

F

FIGURE 7-3

Continued **E,F:** A rotator cuff repair is performed.

ued through the deltoid. The rotator cuff and its bursa in the subacromial space are immediately encountered. Again, the humeral neck, greater tuberosity, rotator cuff, and even the long head of the biceps, to some degree, can be accessed from this approach. Care needs to be taken to avoid injuring the axillary nerve or detaching an excessive amount of deltoid.

The posterior approach offers access to the posterior and inferior aspects of the glenohumeral joint. In the trauma scenario, open reduction and internal fixation of the glenoid, scapular body, and sepsis drainage can be provided. Depending on the amount of exposure required, the deltoid can be split rather than detached. The interval between the deltoid muscle and the inner lying infraspinatus muscle is identified next. The internervous interval between the infraspinatus and the teres minor is next identified and is usually developed with blunt finger dissection. Some surgeons prefer to use the interval between the two heads of the infraspinatus. By retracting each of these muscles, the inferior and posterior aspects of the glenoid can be reached.

If the joint needs to be explored, incise it longitudinally close to the scapular edge. Care needs to be taken to protect the axillary nerve as it runs in the quadrangular space beneath the teres minor. The other nerve that can potentially be injured is the suprascapular nerve as it passes around the base of the spine of the scapula and runs from the supraspinatus fossa to the infraspinatus fossa. Damage to this can cause loss of innervation to the supraspinatus and infraspinatus muscles. Excessive retraction of the infraspinatus medially can result in neurapraxia. Finally, the posterior circumflex humeral artery runs with the axillary nerve in the quadrangular space beneath the inferior border of the teres minor; and again, if the dissection is performed too low, the structure can be injured.

POSTOPERATIVE MANAGEMENT

The shoulder is a complex joint and will rapidly become stiff. Ideally, adequate motion is needed for optimum function of the extremity for the patient. Rehabilitation depends on type of injury, stability of repairs, and amount of soft tissue injury. In most cases, the three-phase system developed by Hughes and Neer will suffice. The first phase incorporates passive-assistive exercises. Active and early resistive exercises are started in the second phase. Finally, the third phase is a program dedicated to stretching and strengthening exercises. In general, these exercises are performed three to four times per day for 20 to 30 minutes. In the first phase, it is not uncommon for pain medication to be used. Working with a skilled physical therapist can improve patient compliance and outcome.

Phase one is started in the early posttraumatic period. If there is secure fixation of the underlying injuries, passive exercises may be begun 24 to 72 hours after the index procedure. The surgeon must be careful not to forget about the elbow, wrist, and fingers. If these are neglected, permanent stiffness can result in these joints, and the extremity is at risk for complex regional pain syndrome (hand-shoulder syndrome). The first exercise usually consists of the pendulum or Codman's type in which the arm is rotated both outwardly and inwardly in small circles. Next, the supine external rotation with a stick exercise is used. The elbow and distal humerus must be supported with either a towel or sheets. A 20-degree shoulder abduction can facilitate performing this exercise. Gentle pulley exercises can be added to the regimen as well as extension. In general, isometrics are not started until there is evidence of some fracture healing.

Phase two exercises involve active, gentle resistive, and stretching programs. Supine active forward elevation is the first one because the effects of gravity are reduced by making the elevation easier. The patient then can be progressed to doing this exercise in a standing or sitting position. A stick in the unaffected arm can assist the involved arm with this maneuver. TheraBands can be used to strengthen the internal and external rotators as well as the anterior, middle, and posterior aspects of the deltoid. These are usually done in repetitions of 10 to 15 per session. Wall climbing exercises with stretching are also performed. Internal rotation can be one of the most difficult aspects of motion to regain in the shoulder, and the patient can work on assisting the affected extremity with the unaffected one by trying to have the hand crawl up the back of the patient.

Phase three exercises are started after solid evidence of fracture healing. The rubber strips may be replaced by rubber tubing to increase resistance. Continued aggressive stretching is performed. Light weights are usually tolerated at this time. Weights start at 1 lb and are increased in 1-lb increments, usually stopping at 5 lb. If there is significant pain with the weight, then these should be discontinued as strength can generally recover with functional activity.

COMPLICATIONS

Postoperative Complications

Postoperative complications, as previously mentioned, include neurovascular injury and soft tissue loss. In the traumatized shoulder, the usual anatomic landmarks may be distorted or absent. This makes it imperative that surgeons take their time and appropriately identify neurovascular structures and internervous planes when possible. Other factors such as hardware loosening and infection can occur. In the event of excessive soft tissue loss, flap coverage may be required (see Chapter 8). Free flaps such as a latissimus or anterolateral thigh flap can be considered depending on the need for muscle versus subcutaneous and cutaneous layers. With pinning techniques, pin migration can be a problem and has been reported in the literature.

In general, complications can be broken down into vascular injury, brachial plexus injury, chest injury, myositis ossificans, frozen shoulder, avascular necrosis, nonunion and malunion, and complex regional pain syndrome. Fortunately, vascular injuries are infrequent, but they can occur and can result in loss of the extremity. Injury of the axillary artery represents about 6% of all arterial traumas and usually occurs secondary to fractures of the proximal humerus. It can be seen in older individuals with significant atherosclerosis as the vessel may tear secondary to dislocation or blunt trauma. The most common site of injury to the axillary artery is proximal to the take-off of the anterior circumflex artery. It is important to check the radial pulse, but this is no guarantee that arterial injury has not occurred. Other signs to look for include an expanding hematoma, pallor, and paresthesias. Missed arterial injuries can result in gas gangrene, amputation, and compressive neuropathies at the brachial plexus leading to permanent nerve palsies. If three is any suspicion, angiography should be performed immediately.

Brachial Plexus Injuries

Brachial plexus injuries can occur after proximal humerus fractures. This has been reported to have an incidence of 6.1%. Isolated injury to the axillary nerve is not uncommon and has been reported, but any or all components of the brachial plexus can be involved. It is, thus, extremely important to evaluate the patient initially and document any compromise in skin sensation and motor function. If a nerve injury is clinically suspected, it should be carefully followed, and electromyography and nerve conduction velocity studies should be used to monitor for progression or failure of healing. Nerve injuries that fail to show improvement clinically and electrically may need to be explored.

Chest Injury to the Thoracic Cavity

Chest injury to the thoracic cavity can occur after fractures and trauma to the shoulder. There have been reports of intrathoracic dislocation of the head with surgical neck fractures of the humerus, as well as pneumothorax and hemathorax associated with the trauma that resulted in the proximal humerus fracture.

Frozen Shoulder

Frozen shoulder is extremely common after any type of injury or surgery to the shoulder. Even with implementation of well-organized and carefully monitored physical therapy, adhesive capsulitis can develop. Fortunately, most cases of adhesive capsulitis respond to programs of exercise and stretching. In those that fail to improve after 4 to 6 months, manipulation and lysis of adhesions can be considered. There is a risk of refracture, however. Painful and impinging hardware can also result in shoulder motion limitations; if the patient desires, once fracture union is obtained, the hardware may be removed.

Myositis Ossificans

Myositis ossificans is known to occur after fracture dislocations. It can also occur in head-injured patients. It is more commonly seen when there is a chronic unreduced fracture dislocation. Avascular necrosis of the humeral head can occur with shoulder trauma. This is more common in three- and four-part fractures, but can occur with any type of injury about the shoulder, including soft tissue injuries. Excessive periosteal stripping and excessive soft tissue dissection may also result in this complication. Nonunions and malunions can occur with any type of fracture and these may result from fractures about the shoulder. Their treatment goes beyond the purpose of this chapter.

Complex Regional Pain Syndrome

This entity, formerly known as reflex sympathetic dystrophy and before that as hand-shoulder syndrome, is cited to affect from 10% to 30% of patients who have shoulder trauma that required surgery. Soft tissue and bony injury can result in this pathologic process marked chronic pain. The patients do not necessarily have to have any type of penetrating or open trauma. The treatment of complex regional pain syndrome is early recognition of the problem, sympathetic blocks, Neurontin, and aggressive therapy. Complex regional pain syndrome can occur in any setting with light or aggressive therapy and minimal or extensive trauma. Once the condition is recognized, treatment should be initiated. If there is any question, quantitative sudomotor axon reflex testing may be helpful.

RECOMMENDED READING

Blom S, Dahlback LO. Nerve injuries in dislocations of the shoulder joint and fractures of the neck of the humerus: a clinical and electromyographic study. *Acta Chir Scand.* 1970;136:461–466.

Hughes M, Neer CS II. Glenohumeral joint replacement and postoperative rehabilitation. *Phys Ther.* 1975;55:850–858.

Linson MA. Axillary artery thrombosis after fracture of the humerus. *J Bone Joint Surg.* 1980;62A:1214–1215.

Neer CS II. Displaced proximal humeral fractures. Part I. Classification and evaluation. *J Bone Joint Surg.* 1970;52A:1077–1089.

Neer CS II. Displaced proximal humeral fractures: Part 2. Treatment of three-part and four-part displacement. *J Bone Joint Surg.* 1970;52A:1090–1103.

8 Rotational Flaps for Rotator Cuff Repair

Emilie V. Cheung and Scott P. Steinmann

INDICATIONS/ CONTRAINDICATIONS

Massive soft tissue tears of the rotator cuff pose significant challenges to the shoulder surgeon. Although most tears can be successfully repaired in a primary fashion, some massive tears of the rotator cuff are termed irreparable, either due to their severely contracted state or simply because of their size. Cofield has defined the term massive rotator cuff tear as greater than 5 cm, whereas others have defined it as involvement of at least two tendons.

Chronic tears, commonly seen in older patients, have evidence of attritional changes in both the tendon substance and the muscle fibers. This has been termed fatty degeneration by Gerber and can be best characterized and graded based on its appearance on T1 weighted magnetic resonance imaging (MRI) of the shoulder in the oblique sagittal plane. The presence of fatty degeneration of the musculotendinous unit may compromise the results of even a seemingly successful repair due to poor tissue quality and limited regenerative capacity. The limitations of successful tendon repair are thus a function of the length of time since injury, the degree of tissue contraction, and extent of fatty degeneration.

Management of such tears often begins with conservative management. If this fails, surgical management may include debridement of the cuff tear, which may result in satisfactory pain relief, but will not restore strength or function. Partial repair may be possible in some instances, but this does not restore normal function. Other options include allograft or synthetic tendon augmentation, but these have met with varying success in the literature.

Long-standing rotator cuff tears result in altered kinematics of the glenohumeral joint, and rotator cuff tear arthropathy may eventually develop as a painful end-stage condition. Hemiarthroplasty can be a reasonable option in patients who have an intact coracoacromial arch limiting anterior superior escape of the humeral head. The reverse shoulder prosthesis has recently been shown to be an effective treatment option for patients with irreparable rotator cuff tears and anterior superior instability of the humeral head. At mid-term follow-up, improvements in range of motion and pain relief have been reported in the majority of cases. However, this is generally reserved for select indications in an elderly patient. The long-term results of this prosthesis have yet to be determined.

A patient who has had a previously failed massive rotator cuff repair may be challenging to treat. Tendon transfers are another option for salvaging massive rotator cuff defects. They have the distinct advantage in their ability to restore strength, in addition to providing pain relief. Local tendon transpositions historically have included superior subscapularis, teres minor, and teres major transfers. Deltoid flap reconstruction has also been reported. Our preferred method of tendon transfer for posterior superior rotator cuff tears is the latissimus dorsi transfer.

Gerber et al described the procedure of latissimus dorsi transfer as an option for the treatment of massive posterior superior rotator cuff defects in 1988. This procedure has been shown to restore an active external rotation and forward flexion moment at the shoulder, which are the primary functional deficits for this type of massive rotator cuff tear.

Latissimus transfer in cases of a failed previous rotator cuff tear results in overall improvement in function and pain relief, but is generally inferior to that observed after a primary transfer. A comparative analysis on the results of latissimus dorsi transfer for primary irreparable rotator cuff tears, versus for salvage reconstruction for a failed previous rotator cuff repair was performed by Warner and Parsons. Patients' satisfaction and function were superior in primary latissimus dorsi transfer when compared with patients undergoing salvage reconstruction of failed previous rotator cuff repairs.

Subscapularis tendon ruptures occur less frequently than supraspinatus and infraspinatus ruptures. However, they can occur in isolation, during anterior shoulder dislocation, or an as extension of a massive rotator cuff tear. Our preferred method of tendon transfer for irreparable subscapularis tendon tears is the pectoralis major transfer. Combined latissimus dorsi transfer with pectoralis major transfer may be indicated in massive rotator cuff deficiency involving both the posterior superior cuff and the subscapularis.

The primary indication for latissimus dorsi transfer is the loss of active external rotation due to an irreparable tear of the posterior superior rotator cuff. The patient is dissatisfied with increased functional demands, which are beyond the limitations of conservative treatment.

The primary indication for pectoralis major tendon transfer is irreparable rupture of the subscapularis, characterized by retraction of the musculotendinous unit to the glenoid, and fatty infiltration of the muscle. In a patient with posterosuperior rotator cuff tear with extension of the defect into the subscapularis, isolated latissimus transfer is contraindicated unless there is either concomitant repair of the subscapularis, or transfer of the pectoralis major, to compensate for subscapularis dysfunction.

PREOPERATIVE PLANNING

We begin with the history and physical examination, which are essential in diagnosis and assessment of the nature of the rotator cuff tear. Often, the patient complains of pain or dysfunction with an insidious onset. Other times, the patient complains of fatigue during forward elevation or external rotation of the shoulder. No history of trauma can be recalled and the symptoms have been chronic over months or years, which leads us to believe that the etiology is attritional. Thus, we suspect poor tendon quality and the possibility of an irreparable tear.

The physical examination of the shoulder begins by inspection of both shoulders. Deformity associated with anterior superior escape of the humeral head indicates anterosuperior rotator cuff tear, which is a contraindication for latissimus transfer. Spinati muscle atrophy is noted, and often indicates an irreparable rotator cuff tear is present. A defect of the deltoid is a relative contraindication for this procedure. Manual motor testing of shoulder forward elevation, abduction, external rotation, and internal rotation are recorded.

The *hornblower's sign*, or external rotation lag sign (discrepancy between active and passive external rotation of greater than 30 degrees), is important to recognize. A positive sign is highly suggestive of a massive rotator cuff tear, amenable to latissimus dorsi transfer.

Another physical examination finding that is important to recognize is the *lift-off test* (the inability to actively lift the dorsum of the hand off from a resting position on the lower back), or *belly press test* (the inability to actively maintain the elbow anterior to the midline of the trunk as viewed from the side). An inability to perform these maneuvers is highly suggestive of involvement of the subscapularis in the rotator cuff tear. If a subscapularis tear is present and determined irreparable, then a pectoralis major transfer should be performed in conjunction with the latissimus transfer.

Active and passive range of motion in forward elevation, external rotation, and internal rotation are documented. Loss of passive external rotation and forward elevation is a contraindication to this procedure. Active range of motion is also measured. Patients need to be able to achieve active forward elevation to 90 degrees to be candidates for the procedure. If the patient has pseudoparalysis and minimal forward elevation, the procedure will fail. The main goal of the procedure is to promote active external rotation to eliminate the hornblower's sign and enable the patient to reach the top of the head.

It should be noted that some patients with massive cuff tears are amenable to conservative treatment, and eventually may experience minimal pain and satisfactory function, especially in the elderly population. Latissimus dorsi transfer is more commonly performed in those individuals with higher functional demands.

Imaging studies are useful for assessing the patient who is suspected of having a painful, torn rotator cuff, unresponsive to conservative treatment. Our standard radiographic views include a true anteroposterior (AP) view of the shoulder and an axillary view. The true AP view best demonstrates superior migration of the humeral head in the context of massive rotator cuff tears. The acromiohumeral distance (ACHD) is measured on this view. A normal ACHD value is 10.5 mm. An ACHD value of 7 mm or less suggests an irreparable tear of the infraspinatus and is a strong indicator to consider a latissimus dorsi transfer, in the context of the previously mentioned physical examination findings. The true AP and axillary views demonstrate degenerative changes of the glenohumeral joint, which would be a contraindication to tendon transfer.

Magnetic resonance imaging is commonly performed at our institution in patients with suspected large rotator cuff tears in whom we are considering surgical treatment. It is useful for assessing not only the size of the tear, but the degree of muscle atrophy and the degree of fatty degeneration. Advanced fatty degeneration and a massive tear indicate a low likelihood of successful repair, but may be considered for latissimus dorsi transfer with or without pectoralis major transfer. In many patients with massive rotator cuff tears, we are able to repair the rotator cuff tear arthroscopically. Therefore, in almost all patients who are candidates for a latissimus dorsi transfer, we recommend an attempted arthroscopic repair as the initial surgical procedure.

LATISSIMUS DORSI TRANSFER

Surgery

The patient is placed in the lateral decubitus positioning with all bony prominences well-padded. The superior approach for rotator cuff repair in Langer's lines is used. Skin flaps are raised. The deltoid is split in line with its fibers or as an alternative if greater exposure is desired; the deltoid can be reflected from the acromion with a bone chip using an osteotome (Fig. 8-1). A subacromial retractor is placed to visualize the rotator cuff defect. Excise the subacromial bursa for optimal visualization. If the tear is determined to be irreparable, proceed with latissimus dorsi tendon transfer.

A second skin incision is placed along the posterior aspect of axilla, along the lateral border of the latissimus (Fig. 8-2). Skin flaps are created. The latissimus and teres major muscles are visualized (Fig. 8-3). Dissecting distally, identify the latissimus and teres major tendons, which are in intimate contact (Fig. 8-4). The latissimus tendon is very thin as you follow its insertion into the axilla (Fig. 8-5). The teres major tendon can be transferred with the latissimus tendon if the subscapularis is intact and if the patient has extreme weakness. However, the teres major is a bulky muscle with poor excursion. It is difficult to pass both muscles under the acromion, and often the teres major will not reach the superior aspect of the humeral head.

The latissimus tendon should be released directly off of the bone to achieve greatest length. This is best done with electrocautery (Fig. 8-6). Palpation of the radial nerve is helpful at this stage to note its location and lessen the chance of nerve injury. Note that the latissimus tendon is tendinous, without muscular fibers at its humeral attachment site. In contrast, the teres major tendon is very short, and the musculotendinous unit is very muscular at its attachment on the humerus. Internal rotation of the arm helps to bring the insertion site into view and allows for easier dissection. However, when the arm is internally rotated, the axillary and radial nerves are brought closer to the latissimus dorsi insertion, and care must be taken with this exposure and arm positioning (Fig. 8-7).

Locking nonabsorbable sutures are placed into the distal end of the latissimus tendon, with four tails left distally for tying at the end. This step may be repeated for the distal end of the teres major tendon. Ensure the muscles are gliding freely with adequate excursion. The neurovascular pedicle of the latissimus enters anteriorly, about 10 to 15 cm from its musculotendinous junction.

Identify the teres minor, triceps, and deltoid. Pass a Kelly clamp from the superior incision, over teres minor, and underneath deltoid, to exit through the inferior incision, by blunt dissection. The sutures are placed into the clamp, and the latissimus tendon is pulled up into the superior wound, over the superior posterior aspect of the humeral head (Fig. 8-8). The teres major can be passed similarly. A rongeur is used to remove residual soft tissue from the posterior superior aspect of the greater tuberosity, which will receive the transferred tendon ends. Pass the sutures through bone with a free curved needle, and tie over a bony bridge or use suture anchors (Fig. 8-9). A strong repair is required since there will be a lot of tension on the repair. It is often helpful to tie the sutures over a small metal

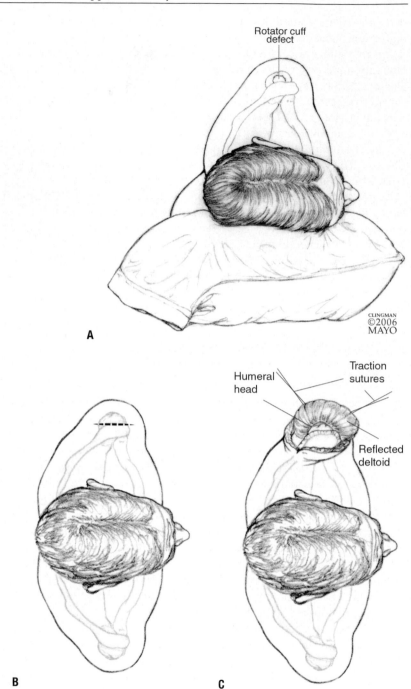

FIGURE 8-1

A: The patient is placed in the lateral decubitus position with all bony prominences well padded. **B:** The superior approach for rotator cuff repair in Langer's lines is used. **C:** The deltoid is split in line with its fibers, or as an alternative if greater exposure is desired, the deltoid can be reflected from the acromion with a bone chip using an osteotome.

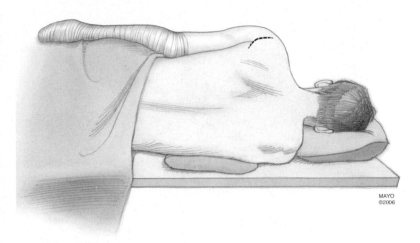

FIGURE 8-2

The second skin incision is placed along the posterior aspect of axilla, along the lateral border of the latissimus.

MAYO
©2006

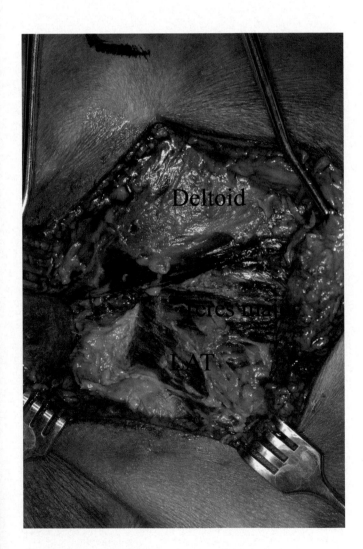

FIGURE 8-3

The latissimus and teres major muscles are visualized inferior to the deltoid muscle.

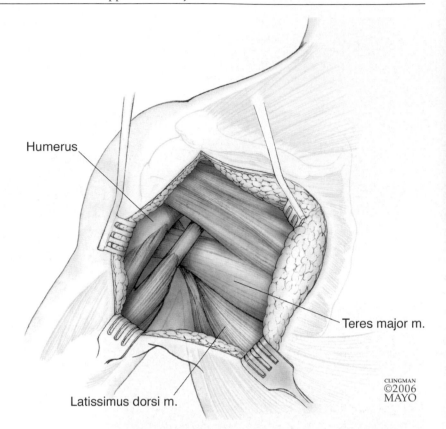

Humerus

Teres major m.

Latissimus dorsi m.

CLINGMAN
©2006
MAYO

FIGURE 8-4

Dissecting distally, identify the latissimus and teres major tendons, which are in intimate contact. Note that the deltoid muscle has been removed for illustrative purposes.

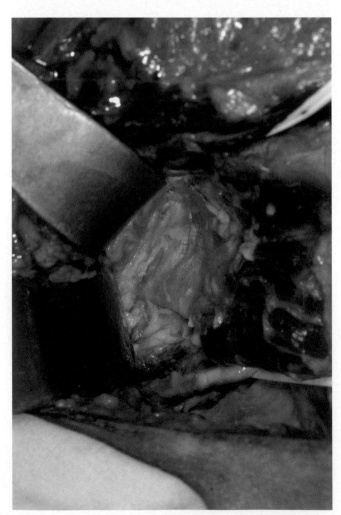

FIGURE 8-5

The latissimus tendon is very thin, as you follow its insertion site into the axilla.

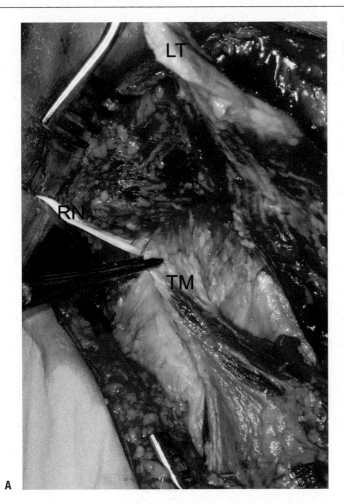

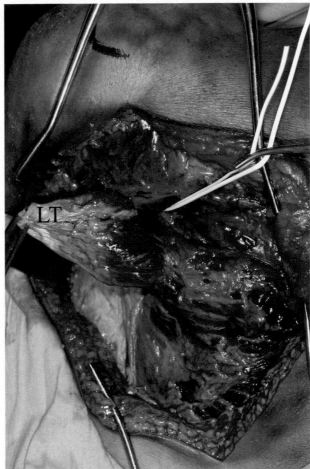

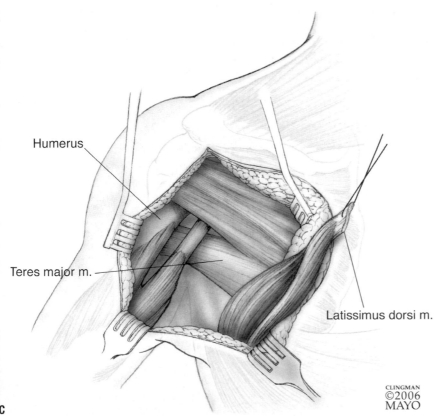

CLINGMAN
©2006
MAYO

FIGURE 8-6

A: The teres major tendon (TM), held with the forceps, can be transferred with the latissimus tendon if the subscapularis is intact and if the patient has extreme weakness. Note the radial nerve is identified in this photograph with the white vessel loop. **B:** The latissimus tendon should be released directly off of the bone to achieve greatest length. **C:** The latissimus tendon has been released. Note that the deltoid muscle has been removed for illustrative purposes.

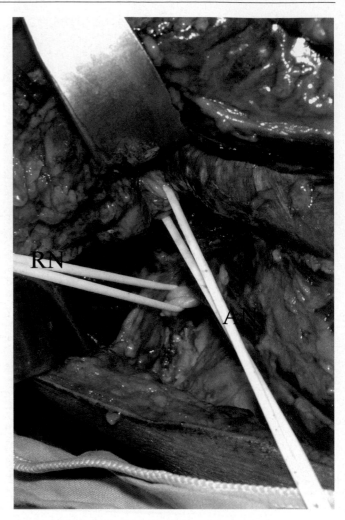

FIGURE 8-7

The axillary and radial nerves have been identified for illustrative purposes.

or absorbable washer. Suture the border of subscapularis and rotator interval to the transferred tendon. The goal is to have a strong mechanical repair, and not necessarily a watertight repair.

The deltoid with its bony attachment is repaired back to the acromion with nonabsorbable sutures. The wound is closed in layers over a drain.

Postoperative Management

The arm is placed into a pillow sling for 6 weeks to remove tension from the repair. During this period, passive flexion and external rotation are performed with the arm in the brace. Internal rotation is prohibited to prevent stress on the tendon repair. Specific training with a physical therapist is helpful to retrain the transferred musculotendinous unit to contract during active external rotation and forward flexion of the shoulder. The ability to gain voluntary control of the transferred latissimus is variable, and in many instances probably functions as an interposition. Many patients will be able to actively recruit the muscle during external rotation and forward flexion after 6 months.

Complications

Complications after latissimus dorsi transfer have been rare. Rupture of the transferred tendon has been reported. Ensuring that the tension of the repair is not due to under-excessive tension, protection of the repair with the splint, and avoiding active internal rotation for 6 weeks should prevent this complication. Refixation of the transferred tendon may be attempted.

Temporary axillary and radial nerve palsy has also been reported and perhaps avoided by careful surgical dissection and avoiding exuberant retraction of the deltoid fibers during exposure.

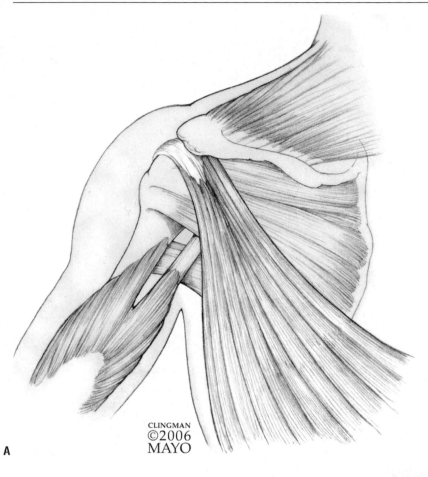

CLINGMAN
©2006
MAYO

A

FIGURE 8-8

A–C: The latissimus tendon has been passed under the posterior deltoid, up into the superior wound, and over the superior posterior aspect of the humeral head (HH). The teres major can be passed similarly. Note that the deltoid muscle has been removed for illustrative purposes.

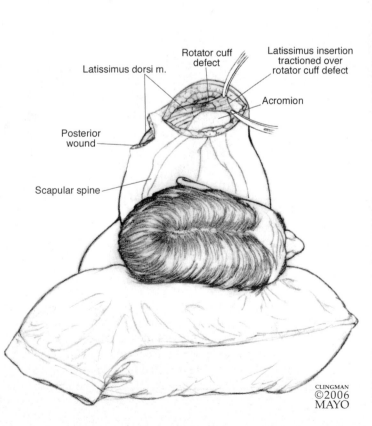

Rotator cuff defect

Latissimus insertion tractioned over rotator cuff defect

Latissimus dorsi m.

Acromion

Posterior wound

Scapular spine

CLINGMAN
©2006
MAYO

B

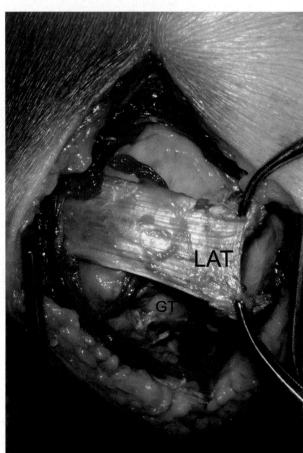

LAT

GT

C

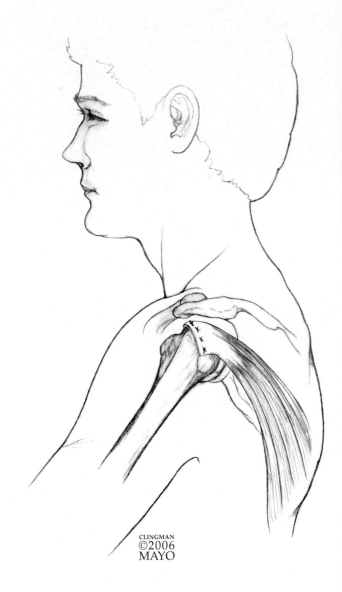

FIGURE 8-9

The tendon is tied over a bony bridge at the greater tuberosity.

CLINGMAN
©2006
MAYO

PECTORALIS MAJOR TENDON TRANSFER

Surgery

Standard beach-chair positioning is used for this surgery. A deltopectoral approach is made, and skin flaps are created (Fig. 8-10). The torn subscapularis musculotendinous unit is mobilized by releasing adhesions from the base of the coracoid, the brachial plexus, and the subscapularis fossa. A repair of the subscapularis is attempted by placement of modified Mason-Allen sutures in the remaining tendon and fascial tissue using nonabsorbable suture. The repair to the lesser tuberosity should be made with the arm in neutral rotation, if possible.

If repair is not possible, a pectoralis transfer is performed. Through the deltopectoral approach, the conjoint tendon, the tendon of the pectoralis major, and the anterior surface of the humeral head are exposed (Fig. 8-11). The tendon of the pectoralis major is exposed over its full length at the humerus, and the superior one-half to two-thirds of the tendon (depending on the size of the defect) is detached from the humerus (Fig. 8-12). The clavicular portion of the pectoralis major is taken for the transfer, and is bluntly dissected over a length of about 10 cm from the sternal portion of the pectoralis major, which remains intact. Modified Mason-Allen sutures are placed in the tendon using nonabsorbable suture (see Fig. 8-12).

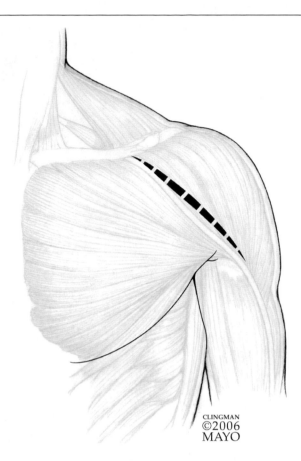

CLINGMAN
©2006
MAYO

FIGURE 8-10

A deltopectoral incision is made.

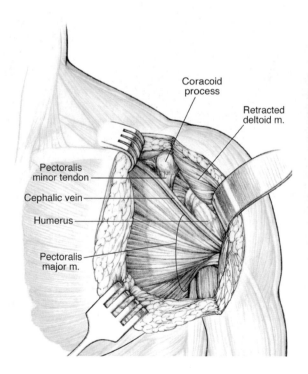

Coracoid
process

Retracted
deltoid m.

Pectoralis
minor tendon

Cephalic vein

Humerus

Pectoralis
major m.

A

FIGURE 8-11

A,B: Through the deltopectoral approach, the conjoint
tendon, the tendon of the pectoralis major, and the anterior
surface of the humeral head are exposed.

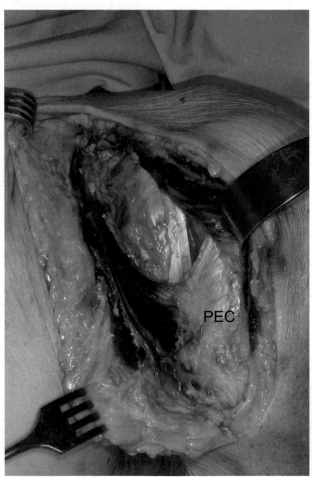

PEC

B

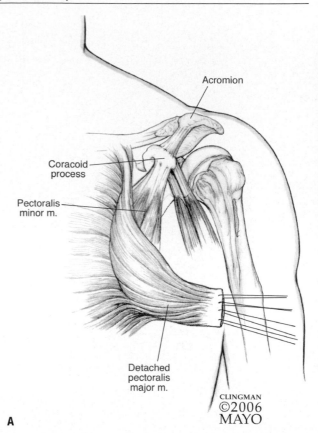

FIGURE 8-12

A: The tendon of the pectoralis major is exposed over its full length at the humerus, and the superior one-half to two-thirds of the tendon (depending on the size of the defect) is detached from the humerus. **B:** Locking sutures have been placed into the pectoralis major tendon.

A

CLINGMAN
©2006
MAYO

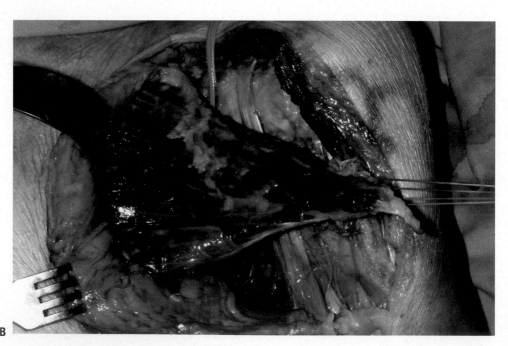

B

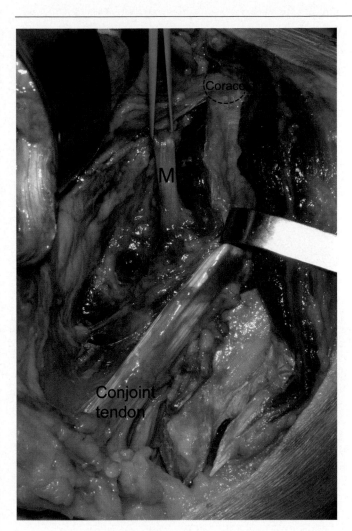

FIGURE 8-13

The musculocutaneous nerve has been identified with the blue vessel loop, between the conjoined tendon and the pectoralis major, about 5 cm distal to the coracoid.

The musculocutaneous nerve is identified by palpation, in the interval between the conjoined tendon and the pectoralis minor (Fig.8-13). A reinsertion site for the pectoralis major tendon at the medial aspect of the lesser tuberosity is prepared with a rongeur. Using curved forceps, the pectoralis major muscle is advanced behind the conjoined tendon in front of the musculocutaneous nerve, and the tendon is attached to the lesser tuberosity using transosseous repair, with the arm in neutral rotation (Fig. 8-14). The musculocutaneous nerve is palpated within the space between muscles to confirm that there is no tension on the nerve. If tension is found, the size of the muscle belly should be reduced. The supraspinatus is sutured to the proximal border of the pectoralis major tendon to close the rotator interval, if possible. In most patients, the tendon should be long enough to permit at least 30 degrees of external rotation of the arm after the tendon has been sutured to the lesser tuberosity. The conjoined tendon has been noted to arch forward slightly.

A proximal biceps tenodesis or release may be performed, depending on the presence of tendinopathy. Acromioplasty is not performed if the patient has an isolated subscapularis tear, or if the patient has a high likelihood of postoperative anterosuperior subluxation.

Postoperative Management

A sling is worn for 6 weeks postoperatively, and passive range-of-motion exercises are performed within the safe range of motion found intraoperatively starting on postoperative day 1. External rotation to neutral is allowed. Active range-of-motion exercises in all directions, including external rotation, are begun at 6 weeks postoperatively. Full loading is allowed at 12 weeks postoperatively.

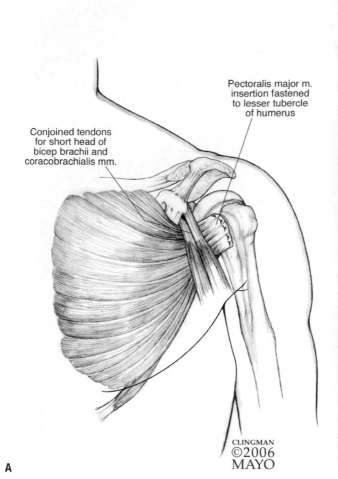

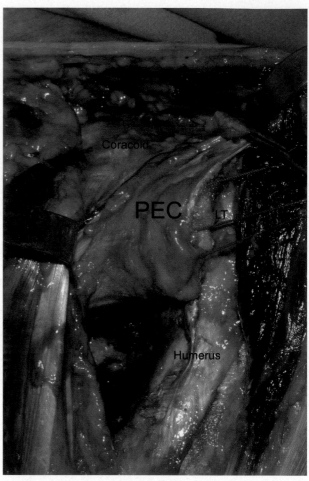

FIGURE 8-14

A: The pectoralis major muscle is advanced behind the conjoined tendon in front of the musculocutaneous nerve. For illustrative purposes, the inferior half of the pectoralis tendon is not shown. **B:** The tendon is attached to the lesser tuberosity using transosseous repair, with the arm in neutral rotation. For illustrative purposes, the inferior half of the pectoralis tendon is not shown.

Complications

Avulsion of the transferred pectoralis major tendon has been reported as a potential complication by Jost et al. This can be diagnosed clinically and by MRI, and has been treated with refixation of the transfer. Postoperative infection is another rare complication that should be treated with open irrigation, debridement, and a 6-week course of antibiotics. In very thin patients, a slightly more prominent anterior bulging of the anterior deltoid may be seen when compared to the other side.

RECOMMENDED READING

Aldridge JM, Atkinson TS, Mallon WJ. Combined pectoralis and latissimus dorsi transfer for massive rotator cuff deficiency. *J Shoulder Elbow Surg.* 2004;13:621–629.

Cleeman E, Hazrati Y, Auerbach JD, Stein K, Hausman M, Flatow E. Latissimus dorsi tendon transfer massive rotator cuff tears: a cadaveric study. *J Shoulder Elbow Surg.* 2003;12:539–543.

DeOrio JK, Cofield RH. Results of a second attempt at surgical repair of a failed initial rotator cuff repair. *J Bone Joint Surg.* 1984;66(4):563–567.

Gerber C, Vinh TS, Hertel R, Hess CW. Latissimus dorsi transfer for the treatment of massive tears of the rotator cuff. A preliminary report. *Clin Orthop.* 1988;232:51–61.

Gerber C. Latissimus dorsi transfer for the treatment of irreparable tears of the rotator cuff. *Clin Orthop.* 1992;275:52–160.

Jost B, Puskas GJ, Lustenberger A, Gerber C. Outcome of pectoralis major transfer for the treatment of irreparable subscapularis tears. *J Bone Joint Surg.* 2003;85A:1944–1951.

Resch H, Ritter E, Matschi W. Transfer of the pectoralis major muscle for the treatment of irreparable rupture of the subscapularis tendon. *J Bone Joint Surg.* 2000;82A:372–381.

Warner JJP, Parsons IM. Latissimus dorsi tendon transfer: a comparative analysis of primary and salvage reconstruction of massive, irreparable rotator cuff tears. *J Shoulder Elbow Surg.* 1999;10:514–521.

9 Surgical Exposure of the Elbow Following Bony and Soft Tissue Trauma

Emilie V. Cheung, Nathan A. Hoekzema, and Scott P. Steinmann

INDICATIONS/CONTRAINDICATIONS

The soft tissue surrounding the elbow is thin and pliable, yet durable enough to withstand constant flexion and extension. Optimal functional recovery in traumatic elbow injuries requires early and, in many cases, immediate motion. Skin slough, delayed healing, and dehiscence of skin flaps following treatment of elbow fractures can adversely affect elbow rehabilitation, delaying motion and increasing the risks of infection and nonunion. Properly planned incisions can allow for excellent exposure of the elbow while maximizing skin flap vascularity, minimizing the risks of postoperative wound complications.

Surgical exposures of the elbow typically involve a 'universal' posterior incision. This allows circumferential access by the creation of full-thickness skin flaps medially and laterally as needed. This allows for all intraoperative possibilities and avoids the creation of skin bridges if further surgery is needed in the future. Alternatively, separate medial and lateral skin incisions may be performed for isolated medial and lateral exposure. Prior surgical procedures should be carefully noted preoperatively. Previous incisions may need to be incorporated in order to avoid creating narrow skin bridges which are susceptible to skin necrosis and potential wound complications.

SURGERY

Patient Positioning

In our practice, the patient is routinely placed in the supine position with a small stack of towels placed underneath the ipsilateral scapula, and the arm draped across the chest after sterile preparation. The operating table should be slightly tilted away from the surgeon to help with visualization and exposure. This positioning is optimal for fixation of distal humeral fractures, radial head fractures, and medial or lateral ligament reconstruction. For medial ligament or coronoid fracture fixation, the supine position is used, but a sterile Mayo stand is utilized to position the arm more accurately for medial elbow exposure. Intraoperative fluoroscopy, if indicated, is placed on the ipsilateral side, and the elbow may be brought out laterally from the chest for the fluoroscope intermittently during the procedure. A sterile tourniquet is usually used in all elbow approaches. This allows for ease of removal if more proximal exposure of the humerus is needed. Hip rests or a bean bag may provide additional stability.

Posterior Approaches

Indications

- Triceps repair
- Combined medial and lateral approach
- Distal humerus ORIF
- Total Elbow Arthroplasty

Contraindications

Prior medial or lateral incisions.

Incision   The bony landmarks, including the olecranon process and the subcutaneous border of the proximal ulna, are marked (Figs. 9-1 to 9-6). The incision starts about 5 centimeters proximal to the olecranon process centered on the triceps tendon. It is then taken distally to either the lateral or medial side of the olecrenon, according to surgeon preference, and finishes distally following the subcutaneous border of the ulna. Full-thickness skin flaps are then developed, kept as thick as possible with the deep plane being the triceps fascia and epitenon proximally, and the forearm fascia and ulnar periosteum distally. If most of the surgical procedure will be on the medial side of the elbow, then the posterior incision should be placed to that side. Likewise, if a radial head fracture is being exposed, then the posterior incision should be made on the lateral side of the olecranon. If one chooses to err on the medial side of the olecranon, the incision should not be placed directly over the cubital tunnel, to avoid injuring the ulnar nerve.

Deep Dissection   The ulnar nerve is most easily found proximally between the medial intermuscular septum and the medial head of the triceps muscle. If the nerve is going to be transposed, it should be freed from proximal to distal in order to minimize damage to the nerve branches. Articular branches usually need to be sacrificed, but the first motor branch should be identified, mo-

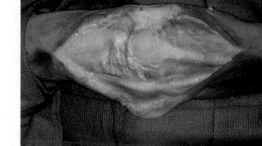

FIGURE 9-1

The skin is incised posteriorly with full thickness flaps raised as needed.

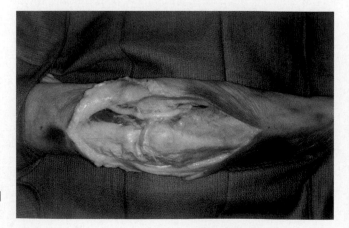

FIGURE 9-2

The ulnar nerve is carefully released from the cubital tunnel.

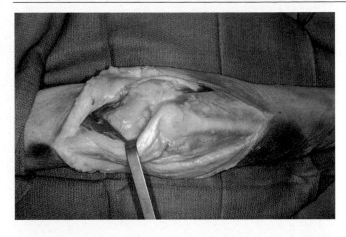

FIGURE 9-3

The medial and lateral sides of the triceps muscle are released in order to fully visualize the posterior fossa and the ulnohumeral articulation.

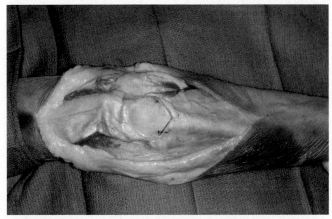

A

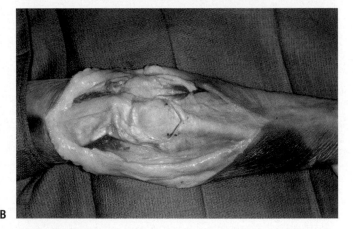

B

FIGURE 9-4

A,B: The olecranon osteotomy is best located at the small area of olecranon that is devoid of cartilage. A lap sponge may be threaded between the humerus and ulna to avoid inadvertent cartilage damage. The osteotomy is started with a reciprocating saw and then finished with an osteotome. Hardware may be predrilled to facilitate final osteotomy repair.

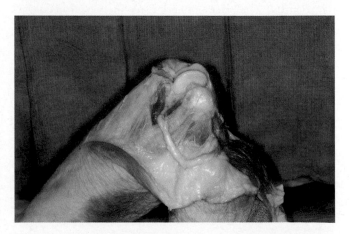

FIGURE 9-5

The osteotomied olecranon is retracted with the triceps tendon demonstrating near full visualization of the articular spool.

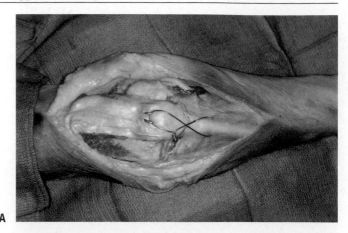

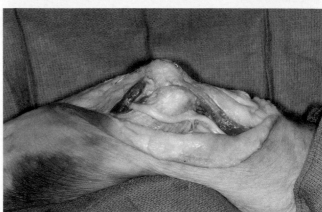

FIGURE 9-6

A,B: The completed tension band repair. The bent K-wires will then be sunk beneath the triceps tendon and the tendon repaired over them to minimize pin backout.

bilized, and preserved. The leading edge, about 1 cm, of the distal medial intermuscular septum is removed to prevent tethering of the nerve after being anteriorly transposed. The nerve is then placed into a subcutaneous pocket anterior to the medial epicondyle. A suture is placed in the subcutaneous tissue and secured to the fascia to create a sling and prevent posterior subluxation of the nerve. If the nerve is not going to be transposed, care should be taken to avoid destabilizing the nerve in the cubital tunnel by leaving the soft tissue constraints of Osborne's fascia intact.

Olecranon Osteotomy   An olecranon osteotomy may be performed to gain full visualization of the articular surface of the distal humerus.

After identification and protection of the ulnar nerve, a capsulotomy is made at both the medial and lateral sides of the olecranon at the apex of the greater sigmoid notch to locate the olecranon "bare area." This is the area of the olecranon where the articular cartilage narrows and is the optimal location for the osteotomy. A lap sponge may be threaded under the olecrenon to protect the distal humeral articular cartilage from inadvertent damage. The osteotomy is created in a Chevron configuration, with the apex usually pointed distally using an oscillating saw. The saw is used for one-third of the bone cut, the second third is made with an osteotome, and the last third is cracked or fractured open with an osteotome to create the completed osteotomy. Once the osteotomy has been made, the anconeus needs to be taken off the lateral side of the olecranon fragment. Transection of the anconeus will denervate it. To avoid this problem, one technique is an anconeus flap transolecranon approach (AFT) which involves detaching the anconeus as a flap distally to proximally until the osteotomy site is reached. The osteotomy is then performed and the olecranon fragment and the anconeus are retracted proximally together to expose the distal humerus. Alternatively, the anconeus may be elevated from the proximal fragment of the olecranon osteotomy and elbow region with its distal attachment on the ulnar shaft left intact. The anconeus is then retracted laterally while the proximal fragment of the olecranon osteotomy is retracted proximally, which allows ample visualization of the distal humerus. The osteotomy site has been reported to heal reliably with few complications.

It is advantageous to place the hardware on the proposed olecranon fragment (if using a cannulated screw or Kirschner wires) prior to making the osteotomy so that the tract of the hardware is created anatomically, which will facilitate optimal alignment of the osteotomy site at the end of the procedure. We use either two Kirschner wires or a 6.5 or 7.6 mm cannulated screw and washer, with an 18 gauge tension band wire. The drill hole for placement of the wire is placed at an equal distance from the olecranon osteotomy as the distance of the osteotomy site to the tip of the olecranon. The osteotomy should be repaired by advancing the K-wires into the anterior ulnar cortex distal to the coronoid. After the K-wires have reached the anterior cortex, they are backed out about 5 mm and bent 180 degrees and tapped back until buried under the triceps tendon. The triceps may then be sutured over the wires to discourage backing out. Alternatively, a precontoured olecranon plate may be utilized for fixation.

Bryan-Morrey triceps reflecting approach   After identification and protection of the ulnar nerve, a periosteal elevator is used to dissect the triceps muscle, including the medial and lateral margins of the triceps muscle, from the posterior humeral cortex. The triceps tendon is sharply dissected through Sharpey's fibers directly off of the olecranon starting medially and extending laterally. It is helpful to use a Beaver blade scalpel to sharply dissect the triceps tendon off of bone. The fascial overlying Kocher's interval is identified and longitudinally split. The triceps tendon and anconeus should be reflected medially to laterally, ending at Kocher's interval. The triceps may be removed with a thin wafer of bone as well, but this is not our standard practice. At the end of the procedure, the triceps tendon is repaired back to the olecranon using two transosseous drill holes placed in a cruciate configuration and one additional drill hole placed in a transverse orientation with nonabsorbable suture. The repair should be protected postoperatively by avoiding active elbow extension against resistance for a minimum of 6 weeks.

Van Goerder approach   After identification and protection of the ulnar nerve, the triceps tendon is identified several centimeters proximal to its insertion on the olecranon and a Chevron-shaped transection of the tendon is performed with the apex proximal. This is repaired at the end of the procedure with nonabsorbable suture. The repair should be protected postoperatively by avoiding active elbow extension against resistance, and avoiding passive stretching in positions of terminal elbow flexion for a minimum of 6 weeks.

TRAP approach   The trans-anconeus pedicle flap (TRAP) approach requires a longer skin incision distally along the subcutaneous border of the ulna. The anconeus muscle is identified along the lateral aspect of the subcutaneous border of the ulna, and released by sub-periosteal dissection from its insertion on the ulna. The muscle is released in its entirety distally to proximally. It is reflected proximally to afford visualization of the distal humerus.

Medial Approach

Indications

- Ulnar nerve pathology
- Capsular release for stiffness
- Need to preserve the lateral ulno-humeral ligamentous complex

Contraindications

- Need for access to radial head or lateral ligaments

Incision   The medial exposure can use either the posterior or medial-posterior skin incision (Figs. 9-7 and 9-8). Once again, the skin incision can be tailored to work with need for exposure of other structures or existent scars from prior exposures.

Identification of the ulnar nerve is necessary for an adequate and safe medial exposure. The nerve should be identified proximally and subsequent dissection carried distally. In revision surgery and cases with a prior transposition, it is especially helpful to identify the nerve in a normal area prior to the dissection from scarred tissue. Once the nerve is safely identified, the medial supracondylar ridge is palpated along with the overlaying medial intermuscular septum. The medial antebrachial cutaneous nerve will be found on the fascia anterior to the septum. This should be protected to avoid postoperative neuroma formation.

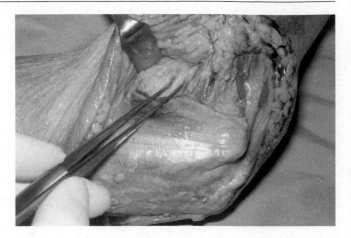

FIGURE 9-7

A skin incision is made and the subcutaneous fat is elevated from the forearm fascia. Care is taken to protect the medial antebrachial cutaneous nerve that lies in the subcutaneous adipose tissue.

The medial intermuscular septum is identified along with the medial supracondylar ridge. The brachial fascia is incised along the anterior aspect of the septum and the flexor-pronator group is released from the supracondylar ridge. Distally the flexor group is split leaving the posterior aspect of the flexor carpi ulnaris in place. The muscle group can be elevated off the anterior capsule and extend all the way across to the lateral aspect of the joint. A cuff of tissue may be left on the ridge, so that the muscle group can be repaired at the end of the procedure. The dissection is subperiosteal, deep to the brachialis so that the brachial artery and median nerve are protected.

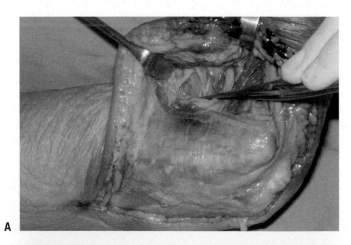

A

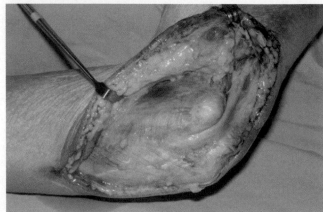

FIGURE 9-8

A,B: The median nerve is found lateral and deep to the flexor pronator group with the lateral antebrachial cutaneous nerve even more lateral.

B

Medial Coronoid Approach

Indications

● Fixation of coronoid fractures

Incision   The medial coronoid can be easily exposed through the floor of the cubital tunnel (Figs. 9-9 to 9-13). The posterior or medial approach is used to expose the ulnar nerve. The nerve is gently dissected and may be anteriorly transposed as previously described. It may be secured to a fasciocutaneous sling during fracture fixation to avoid excessive manipulation and inadvertent traction during the procedure. The nerve may be left in place if there are no concerns for neuropathy and as long as it is not destabilized. The two heads of the flexor carpi ulnaris (FCU) are split. The anterior half is retracted anteriorly, and the posterior half is retracted posteriorly in order to expose the coro-

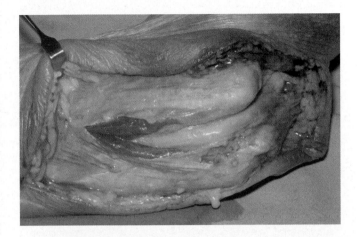

FIGURE 9-9

The ulnar nerve is released from the cubital tunnel in the standard fashion, taking care to split the FCU between the two heads. In this photograph, Osborne's ligament overlying the cubital tunnel has been released.

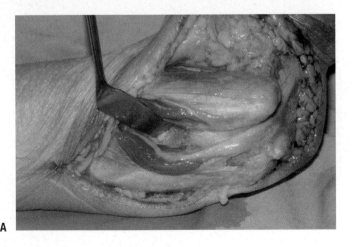

FIGURE 9-10

A–C: The nerve is gently retracted posteriorly and the ulnar head of the FCU is carefully dissected off of the medial collateral ligament (MCL), exposing the coronoid.

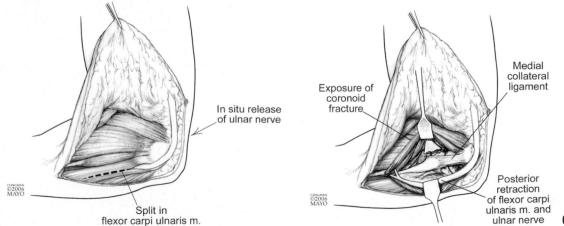

In situ release of ulnar nerve

Split in flexor carpi ulnaris m.

Exposure of coronoid fracture

Medial collateral ligament

Posterior retraction of flexor carpi ulnaris m. and ulnar nerve

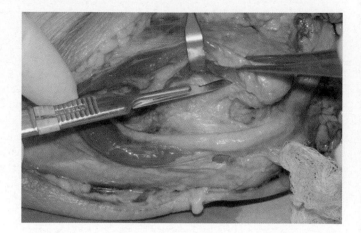

FIGURE 9-11

The medial collateral ligament is nearly fully visualized by peeling the humeral head of the FCU laterally and superiorly.

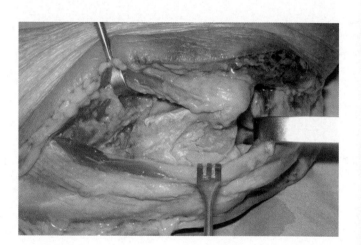

FIGURE 9-12

Utilizing the full extent of this exposure affords access to the coronoid, the medial collateral ligament, and even limited access to the posterior fossa.

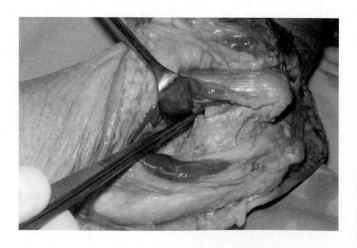

FIGURE 9-13

Entire coronoid may be seen. A full view of the MCL can be achieved including the medial epicondyle as well as the sublime tubercle.

noid. The anterior band of the medial collateral ligament (MCL) is usually attached to a large anteromedial coronoid fragment. Care should be taken not to detach the ligament from this fragment. If the capsular attachments are intact, the surgeon can judge fracture reduction based on realignment of the metaphyseal fracture fragments. The dissection of the flexor carpi ulnaris muscle fibers from the medial collateral ligament should start distally and the muscle should be brought proximally to avoid damaging the ligament and potentially destabilizing the elbow. The insertion of the MCL on the sublime tubercle should be evident. The coronoid will be in the deep portion of the wound, anterior to the ligament.

Alternatively, if there is a large coronoid fragment, the FCU may be reflected anteriorly using subperiosteal dissection from the proximal ulna including the flexor-pronator mass proximally, as described by Taylor and Scham. Care must be taken to protect the ulnar nerve, which may need to be transposed when this approach is used.

Lateral Approaches

Indications

- Radial head ORIF, resection, or replacement
- Lateral epicondylitis debridement
- Repair of lateral ulnocollateral ligament
- Release of contractures

Contraindications

- The need to approach medial pathology
- Ulnar nerve involvement
- Medial humeral condyle fractures

Incision   The lateral approach to the elbow has become a standard means to gain access to the elbow joint (Figs. 9-14 to 9-22). The deep lateral approach was initially described by Kocher in 1911 and has been subsequently modified by Cohen, Hastings, and Morrey in its extensile exposure to preserve the lateral collateral annular ligament complex.

There are several different variations of the lateral exposure. The direct lateral, the LCL preserving, Kocher's approach, and the Mayo Modification have all been described. The general principle and anatomic intervals, however, are the same and are described here.

This approach to the radial head splits the lateral annular ligament complex and stays anterior to the lateral ulnar collateral ligament. The skin incision is placed either as a posterior incision with a large full-thickness lateral flap, or the incision is placed along the lateral epicondyle over the radial head to the lateral aspect of the ulna. Skin flaps are created over the antebrachial fascia.

Kocher's interval   The interval between the extensor carpi ulnaris (ECU) and the anconeus is identified. The fascia is incised from the lateral epicondyle distally following the junction of the ECU and anconeus. Care is taken to elevate the ECU anteriorly and the anconeus posteriorly. The capsule is incised along the anterior border of the lateral ulnocollateral ligament, about 1 cm above

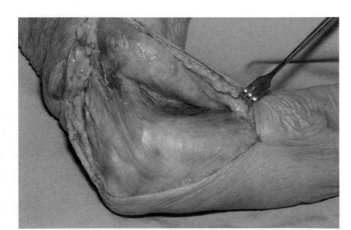

FIGURE 9-14

A lateral or posterior skin incision may be used. The skin and subcutaneous tissues are carefully removed from the investing fascia. Special attention should be taken to avoid damage to the lateral antebrachial cutaneous nerve, which will travel within the fat at the distal aspect of this incision.

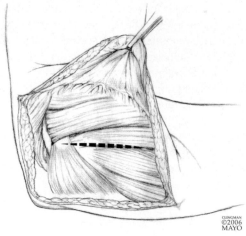

**Incision in common
extensor tendon**

FIGURE 9-15

An alternative to the Kocher's approach is to split
the common extensor group at the equator of the
radiocapitellar joint. This decreases the likelihood
of disrupting the lateral collateral complex.

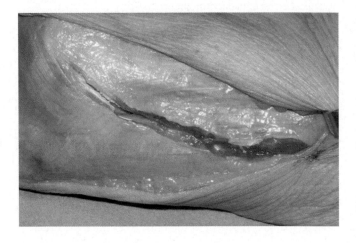

FIGURE 9-16

A traditional Kocher incision is
made between the anconeus and the
extensor carpi ulnaris (ECU). Care
is taken to develop this interval
between the lateral collateral
ligament complex (LCL) and the
ECU.

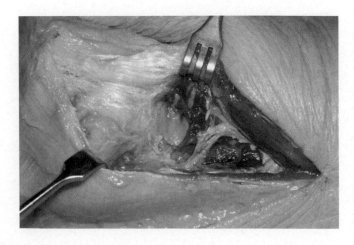

FIGURE 9-17

The extensor origin is dissected
from the LCL.

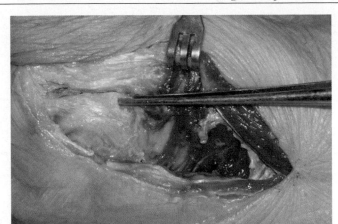

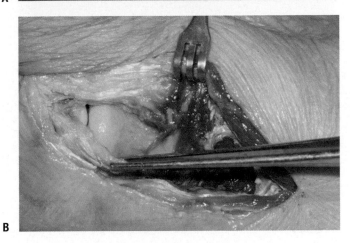

FIGURE 9-18

A,B: The capsule is incised anterior to the equator of the radial head in order to preserve the LCL complex.

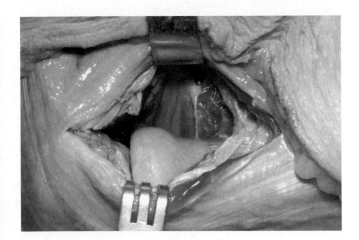

FIGURE 9-19

Excellent exposure of the radial head and neck is achieved. When retracting the anterior structures, pronating the forearm will reduce tension on the posterior interosseous nerve.

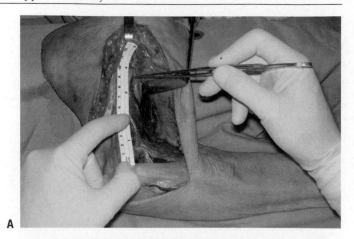

A

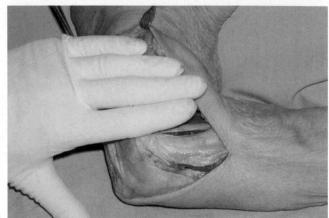

B

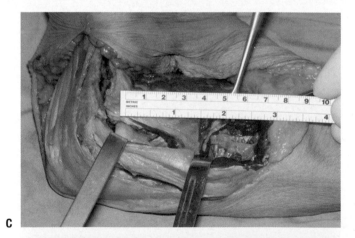

C

FIGURE 9-20

A–D: The radial nerve can be found proximally as close as 4 fingerbreadths (9 cm) proximally from the lateral epicondyle. The safe zone for the PIN is within 2 fingerbreadths (4 cm) distal of the radial head.

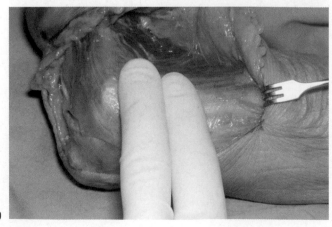

D

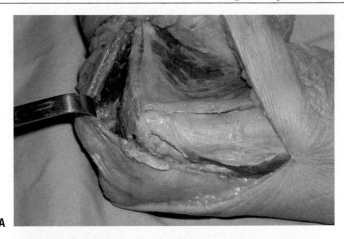

A

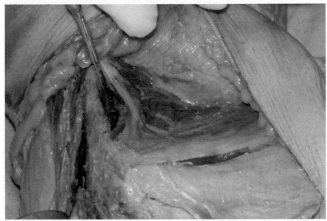

B

FIGURE 9-21

A,B: The lateral approach can be extended by continuing the dissection proximally on both the anterior and posterior side of the lateral humerus. Once again, one must be mindful of the LCL origin at all times.

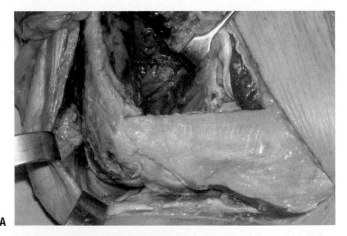

A

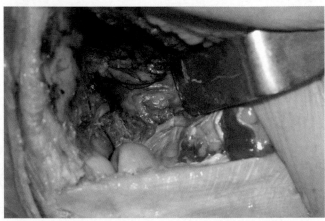

B

FIGURE 9-22

A,B: The brachioradialis is elevated anteriorly allowing for full visualization, even of the coronoid.

the crista supinatorius. Care should be taken during this dissection in order to preserve the lateral collateral ligamentous complex, and avoid destabilizing the elbow.

This exposure can then be extended both proximally and distally as in the case of a lateral ulnar collateral ligament reconstruction. The proximal dissection is achieved by elevating the common extensor tendon off the supracondylar ridge. The radial nerve is usually found proximally as close as 4 finger breadths (8 cm) above the lateral epicondyle, or on average (10 cm) in men from the articular surface. Distally, the posterior interosseus nerve will be found in the area of the radial neck about 2 finger breadths (4 cm) distal to the radiocapitellar joint.

POSTOPERATIVE MANAGEMENT

Elbow rehabilitation is determined by fracture stability and concomitant ligamentous injury.

COMPLICATIONS

Flap necrosis, dehiscence, and wound infection are complications of any surgical incision surrounding the elbow. If the skin has been significantly traumatized prior to elbow exposure, skin slough and partial flap loss should be suspected and early wound examination should be performed to prevent wound infection. Many times partial skin loss may be treated with local wound care and dressing changes; however, if underlying vital structures are exposed, alternative means of wound closure must be considered. For exposed hardware, prosthesis, or nerve we favor aggressive wound debridement and early coverage with either the anconeus, a pedicled radial forearm fasciocutaneous flap, or latissimus flap.

RECOMMENDED READING

Cohen MS, Hastings H. Posttraumatic contracture of the elbow. Operative release using a lateral collateral ligament sparing approach. *J Bone Joint Surg Br.* 1998;80(5):805–812.

Hotchkiss RN: Elbow contracture. In: Green DP, Hotchkiss RN, Pederson WC, eds. *Green's operative hand surgery.* Philadelphia: Churchill-Livingstone, 1999:667–682.

O'Driscoll SW. The triceps-reflecting anconeus pedicle (TRAP) approach for distal humeral fractures and nonunions. *Orthop Clin North Am.* 2000;31(1):91–101.

Ring D, Gulotta L, Chin K, et al. Olecranon osteotomy for exposure of fractures and nonunions of the distal humerus. *J Orthop Trauma.* 2004;18(7):446–449.

Ring D. Fractures of the coronoid process of the ulna. *J Hand Surg Am.* 2006;31(10):1679–1689.

Smith FM. *Surgery of the elbow.* 2nd ed. Philadelphia: W.B. Saunders Co.; 1972.

Taylor TKF, Scham SM. A posteromedial approach to the proximal end of the ulna for the internal fixation of olecranon fractures. *J Trauma.* 1969;9:594–602.

Tornetta P 3rd, Hochwald N, Bono C, et al. Anatomy of the posterior interosseous nerve in relation to fixation of the radial head. *Clin Orthop Relat Res.* 1997;(345):215–218.

Uhl RL, Larosa JM, Sibeni T, et al. Posterior approaches to the humerus: when should you worry about the radial nerve? *J Orthop Trauma.* 1996;10(5):338–340.

10 Radial Forearm Flap for Elbow Coverage

Kodi K. Azari and W. P. Andrew Lee

INDICATIONS/CONTRAINDICATIONS

Soft tissue defects involving the posterior aspect of the elbow are not uncommon and can be challenging to manage. Tissue defects can be from trauma, burns, post-oncologic resection, pressure ulcers, extravasation injury, chronic bursitis, or chronic infection (4,7,15). In addition, elbow prosthetic devices can be exposed with devastating consequences. The goals of treating posterior elbow soft tissue defects is to provide wound closure, decrease the risk of infection, decrease edema, and allow the initiation of early rehabilitation (2,12). The soft tissue reconstruction must be aesthetically acceptable, durable, and elastic enough to allow for the constant unhindered movement of skin over the olecranon with elbow flexion and extension (7).

Many soft tissue reconstructive options exist and must be tailored to the needs of the patient's wound characteristics. Superficial wounds can be addressed by primary wound closure. Wounds with exposed "white structures" such as tendons, neurovascular structures, bone, and joint will necessitate flap coverage (9). Available flap options include regional muscle and musculocutaneous flaps, distant staged pedicle flaps, and microvascular free tissue transfer (8). Although these flaps are useful for elbow soft tissue coverage, they can carry significant morbidity. For example, regional muscle and musculocutaneous flaps necessitate the harvesting of a functional muscle; distant pedicle flaps (such as the groin or thoracoepigastric flap) require the binding of the extremity to the flank for several weeks with significant discomfort and ensuing stiffness; and free flaps introduce the added complexity of microsurgery and prolonged surgical time (4,8). Because of the liabilities of the previously mentioned flaps, local fasciocutaneous flaps have gained popularity (10), of which the proximally based radial forearm flap is the recognized workhorse for elbow soft tissue coverage (8).

The radial forearm flap is composed of the skin, subcutaneous fat, and fascia that, if needed, can be elevated to include the entire volar surface of the forearm (13) (see Fig. 10-2). This is a reliable flap with a rich arterial supply from the septocutaneous perforator branches of the radial artery (see Fig. 10-3). The deep venous drainage for the flap is provided by the paired venae comitantes that run parallel with the radial artery and the superficial venous drainage is by branches of the cephalic vein. The radial forearm flap is versatile because it may be transposed either in the radial or ulnar direction and can be made sensate by encompassing the cutaneous nerves of the forearm. Furthermore, this flap can provide stable soft tissue coverage while still preserving elbow range of motion.

Contraindications to the use of the radial forearm flap include any injury to the radial artery, severe forearm soft tissue injuries, and inadequate collateral flow to the hand and thumb. A possible relative contraindication is recent cannulation of the superficial venous system of the upper extremity, as this may result in venous thrombus formation in the flap and subsequent venous congestion (5).

PREOPERATIVE PLANNING

Preparation of the Wound Bed

In cases of complex elbow wounds, it is extremely important to gain control over the wound before definitive soft tissue reconstruction. Osseous injuries and dislocations need to be stabilized with appropriate internal or external fixation and ligament reconstruction. When soft tissue injuries are present, it is mandatory to perform serial debridement of devitalized tissues until only viable tissues remains. Infections require appropriate debridement and culture-specific antibiotic coverage. It should be noted that meeting the above requisites as quickly as possible will allow for earlier definitive vascularized wound coverage with radial forearm flap and thus afford a more successful functional outcome.

Assessment of the Arterial Vascularity of the Hand

It is imperative to assess the arterial vascularity of the hand by performing a modified Allen's test before performing the radial forearm flap. A modified Allen's test is performed by occluding the radial artery at the wrist crease and evaluating the perfusion of the digits using a hand-held pencil Doppler. In particular, one must ensure that there are Doppler signals to the thumb digital arteries once the radial artery is occluded. If the modified Allen's test shows evidence of vascular insufficiency, then one must be prepared to reconstruct the arterial tree using a saphenous vein graft or choose a soft tissue reconstruction technique other than the proximally based radial forearm flap.

SURGERY

Patient Positioning

For optimal position, patients are placed supine on the operating room table. The entire upper extremity from axilla to hand is prepped and draped in standard surgical fashion, and a sterile proximal arm tourniquet applied.

Technique

The course of the radial artery is marked by drawing a line from the center of the anticubital fossa to the radial border of the proximal wrist crease (where the radial artery pulse is palpable) (Fig. 10-1). A skin island that is the shape and slightly larger than the periolecranon defect is designed and centered along the central axis of the radial artery (Fig.10-2). The limit of the flap width is the radial and ulnar borders of the volar forearm and can extend from the antibrachial fossa to a few centimeters proximal to the distal wrist crease. The exact position of the flap is determined by a using a nonstretchable template with the antibrachial fossa as the pivot point of the vascular leash (Fig. 10-3).

Usually, the distal incision is made first and the radial artery and accompanying venae comitantes that reside between the flexor carpii radialis (FCR) and brachioradialis (BR) tendons are isolated and divided. The cephalic vein, which lies radial to the brachioradialis tendon, is also isolated and divided.

FIGURE 10-1

The course of the radial artery and venae comitantes is marked by drawing a line from the center of the anticubital fossa to the radial border of the proximal wrist crease.

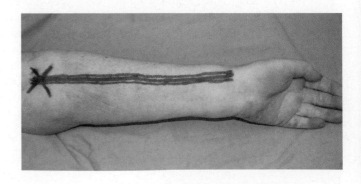

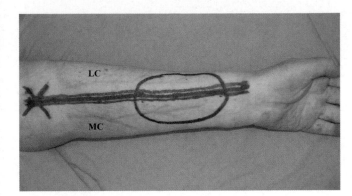

FIGURE 10-2

A skin island that is the shape and slightly larger than the periolecranon defect is designed and centered along the central axis of the radial artery. The medial cutaneous (MC) or lateral cutaneous (LC) nerves of the forearm can be included in the skin paddle to form an innervated neurosensory flap.

The proximal incision of the flap is made and the radial artery is identified between the FCR and BR. Care should be taken not to injure the cephalic vein (or the medial or lateral cutaneous nerves if the radial forearm flap is designed as an innervated neurosensory flap) (see Fig. 10-2). Next, the ulnar incision is made and carried to the tissue plane deep to the deep forearm fascia. This subfascial plane is developed and the flap is raised from ulnar to radial off the underlying flexor carpii ulnaris, flexor digitorum sublimus, palmaris longus, and flexor carpii radialis muscles. It is imperative to preserve the paratenon of the tendons to allow skin graft coverage of the flap donor site. The dissection is carried ulnarly until the radial border of the FCR. At this important juncture the intermuscular septum carrying the septocutaneous branches of the radial artery is identified and carefully preserved (Fig. 10-4).

The radial border incision is made and the subfascial dissection is carried ulnarly. The brachioradialis muscle is retracted laterally allowing for the identification of the radial artery, intermuscular septum, and superficial radial sensory nerve. In the upper border of the flap, the cephalic vein is located and integrated in the flap for added venous drainage. The flap is next elevated and the radial artery, venae comitantes, cephalic vein, and medial or lateral cutaneous nerves (for an innervated sensory flap) are dissected proximally to an appropriate pivot point that allows for a tension free flap transfer (Fig. 10-5).

The tourniquet is released and the vascularity of flap is ascertained. In cases where large flaps are required, the perfusion of the peripheral flap skin can be evaluated by the administration of intravenous fluorescein. Initially a small test dose of 100 mg is given, and the patient's vital signs are closely monitored for 20 minutes. If there is no evidence of hemodynamic instability, then the full dose of 10 mg/kg is administered and the skin paddle evaluated 10 minutes later under ultraviolet light (Wood's lamp). The extreme areas of the flap that appear dark and do not fluoresce are sharply trimmed.

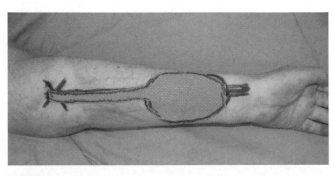

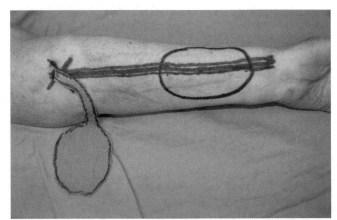

A B

FIGURE 10-3

A,B: The exact position of the skin paddle is established by a using a nonstretchable template with the antibrachial fossa as the pivot point of the vascular leash.

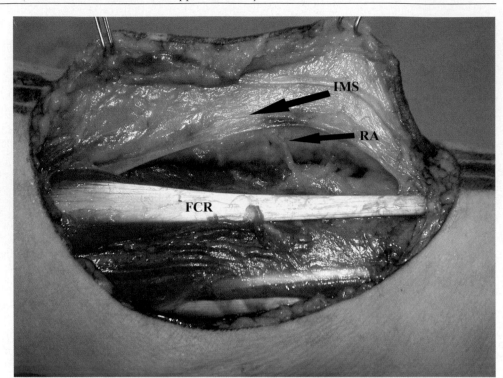

FIGURE 10-4

View from an ulnar to radial subfascual dissection demonstrating the radial artery (*RA*), intermuscular septum (*IMS*) through which septocutaneous perforator branches of the radial artery traverse, and flexor carpii radialis tendon (*FCR*).

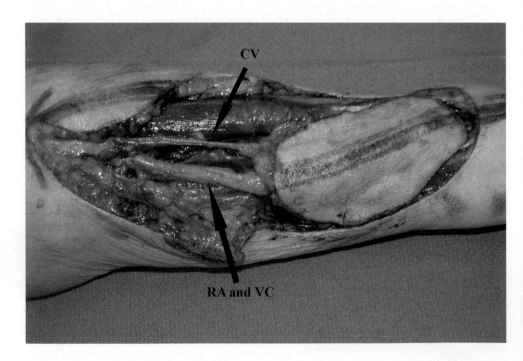

FIGURE 10-5

This figure demonstrates a flap that has been dissected proximally to an appropriate pivot point that will allow a tension free flap transfer. Note the vascular pedicle containing the radial artery (*RA*) and venae comitantes (*VC*). The cephalic vein (*CV*) was included in this flap for venous drainage augmentation.

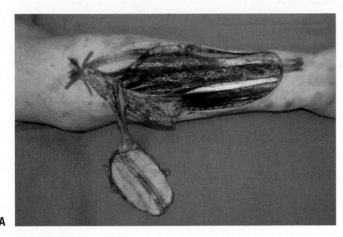
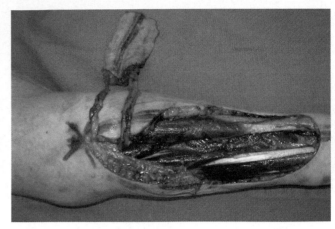

A   **B**

FIGURE 10-6

Once the vascular pedicle is dissected to an appropriate pivot point, the flap can be transposed to the posterior elbow region from either an ulnar **(A)** or radial **(B)** direction.

When certain that the flap is well perfused, the flap is transferred from either an ulnar or radial direction through a subcutaneous tunnel to the elbow and inset with interrupted suture (Fig. 10-6). After obtaining meticulous hemostasis, we routinely attempt to cover the exposed tendons with local flexor tendon muscle bellies and soft tissues. This is followed by unmeshed split-thickness skin graft coverage of the entire donor site (Fig. 10-7).

A case of a proximally based neurosensory radial forearm flap for soft tissue reconstruction of the periolecranon region is illustrated in Figure 10-8.

POSTOPERATIVE MANAGEMENT

Immobilization and elevation are absolutely critical in the postoperative management of elbow reconstruction with the radial forearm flap. A nonconstricting and bulky above-elbow splint (including fingers) is applied with a window cut out for accessibility and inspection of the flap. The elbow is held at 90 degrees, and the digits are placed in the position of safety. The digits are immobilized to prevent shear forces on the forearm donor site skin graft by tendon excursion. To help decrease postoperative edema and the possibility of the patient exerting pressure on the flap while asleep, the arm can be hung from an intravenous fluid pole. For the first 3 postoperative days, the flap is evaluated on a frequent (every 4 to 8 hr) basis for capillary refill and the absence of venous congestion. The splint and the donor site bolster are removed on postoperative day 5 when capillary inosculation of the skin graft has occurred. Thereafter, a soft dressing is applied and the skin graft and flap

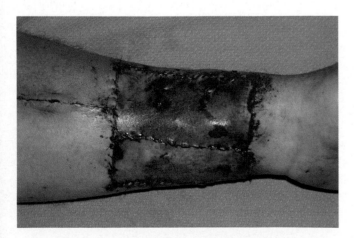

FIGURE 10-7

The forearm donor site is covered with an unmeshed split-thickness skin graft.

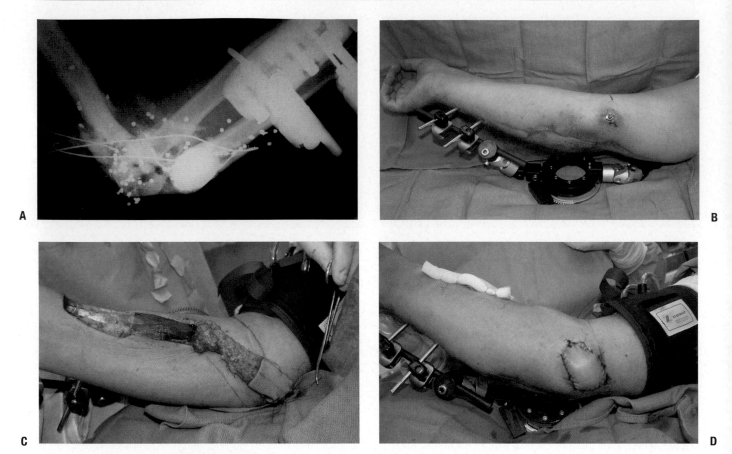

FIGURE 10-8

A 32 year old male with significant injury to the elbow from a shotgun assault. Following appropriate bone stabilization with external and internal fixation **(A)** he developed wound dehiscence and hardware exposure **(B)**. An innervated neurosensory radial forearm flap was designed incorporating the medial cutaneous nerve of the forearm **(C)** and inset through a subcutaneous tunnel **(D)**.

suture lines are kept moist with bacitracin ointment. Digital and elbow range of motion are gently begun and progressively increased.

RESULTS

Case reports of soft tissue reconstructions about the elbow region can be found in the medical literature. Hallock (6) described two cases of chemotherapy extravasation and exposure of hardware with successful healing following radial forearm flap. Thornton (13) reported a case of olecranon osteoradionecrosis treated with the radial forearm flap resulting in early elbow range of motion and complete healing. Small and Miller (11) present three cases in elderly patients to illustrate the utility of the radial forearm flap. One patient had an established infection with radial head and lateral epicondyle ischaemia. Despite aggressive treatment this patient died 32 days postoperatively from sepsis. Another patient with a crush injury developed an ankylosed elbow that was free of pain and infection. Meland (7) reported successful pedicled radial forearm flap coverage for three patients with recalcitrant about the elbow defects in whom one or more previous flaps had failed. Tizian (15) reported the use of proximally based radial forearm flap in 14 patients. All patients showed complete healing of the periolecranon region and forearm donor site with unrestricted elbow range of motion. In a recent comparative review by Chondry and colleagues, the radical forearm flap provided excellent coverage of moderate size defects of the elbow. The flap was associated with fewer complications when compared to the pedicled latissimus dorsi flap (1).

COMPLICATIONS

A major, yet rarely encountered complication of the radial forearm flap is ischemia of the hand. A meticulous preoperative Doppler examination of the hand using the modified Allen's test should identify patients who are at risk. However, if arterial insufficiency of the hand is encountered once the flap is elevated, the radial artery needs to be reconstructed using an interposed vein graft. A great saphenous vein graft anastomosed end-to-side proximally and end-to-end distally is the authors preferred method.

Other major complications include flap ischemia and congestion. In both of these instances careful evaluation of the flap is mandatory to ensure that the subcutaneous tunnel is adequate, the skin paddle is not under excessive tension or external pressure, and there is no undue stretching or twisting of the vascular pedicle.

Donor site problems are one of the most common complications of the radial forearm flap. These complications can include hypertrophic scarring, poor skin graft take, and tendon loss (3,14). As mentioned previously, it is imperative to preserve the flexor tendon paratenon and attempt to cover exposed tendons such as the FCR with local muscle bellies and soft tissue advancement. If there is inadequate skin graft take and tendon exposure, local dressing changes with saline-dampened gauze are initiated to prevent tendon desiccation until the wound healing by secondary intention is complete. In rare cases, secondary flaps may be required to cover exposed tendons in the forearm. Other reported donor site complications can include injury to the radial sensory nerve or hand swelling and stiffness (14).

CONCLUSION

Soft tissue defects of the posterior elbow are not uncommon and can often be difficult to reconstruct. Although a multitude of reconstruction options are available, each patient needs to be individualized. The advantages of the pedicled radial forearm fasciocutaneous flap for the management of elbow defects include ipsilateral donor site and scar, relatively simple dissection, long vascular pedicle that allows a wide arc of rotation, ability to make into a neurosensory flap by including forearm cutaneous nerves, no requirement for microsurgical expertise, ease of postoperative limb positioning, and highly reliable and vascularized tissue that is an excellent option even in the setting of osteomyelitis (7).

RECOMMENDED READING

Mathes S, Nahai F. *Reconstructive Surgery: Principles, Anatomy, and Technique.* New York: Churchill Livingstone, 1997.

REFERENCES

1. Chondry AH, Moran SL, Li S, et al. Soft tissue coverage of the elbow: an outcome analysis and reconstructive algorithm. *Plast Reconstr Surg.* 2007;119:1852.
2. Davalbhakta AV, Niranjan NS. Fasciocutaneous flaps based on fascial feeding vessels for defects in the periolecranon area. *Br J Plast Surg.* 1999;52:60.
3. Fenton OM, Roberts JO. Improving the donor site of the radial forearm flap. *Br J Plast Surg.* 1985;38:504.
4. Frost-Arner L, Bjorgell O. Local perforator flap for reconstruction of deep tissue defects in the elbow area. *Ann Plast Surg.* 2003;50:491.
5. Hallock GG. Caution in using the Chinese radial forearm flap. *Plast Reconstr Surg.* 1986;77:164.
6. Hallock GG. Island forearm flap for coverage of the antecubital fossa. *Br J Plast Surg.* 1986;39:533.
7. Meland NB, Clinkscales CM, Wood MB. Pedicled radial forearm flaps for recalcitrant defects about the elbow. *Microsurgery.* 1991;12:155.
8. Orgill DP, Pribaz JJ, Morris DJ. Local fasciocutaneous flaps for olecranon coverage. *Ann Plast Surg.* 1994;32:27.
9. Russell RC, Zamboni WA. Soft tissue reconstruction. Coverage of the elbow and forearm. *Orthop Clin North Am.* 1993;24:425.
10. Sherman R. Soft-tissue coverage for the elbow. *Hand Clin.* 1997;13:291.
11. Small JO, Millar R. Radial forearm flap cover of the elbow joint. *Injury.* 1988;19:287.
12. Stevanovic M, Sharpe F, Itamura JM. Treatment of soft tissue problems about the elbow. *Clin Orthop Relat Res.* 2000;370:127.
13. Thornton JW, Stevenson TR, VanderKolk CA. Osteoradionecrosis of the olecranon: treatment by radial forearm flap. *Plast Reconstr Surg.* 1987;80:833.
14. Timmons MJ, Missotten FE, Poole MD, et al. Complications of radial forearm flap donor sites. *Br J Plast Surg.* 1986;39:176.
15. Tizian C, Sanner F, Berger A. The proximally pedicled arteria radialis forearm flap in the treatment of soft tissue defects of the dorsal elbow. *Ann Plast Surg.* 1991;26:40.

11 Pedicled and Free Latissimus Flap for Elbow and Forearm Coverage

Kenji Kawamura and Kevin C. Chung

INDICATIONS/CONTRAINDICATIONS

The latissimus dorsi (LD) has proven to be a reliable muscle in the coverage of soft tissue defects about the shoulder and elbow. Familiarity with this muscle and its application in cases of trauma is essential for all upper extremity surgeons. The major arterial inflow and venous outflow for the LD flap is based on the thoracodorsal artery and venae comitantes. The average diameter of the thoracodorsal artery is 2.5 mm, and that of venae comitantes is 3.0 mm. The average length of maximum vascular pedicle is 12 cm, which can be obtained by dissecting the thoracodorsal vessels toward the proximal axillary artery and vein.

The indication for the use of the LD flap to the elbow and forearm is to cover a large skin and soft tissue defect that cannot be managed with local flaps. In cases in which vital muscle structures were damaged, the LD flap can provide coverage of soft tissue defects, as well as functional muscle transfer to restore of elbow, wrist, and finger motion. Unstable soft tissue coverage over elbow fracture or recalcitrant infection around the elbow may also be amenable to the LD flap because this flap provides well-vascularized tissue that can seal dead spaces and increase blood flow to the local environment.

The pedicled LD flap can cover the forearm up to approximately 8 cm distal to the olecranon when transposed anteriorly, and about 6 cm distal to the olecranon when transposed posteriorly. Soft tissue defects over 8 cm distal from the olecranon are not suitable for the pedicled LD flap transfer, and if this muscle is to be used, the free LD flap transfer should be considered.

Contraindications for flap use include previous injury to the muscle or pedicle, such as in cases of previous thoracotomy, axillary arterial injury, or in some cases, axillary lymphadenectomy. Breast cancer surgery may injure the nerve or arterial supply to the LD muscle, rendering it fibrotic and inadequate for transfer. In such patients, palpation of a contracting LD muscle usually verifies an uninjured nerve and vascular pedicle.

The LD muscle functions as an expendable adductor, extender, and internal rotator of the arm. These functions are essential for activities of daily living for patients with contralateral shoulder girdle paralysis or extremity paralysis from spinal cord injury. One must be careful in evaluating the impact of removing the LD muscle in these situations. In general, one should not use the LD muscle for soft tissue coverage in these patients because of functional requirements.

PREOPERATIVE PLANNING

The LD flap can be harvested as not only a muscle flap but also a musculocutaneous flap. Muscle flap covered with skin graft is less bulky and can seal deep defects, however, musculocutaneous flap gives better aesthetic reconstruction because the skin paddle can conform to the skin texture of the upper arm. When a LD musculocutaneous flap is applied, it is recommended that the skin paddle is designed several centimeters superior to the muscle origin at the iliac crest to avoid the risk of skin paddle necrosis because the blood supply of the subcutaneous tissue near the origin is inconsistent. When greater flap reach is required, a portion of the skin paddle may be designed over the inferior margin of the muscle. This technique can facilitate a greater distal coverage of the forearm when the pedicled LD musculocutaneous flap is rotated. The entire skin paddle can survive if enough musculocutaneous perforators are included in the proximal portion of the skin paddle design.

The arc of transposition of the LD flap depends on the location of the wound. When defects are present in the posterior aspect of the elbow and forearm, posterior arc transposition of the pedicled LD flap is recommended. Similarly, when defects are present in the anterior aspect, anterior arc transposition is recommended.

It is important to assess the strength of the LD muscle preoperatively when the LD flap is used for simultaneous soft tissue coverage and functional restoration. When a soft tissue defect is caused by a trauma, particularly associated with a motorcycle accident, the LD muscle may be paralyzed by brachial plexus injury. If the paralyzed LD muscle is planned to be used as a functional transfer, reinnervation of the LD muscle by another motor nerve, for example, intercostal nerve or accessory nerve, can be performed during operative procedures. LD muscle previously paralyzed by neurologic disorders can only be used for soft tissue coverage and should not be used for functional muscle transfer.

Preoperative angiography of the injured upper extremity will help plan for free LD flap transfer. The free flap transfer may require a more proximal vessel dissection, vein grafting, and end-to-side anastomoses in cases with a potential disruption of the recipient vessels.

For aesthetic consideration at the donor site, it is important to ask for the patient's clothing preference preoperatively for planning the skin incision. For example, a transverse incision along the bra line is recommended to conceal the donor site scar for a woman, but an oblique incision may be suitable for a patient who likes to wear backless dresses. Furthermore, the endoscopic harvesting technique may be preferred for children, those who are prone to hypertrophic scars, and for other aesthetic considerations.

SURGERY

The patient, under general anesthesia, is placed in the lateral decubitus position. The injured upper limb and ipsilateral hemithorax caudal to the iliac crest are prepped and draped. The injured upper limb is supported on a sterile Mayo stand with a 90-degree abduction position of the shoulder (Fig. 11-1A). The lateral buttock and thigh are also prepared for skin grafting if necessary. A beanbag or axillary roll with padding is placed on the opposite axilla to protect the dependent shoulder in the decubitus position, and all other pressure points are also carefully padded.

In cases of traumatic defects, the wounds are again thoroughly debrided before the flap procedure is performed. When a LD musculocutaneous flap is applied, the skin paddle that includes the perforators arising from the branch of the thoracodorsal artery is designed on the LD muscle. There is a longitudinal row of perforators 2 to 5 centimeters from the lateral border of the LD muscle, which can be easily identified with a Doppler blood flowmeter. The largest skin paddle that can be moved safely is 20 × 15 cm, however, primary closure is only possible with skin paddles 8 cm in width.

The procedure is performed with ×2.5 loupe magnification. The incision usually begins at the posterior aspect of the axilla angled along the anterolateral border of the latissimus dorsi muscle and extends inferiorly to the iliac crest. An aesthetic incision in a woman is designed in a transverse incision along the bra line. The LD muscle is dissected medially to the paraspinous muscle and caudally to the lumbosacral fascia. The origin of the muscle is detached from the thoracic and lumbar vertebra, posterior ribs, and lumbosacral fascia. The flap is elevated superiorly toward the axilla to separate the undersurface of the muscle from the chest wall. Perforators from the intercostal and lumbar arteries are clipped. The neurovascular pedicle, which includes the thoracodorsal artery, venae comitantes, and nerve, is identified more proximally on the undersurface of the muscle. The tho-

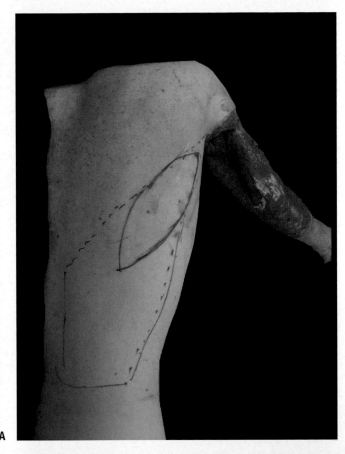

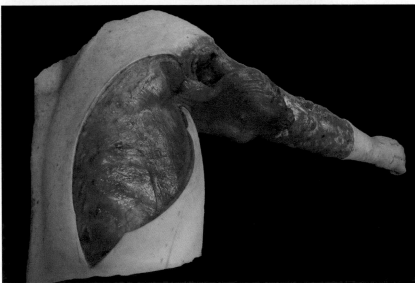

FIGURE 11-1

A: The patient was placed in the lateral decubitus position with the injured upper limb on a sterile Mayo stand with a 90-degree abduction position of the shoulder. **B:** A pedicled latissimus dorsi muscle flap was harvested and rotated posteriorly to the upper arm. A skin paddle was excised for contouring the flap on the arm. It is difficult to design a skin paddle to fit the wound geometry and it is simpler to just use the muscle only and cover with skin graft. *(Continued)*

racodorsal vessels are carefully dissected toward the proximal axillary artery. The circumflex scapular vessels and the serratus anterior and teres major branches are ligated to allow maximal pedicle length. Leaving the thoracodorsal nerve intact may be considered when the flap is transferred on the pedicle, even though the flap is not used as a functional transfer. Retaining innervation minimizes postoperative muscle atrophy and will maintain muscle thickness and durability. This consideration is particularly important for distal elbow coverage when the thin muscle near the origin of the LD muscle at the iliac crest maintains its bulk.

After the dissection of the neurovascular pedicle has been completed, the insertion of the LD muscle at the humerus is divided. Additional distal coverage with the pedicled LD flap can be obtained

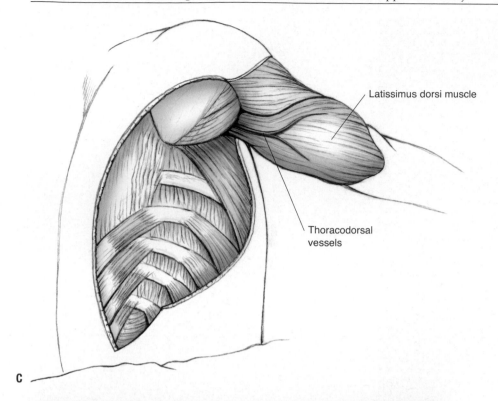

C

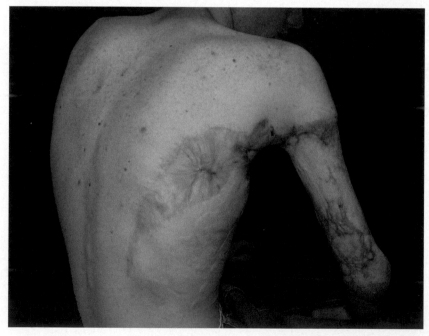

D

FIGURE 11-1

Continued **C:** Schematic drawing of a pedicled latissimus dorsi muscle transfer based on Figure 11-1B. **D:** Complete wound healing at 3 months postoperatively.

by releasing its insertion from the intertubercular grooves of the humerus. When the LD flap is transferred as a free flap, vascular pedicle is divided at the juncture with the axillary artery and vein to obtain the maximum pedicle length. The thoracodorsal nerve is also divided at its proximal point when the flap is used as a functional transfer. When the LD flap is transposed to the elbow and forearm defects, the muscle can be positioned along its path by incising intervening skin or can pass under a subcutaneous tunnel (see Fig. 11-1B,C). The subcutaneous tunnel may be useful in situations when the defect size is relatively small and the transposed small muscle can be tailored to pass easily through the tunnel. But for large muscle, the subcutaneous tunnel may compress the vascular pedicle and the intervening skin should be incised to allow a tension-free passage.

The muscle is sutured to the subcutaneous tissue in the proximal portion of the wound to prevent tension on the pedicle. For functional muscle transfer, muscle tension is critical. For elbow flexor reconstruction, the length of the transferred muscle is adjusted so that the elbow remains at 100 degrees flexion and the forearm is held in complete supination after both ends are sutured. By extending the muscle with strips of fascia lata, finger flexion or extension can also be restored.

Split-thickness skin graft is applied as needed for the transposed muscle or over the donor site (see Fig. 11-1D). Two silastic drains are placed at the donor site, and one is placed below the transposed muscle. Before closure of the donor site, fibrin sealant may be used to reduce seroma formation over the back.

When a free LD flap transfer is used for coverage of a forearm defect (Fig. 11-2A), dissection of recipient vessels should be performed before harvesting the flap to confirm the necessary length of the pedicle. A large LD muscle flap is suitable to cover a forearm defect because the flat configuration of the LD muscle allows it to be wrapped around the forearm. The LD muscle is a versatile muscle for coverage of a complex wound whereby the geometry of the wound requires two separate flaps. Splitting of the LD muscle is helpful in this situation. The thoracodorsal vessels usually bifurcate into medial and lateral branches just after entering the LD muscle. The LD muscle can be split longitudinally into halves based on these two branches. Splitting the LD muscle provides two flaps to coverage different wounds on the forearm (see Figs. 11-2B,C).

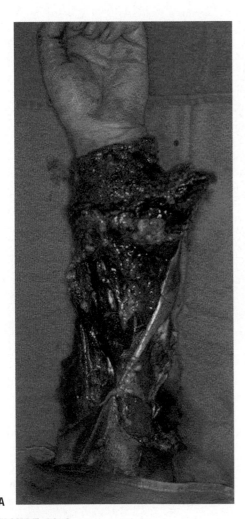 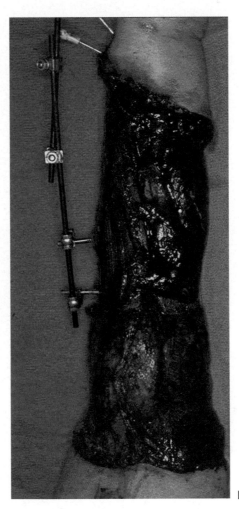

A   B

FIGURE 11-2

A: Crush injury of the forearm. **B:** The latissimus dorsi muscle was split longitudinally into halves by identifying the arterial pedicles. One half was used to cover the soft tissue defect over the posterior elbow, and the other half was used to cover the exposed bone at the wrist and exposed tendons. The thoracodorsal artery was anastomosed to the brachial artery using an end-to-side technique, and the thoracodorsal vein was anastomosed to the brachial concomitant vein with an end-to-end technique. *(Continued)*

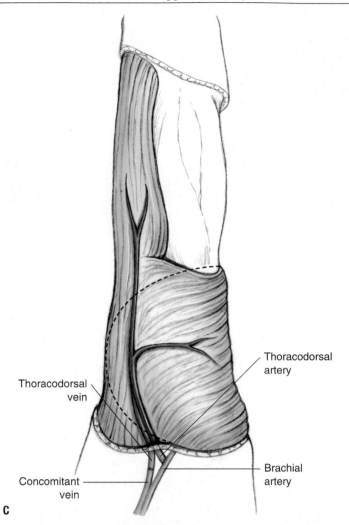

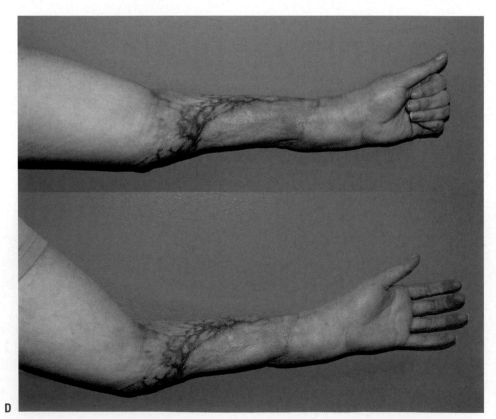

FIGURE 11-2

Continued **C:** Schematic drawing of a free latissimus dorsi muscle transfer based on Figure 11-2B. **D:** Complete wound healing at 4 months postoperatively. There are no limitations of finger motions. *(Continued)*

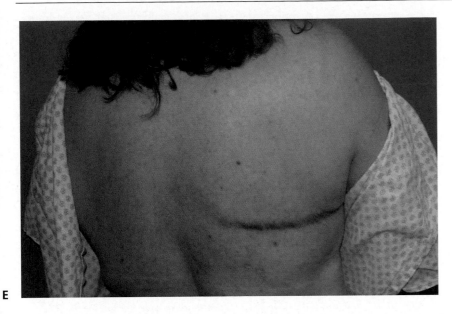

E

FIGURE 11-2

Continued **E:** Donor site scar resulting from an aesthetic transverse incision along the bra line.

POSTOPERATIVE MANAGEMENT

During the first 48 hours after the operation, flap circulation is closely monitored by direct observation of the flap, which includes color, temperature, capillary refilling time, and bleeding of the flap. A Doppler blood flowmeter is useful to examine the arterial flow into the flap. If there is concern about the arterial inflow or venous outflow, the pedicle should be reexamined and the wound reexplored. Kinking and tension on the pedicle must be relieved to prevent total necrosis of the muscle. Postoperative hematoma can also compromise venous outflow.

The drain at the donor site must remain in place for 2 to 3 weeks to prevent seroma formation. Application of fibrin sealant in the donor site may reduce seroma formation, but the drains should remain in place until drainage is minimal, usually less than 25 mL/day. Compression of the donor site by thoracic elastic bandages may be effective to enhance sealing of the wound. When a seroma is diagnosed, needle aspiration is performed. Small seromas (<100 mL) may resorb spontaneously, but a large seroma needs serial aspirations.

The elbow is immobilized at 90 degrees of flexion, and the shoulder is adducted for 3 weeks after the operation to avoid wound dehiscence and tension on the pedicle. During this period, finger and wrist exercises are actively practiced (see Fig. 11-2D). After splint removal, elbow and shoulder range of motion exercises are started. The goal of physiotherapy is to recover the full range of motion of the elbow and shoulder.

COMPLICATIONS

Donor site seroma or hematoma is the most commonly encountered complication at the donor site following harvest of the LD flap. Seromas can be relieved with frequent needle aspirations, but hematomas must be drained immediately to avoid secondary donor site complications relating to wound dehiscence or skin necrosis.

Scarring over the donor site is inevitable, but can be easily covered by clothing. Planning the skin incision and endoscopic harvesting technique can reduce back scar problems (see Fig. 11-2E).

Total flap necrosis is a rare complication with the LD flap method. However, partial flap necrosis at the distal portion may occur because of inconsistent blood supply to the lower third of the LD muscle. Bleeding at the distal end of the LD flap should be checked when the flap is elevated. Kinking and tension on the pedicle can cause disturbance of flap circulation and must be recognized immediately. It is also important to note potential ischemia of the transferred muscle caused by subcutaneous tunnel compression.

Power and endurance of shoulder extension and adduction may be weakened in the absence of the LD muscle. The weakness is not noticeable in most patients and will recover within a few months after removal of the LD muscle because the synergistic shoulder muscles such as teres major, pectoralis major, and subscapularis substitute the function of the LD muscle.

Hyperabduction of the arm during the operation may cause iatrogenic brachial plexus injury, which is reversible within several weeks. Care must be taken to avoid prolonged shoulder abduction during the operative procedure.

Lumbar hernia after the latissimus dorsi flap is an extremely uncommon complication and it may be misdiagnosed as lumbar seromas. Lumbar hernia can be avoided by preserving of the fascia underlying the distal latissimus dorsi aponeurosis.

RECOMMENDED READING

Adams WP Jr, Lipschitz AH, Ansari M, et al. Functional donor site morbidity following latissimus dorsi muscle flap transfer. *Ann Plast Surg*. 2004;53:6–11.

Axer A, Segal D, Elkon A. Partial transposition of the latissimus dorsi. A new operative technique to restore elbow and finger flexion. *J Bone Joint Surg*. 1973;55A:1259–1264.

Brones MF, Wheeler ES, Lesavoy MA. Restoration of elbow flexion and arm contour with a latissimus dorsi myocutaneous flap. *Plast Reconstr Surg*. 1982;69:329–332.

Chang LD, Goldberg NH, Chang B, et al. Elbow defect coverage with a one-staged, tunneled latissimus dorsi transposition flap. *Ann Plast Surg*. 1994;32:496–502.

Cho BC, Lee JH, Ramasastry SS, et al. Free latissimus dorsi muscle transfer using an endoscopic technique. *Ann Plast Surg*. 1997;38:586–593.

Fisher J, Wood MB. Late necrosis of a latissimus dorsi free flap. *Plast Reconstr Surg*. 1984;74:274–281.

Freedlander E. Brachial plexus cord compression by the tendon of a pedicled latissimus dorsi flap. *Br J Plast Surg*. 1986;39:514–515.

Hovnanian AP. Latissimus dorsi transplantation for loss of flexion or extension at the elbow. A preliminary report on technic. *Ann Surg*. 1956;143:493–499.

Jamra FNA, Akel S, Shamma AR. Repair of major defects of the upper extremity with a latissimus dorsi myocutaneous flap: A case report. *Br J Plast Surg*. 1981;34:121–123.

Jutte DL, Rees R, Nanney L, et al. Latissimus dorsi flap: A valuable resource in lower arm reconstruction. *South Med J*. 1987;80:37–40.

Katsaros J, Gilbert D, Russell R. The use of a combined latissimus dorsi-groin flap as a direct flap for reconstruction of the upper extremity. *Br J Plast Surg*. 1983;36:67–71.

Lin CH, Wei FC, Levin LS, et al. Donor-site morbidity comparison between endoscopically assisted and traditional harvest of free latissimus dorsi muscle flap. *Plast Reconstr Surg*. 1999;104:1070–1077.

Logan AM, Black MJM. Injury to the brachial plexus resulting from shoulder positioning during latissimus dorsi flap pedicle dissection. *Br J Plast Surg*. 1985;38:380–382.

MacKinnon SE, Weiland AJ, Godina M. Immediate forearm reconstruction with a functional latissimus dorsi island pedicle myocutaneous flap. *Plast Reconstr Surg*. 1983;71:706–710.

Medgyesi S. A successful operation for lymphodema using a myocutaneous flap as a "wick." *Br J Plast Surg*. 1983;36:64–66.

Moon HK, Dowden RV. Lumbar hernia after latissimus dorsi flap. *Plast Reconstr Surg*. 1985;75:417–419.

Mordick TG II, Britton EN, Brantigan C. Pedicled latissimus dorsi transfer for immediate soft-tissue coverage and elbow flexion. *Plast Reconstr Surg*. 1997;99:1742–1744.

Mutaf M, Ustuner ET, Sensoz O. Intra-operative tunnel expansion to prevent tunnel compression following latissimus dorsi muscle transfers. *J Hand Surg*. 1993;18B:446–448.

Rogachefsky RA, Aly A, Brearley W. Latissimus dorsi pedicled flap for upper extremity soft-tissue reconstruction. *Orthopedics*. 2002;25:403–408.

Sadove RC, Vasconez HC, Arthur KR, et al. Immediate closure of traumatic upper arm and forearm injuries with the latissimus dorsi island myocutaneous pedicle flap. *Plast Reconstr Surg*. 1991;88:115–120.

Schottstaedt ER, Larsen LJ, Bost FC. Complete muscle transposition. *J Bone Joint Surg*. 1955;37A:897–919.

Schwabegger A, Ninkovic M, Brenner E, et al. Seroma as a common donor site morbidity after harvesting the latissimus dorsi flap: Observations on cause and prevention. *Ann Plast Surg*. 1997;38:594–597.

Silverton JS, Nahai F, Jurkiewicz MJ. The latissimus dorsi myocutaneous flap to replace a defect on the upper arm. *Br J Plast Surg*. 1978;31:29–31.

Stevanovic M, Sharpe F, Thommen VD, et al. Latissimus dorsi pedicle flap for coverage of soft tissue defects about the elbow. *J Shoulder Elbow Surg*. 1999;8:634–643.

Uhm K, Shin KS, Lee YH, et al. Restoration of finger extension and forearm contour utilizing a neurovascular latissimus dorsi free flap. *Ann Plast Surg*. 1988;21:74–76.

Weinrach JC, Cronin ED, Smith BK, et al. Preventing seroma in the latissimus dorsi flap donor site with fibrin sealant. *Ann Plast Surg*. 2004;53:12–16.

Zancolli E, Mitre H. Latissimus dorsi transfer to restore elbow flexion. *J Bone Joint Surg*. 1973;55A:1265–1275.

12 Fasciotomies for Forearm and Hand Compartment Syndrome

Jeffrey B. Friedrich and Alexander Y. Shin

INDICATIONS/CONTRAINDICATIONS

Indications

The chief indication for forearm and/or hand fasciotomies is essentially any suspicion that the patient has a forearm or hand compartment syndrome. The diagnosis of upper extremity compartment syndrome is made with a combination of clinical examination and objective diagnostic measurements. The clinical examination findings for upper extremity compartment syndrome traditionally have been taught as the five "P's" which include pain in the forearm and hand, increased pain with passive extensive extension of the fingers, pallor, pulselessness, and paresthesias. However, one must note that not all of these criteria need be present to determine that a patient has compartment syndrome. In fact, pulselessness can be a very late or nonexistent finding in the patient who has a compartment syndrome. Therefore, reliance on these five P's should also be balanced with other clinical examination findings as well as objective diagnostic findings. In addition to the criteria mentioned, the forearm and hand suffering from compartment syndrome will typically be very tense and swollen and can often have signs of trauma from the inciting injury, if that is the cause of the compartment syndrome. Skin changes such as blistering and a "shine" due to significant swelling are common findings as well (Fig. 12-1).

Compartment syndrome can be caused by extrinsic pressure such as casts or splints, and this possibility should be factored into the diagnostic algorithm. The first step in evaluation with a patient who is in a cast or splint is removal or loosening of the immobilization device. Other scenarios in which the physician should suspect the development of compartment syndrome include crush injuries, supracondylar humerus fractures, two-bone forearm fractures, and any situation where there has been a period of ischemia followed by reperfusion, such as brachial arterial injury, upper arm replants, or a comatose patient who has been found with the arm in compression.

Objective data are obtained to help corroborate the diagnosis of compartment syndrome, usually in the form of intracompartmental pressure measurements. These can be taken by a variety of techniques including saline infusion pressure transducers, slit or wick catheters, or even arterial pressure monitors. There are newer diagnostic tools to diagnose compartment syndrome including near-infrared spectroscopy, electromyography, myotonometry, and laser Doppler; however, these modalities are, at this point, experimental and can only be used as correlative measures at best.

If compartment syndrome is suspected, it is essential that intervention be implemented quickly to lessen injury to the underlying muscles and nerves. Increased pressure on muscle can lead to irreversible ischemia and eventual necrosis. Late sequeli of untreated compartment syndrome of the forearm produces contractures of the volar forearm commonly known as Volkmann's ischemic con-

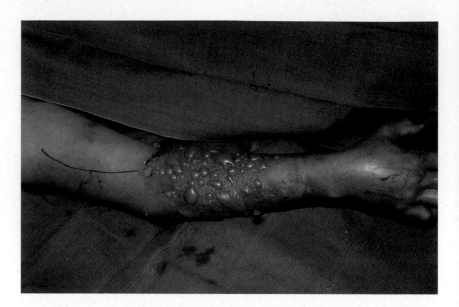

FIGURE 12-1

Patient with forearm compartment syndrome demonstrating typical cutaneous findings including tense swelling and blistering.

tracture. In general, prompt administration of surgical decompression of the forearm compartment will adequately treat the forearm compartment syndrome and leave a patient with minimal residual dysfunction.

Contraindications

While one can argue that hemodynamic instability would be a relative contraindication to upper extremity fasciotomies, it is recommended that this not be viewed as an absolute contraindication, and that once the patient is stabilized, the surgical team proceeds with forearm and/or hand fasciotomies at the earliest available time. In the worst-case scenario, fasciotomies can be performed at the bedside in the intensive care unit. In general, upper extremity compartment syndrome is an emergency and there should be no absolute contraindications to this procedure.

PREOPERATIVE PLANNING

When planning for surgical intervention for upper extremity compartment syndrome, the previously mentioned diagnostic modalities should be used to document increased forearm or hand pressures. In addition, if it is thought that the patient has developed a compartment syndrome in the setting of external compression including splints or casts, these devices should be loosened or removed immediately to help diagnose the cause of the patient's symptoms as well as provide some measure of relief from the compressive insult. Often, the removal or loosening of a cast can provide adequate treatment; but even if the patient does show resolution of symptoms, practitioners are encouraged to remain vigilant and continue to closely monitor the patient's extremity until there has been a total resolution in symptoms. Other planning should include early notification of anesthesia and operating room staff and the availability of blood for transfusion if it is indicated during the surgical procedure.

In some cases coagulopathy can contribute to or be the sole cause of compartment syndrome. Excessive bleeding following fracture reduction or continued bleeding following surgery can lead to increased compartmental pressures. If a bleeding dyathesis is suspected, appropriate steps should be taken to correct the deficiency before operative intervention.

SURGERY

Patient Positioning

Once anesthetized, the patient should be positioned in a way that affords adequate access to the entire affected upper extremity for both surgeon and assistant. This includes turning the operating table at a right angle to the anesthesia provider and placing the affected upper extremity on an arm board that is attached to the operating room table. Good lighting is essential, especially because the viability of the muscles in the forearm and hand needs to be assessed at the time of fasciotomy. While pneumatic tourniquets are frequently used for upper extremity surgery, they should not be used for a forearm fasciotomy because, as stated previously, the perfusion of the affected forearm musculature must be assessed at the time of fasciotomy.

Technique for Fasciotomy of Forearm

The classic teaching of forearm fasciotomies includes two incisions, one on the volar aspect and one on the dorsal aspect of the forearm. In general, both volar forearm compartments (superficial and deep) are decompressed via the volar incision while the dorsal compartment and the mobile wad can be adequately decompressed via the dorsal incision. A variety of incisions on the volar forearm has been proposed and has even been studied in cadavers. Ulnar sided incisions have been shown to be the safest approach to both superficial and deep volar forearm compartments, providing adequate visualization while avoiding injury to the radial artery and median nerve. Typically, the volar forearm incision extends from the antecubital fossa down to the wrist. The most common design is that of a sigmoid incision. The incision is marked beginning on the medial aspect of the elbow just anterior to the medial epicondyle, curving radially along the mid-forearm, curving back to the distal ulnar side of the forearm, and finally coming along the distal wrist crease to approximately the level of the carpal tunnel (Fig. 12-2). The purpose of this design is to, in theory, offer protection for the median nerve once decompression has been performed. The radially-based flap in the distal forearm will provide this median nerve protection even with marked edema and gaping of the wound. Once the skin incision is marked, it is incised with a scalpel. The dissection is further carried down through the subcutaneous tissues with either electrocautery or scissor dissection. Once the antebrachial fascia of the volar forearm is visualized, the fascia is incised with curved tenotomy-type scissors. The fascial division should be extended proximally and distally until the entire superficial volar forearm compartment is decompressed. Once the fascia is open, the viability of the musculature must to be assessed. If compartment syndrome is detected early and fasciotomy is employed in a rapid manner, there will typically not be any visible muscle necrosis. If, after observing the musculature for several minutes there is no reperfusion, or there is distinct necrosis of any of the forearm muscles, consideration should be given to muscle debridement at that time.

At this point only the superficial volar forearm compartment has been decompressed and the operating surgeon must then decompress and observe the musculature of the deep volar compartment as this is the area most frequently affected during a forearm compartment syndrome (Fig. 12-3). The deep volar compartment is approached through the interval between the flexor digitorum superficialis (FDS) and the flexor carpi ulnaris (FCU). The FDS muscle belly is retracted radially and the FCU muscle belly is retracted ulnarly; this allows visualization of the deep compartment and protects the median nerve and ulnar neurovascular bundle. The deep volar fascia is opened along the entire length of the flexor digitorum profundus (FDP) and flexor pollicis longus (FPL) muscle bellies. Once the fascia is incised, the muscles will quite often appear edematous and will herniate from their respective compartments. The viability of these muscles must also be assessed at the time of the procedure. Consideration should be given to excision of any distinctly necrotic muscle at the time of fasciotomy, as this can become a nidus for infection if left in situ.

Some authors believe that decompression of the volar forearm compartments will secondarily lead to adequate decompression of the dorsal forearm compartment as well as the mobile wad. However, if one is planning to take this approach it is strongly advised that compartmental pressure readings of the dorsal forearm compartment as well as the mobile wad be taken intraoperatively to con-

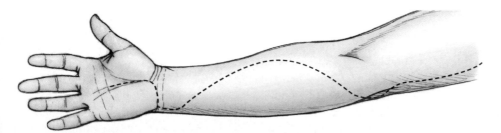

FIGURE 12-2

Incision pattern for fasciotomies of the forearm and carpal tunnel. (Adapted from Gulgonen A. Compartment syndrome. In: Green, et al, eds. *Green's operative hand surgery.* 5th ed. Philadelphia: Elsevier; 2005. With permission.)

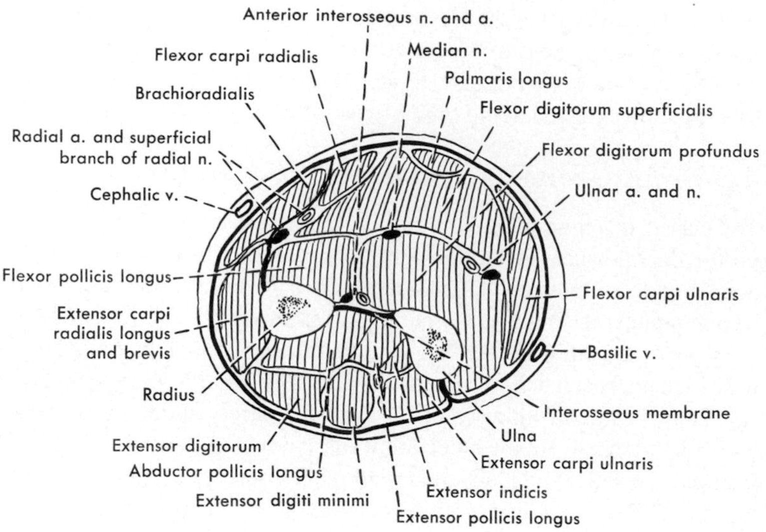

FIGURE 12-3

Cross-sectional anatomy of the mid-forearm. Note the deep position of the flexor pollicis longus and flexor digitorum profundus adjacent to the radius, ulna, and interosseus membrane. This deep position against the rigid skeleton makes these muscles particularly vulnerable to damage due to compartment syndrome (used by permission of Mayo Foundation).

firm that decompression of the volar side of the forearm has indeed led to adequate decompression of the dorsal forearm.

After completing the volar forearm decompression, the dorsal side is now approached. The incision of the dorsal forearm is in linear fashion over the midline of the forearm dorsum. Again, this is incised with a scalpel and carried down through the subcutaneous tissue with either electrocautery or scissor dissection. The dorsal forearm fascia is incised typically with tenotomy scissors along the length of the extensor muscle bellies both proximally and distally. Once the musculature of the dorsal forearm compartment has been assessed, one must then dissect in the subcutaneous plane in the radial direction to access the mobile wad. It is here that the fascia over the brachioradialis and the radial wrist extensors (extensor carpi radialis brevis and longus) is incised with scissors and, again, the musculature is assessed.

Technique for Fasciotomy of the Hand

The hand has seven compartments: the thenar, hypothenar, carpal tunnel, and four interosseus compartments. Fortunately, all seven compartments can be decompressed with only four incisions. The carpal tunnel is opened in continuity with the forearm fasciotomy. The forearm incision is carried transversely within the wrist crease to the division of the thenar and hypothenar mounds. Here the incision is carried distally to the distal point of the transverse carpal ligament (see Fig. 12-2). After dividing the skin and subcutaneous tissues, the transverse carpal ligament is divided with scissors or a scalpel, all while continually protecting the median nerve.

The thenar and hypothenar compartments are decompressed next. These incisions are made at the border of the glabrous and hair-bearing skin of the thenar and hypothenar eminences, respectively, and are approximately 3 to 4 cm long. Once the skin and fat is opened, the fascias of these compartments are also opened with spreading scissor dissection.

Finally, the four interosseus compartments can be opened with two incisions on the dorsum of the hand. These incisions are centered over the index and ring finger metacarpal bones, and are 3 to 4 cm long. After making the index metacarpal incision, scissors are used to spread radially to open the first interosseus compartment and ulnarly to open the second interosseus space. Similarly, one enters the ring metacarpal incision to spread radially into the third interosseus compartment and ulnarly into the fourth interosseus compartment (Fig. 12-4).

At this point all of the compartments of the forearm and hand have been adequately decompressed. Primary closure is usually not possible, and not advised. One should consider delayed primary closure of the forearm and hand wounds following resolution of the patient's compartment syndrome, stabilization of the patient, and assurance that there is no underlying muscle necrosis or signs of infection. Delayed primary closure can be undertaken from 1 to 7 days following a fasciotomy, depending on the health of the patient and status of the underlying tissue. Temporary retention sutures or running elastic sutures (the "Jacob's ladder" or "Roman sandal") can be placed in the wound to provide some skin approximation (Fig. 12-5), but it is not advised that full closure be

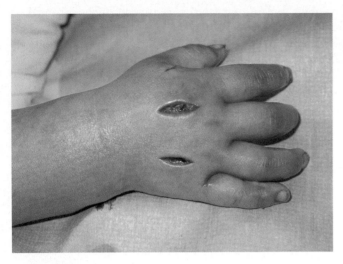

FIGURE 12-4

Two dorsal hand incisions placed over the index and ring metacarpals for decompression of the interosseus musculature of the hand.

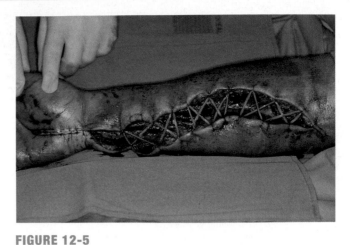

FIGURE 12-5

Partial coaptation of forearm fasciotomy wound edges using the "Roman sandal" method. Vessel loops or rubber bands are weaved across the wound to bring the skin edges closer while allowing for some expansion due to postoperative edema.

attempted at this time as this can essentially recreate a compartment syndrome due to a tight skin envelope. Another acceptable method of wound temporization is application of a negative pressure dressing, which has the dual benefit of wound fluid evacuation and prevention of further skin edge retraction.

Following initial fascial release, repeat examination under anesthesia is recommended at 24 to 48 hours; this allows the surgeon to verify that all necrotic muscle has been removed. If extremity edema has subsided, the skin may be closed with delayed primary closure. If there is any concern that closure is "tight" or that closure could recreate a compartment syndrome, a "Jacob's ladder" or negative pressure dressing is reapplied to the wound and the patient is scheduled for surgical re-evaluation in 24 to 48 hours. Delayed primary closure of both palmar and dorsal wounds may be impractical in cases where the antecedent trauma has been significant. In such cases, skin grafting may be carried out over exposed muscle bellies to expedite wound coverage and patient rehabilitation (Fig. 12-6).

POSTOPERATIVE MANAGEMENT

Postoperatively, the patient's forearm wounds should be dressed with nonadherent gauze. We most commonly use gauze impregnated with either petroleum or antibiotics to prevent wound desiccation. The patient should also be placed in a plaster or thermoplastic splint that covers the entire length of the forearm and places the hand in an intrinsic-plus position. One must take great care with the placement of this splint or cast as it can itself cause a compartment syndrome and lead to further muscle

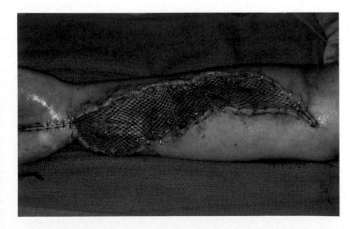

FIGURE 12-6

Forearm fasciotomy wound immediately following skin grafting.

damage despite adequate decompression of the forearm and hand compartments. In the several days between fasciotomy and wound closure, adequate wound care should be ensured. This is performed with frequent dressing changes and either whirlpool or pulse lavage type irrigation. At this time it is also wise to instruct the patient in hand motion exercises. The chief reason for these exercises is to ensure that the patient's range of motion remains relatively stable and that tendon gliding continues, especially with the flexor tendons at the wrist level.

COMPLICATIONS

As with any surgery, bleeding and hematoma are possible, especially in a forearm fasciotomy in which no tourniquet is used intraoperatively. Any open wound is prone to infection, and good wound care should be instituted to prevent this problem. Finally, the most dreaded complication of forearm fasciotomy is continued muscle necrosis and eventual fibrosis despite forearm fasciotomies. In general, this will likely not occur with adequate decompression. As stated previously, the most likely reason for continued muscle necrosis following this operation is inadequate decompression of the forearm and hand compartments.

RESULTS

In general, adequate decompression of the compartments of the forearm and hand will allow resolution of the compartment syndrome and will lead to an outcome in which the patient has no or minimal residual dysfunction, although this general scenario is not without exceptions. Most frequently, the cause of muscle necrosis and subsequent fibrosis following forearm fasciotomy is due to incomplete fasciotomy. Therefore, care must be taken intraoperatively to fully extend the fasciotomy proximally and distally, thereby decompressing the full length of all the affected muscle bellies. Following fasciotomy, patients will require diligent wound care to ensure that the wounds remain clean so that they will be ready for either delayed primary closure or skin grafting.

RECOMMENDED READING

Del Pinal F, et al. Acute hand compartment syndromes after closed crush: a reappraisal. *Plast Reconstr Surg.* 2002;110(5):1232–1239.

Elliott KG, Johnstone AJ. Diagnosing acute compartment syndrome. *J Bone Joint Surg Br.* 2003;85(5):625–632.

Gelberman RH, et al. Compartment syndromes of the forearm: diagnosis and treatment. *Clin Orthop Relat Res.* 1981;161: 252–261.

Gulgonen A. Acute compartment syndrome. In: Green, et al, eds. *Green's operative hand surgery.* Philadelphia: Elsevier;2005:1986–1996.

McQueen MM, Gaston P, Court-Brown CM. Acute compartment syndrome. Who is at risk? *J Bone Joint Surg Br.* 2000;82(2):200–203.

Naidu SH, Heppenstall RB. Compartment syndrome of the forearm and hand. *Hand Clin.* 1994;10(1):13–27.

Tsuge K. Treatment of established Volkmann's contracture. *J Bone Joint Surg Am.* 1975;57(7):925–929.

13 Soft Tissue Interposition Flaps in the Management of Heterotopic Ossification and Proximal Radioulnar Synostosis

Douglas P. Hanel and Seth D. Dodds

INDICATIONS/CONTRAINDICATIONS

Heterotopic ossification of the elbow with loss of motion can be severely debilitating. The functional arc of elbow motion spans from 30 to 130 degrees of flexion and from 50 degrees of pronation to 50 degrees of supination. Limitations to this functional arc significantly impair the ability to perform activities of daily living. Cases of elbow ankylosis or radioulnar synostosis further minimize use of the affected extremity. Once heterotopic ossification has developed and constricts motion, it is nearly impossible to regain the lost motion with conservative measures, such as physical therapy, dynamic splinting, radiation therapy, or medication.

Surgical resection of heterotopic bone about the elbow should be considered in patients who present with an unacceptable loss of flexion/extension or pronation/supination. Excision is also warranted in cases of neurovascular impingement caused by ectopic bone. In cases of proximal radioulnar synostosis or even radial head excision, interposition materials can be used to cover exposed bone surfaces.

While options for soft tissue interposition include silicone sheeting, fat graft, and free adipofascial flaps, pedicled myofascial flaps and allograft fascia lata have become increasingly popular. The pedicled anconeus myofascial flap is an ideal choice in those cases approached posterolaterally, whereas the pedicled brachioradialis muscle flap passed through the interosseous membrane is best suited for those cases approached from an anterior exposure. The soft tissue interposition acts as a barrier to the formation of recurrent heterotopic calcification and allegedly decreases pain with pronation and supination. It is suggested, though unproven, that pedicled graft tissue has greater potential for sustained viability when judged against nonvascularized tissue transfers, such as subcutaneous fat or an adipose fascial graft. When properly fixed to the underlying bone, these pedicled flaps can sustain aggressive postoperative range-of-motion exercises that might dislodge less robust tissue such as fat alone or adipose-fascial grafts. We prefer the anconeus muscle pedicle flap when available and tensor fascia lata allograft when the anconeus is not available or not large enough.

Historically, contraindications to excision of heterotopic bone with or without soft tissue interposition flaps included immature ossification and an unreliable soft tissue envelope. In the past decade there have been a number of reports documenting the efficacy of early excision of heterotopic bone. It is our experience that patients suffer less soft tissue contracture and have superior function with early release of a stiff elbow. The recurrence of heterotopic bone in the posttraumatic setting has not been shown to be predicated on the timing of the excision. Outcomes of surgical excision, however, will be threatened by a poor soft tissue envelope. Once the posttraumatic or post-burn wounds have healed, soft tissue swelling has abated, and nerve recovery has plateaued, patients may safely undergo elbow contracture release.

Contraindications to pedicled soft tissue interposition flaps depend on the specific muscle selected. For an anconeus muscle interposition, previous traumatic or surgical disruption of its primary vascular supply (the medial collateral artery from the profunda brachii) jeopardizes the viability of the raised muscle flap. The brachioradialis "wrap around" flap should not be raised if there is a nonfunctioning biceps brachii or brachialis, as the brachioradialis provides assistance with elbow flexion as well as supination when the forearm is fully pronated. Assuming that the arm and forearm musculature is intact, using the anconeus or brachioradialis as a pedicled interposition flap causes little functional loss.

PREOPERATIVE PLANNING

Before operative release and soft tissue interposition, patients must be carefully evaluated. The history should focus on the primary complaint. Patients must verbalize appropriate frustration with their disability from elbow stiffness to warrant release. It is also imperative that patients demonstrate the willingness and capacity for intensive rehabilitation. If the presenting complaint is predominantly pain, then contracture release will be futile. A focused surgical history needs to be elicited. Previous injuries and surgeries of the involved extremity offer critical information about the status of osseous and cartilaginous structures as well as the elbow's soft tissue envelope. Operative reports from previous surgeries help understand the integrity and location of possibly transposed neurovascular structures.

Elbow range of motion, stability, pain, and functional ability are assessed. The Mayo Elbow Performance Score serves as a summary of these findings. In addition, the examination includes assessment of forearm rotation and wrist and hand function. If there is physical evidence of nerve dysfunction, electrodiagnostic studies should be obtained to confirm the location of compression and to act as a baseline of nerve function. All of our patients have had previous surgeries, and as such, a careful assessment of incisions about the elbow with regard to the palpable and radiographic location of heterotopic ossification is essential. The integrity of the skin and subcutaneous tissues should be evaluated. Lingering soft tissue swelling, edema, or erythema may all point to additional diagnoses to be contended with before deciding on heterotopic bone excision.

Standard radiographs of the elbow are obtained with oblique views to improve visualization of ectopic ossification. We routinely perform computed tomography (CT) on cases of elbow heterotopic ossification where the congruity of the articular surface is in question and in all cases with proximal radioulnar synostosis. An axial CT scan with coronal and sagittal reformatted images is currently the most helpful method to visualize the location and extent of a bony bridge between the radius and ulna (Figs. 13-1 and 13-2). Vascular study of the elbow and proximal forearm should be considered if there are concerns about the integrity of the regional blood supply, especially in cases of pedicled soft tissue interposition. Unless there are specific historical or physical findings suggesting potential or indolent infection, we limit blood studies to those required for a prolonged general anesthetic.

The timing for intervention is somewhat nebulous and is certainly directed by physician bias. We do not believe there is sufficient scientific evidence to suggest that nuclear medicine scans or blood alkaline phosphatase levels are beneficial in the assessment or timing of surgical intervention. In reviewing the literature and comparing our experience, it would appear that waiting for fracture heal-

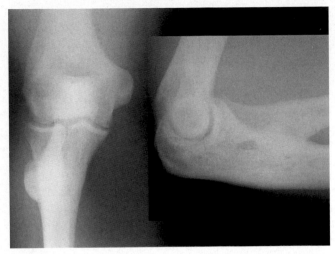

FIGURE 13-1

The anteroposterior and lateral elbow radiographs of a 42-year-old power lifter 8 weeks after a single incision repair of distal biceps tendon rupture. The forearm is ankylosed in mid pronation-supination.

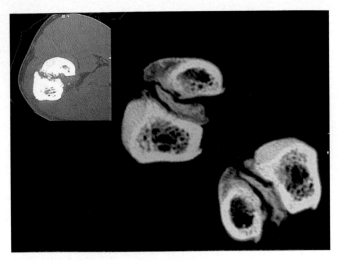

FIGURE 13-2

Coronal CT image reveals the extent of heterotopic bone involvement in the region of the bicipital tuberosity.

ing and ectopic bone maturation, defined as well-delineated borders, is the most commonly used parameters. This would suggest that operative intervention be carried out 4 to 12 months after injury.

Excision of heterotopic ossification and soft tissue flap interposition does not require a great deal of special equipment. We have listed a few items that facilitate operative intervention and postoperative rehabilitation in Table 13-1. In addition to the tools listed in the table, we have the following items readily available: a hinged fixator, radial head prosthetics, allograft tendon for ligament reconstruction, allograft fascia lata if local interposition material is not available, and a total elbow arthroplasty set when all else fails and the patient is the appropriate age.

SURGERY

Patient Positioning

Operative approach and patient positioning are determined by previous incisions, location of heterotopic bone or synostosis, and shoulder mobility. While many surgeons prefer to operate on the elbow with the affected extremity positioned across the patient's supine chest, we prefer to position

TABLE 13-1. Soft Tissue Interposition Flaps for Elbow Heterotopic Ossification: Operative Equipment	
Standard Equipment	**Optional Equipment**
Sterile tourniquet	Fluoroscopy
Retractors, thyroid type	Hardware removal instruments
(long and narrow)	Total elbow arthroplasty
Lamina spreader	Lidocaine infusion pump
Vessel loops	Continuous passive motion machine
Rongeurs	Postoperative radiation therapy
(including Kerrison and pituitary)	Static progressive vs. dynamic splinting
Osteotomes and curettes	
Suture anchors	
Hinged elbow distractor	
Tensor fascia lata allograft	
Closed suction drain	

the patient with the affected extremity abducted onto a radiolucent table. The extremity is draped free up to the clavicle. If the shoulder is mobile, external rotation will present the medial and anterior aspects of the elbow while internal rotation presents the lateral and posterior elbow. The flexibility to effortlessly alternate between lateral and medial approaches facilitates complete excision of heterotopic bone about the elbow.

Technique

Exposure   We do not use tourniquets for these cases. They are a detriment to tissue mobilization, mask small arterial bleeding, and lead to venous engorgement during prolonged cases. The initial increase in bleeding at the time of incision is mitigated by injecting the proposed incision with 0.25% bupivacaine and 1/200,000 dilute epinephrine solution. The incision is delayed 7 to 10 minutes to allow the epinephrine to affect local capillaries.

It is our preference to use a posterior skin incision for elbow release surgery. This window allows a "global" approach to the elbow and can be used to access the medial, lateral, and anterior sides of the joint. The skin incision is typically straight, passing 2 cm medial or lateral to the tip of the olecranon, but may be curvilinear to incorporate previously placed posteromedial or posterolateral surgical scars. Depending on the required heterotopic bone excision or hardware removal, the incision may extend from the proximal arm to the distal forearm. This dissection avoids injury to both the medial and the lateral brachial cutaneous nerves, preserving sensibility to the proximal forearm.

When employing this approach, it is critical to create thick soft tissue flaps. The skin incision is carried down to and includes the triceps fascia proximally and the extensor fascia of the forearm distally. This effectively creates robust fasciocutaneous flaps that can be elevated circumferentially about the elbow. The extent of elevation is dictated by the location of the joint involvement. If there is medial joint involvement, as determined by CT scan, or ulnar nerve symptoms, we address these first. If there is no involvement we go directly to the lateral elbow and proximal forearm. The dissection is carried to the medial intermuscular septum, and the ulnar nerve is identified as it passes from the anterior to the posterior compartment approximately 8 to 10 cm proximal to the medial epicondyle. Even if the ulnar nerve has been "transposed anteriorly" in previous procedures, we believe that it is critical to identify the entire medial intermuscular septum, and follow it to the humerus (Fig. 13-3). In cases in which the medial intermuscular septum has been excised in part or in whole, the dissection follows the medial border of the triceps until the humerus is encountered. When the ulnar nerve is found, it should be mobilized from the cubital tunnel, preferably with a small cuff of medial triceps to protect the nerve's vascular supply. The nerve is followed into the forearm until disappeared deeply between the heads of the flexor carpi ulnaris. Any tight scar or fascial bands crossing the nerve in this dissection are divided. The medial intermuscular septum is removed in its entirety. By following the ulnar nerve proximally in the arm, the median nerve and its accompanying brachial artery can be located along the anterior margin of the intermuscular septum. Alternatively, in arms that are not densely scarred the median nerve and brachial artery can be identified in the distal arm superior to the leading edge of the pronator teres origin as it runs medial to the substance of the biceps and brachialis muscles and just beneath the fibers of the bicipital aponeurosis. Excision of heterotopic bone involving the medial posterior and anterior elbow joint is conducted and described in greater detail in the next section.

Next, the lateral side of the elbow and involvement of the proximal forearm are addressed. In cases of anterolateral heterotopic ossification, the radial nerve is identified at mid-arm and followed distally. This is done by elevating the lateral flap in the same tissue plane as the medial dissection, between the muscular investing fascia and the muscle belly of the triceps. When the lateral intermuscular septum is encountered, the radial nerve should be identified and protected. Identifying the radial nerve in a scarred bed can be daunting. We therefore use the following strategies. First, inspect the undersurface of the flap; frequently the posterior antebrachial cutaneous branches of the radial nerve to arm and forearm are visible. These branches can be followed proximally into the lateral intermuscular septum where they are found to take off from the radial nerve proper (Fig. 13-4). If this landmark is not readily available, our second approach is to dissect the distal portion of the flap toward the lateral epicondyle. On reaching the lateral intermuscular septum, the dissection is directed cephalad. The triceps muscle belly is freed from the posterior aspect of the intermuscular septum. Small vessels and nerves seen entering the triceps muscle should be followed proximally; they will lead to the radial nerve proper. If these markers fail to lead to the nerve, cautiously proceed along the posterior intermuscular septum. Somewhere between 6 and 10 cm proximal to the tip of

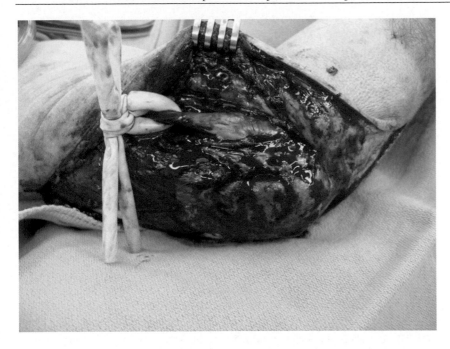

FIGURE 13-3

This previously "transposed ulnar nerve" sits directly on the medial epicondyle. It is essential to identify and protect the ulnar nerve before proceeding with capsular and heterotopic bone resection.

the lateral epicondyle, the nerve will be encountered passing along the spiral groove to pass through the lateral intermuscular septum to enter the anterior aspect of the arm. Once the radial nerve is identified, the lateral intermuscular septum is removed and the nerve followed distally. At the level of the elbow, the nerve is easily followed into the internervous plane between the proximal aspect of the brachioradialis and the distal aspect of the brachialis. Simple blunt dissection between these two muscles just superior to the joint line will reveal the radial nerve before it dives under the supinator more distally.

Excision of Heterotopic Bone   The excision of heterotopic bone and the scarred joint capsule follows. Anterior heterotopic bone frequently resides in the distal aspect of the brachialis muscle. It can extend medially and laterally encasing the collateral ligaments or even neighboring neurovascular structures. If a medial approach is chosen, entrance to the joint capsule and distal aspect of the brachialis can be achieved by exploiting the internervous plane between the ulnar innervated

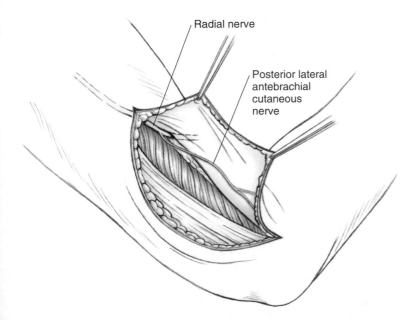

Radial nerve

Posterior lateral antebrachial cutaneous nerve

FIGURE 13-4

The posterior antebrachial cutaneous nerve is identified distally and followed proximally into the lateral intermuscular septum. This cutaneous nerve leads to the radial nerve proper. The radial nerve proper can then be followed from into the anterior compartment of the arm.

flexor carpi ulnaris and the median innervated palmaris longus, flexor carpi radialis, and pronator teres. Alternatively, the flexor-pronator muscle mass can be sharply elevated off the medial epicondyle, carefully preserving the underlying anterior band of the medial collateral ligament. In severely contracted elbows, this exposure affords uncompromised visualization of the anterior capsule and crossing neurovascular bundle. This elevated myofascial flap can be reattached to the medial epicondyle with multiple suture anchors or sutured down to the epicondyle through bone tunnels. If the flexor-pronator mass is released, consideration can be given to submuscular transposition of the ulnar nerve.

The anterolateral aspect of the elbow is approached next. If there is complete elbow flexion and extension, the dissection is directed toward the posterolateral forearm. In cases in which the anterior joint needs to be exposed, one of three intervals is used (Fig. 13-5). The first approach, and in our experience the most frequently used, elevates the proximal most portion of the muscle taking origin from the medial epicondyle, usually the brachioradialis and a portion of the extensor carpi radialis longus. The dissection is carried medially, sweeping the brachialis from the front of the humerus. The interval between this muscle and the anterior joint capsule is developed. Heterotopic bone, if encountered, is dissected with blunt-tipped elevators and left attached to the anterior joint structures. If the relationship between these structures and the radial nerve is doubtful, the nerve is again identified in the distal arm and followed into the area of joint dissection. Under direct visualization, a blunt right-angled retractor is placed in the interval between the anterior joint dissection and the more superficially located muscle and nerve. The dissection stops distally when the coronoid process is encountered or the heterotopic bone becomes confluent the forearm bones. The entire anterior joint capsule and the heterotopic bone are removed. The coronoid fossa is cleared of soft tissues. Two other approaches to the anterolateral elbow consist of developing the interval between the anconeus and extensor carpi ulnaris, or the interval between the extensor carpi radialis brevis origin and the extensor digitorum communis. Both dissections allow easy access to the joint capsule overlying the radial head and neck. The capsular, radial, and annular portion of the lateral collateral ligament complex can be reflected or excised to expose the joint. The ulnar portion of the lateral collateral ligament, if not encased in ectopic bone, should be preserved (Fig. 13-6). More often than not, elevation of the lateral elbow complex from the ulna it is necessary. The ligamentous attachments will be reconstructed after the ectopic bone has been excised. If visualization of the anterior joint capsule is insufficient with these intermuscular approaches, the origin of the brachioradialis and extensor carpi radialis longus is elevated as described previously.

The posterior elbow joint is approached from the lateral side by elevating the triceps muscle from the lateral column of the distal humerus and developing the interval between triceps muscle and the posterior joint capsule. The triceps muscle insertion onto the olecranon is preserved. The posterior capsule, the contents of the olecranon fossa, and any bony impediments to elbow motion arising from theses posterior structures are debrided.

Proximal Radioulnar Synostosis Takedown In cases in which pathology is limited to the proximal radioulnar joint in the vicinity of the bicipital tuberosity, the synostosis may be approached by sweeping the entire anconeus and ulnar origin of the extensor carpi ulnaris complex off of the

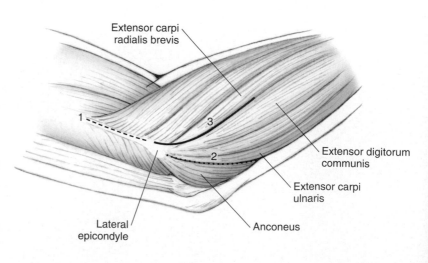

FIGURE 13-5

Three intervals used to approach the anterior lateral elbow. (1) Partial elevation of the muscles taking origin from the lateral epicondyle, the brachioradialis, and cephalad portion of the extensor carpi ulnaris. (2) Anconeus and extensor carpi ulnaris. (3) Extensor carpi radialis brevis and extensor digitorum communis.

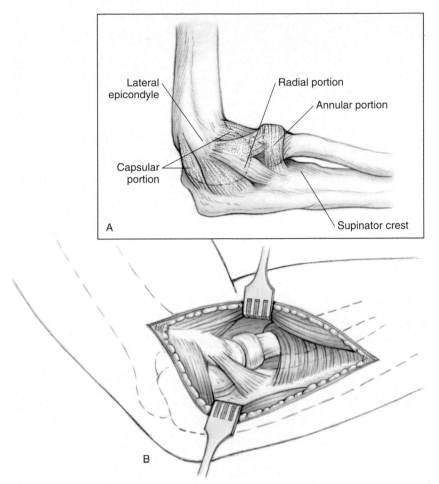

FIGURE 13-6

A: Lateral collateral ligament complex of the elbow consisting of the capsular, radial, and annular portions (*stippled*) removed to expose the lateral elbow articulations. **B:** The stippled portion of Figure 13-6A has been removed, exposing the radial head and neck, and the distal humerus. Preserving the ulnar portion of lateral collateral ligament (*shaded area*), when possible, preserves elbow stability.

posterolateral edge of the proximal ulna (Fig. 13-7A–C). The dissection along the proximal ulna is carried along the radial edge to the base of the synostosis and followed along the interosseous space until the radius is encountered. If the forearm can be pronated, there should be no danger to the posterior interosseous nerve. A pronated forearm allows the posterior interosseous nerve to lay anteriorly and medially protected in the substance of the supinator muscle. However, a supinated forearm does just the opposite. In cases where the forearm is ankylosed in supination, consideration should be given to locating the posterior interosseous nerve before the posterior dissection. This usually requires an anterior incision immediately adjacent to the ulnar border of the brachioradialis. The radial nerve is found in the interval between the brachioradialis and brachialis muscle and followed distally until it is seen to divide into the posterior interosseous nerve (PIN) and the superficial branch of the radial nerve. The PIN is followed distally into the supinator muscle. The arcade of Frohse is divided along with fibrosed muscle and scarred tissue that could lead to potential compression injury during the dissection. The posterior dissection is then resumed.

Once the anconeus is elevated, tissue retraction is maintained by broad right-angled retractors or broad Homan retractors. Narrow lever arm type retractors are avoided. Although anecdotal, it is thought that narrow retractors place excessive pressure on adjacent neurovascular structures, especially the PIN.

Synostosis resection proceeds using a combination of small rongeurs, osteotomes, and Kerrison rongeurs. Small lamina spreaders help retract the proximal radius and proximal ulna, opening up the space between. Once the synostosis has been released and there is freedom between the two bones, the lamina spreader offers greater direct visualization of remaining ectopic bone. The synostosis can now be excised down to the native cortices of the proximal radius and proximal ulna. It is imperative that the exposed bony surfaces be debrided to a smooth surface. Sharp edges combined with forearm rotation will penetrate and disrupt interposition flaps.

Intraoperative radiography is used to demonstrate the thoroughness of the ectopic bone excision. On completion of the resection, the surgical field is irrigated with 3 L of normal saline. Bleeding

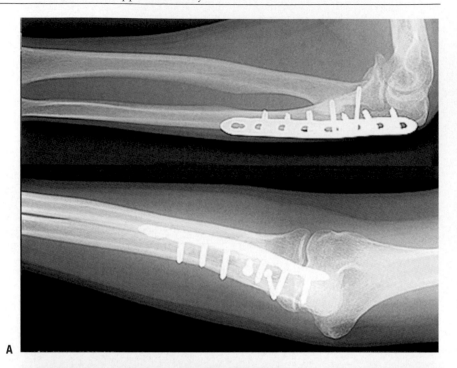

A

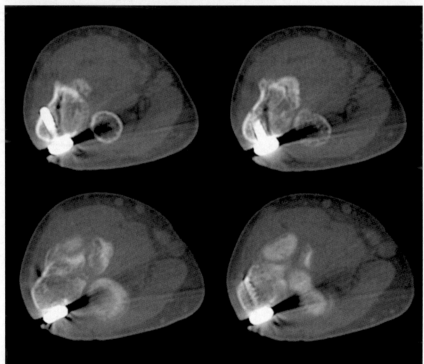

FIGURE 13-7

A: This patient developed a radioulnar synostosis after treatment of a Monteggia fracture. **B:** The CT scans demonstrate the location of the synostosis adjacent to the bicipital tuberosity. *(Continued)*

B

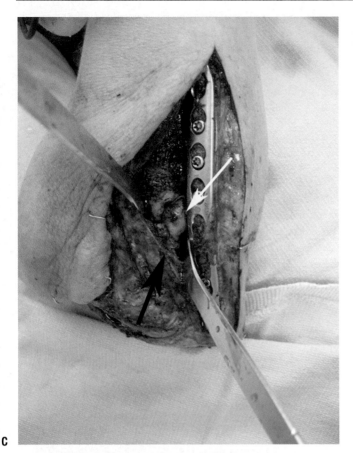

C

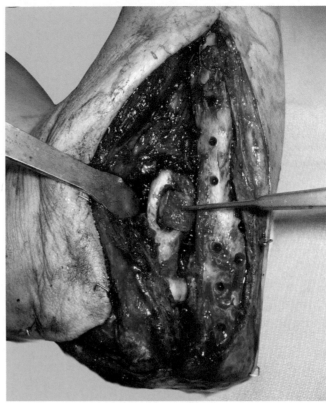

E

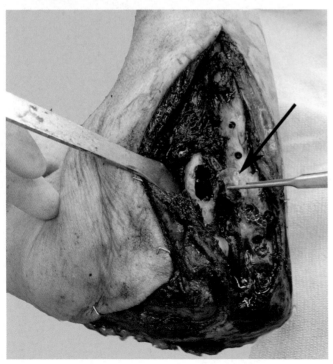

D

FIGURE 13-7

Continued **C:** The entire anconeus and extensor carpi ulnaris complex have been elevated from the ulna (*dark arrow*), exposing the bridge of heterotopic bone between the radius and ulna (*light arrow*). **D:** The synostosis encased the bicipital tuberosity and tendon. The ectopic bone was removed, and the tendon left attached to a block of heterotopic bone (*dark arrow*). The resection exposed the medullary canal of the radius. The fixation plate was removed. **E:** The medullary canal is packed with allograft bone chips to minimize extrusion of marrow content. The biceps tendon and attached bone block are pushed into the medullary canal and secured with a stout nonabsorbable points in soft tissues are coagulated, and bleeding points in exposed bone are sealed with bone wax. If the medullary canal of either the radius or ulna is breached, the hole is packed with allograft bone graft soaked in thrombin. This stops the marrow content from flowing into the operative field (see Fig. 13-7D,E).

Interposition Material   Even with meticulous technique, the proximity of the proximal radius and ulna to each other makes these structures prone to recurrent synostosis. Some type of interposition material is a useful preventative adjunct. Three techniques are discussed in the following section. Each of these procedures is preceded with copious irrigation of the synostosis site and diligent hemostasis as described previously.

Pedicled Anconeus Myofascial Flap Interposition   The anconeus myofascial flap receives its blood supply from the collateral circulation about the elbow, predominantly the medial collateral artery (MCA) branch of the profunda brachii artery and venae commitantes (Fig. 13-8). The muscle is elevated from the posterior lateral border of the ulna, usually in a distal to proximal direction. The distal edge starts roughly at the junction of the proximal and mid one-third of the fore-

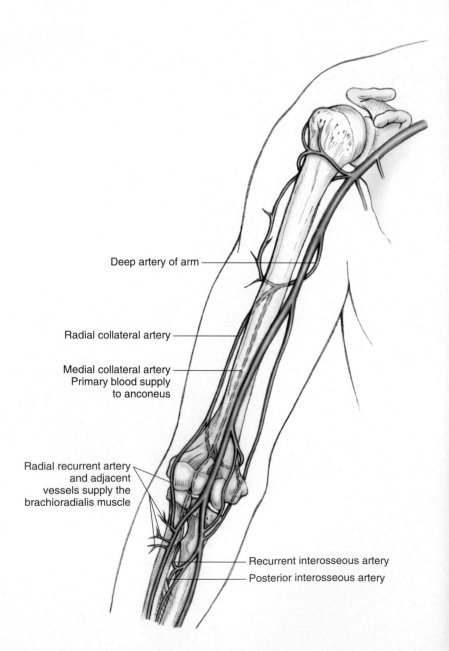

FIGURE 13-8

The arterial anatomy of the distal arm. The medial collateral artery (MCA), a branch of the profunda brachii, is the primary blood supply to the anconeus. The radial recurrent artery (RRA), a branch of the radial artery, and small arterial branches within 3 cm of the RRA, provide the primary blood supply to the brachioradialis muscle.

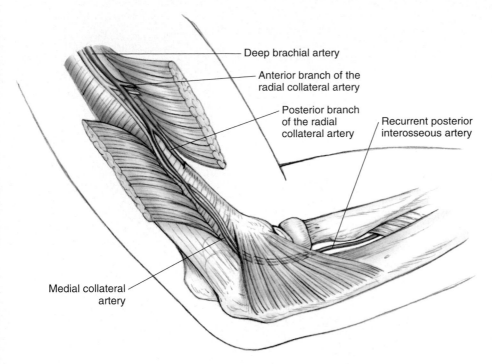

FIGURE 13-9

In addition to the medial collateral artery (MCA), the anconeus receives blood supply distally from the recurrent posterior interosseous artery (RPIA). These vessels (the MCA and RPIA) frequently form an anastomosis on the deep surface of the anconeus. The RPIA is frequently sacrificed in the process of elevating this flap. (From Schmidt CC, Kohut GN, Greenberg JA, Kann SE, Idler RS, Kiefhaber TR. The anconeus muscle flap: its anatomy and clinical application. *J Hand Surg Am.* 1999;24(2):359-369. With permission.)

arm. A stout septum separates this muscle from the flexor carpi ulnaris. Identification of this septum and the anconeus itself may be difficult if previous surgery or initial trauma has injured the muscle. In these cases, an alternative material may be required.

Elevation of the flap is carried up to the lateral epicondyle until sufficient freedom exists to permit mobilization of the tissue's leading edge to the distal extent of the synostosis. By protecting the proximal origin and the lateral fascial attachments of the triceps, the medial collateral artery of the elbow can be preserved. The anconeus also receives blood supply distally from the recurrent posterior interosseous artery (RPIA). These vessels (the MCA and RPIA) frequently form an anatomosis on the deep surface of the anconeus (Fig. 13-9). The RPIA is usually sacrificed in the process of removing the synostosis or in elevating this flap.

The distal end of the anconeus flap is attached to the ulnar edge of the biceps tuberosity while the forearm is placed in full pronation. Sutures alone or suture anchors placed into the proximal radius or biceps tendon secure the anconeus flap with mattress or Bunnel locking stitches. Now, as the forearm is supinated, the anconeus will be drawn into the proximal radioulnar space where the synostosis previously lay—creating a thin, pedicled interposition flap of viable muscle and fascia (Fig. 13-10).

The utility of the anconeus myofascial interposition flap has recently been expanded by Morrey and Schneeberger to include soft tissue interposition between the capitellum and the proximal radius in cases of radial head excision or failed radial head arthroplasty (Fig. 13-11). Three interposition options are described: type I, interposition at the radiocapitellar joint; type II, the muscle is brought

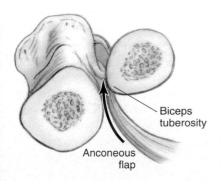

FIGURE 13-10

With the forearm placed in full pronation, the distal end of the anconeus flap is attached to the ulnar edge of the biceps tuberosity (BT) with a suture anchor or direct stitch into the biceps tendon. As the forearm is supinated (*arrow*), the anconeus will be drawn into the proximal radioulnar space.

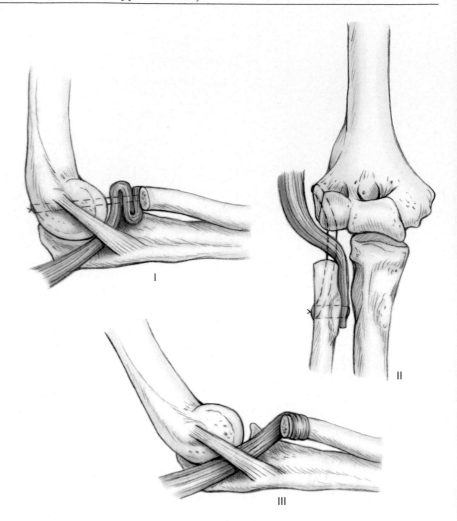

FIGURE 13-11

Three interposition options for the anconeus flap after radial head resection: type I, radiocapitellar joint: type II, radiocapitellar and proximal radioulnar joint; and type III, proximal radioulnar wrap. (From Morrey BF, Schneeberger AG. Anconeus arthroplasty: a new technique for reconstruction of the radiocapitellar and/or proximal radioulnar joint. *J Bone Joint Surg Am.* 2002;84-A(11):1960–1969. With permission.)

posterior to the intact fibers of the ulnar portion of the lateral ulnar collateral ligament and interposed between radiocapitellar and proximal radioulnar joint; and type III, proximal radioulnar wrap. In each type of interposition, the muscle is secured with stout suture placed through drill holes.

Distally based anconeus myofascial flaps composed of anconeus and some neighboring extensor carpi ulnaris have been described. This flap depends on an intact RPIA for its blood supply, a small vessel that is easily injured during the initial fracture fixation or during resection of a synostosis. Distally based anconeus flaps may have application in the management of soft tissue defects not associated with elbow fractures such as burns or skin avulsion but should be used with caution in the setting of synostosis resection.

The proximally based anconeus pedicle flap can also be used to provide soft tissue coverage of small defects about the traumatized elbow. Three areas where this muscle will reach is the lateral epicondyle, the posterior surface of the olecranon, and the distal radial aspect of the triceps insertion into the olecranon. The muscle is elevated, rotated over the defect, and covered with split thickness skin grafts.

Pedicled Brachioradialis Myofascial Flap Interposition   The brachioradialis interposition flap is useful when resection of a radioulnar synostosis is performed through a combined anterior and posterior approach. The posterior incision and approach is the same as described previously: the anconeus-extensor carpi ulnaris interval is developed, the supinator sharply elevated from the ulna, and the synostosis excised. The anterior approach is conducted through a longitudinal incision made along the ulnar border of the brachioradialis, from the elbow flexion crease to the distal forearm. The superficial branch of the radial nerve is located in the distal forearm and carefully dissected from the undersurface of the brachioradialis. This nerve is followed proximally into the cephalad region of antecubital fossa where it is found to branch from the radial nerve. At this level the radial nerve branches to the brachioradialis, and extensor carpi radialis muscle may be encountered and is protected. Most important, the posterior interosseous nerve branch is identified and followed into the substance of the supinator muscle. The stout fibers on the leading edge of the supinator, the arcade of Frohse, are a potential source for compression during the remainder of the procedure and are divided. Simultaneously with the dissection of the radial nerve, the radial artery and its branches to the lateral elbow are encountered and protected. The largest of these branches, the radial recurrent artery, is found crossing from ulnar to radial, just distal to the biceps tendon (see Fig. 13-8). Care is taken to preserve not only the radial recurrent artery, but also the branches of the radial artery just distal to the radial recurrent artery. While the proximal aspect of the brachioradialis muscle belly is vascularized by the radial recurrent artery, the distal aspect of the muscle receives its blood supply from the arborization of the radial artery approximately 3 cm distal to the radial recurrent artery. In this dissection the median nerve and the ulnar artery are shielded by the medially retracted flexor-pronator muscle mass on the ulnar aspect of the proximal forearm.

Once these pertinent neurovascular structures are dissected free and protected, attention can be turned to the synostosis excision. Typically, the heterotrophic bone is found within or deep to the supinator muscle as it extends between the proximal radius and ulna. This anterior approach is helpful to visualize and debride the full extent of bridging bone in complex or revision cases of synostosis resection. After the synostosis has been taken down and the exposed bone edges covered with bone wax, the pedicled brachioradialis myofascial interposition flap is raised (see Fig. 13-12).

The tendon of the brachioradialis is divided and the muscle raised from distal to proximal. The previously identified neurovascular structures are left intact. Although the muscle can be released proximally from its origin on the lateral epicondyle and lateral intermuscular septum, this is usually not necessary; the muscle typically provides enough length for interposition between the proximal radius and ulna.

The muscle is interposed between the radius and ulna from anterior to posterior and secured in one of two ways. The first is to secure muscle to the posterior surface of the fully supinated radius using suture anchors or drill holes. When the forearm is pronated, the muscle is advanced into the interosseous space. The second method, introduced by Diego Fernandez, wraps the muscle around the proximal radius, deep to the superficial branch of the radial nerve, and is sutured to itself with locking sutures. Passing the stitches through the muscle fascia as well as through some of the tendonous fibers optimizes the fixation of this interposition flap to the bone.

In addition to being used for an interposition material, the brachioradialis can be used as a myofasciocutaneous flap to provide coverage for medium-sized elbow defects. The skin over the brachioradialis, centered on the radial recurrent artery, may be harvested up to 2 to 3 cm in width and 6 to 10 cm in length from proximal to distal. A narrow skin paddle permits primary closure of the donor site. Alternatively, the muscle alone can be elevated, inset, and split thickness skin graft is applied over it. The brachioradialis flap can be safely rotated to reach soft tissue defects involving the antecubital fossa, the volar one-third of the forearm, and the posterolateral aspect of the elbow between the lateral epicondyle and the olecranon.

Tensor Fascia Lata Interposition   There are certainly cases of heterotopic ossification and radioulnar synostosis in which transposing a local muscle flap may be difficult or impossible. Most frequently these are cases in which the anconeus was injured during the initial traumatic event and where the extensive dissection of the brachioradialis muscle and additional scars are avoidable. In such circumstances, an alternative approach is to use tensor fascia lata (TFL) for interposition. Autograft TFL has the advantage of biocompatibility but the marked disadvantage of donor site morbidity including superficial nerve injury, additional site of scarring, and asymmetry of the thigh secondary to muscle herniation. Given the potential complications and the reality that the interposition graft (whether autograft or allograft) is not living tissue after harvest, we have abandoned the use of autograft TFL in favor of allograft.

The technique is straightforward. Following synostosis exposure and resection, the tensor fascia lata allograft is shaped to cover the exposed bone. A graft 10 to 12 cm long and 4 to 5 cm wide is required in most cases. The tensor fascia lata graft is wrapped around the most accessible bone, usually the ulna, and sutured into place using absorbable sutures (see Fig. 13-13). With a complete wrap, the graft can simply be sutured to itself or neighboring soft tissues to maintain its position. Another technique is to suture the graft to the exposed surface of the ulna, interpose it between the radius and ulna, securing to the exposed surface of the fully pronated radius with suture anchors. As the forearm supinates, the graft follows the radius and provides an effective barrier to reformation of the synostosis. The TFL, once secured to the underlying bone, creates an intact, but not water tight, sleeve

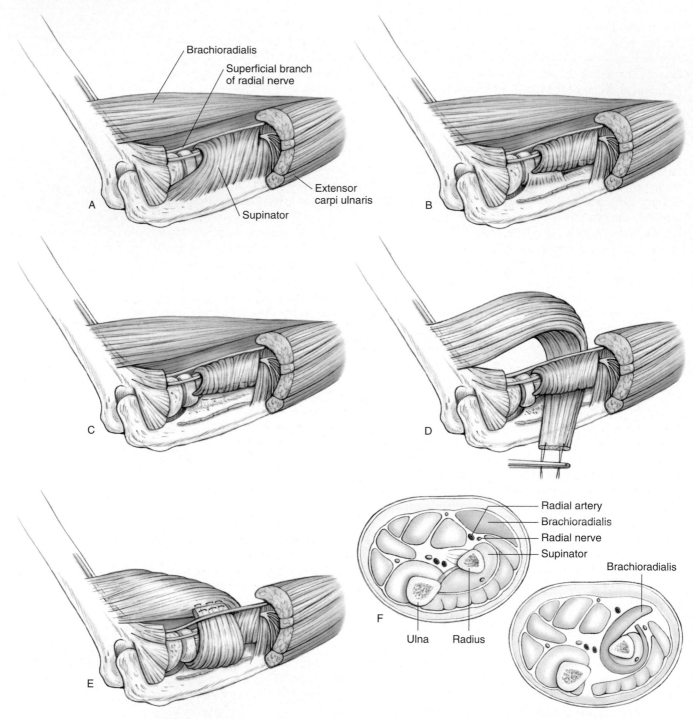

FIGURE 13-12

A: Posterior lateral approach (Kocher). Through a separate incision, the interval between the anconeus and extensor carpi ulnaris is developed. **B:** The supinator is sharply elevated off of the ulna exposing the radioulnar synostosis. **C:** The synostosis is removed and if necessary the interosseous ligament-membrane is excised. **D:** A separate anterior incision runs just ulnar to the brachioradialis muscle. The tendon is divided distally, the superficial branch of the radial nerve is separated from the under belly of the muscle, and the vascular bundles entering the muscle in the proximal forearm are preserved. The muscle is passed through the interosseous space created by the resection. **E:** The tail of the muscle is brought deep to the radial nerve and sutured to the proximal muscle belly. **F:** Cross-section of the forearm. Note the muscle passes radial to the radial artery in the mid forearm, distal to the biceps tendon and deep to the superficial branch of the radial nerve. (From Fernandez DL, Joneschild E. "Wrap around" pedicled muscle flaps for the treatment of recurrent forearm synostosis. *Tech Hand Up Extrem Surg.* 2004;8(2):102–109. With permission.)

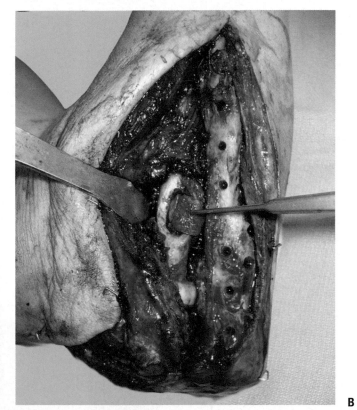

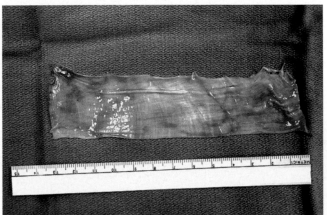

A

B

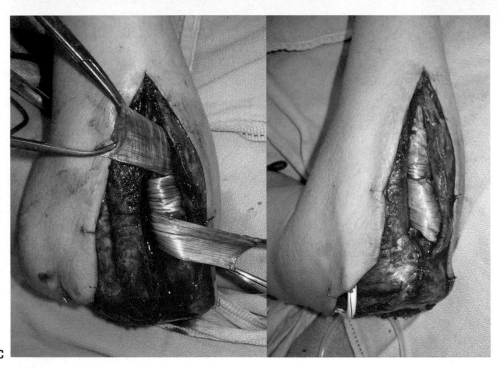

C

FIGURE 13-13

A: This 4 × 14 cm tensor fascia lata allograft will be used as an interposition material. **B:** This is the forearm of the patient shown in Figure 13-7. After synostosis resection, the rough surfaces of the radius and the ulna are prone to reformation of the synostosis. **C:** The tensor fascia lata allograft is wrapped around the ulna and secured with stout absorbable sutures. *(Continued)*

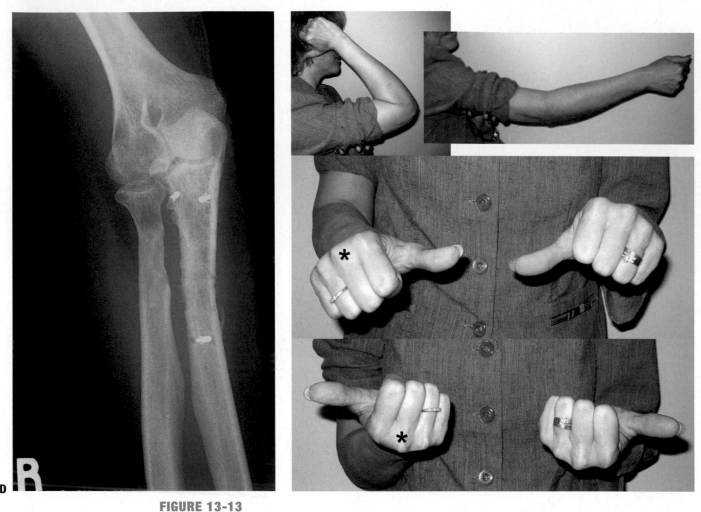

FIGURE 13-13

Continued **D:** Radiographs of the elbow 6 months postoperatively. **E:** Range of motion 6 months postoperatively.

around the proximal aspect of one of the forearm bones. The goals of this type of fascial interposition are twofold: to provide painless forearm rotation and to act as a barrier to future bridging heterotopic bone.

Closure   After heterotopic bone excision from an elbow, medial or lateral instability frequently arises. If the collateral ligaments have been excised, they should be reconstructed. Allograft tendon provides an alternative to harvesting autogenous palmaris longus or plantaris for these patients. Using either form of collagen, a tendon reconstruction can be performed with a combination of suture anchors and bone tunnels. Care should be given to reconstructing the anterior band of the medial collateral ligament and the ulnar band of the lateral collateral ligament, as these ligaments have been shown to be instrumental in the maintenance of elbow stability. If stability cannot be achieved with ligamentous reconstruction, a dynamic external fixator or dynamic traction fixator should be applied.

Closed suction drains anterior and posterior to the elbow joint are an integral part of minimizing postoperative swelling and hematoma formation. It is not necessary to place a drain in the site of a synostosis takedown, but it should be placed deep to the fascial layer. Before closing the deep soft tissues, a lidocaine or bupivacaine continuous infusion pump may be placed to help maximize postoperative pain control (in cases in which axillary catheters are not used). The catheter for a bupivacaine infusion pump should be placed in a soft tissue layer or location separate from that of the closed suction drains. Divisions in the intermuscular septi do not need to be sutured, but muscle attachments to the distal humerus or proximal ulna should be repaired. For origins and insertions of muscle about the medial and lateral elbow, suture anchors provide sufficient stability for the bony reattachment. If the medial, flexor-pronator muscle mass has been elevated, consideration can be made to submuscular transposition of the ulnar nerve. Otherwise, a simple subcutaneous transposition maintained with a small strip of flexor-pronator fascia frequently will suffice. The fascial layer may be repaired with absorbable suture in a running or interrupted fashion. Subcutaneous and skin closure follows. The skin closure should not be under tension, nor should it be so tight as to prevent egress of drainage when early motion is initiated.

POSTOPERATIVE MANAGEMENT

Surgical outcomes of heterotopic bone excision and interposition soft tissue flaps weigh heavily on the patient's postoperative rehabilitation. The affected upper extremity is immobilized in a soft dressing to allow immediate motion. An axillary block catheter placed by the anesthesia team can provide substantial pain relief in the immediate postoperative setting. When such a catheter cannot be placed, we have used continuous bupivacaine infusion pumps to supplement intravenous narcotic pain control.

With adequate analgesia, continuous passive motion of the elbow can be performed in flexion and extension. It is our preference to use a bedside continuous passive motion (CPM) machine for the elbow rather than the more mobile units that provide motion during ambulation. The bedside units tend to maintain a constant position, capitalizing on leverage to impart motion at the patient's elbow. We have not identified a reliable method for continuous passive forearm motion and instead rely on intermittent sessions wherein the extremity is removed from the CPM machine, the elbow flexed 90 degrees, and forearm motion addressed. Resting splints are worn while the patient sleeps at night. The position of the splint is dictated by the particular problems addressed with surgery. For patients with elbow flexion and extension problems, the limb is immobilized in maximum extension and supination. For those patients whose primary problem is forearm motion, the limb is immobilized with elbow flexed 90 degrees and the forearm in maximum supination. Patients are usually discharged on the fourth day postoperatively, and an aggressive home and outpatient therapy program is instituted.

Elbow and forearm specific exercises include active, active-assisted range of motion as well as gentle passive assisted range of motion. To minimize the "trick maneuver" of radiocarpal and intercarpal rotation to augment apparent pronation and supination, the wrist is secured in an immobilizer and a solid object such as a common household tool, a hammer, is grasped tightly in the hand. Doing this directs all pronation and supination efforts to the forearm. When not exercising, the patient should use a static progressive splint, especially at night. The splint is applied an hour before sleep, and the pain associated with initial application should have dissipated enough that sleep will not be interrupted. Dynamic rubber band or spring driven splints are never used. Splinting and exercises are rarely carried out past 6 months postoperatively, as there is usually no change in the range of motion past this date. Anecdotally, however, patients frequently report that even though their range of motion does not change after 6 months, their strength and ease of motion improves up to 2 years postoperatively.

Radiation treatment of the resected bed of heterotopic ossification or synostosis has been shown to be successful in preventing recurrence of ectopic bone. However, no prospective randomized trial has shown this modality to be better than resection alone. As this procedure comes with some inherent risk of wound breakdown, neuritis, and lymphedema, and a remote risk of sarcoma, it should be discussed with the patient preoperatively. We limit radiation therapy to a single dose of 700 cGy within 36 hours of surgery and only in those patients in whom there was ankylosis of the proximal radioulnar joint. All patients are given ketorolac 30 mg IV daily for the 4 days; beyond that, nonsteroidal anti-inflammatory medicines are not used.

COMPLICATIONS

While the release of a stiff or ankylosed elbow can provide dramatic improvement in a patient's upper extremity function, the procedure is not without its complications. It is a high-risk operation which requires strong appreciation for the anatomy of the elbow and traversing neurovascular structures. Nerve injury from retraction or surgical dissection is possible and can be minimized with frequent assessment of nerve location as well as limiting the time and rigorousness of retraction on a nerve. Loss of fixation of the interposition material can be avoided by careful suture fixation into muscle as well as fascia.

Certainly, the most frequent complication of this procedure is recurrence of the heterotopic bone. In many cases new calcifications arise on postoperative radiographs well into the rehabilitation period. If the physical examination demonstrates no signs of motion loss, these ectopic calcifications are clinically insignificant and don't require routine followup. Some motion loss from the gains made intraoperatively can be expected. But a majority of patients who actively participate in their daily motion exercises will maintain a functional arc of motion and achieve an optimal outcome.

RECOMMENDED READING

Alonso-Llames M. Bilaterotricipital approach to the elbow. Its application in the osteosynthesis of supracondylar fractures of the humerus in children. *Acta Orthop Scand.* 1972;43(6):479–490.

Bell SN, Benger D. Management of radioulnar synostosis with mobilization, anconeus interposition, and a forearm rotation assist splint. *J Shoulder Elbow Surg.* 1999;8(6):621–624.

Cohen MS, Hastings H II. Post-traumatic contracture of the elbow. Operative release using a lateral collateral ligament sparing approach. *J Bone Joint Surg Br.* 1998;80(5):805–812.

Dowdy PA, Bain GI, King GJ, et al. The midline posterior elbow incision. An anatomical appraisal. *J Bone Joint Surg Br.* 1995;77(5):696–699.

Failla JM, Amadio PC, Morrey BF. Post-traumatic proximal radio-ulnar synostosis. Results of surgical treatment. *J Bone Joint Surg Am.* 1989;71(8):1208–1213.

Fernandez DL, Joneschild E. "Wrap around" pedicled muscle flaps for the treatment of recurrent forearm synostosis. *Tech Hand Upper Extremity Surg.* 2004;8:102–109.

Garland DE. A clinical perspective on common forms of acquired heterotopic ossification. *Clin Orthop Relat Res.* 1991(263):13–29.

Hastings H II, Graham TJ. The classification and treatment of heterotopic ossification about the elbow and forearm. *Hand Clin.* 1994;10(3):417–437.

Hurvitz EA, Mandac BR, Davidoff G, et al. Risk factors for heterotopic ossification in children and adolescents with severe traumatic brain injury. *Arch Phys Med Rehabil.* 1992;73(5):459–462.

Jones NF, Esmail A, Shin EK. Treatment of radioulnar synostosis by radical excision and interposition of a radial forearm adipofascial flap. *J Hand Surg Am.* 2004;29(6):1143–1147.

Jupiter JB, Ring D. Operative treatment of post-traumatic proximal radioulnar synostosis. *J Bone Joint Surg Am.* 1998;80(2):248–257.

Kamineni S, Maritz NG, Morrey BF. Proximal radial resection for posttraumatic radioulnar synostosis: a new technique to improve forearm rotation. *J Bone Joint Surg Am.* 2002;84-A(5):745–751.

McAuliffe JA, Wolfson AH. Early excision of heterotopic ossification about the elbow followed by radiation therapy. *J Bone Joint Surg Am.* 1997;79(5):749–755.

Moritomo H, Tada K, Yoshida T. Early, wide excision of heterotopic ossification in the medial elbow. J *Shoulder Elbow Surg.* 2001;10(2):164–168.

Morrey BF. Surgical treatment of extraarticular elbow contracture. *Clin Orthop Relat Res.* 2000(370):57–64.

Morrey BF, Askew LJ, Chao EY. A biomechanical study of normal functional elbow motion. *J Bone Joint Surg Am.* 1981;63(6):872–877.

Patterson SD, Bain GI, Mehta JA. Surgical approaches to the elbow. *Clin Orthop Relat Res.* 2000(370):19–33.

Ring D, Jupiter JB. Operative release of complete ankylosis of the elbow due to heterotopic bone in patients without severe injury of the central nervous system. *J Bone Joint Surg Am.* 2003;85-A(5):849–857.

Schmidt CC, Kohut GN, Greenberg JA, et al. The anconeus muscle flap: its anatomy and clinical application. *J Hand Surg Am.* 1999;24(2):359–369.

Viola RW, Hanel DP. Early "simple" release of posttraumatic elbow contracture associated with heterotopic ossification. *J Hand Surg Am.* 1999;24(2):370–380.

Viola RW, Hastings H, 2nd. Treatment of ectopic ossification about the elbow. *Clin Orthop Relat Res.* 2000(370):65–86.

PART III
MANAGEMENT OF SOFT TISSUES WITHIN THE HAND AND WRIST

14 Principles of Hand Incisions

Marco Rizzo and William P. Cooney III

INDICATIONS/CONTRAINDICATIONS

Because of the intricate balance of function in the hand and wrist, incisions in this area are unique. In an effort to ensure healing and maintain function, it is important to plan the incisions appropriately. The fingers have well-established approaches that allow for good visualization of deeper structures without compromising healing. Likewise, the hand and wrist are best approached while following basic principles. Poorly placed incisions result in restrictive scarring (Fig. 14-1), which may lead to diminished motion and function. In addition, the limited skin redundancy on the palmar surface of the hand may make delayed closure of edematous wounds difficult. Sound planning of incisions about the hand and wrist will help to avoid some of these difficulties. The purpose of this chapter is to review accepted incision designs for various aspects of the hand and wrist.

PREOPERATIVE PLANNING

Volar Approach to the Fingers

There are several commonly used approaches to the volar aspect of the fingers and thumb. The traditional Bruner incision is the approach that is most common (1). It is a zigzag incision that angles at the flexion creases of the metacarpophalangeal (MP), proximal interphalangeal (PIP), and distal interphalangeal (DIP) joints (Fig. 14-2). As the incision progresses proximally, the flexion creases of the palm are also points of direction changes. The principle is based on the fact that longitudinal incisions across these creases can generate excessive scarring and limit extension. For optimal healing of the flaps, it is best to keep the angles close to 90 degrees. Angles more acute than 60 degrees carry a higher incidence of skin necrosis.

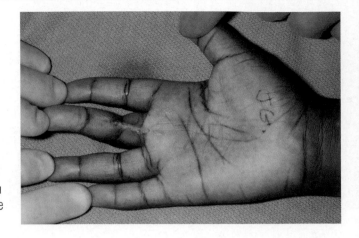

FIGURE 14-1

Example of restrictive scar resulting from straight line incision placed over the flexor surface of the finger.

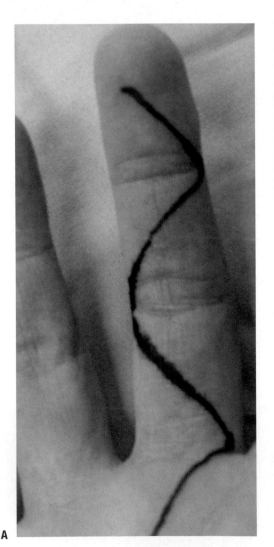

A

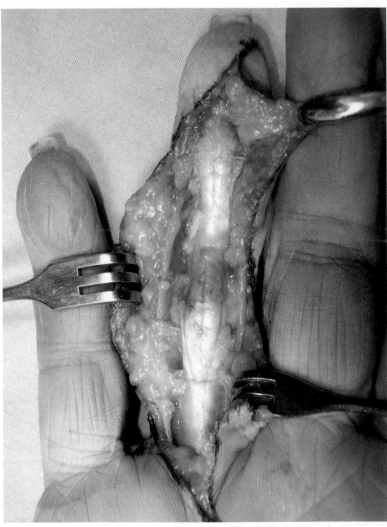

B

FIGURE 14-2

A: Bruner incision approach to the volar aspect of the fingers. The most commonly preferred method of crossing flexion creases is with these undulating angled incisions. **B:** Excellent exposure to the volar aspect of the finger can be achieved. *(Continued)*

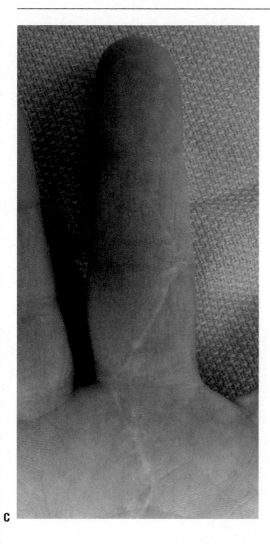

c

FIGURE 14-2

Continued **C:** These scars typically heal nicely.

An alternative to the Bruner incision in the finger is the mid-lateral approach (Figure 3a). It has the advantage of being cosmetically more appealing. The incision is based about the lateral (or medial) side of the finger and the skin is elevated to provide exposure of the underlying tissues. A good way to ensure that the surgeon is not directly over the neurovascular bundles is to connect the incisions at the apex of the flexion creases (Fig. 14-3B). This is also a preferred approach in cases of replantation surgery. Although cosmetically appealing, the challenges of this technique include elevating the skin and ensuring its viability.

In cases of flexion deformity of the fingers such as Dupuytren's contracture, a straight midline incision with z-plasties is an alternative approach to the traditional Bruner incision (Fig. 14-4). This will allow for the elongation of the incision as the flexion deformity is corrected. Angles of 60 degrees help preserve viability at the apex of the skin flap.

Incisions over the distal pulp of the finger, such as is necessary in felons, are best made directly over the area of swelling and induration. These wounds can be loosely closed or allowed to heal via secondary intention. If it appears that the incision may need to be extended proximal to the distal interphalangeal joint, a Bruner incision may be preferred for better exposure.

Dorsal Incisions About the Fingers

The dorsal skin of the hand lacks glaborous connections and has more redundancy, due to the requirements of joint flexion. Because of this redundancy, longitudinal incisions are acceptable. A longitudinal incision allows (Fig. 14-5) for protection of the venous and lymphatic drainage, while giving good visualization of the extensor mechanism (2). Lazy S or curvilinear incisions may also be designed to avoid crossing extension creases (see Fig. 14-5). Incisions over the distal interphalangeal joint can be longitudinal as well, but dissection can be limited due to the nail bed and fold distally. An alternative is the "T" or "H"-shaped incision that allows for visualization of the extensor mechanism and distal interphalangeal joint (Fig. 14-6).

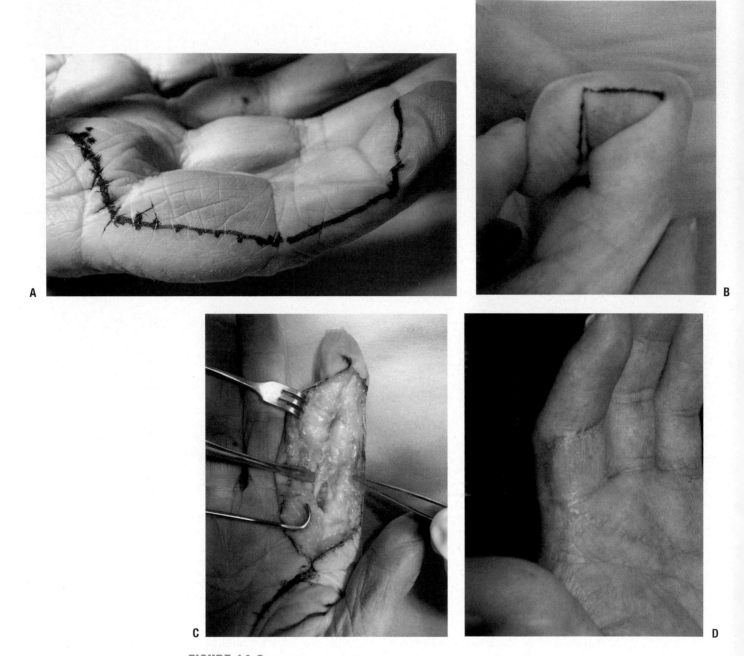

FIGURE 14-3

A: The mid-axial or lateral approach to the fingers. This technique can be a more aesthetic alternative to the Bruner incision. **B:** Care must be taken to connect the incision at the apex of the flexion creases in order to avoid direct dissection over the underlying neurovascular structures and prevent excessive volar scarring. **C:** Although it requires more dissection, excellent exposure can be achieved. **D:** An example of a healed mid-lateral incision.

Volar Incisions About the Hand

Transverse incisions or incisions that parallel the flexion creases offer the best cosmetic results. However, these incisions are perpendicular to the underlying vessels, nerves, and tendons. Therefore, care must be taken when performing these approaches. Incisions for trigger finger releases are a good example (Fig. 14-7). In particular, transverse incisions, in line with the metacarpophalangeal joint flexion crease, at the base of the thumb for A1 pulley release have been found to produce better aesthetic results and result in less restrictive scarring. Traditional longitudinal Bruner-type incisions are commonly tiused and are useful when more exposure is necessary. Again, you want to follow the basic premise of changing directions at the creases to minimize scarring. Wounds or scars

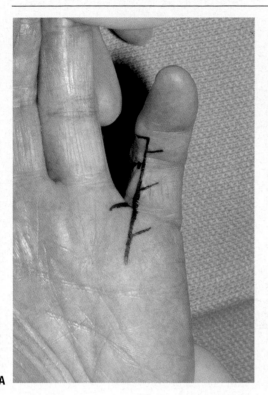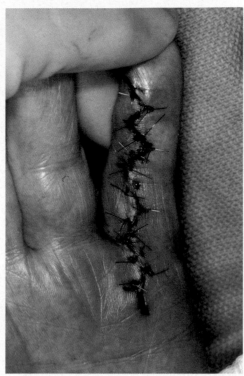

A   B

FIGURE 14-4

A: A longitudinal z-plasty approach to the volar aspect of the finger can be useful in cases of pre-existing flexion contracture, such as in Dupuytren's contracture. **B:** Wound closure is easily achieved with little or no tension with the finger in full extension.

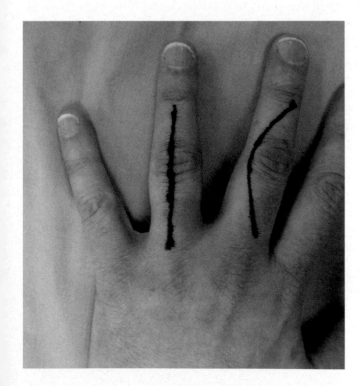

FIGURE 14-5

Two common approaches to the dorsum of the fingers: a straight longitudinal and a more curved longitudinal, which avoids the extension creases.

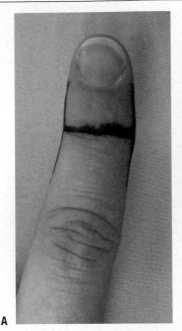

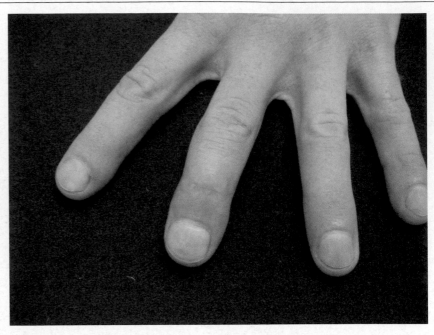

A   B

FIGURE 14-6

A: An "H"-shaped incision over the dorsal aspect of the distal interphalangeal (DIP) joint allows for excellent exposure of the dorsal distal finger. **B:** The wounds typically heal very nicely.

in the web spaces are at risk of developing functionally limiting scars. Depending on the patient, these can sometimes necessitate revision z-plasties and web-space deepening.

In exposing the carpal tunnel, a longitudinal incision, preferably in or in line with the palmar crease, is commonly used. If the incision needs to be extended proximally, Bruner-type zigzag incisions can be made between the distal and proximal wrist flexion creases (Fig. 14-8). These angled incisions are the most common and useful method of crossing flexion creases in the hand and wrist. Care should be taken to stay ulnar to the palmaris longus tendon to avoid injury to the palmar sensory branch of the median nerve.

Dorsal Incisions About the Hand

Longitudinal incision can be successfully used over the dorsum of the hand without the risk of restrictive scarring. Transverse and curvilinear incisions can also be used over the dorsum of the hand if desired. The skin over the dorsum of the hand is mobile and scarring is generally less of a functional problem as the flexor tendons are the dominant force and will minimize the cosmetic and/or functional deficit. Approaches to the carpometacarpal joint can be made longitudinally between the abductor pollicis longus and extensor pollicis brevis tendons, or they can be more radial (along the

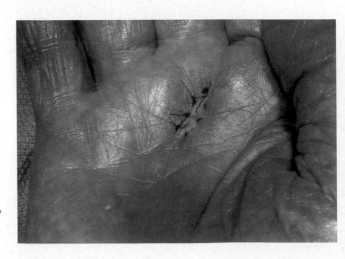

FIGURE 14-7

An incision for trigger finger approach using the palm flexion crease. These can result in cosmetically appealing scars with little or no residual deficit. In cases where greater exposure is necessary, a longitudinal Bruner-type incision is preferred.

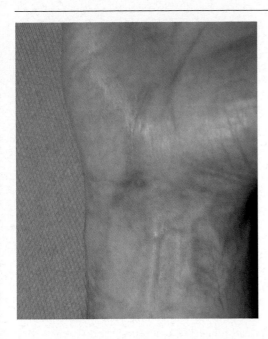

FIGURE 14-8

An extensile carpal tunnel incision. Angulation at the wrist flexion crease will minimize scarring of the wound. By keeping the incision ulnar to the palmaris longus tendon (*dotted line*), injury to the palmar sensory branch of the median nerve can be avoided.

plane of the intersection of the dorsal and volar skin) and extended proximally transversely along the wrist flexion crease, forming a "hockey stick" appearance.

Incisions About the Wrist

Dorsal approaches to the wrist can be longitudinal, transverse, or curvilinear. The tissues on the dorsal aspect of the wrist are redundant and dorsal scarring is not typically a problem. These can include incisions to expose the base of the thumb. Volar incisions to the wrist can be along flexion creases or longitudinal provided the incision changes direction at the flexion creases in a modified Bruner fashion.

Incisions About the Forearm

As we extend proximally, more traditional incisions can be used. If it is a fairly short incision, such as in open treatment of distal radius fractures, a longitudinal incision will suffice (Fig. 14-9). If the incision is extended distally, a Bruner angulation is made at the wrist flexion crease. In cases where extensive exposure is necessary, such as is required in compartment syndrome release, an undulating longitudinal incision works well. If the elbow must be crossed, this is usually done in a lazy S fashion passing to the medial aspect of the anticubital fossa.

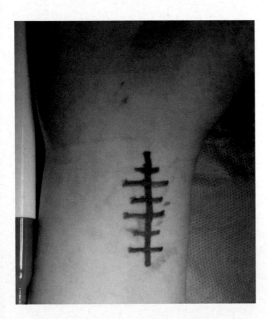

FIGURE 14-9

A longitudinal approach to the distal radius in a case of open reduction and internal fixation of a distal radius fracture. Angulation of the incision can be performed if the incision needs to be extended distally.

Healing by Secondary Intention

In cases such as infection and Dupuytren's contracture, it may be advantageous to leave the wounds at least partially open. These wounds can heal nicely by secondary intention. Modalities such as whirlpool and wound vacuum assisted closure can be helpful in accelerating wound healing as well as minimizing risk of infection. Disadvantages include time to healing and the fact that some patients find the healing process cosmetically unappealing. Unfortunately, functional limitations such as joint contractures can result as rehabilitation is delayed during the wound healing process. However, with good postoperative wound care, this can be an effective way to manage some of the more difficult cases or cases where it is necessary to leave the wounds open (3).

SURGERY

Patient Positioning

Typically, the patient is in a supine position and a hand table is used. A tourniquet is placed in the proximal portion of the arm. We prefer the pressure to be inflated to approximately 250 mm Hg for adults and 200 to 225 mm Hg for children (generally 70–100 mm Hg above the patient's systolic pressure). If the surgery is isolated to the distal aspect of the finger, a finger tourniquet can be placed. In these cases, we routinely also place the upper arm tourniquet which can be used if need be. The entire extremity is prepped. Perioperative antibiotics are administered when indicated.

Technique

Loupe magnification should be used to help avoid injury to important underlying structures. The incision is typically made with a 15-blade knife, taking care to stay perpendicular to the skin and not skiving. The knife can be used to cut the dermis and epidermis. Generally, dissection should proceed from known to unknown or normal to abnormal tissues. Electrocautery, with needle-point cautery, can be used for small veins or vessels. We prefer the use of bipolar cautery. Drains should be liberally used, especially in contaminated wounds or wounds with compromised hemostasis. Options include a small silastic, penrose, or hemovac drain. The drain can be placed without suture so that it can be easily removed postoperatively to not disturb the overlying dressing. Otherwise, drains can be sutured for added protection if the surgeon wants it kept it in for a longer period of time. It is our preference to deflate the tourniquet before wound closure to evaluate hand perfusion as well as hemostasis prior to wound closure. After ensuring adequate hemostasis and viability of the hand, the tourniquet may be reinflated during wound closure. The wounds can be closed in a single layer with a nonabsorbable interrupted 4-0 or 5-0 suture such as nylon or prolene. Either horizontal or vertical mattress sutures can be used. Vertical mattresses are better for everting the skin edges, whereas horizontal mattress sutures allow for less overall sutures. Increased ischemia of the soft tissues can occur with horizontal mattress closure. In young children, an absorbable suture such as catgut or chromic is preferred.

POSTOPERATIVE MANAGEMENT

A thoughtfully applied hand dressing is imperative. Depending on the injury, some period of immobilization is generally recommended. Proper immobilization will allow for the skin and soft tissues to heal with minimal stretch and tension. However, this needs to be balanced with the risk of developing joint contractures. In cases of fracture care, immobilization time is prolonged compared with that for soft tissues. The dressing should be mildly compressive and supportive (Fig. 14-10). Surgeries involving the distal aspects of the digits may be adequately dressed with a tube gauze type of dressing. More proximal reconstructive surgeries will require varying periods of immobilization of the wrist and hand in the position of function. Specifically, with the wrist in mild extension, metacarpophalangeal joints flexed and interphalangeal joints extended. Elective soft tissue procedures such as carpal tunnel releases can be immobilized with the wrist in mild extension and the fingers free to move immediately. Although this is our preference, we acknowledge these can be successfully treated with simply a soft dressing. Drains are discontinued when the wound is dry.

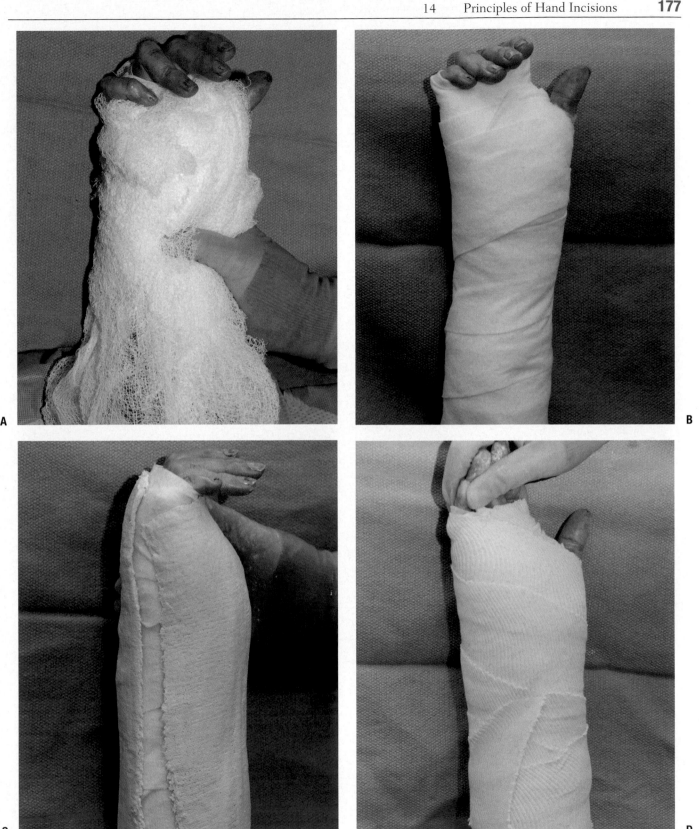

FIGURE 14-10

An example of a compressive dressing in a patient with rheumatoid arthritis who underwent metacarpophalangeal joint arthroplasty. **A:** Following application of xeroform on the incision, fluffs are placed on the volar, dorsal, radial, and ulnar aspects of the wrist and hand. Gauze is lightly placed within the web spaces of the digits. **B:** Abundant cast padding is applied followed by **(C)** plaster. In the immediate postoperative period, we prefer a splint as it will allow for swelling and will compress as the swelling improves. **D:** A bias wrap completes the dressing. In this example, the MP joints need to be immobilized in extension and neutral deviation. If finger motion is not contraindicated, care should be taken not to have the dressing restrict finger motion.

COMPLICATIONS

The most common adverse result of poorly planned incisions is scar contracture (see Fig. 14-1), which can lead to cosmetic and/or functional deficits. More difficult are skin necrosis and subsequent wound healing problems. These can lead to problems such as infection, excessive scar formation, and diminished function. Other less common complications related to inadequate or suboptimal incisions include injury to nerves, arteries, or tendons. However, with good preoperative planning and technique, these complications are usually avoidable.

REFERENCES

1. Bruner JM. The zigzag volar digital incision for flexor tendon surgery. *Plast Reconstr Surg.* 1967;40:571.
2. Graham WP. Incisions, amputations, and skin grafting in the hand. *Orthop Clin North Am.* 1970;1:227.
3. McCash CR. The open palm technique in Dupuytren's Contracture. *Br J Plast Surg.* 1964;17:271.

15 Lateral Arm Flap for Hand and Wrist Coverage

Michael Sauerbier and Goetz A. Giessler

The first description of the lateral arm flap was by Song and coworkers. They used it primarily as a free microvascular flap for small and medium-sized defects in reconstructive procedures of the head and neck. A detailed study by Katsaros et al later popularized it as an extremely versatile, easy to harvest septocutaneous flap with relatively low donor site morbidity. The vascular anatomy is reliable, and the dissection is rather quick and can be performed under regional anesthesia for reconstruction of hand and wrist defects. To date, the flap is used for a wide spectrum of defects all over the body.

The shortcomings of the original lateral arm flap were the flap's bulkiness and a pedicle of moderate length when skin flaps were centered over the middle aspect of the lateral arm. Recent anatomic studies have led to significant modifications in flap design; the skin paddle is now centered over the lower third of the upper arm extending to the lateral epicondyle (extended lateral arm flap). This produces a thin flap with a long pedicle length. The flap may also be used in a reversed fashion (reversed lateral arm flap) or as a pedicled antegrade V-Y flap (extreme lateral arm flap). A pure fascial flap has also been described. The flap may be designed to include vascularized nerve, tendon, and bone. This versatility has made the lateral arm flap a "workhorse" for elective, urgent, and emergency reconstructions of the hand and wrist.

INDICATIONS/CONTRAINDICATIONS

Indications

The lateral arm flap has a wide range of applications for closure of small and medium-sized defects in hand and wrist surgery. The classic fasciocutaneous or fascial flap serves well for reconstruction of the dorsal aspect of the hand or the thumb index web space. Patients with a thin subcutaneous fat layer are the best candidates for the flap because it is soft and easily pliable for complex three-dimensional defects.

For cases of palmar reconstruction, we prefer to use a fascial flap, as the cutaneous lateral arm flap may be too thick. This flap is then covered with a full thickness graft and made sensate by anastomising the posterior cutaneous forearm nerve to the palmar branch of the median nerve. Defects with loss of extensor tendons or metacarpal bone can be closed using a composite lateral arm flap using a distal humeral cortical segment and/or a vascularized triceps tendon graft. For all these indications, the flap has to be used as a free microvascular flap. The pedicle is long enough (see following) for flap positioning around the hand or wrist in many cases. The main alternatives to the lateral arm flap are the (osteo-) cutaneous scapular/parascapular, radial forearm, enterolateral thigh flap, and dorsalis pedis flaps. The specific features of each are provided in Table 15-1.

Contraindications

The free lateral arm flap represents a microsurgical procedure of considerable length. Patients with poor general health who need an elective procedure should be optimized preoperatively; otherwise,

TABLE 15-1.   Comparison of the Lateral Arm Flap to Possible Alternatives for Simple or Composite Reconstructions at the Hand and Wrist

	Lateral Arm Flap	Radial Forearm Flap	Anterolateral Thigh Flap	Scapular Parascapular Flap	Dorsalis Pedis Flap
Max. skin island size (cm)	8 × 25	10 × 20	7 × 25	15 × 28	5 × 8
Max. pedicle length (cm)	11	15	15	10	8
Fascia only	Yes	Yes	—	—	—
Tendon component	Lateral triceps tendon	Palmaris longus, half of the radial carpal flexor	Fascia lata	—	Short toe extensors
Muscle component	—	—	—	Latissimus dorsi, anterior serratus	No
Bone component	Distal humerus	Distal radius	—	Lateral scapular border	2nd metatarsal
Nerve component	Posterior cutaneous forearm nerve	Lateral antebrachial cutaneous nerve	Lateral femoral cutaneous nerve	—	Superficial peroneal nerve
Patient positioning	Supine or lateral prone	Supine or lateral prone	Supine	Lateral prone	Supine

other treatment options should be considered. Previous trauma or surgical procedures in this area, such as plate osteosyntheses of the humerus, probably have destroyed the perforators and are a contraindication. Patients with considerable body fat provide a bulky lateral arm skin flap which is unsuitable for most hand and wrist reconstruction. Using the fasciocutaneous lateral arm flap together with a skin graft can be an option in these cases. The relatively conspicuous scar of the lateral arm flap poses a relative contraindication in female patients. Whenever the donor site cannot be closed primarily, other flap options should be thought of (see previously). Hair transfer may pose a problem in head and neck reconstructions. Likewise, male patients may prove a challenge with hair transfer in hand and wrist reconstructions.

ANATOMY

The skin on the upper lateral arm receives its perfusion by septocutaneous perforators in the lateral intermuscular septum inferior to the tip of the deltoid muscle. They originate from two main branches in the middle of the upper arm between the acromion and the lateral epicondyle originating from the profunda brachii artery. Those main branches are called the anterior and posterior radial collateral arteries (ARCA and PRCA), with the latter having a reliable longitudinal network along the septum to distal arteries. The PRCA is the nourishing artery for the lateral arm flap as it runs close the humerus in the septum between triceps brachii and the brachial muscle. The ARCA branches off between the brachial and brachioradial muscles and is ligated during flap elevation. In rare cases (about 6%), the PRCA is found to be duplicated. On its way distally to the plexus around the elbow, the PRCA gives off three to five septocutaneous perforators serving as feeder vessels for the lateral arm fascia or fasciocutaneous flap. Those surfacing perforators are easily visible during flap dissection. After reaching the subcutaneous plexus, the branches run both anteriorly and posteriorly. In this region, the PRCA anastomoses with the interosseus recurrent artery (between the lateral epicondyle and the olecranon), the recurrent radial artery (anterior to the lateral epicondyle directly above the periosteum), and the inferior ulnar collateral artery to this plexus. These multiple arterial connections allow for distal extension of the skin paddle, which can be harvested up to 12 cm distal to the epicondyle. These anastomoses also allow for the use of the flap in a reverse fashion using one of the perforators from this periarticular plexus.

The venous drainage of the lateral arm flap is by veins of the PRCA together with a rich network of subcutaneous veins including the cephalic vein, which may be included in the anterior part of larger flaps. The cephalic vein does not need to be included in smaller flaps necessarily, but can provide adequate additional venous drainage in larger or composite flaps.

Depending on flap positioning, the overall pedicle length can reach up to 11 cm in the authors' experience, with the artery having a diameter of 2 to 2.5 mm at its proximal origin from the brachial artery.

Bone, tendon, and nerve may be included within the lateral arm flap and used for reconstruction of composite defects. A strip of vascularized bone may be harvested from the distal, epicondylar section of the lateral humerus. Detailed studies have shown one to four nutrient vessels from the PRCA to the bone. These vessels enter the lateral humeral aspect 2 to 7 cm proximal to the lateral epicondyle. Fifty percent of the triceps tendon may also be harvested with the flap, resulting in a maximum tendon graft of 10×2 cm. Gosain et al demonstrated by injection studies that the blood supply to this strip is not via the lateral intermuscular septum, but rather through the triceps muscle. Thus, a cuff of muscle must be included to have a vascularized tendon segment; alternatively, an avascular triceps tendon autograft may be dissected with the flap if one does not wish to violate the triceps muscle. Finally, the posterior cutaneous forearm nerve can be included within the flap allowing for the possibility of a sensate free flap. Harvest of this nerve will result in a strip of distal forearm numbness postoperatively.

PREOPERATIVE PLANNING

Doppler examination can be used for centering the skin paddle over the vascular pedicle. The flap can be harvested in regional anesthesia using a sterile tourniquet (250–300 mm Hg). For a transplantation to the contralateral arm, general anesthesia is adequate. Loupe magnification for flap dissection is strongly recommended (2–4.5 times). The standard lateral arm flap is centered over a virtual axis between the tip of the deltoid muscle and the easily palpable prominence of the lateral epicondyle of the humerus (Fig. 15-1). When marking this axis in patients who are obese or with very mobile skin, the surgeon has to support redundant tissue of the posterolateral upper arm, as gravity might pull the tissues posteriorly, endangering pedicle inclusion. When flap design is continued beyond the lateral epicondyle, the central axis of the flap is continued distally from the lateral epicondyle in the direction of the distal radioulnar joint on the wrist dorsum. Harvesting the flap from the distal humerus and dorsal forearm produces a thinner flap than flaps raised at the mid-humeral level. The reversed or extreme lateral arm flaps have their major indications as a pedicled flap for defect closure around the elbow and proximal forearm.

In planning a composite lateral arm flap, a precise idea about the future positioning of the several components at the recipient site is mandatory. If an osteocutaneous flap is dissected, it should be centered at the distal upper arm, as the receivable bone graft has a maximum length of about 10 cm from the lateral epicondyle proximally. It should not be wider than 25% of the humeral circumference, which is sufficient for most indications at the hand and wrist.

The maximal cutaneous flap area supported by the PRCA on the upper arm varies in size from about 5×10 cm to 8×20 cm. Primary closure is ideal but this is dependent on skin laxity, patient habitus, and general tissue conditions. Preoperative expansion is described in the literature with the expander being placed subfascially and medially to the lateral brachial septum; but this is certainly reserved for rare indications. Flaps less than 6 cm in width can usually be closed primarily.

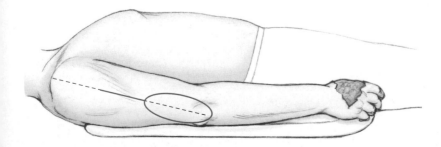

FIGURE 15-1

Planning the axis of a standard lateral arm flap.

SURGERY

Patient Positioning

The patient is placed in the supine or lateral supine position with the extremity on a hand table and the arm draped fully mobile. The tip of deltoid muscle, lateral epicondyle, and dorsal aspect of the radioulnar joint are marked and connected as the flap axis (see Preoperative Planning).

Technique

Dissection is started under tourniquet control. Skin and deep fascia are dissected from the muscles together and the fascia is tacked to the skin by 4-0 resorbable sutures to prevent shear forces on the skin perforaters. In an extended or distal free lateral arm flap, it is likewise important to include the deep fascia together with a small strip of intermuscular fascia. Over the epicondylar prominence, the periosteum should be taken en bloc with the fascia to ensure including the connections to the recurrent radial artery. Retracting the lateral head of the triceps posteriorly, the septum, its attachments to the humerus, the PRCA, and the septocutaneous perforators are visible. Once the posterior exposure is complete, the anterior incision is made and the lateral intermuscular septum is exposed from the anterior. While doing this, the surgeon often encounters the smaller, more oblique oriented septum between the brachial and the brachioradial muscle, which contains the ARCA. The identification of the PRCA perforators is done by carefully flipping the flap over along the axis to look at the lateral septum from both sides, after which all smaller branches from the ARCA are ligated. If the cephalic vein runs through the skin island, it may be dissected out more proximally to have an "emergency run-off" and included in the flap, or left in situ. However, it is not obligatory for a successful lateral arm flap. Now the flap is very mobile and only attached to the septum (Fig. 15-2). A self-retaining retractor now can be inserted. In a fasciocutaneous or purely fascial flap, the periosteum is sharply incised bilaterally to the PRCA and sharply taken off the humerus with a periosteal elevator, as the PRCA often runs very close to it. This implies ligating smaller nourishing branches to the bone in an area of 2 to 7 cm proximal to the lateral epicondyle. The vascular pedicle and the cutaneous nerve then are developed proximally under the deltoid to gain enough pedicle length, which should match with the recipient site situation at this time. Dissecting the cutaneous nerves from the radial nerve has to be done with utmost care to prevent uncontrolled bleeding and hematoma around the nerve. Finally, the tourniquet is released, precise bipolar coagulation is performed, and the flap perfusion is checked. The pedicle is ligated only after proper dissection of the recipient vessels and shortly before microsurgical anastomosis to save ischemia time.

If an osteocutaneous composite lateral arm flap is dissected, the periosteum is not stripped off the bone, but only incised and an oscillating saw used for corticotomy (see Preoperative Planning). The release of the bone segment is carefully finished with a sharp osteotome.

The tendon harvest of a triceps tendon requires identification of the feeding branches from the PRCA into the lateral triceps head. A cuff of muscle is included with the tendon for proper perfusion (see Anatomy).

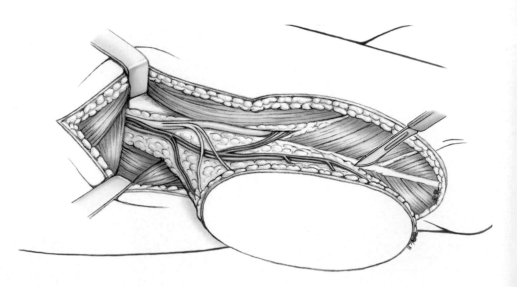

FIGURE 15-2

After the flap is isolated on the septum, the pedicle is followed proximally quite easily.

If the recipient site is prepared properly, the pedicle can be ligated with vessel clips or suture ligation. A suction drain is placed before a double-layered skin closure.

Donor Site Morbidity

Preoperatively, the upper lateral arm can be pinched to check if primary wound closure is possible after removal of the planned skin island. In flaps wider than 8 to 9 cm, primary wound closure is impossible; a skin graft must be applied, and a secondary scar correction or excision after 6 months might be necessary. In the literature, aesthetically unsatisfactory results are reported in about 27% of patients, as even the linear scar is quite visible or can show considerable hypertrophy or pigmentation changes or cause an hourglass-deformity of the upper arm. Early use of silicone sheeting, silicone gel appliance, or intralesional corticoid application should be considered. The sometimes unsightly scar is one of the reasons for restricting the use of the lateral arm flap in female patients.

POSTOPERATIVE MANAGEMENT

At the donor site, early motion of the limb is encouraged, whereas shear forces to the scar should be avoided. Early scar therapy such as with silicone gel, sheet application, or compressive garments has proved to be successful. If an osteocutaneous flap was harvested, the patient should refrain from heavy lifting until 3 months postoperatively. Protective splints might be considered in noncompliant patients. In the case of a triceps tendon segment removal, full weight bearing (e.g., pushups) should not be allowed before 12 weeks postoperatively. If flap healing at the hand and wrist is undisturbed, physiotherapy is begun on the second postoperative day with constant monitoring of flap perfusion. If tendons were reconstructed, special rehabilitation protocols may then be initiated. Compressive gloves are useful after removal of the suture material. Flap thinning or secondary procedures should not be performed until 6 months postoperatively.

COMPLICATIONS

Specific complications of the lateral arm flap are rare and primarily due to poor planning. As it is harvested most often as a fasciocutaneous flap, no attempt should be made to close the fascia postoperatively, as this might lead to a muscular compartment syndrome. Even adapting the fascial edges at the proximal and distal donor site should be avoided, as this might lead to herniation of the triceps through the gap, which is less of a case if only the skin is closed in a two-layered fashion. Hematoma formation can also lead to considerable tension in that area and has to be evacuated surgically. In case of a fracture of the humerus after harvesting a bone graft, open or closed reposition and osteosynthesis should be encouraged to prevent prolonged immobilization of the elbow joint.

Complications with respect to microsurgical routines are no different than those of other free flaps. Extreme pin-cushioning and volume discrepancies due to secondary overall weight gain make flap debulking procedures necessary (e.g., aspiration lipectomy), whereas hair growth can be reduced with laser therapy.

Disturbances in forearm sensitivity (58.7%), lateral epicondylar pain (19.4%), and a hypersensitive donor site (17%) were quoted as long-term complications. To minimize this sensory forearm disturbance, the posterior cutaneous forearm nerve can be dissected carefully out of the flap. Impaired range of motion in the elbow is reported after dissecting a composite flap with a triceps tendon graft, but is a rare complication. Primary or secondary fracture of the humerus following elevation of an osteofasciocutaneous lateral arm flap can be avoided with careful technique (oscillating saw) and removal of only 25% of the lateral cortical circumference. If a neuroma of the posterior cutaneous forearm nerve develops despite division close to the main radial nerve, it should be reexplored, resected, or buried in muscle or bone.

ILLUSTRATIVE CASES

Case 1

An 18-year-old man injured his left wrist with a contaminated butcher knife. Tendons and neurovascular structures were found to be intact. Treatment is demonstrated in Figure 15-3.

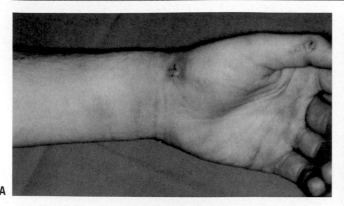

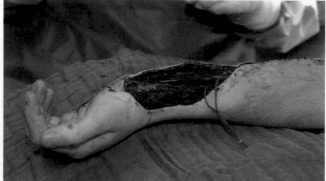

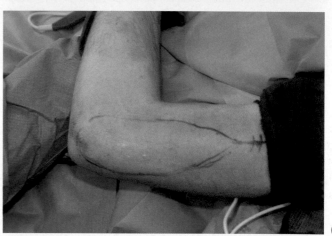

FIGURE 15-3

A: The wound was irrigated and sutured in a small regional hospital. **B:** Two days later the patient developed necrotizing fasciitis and was transferred to our hospital, where the patient underwent two serial debridements with the initiation of antibiotic therapy. The defect now had a size of 12 × 6 cm. The flexor tendons and median nerve were exposed. **C:** A distal, thin lateral arm flap was outlined from the same extremity. **D:** The flap was connected end-to-side to the radial artery and end-to-end to the cephalic vein and sutured into the defect. *(Continued)*

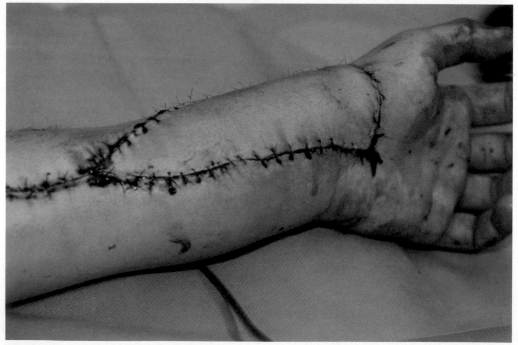

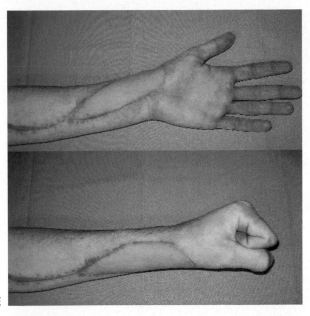

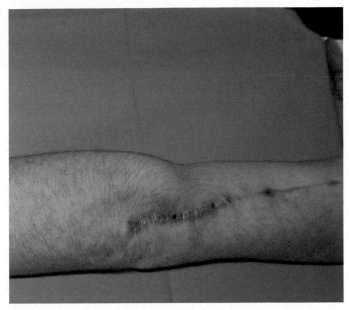

E   F

FIGURE 15-3

Continued **E:** One year postoperative with full range of motion. **F:** Donor site 1 year postoperative. Note the slightly widened scar around the lateral epicondyle.

Case 2

A 70-year-old woman mutilated her left wrist in a suicide attempt and was found 3 days later in her apartment. At the time of presentation, the patient had a large soft-tissue defect in addition to desiccation of the palmar structures. Treatment is demonstrated in Figure 15-4.

Case 3

A combine accident in a 21-year-old man resulted in a rupture of the second extensor digitorum communis, extensor indicis proprius, extensor carpi radialis longus and brevis and extensor pollicis longus tendons, three main branches of the superficial radial nerve, the radial artery and the dorsal wrist capsule, and ligaments and dorsal corticalis of the carpal bones. The whole wound was extremely contaminated with organic debris. Treatment is demonstrated in Figure 15-5.

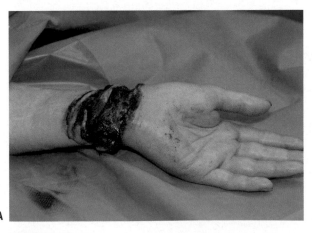

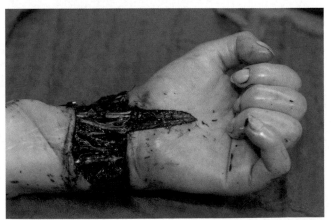

A   B

FIGURE 15-4

A: Intraoperative exploration showed traumatic division of the ulnar artery, median nerve, all superficial and deep flexor tendons, flexor pollicis longus, and flexor carpi radialis and ulnaris tendons. **B:** After a detailed debridement, all functional structures were reconstructed except the superficial flexor tendons, which were resected. Three sural nerve grafts (each 4.5 cm) were interposed; the ulnar artery was reconstructed with a vein graft (6.5 cm). *(Continued)*

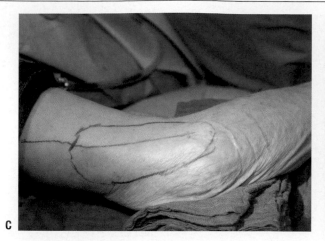

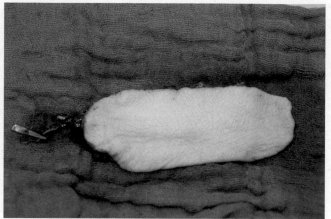

FIGURE 15-4

Continued **C:** A fasciocutaneous, thin lateral arm flap was outlined on the ipsilateral distal upper arm. **D:** The harvested flap had a size of 8 × 4 cm and was anastomosed end-to-end to the radial artery and the cephalic vein. **E:** Result 10 days after the operation. The patient started physiotherapy already on the second postoperative day.

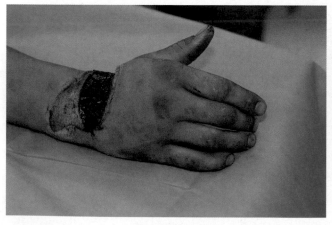

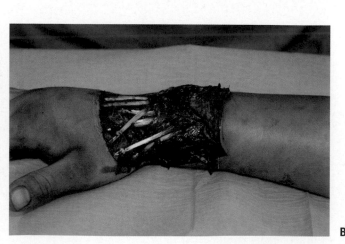

FIGURE 15-5

A: A thorough debridement and irrigation was performed as a first stage. **B:** After debridement, all tendons were sutured and the wound was closed with a free fasciocutaneous ipsilateral lateral arm flap. *(Continued)*

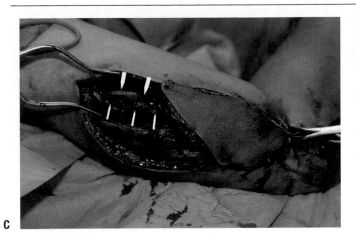

C

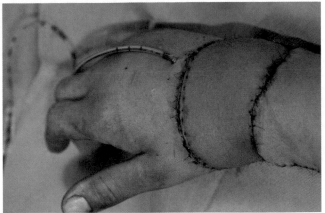

D

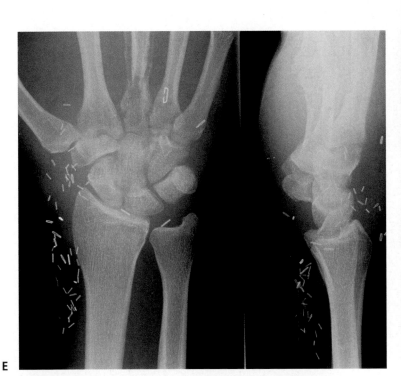

E

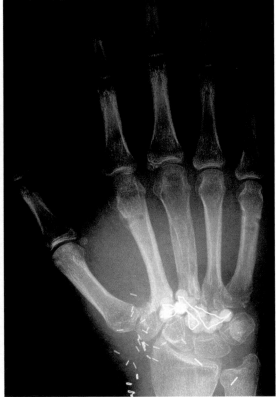

F

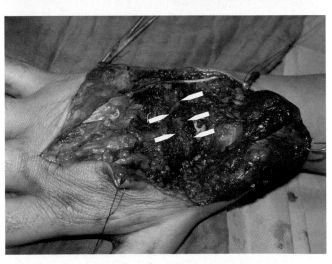

G

FIGURE 15-5

Continued **C:** The pedicle is marked with *thin white arrows*; the radial nerve is indicated by *thick white arrows*. **D:** It was connected end to end to the radial artery and the cephalic vein, respectively. **E:** Unfortunately, a persisting wound infection in the carpus made additional debridements necessary. Antibiotic beads were set into the space and an external fixator was placed. **F:** Finally, the distal carpal row and the bases of the second and third metacarpal bones had to be removed. **G:** A non-vascularized iliac crest bone graft was fixed with K-wires for a carpometacarpal arthrodesis of the second to fifth ray (*white arrows*). *(Continued)*

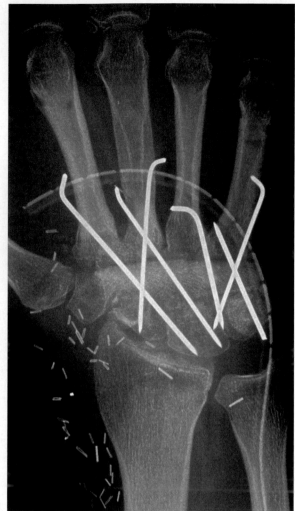

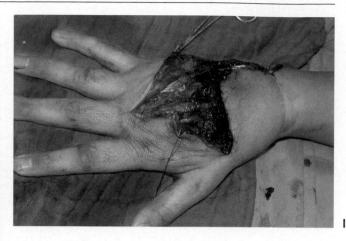

FIGURE 15-5

Continued **H:** Postoperative radiograph. **I:** Due to the infection-related elongated immobilization of the hand, the extensor tendons were severely impaired in their motion, even under the flap, and had to be partially resected and tenolysed. Silicon rods were placed under the flap for a secondary extensor tendon replacement. The flap remained viable and pliable throughout all procedures.

RECOMMENDED READING

Arnez ZM, Kersnic M, Smith RW, et al. Free lateral arm osteocutaneous neurosensory flap for thumb reconstruction. *J Hand Surg Br.* 1991;16(4):395–399.

Arnez Z, Tyler M, Giacomarra V, et al. The radial forearm-lateral arm mega free flap. *Br J Plast Surg.* 1995;48(1):27–29.

Berthe JV, Toussaint D, Coessens BC. One-stage reconstruction of an infected skin and Achilles tendon defect with a composite distally planned lateral arm flap. *Plast Reconstr Surg.* 1998;102(5):1618–1622.

Casoli V, Kostopoulos E, Pelissier P, et al. The middle collateral artery: anatomic basis for the "extreme" lateral arm flap. *Surg Radiol Anat.* 2004;26(3):172–177.

Chen HC, Buchman MT, Wei FC. Free flaps for soft tissue coverage in the hand and fingers. *Hand Clin.* 1999;15(4):541–554.

Coessens BC, Hamdi M. The distally planned lateral arm flap in hand reconstruction. *Chir Main.* 1998;17(2):133–141.

Fodgestam I, Tarnow P, Kalaagi A. Extended free lateral arm flap with preservation of the posterior cutaneous nerve of the forearm. *Scand J Plast Reconstr Surg.* 1996;30:49–55.

Gehrking E, Remmert S, Majocco A. Topographic and anatomic study of lateral upper arm transplants. *Ann Anat.* 1998;180(3):275–280.

Gosain AK, Matloub HS, Yousif NJ, et al.. The composite lateral arm free flap: vascular relationship to triceps tendon and muscle. *Ann Plast Surg.* 1992;29(6):496–507.

Graham B, Adkins P, Scheker LR. Complications and morbidity of the donor and recipient sites in 123 lateral arm flaps. *J Hand Surg Br.* 1992;17(2):189–192.

Haas F, Rappl T, Koch H, et al. Free osteocutaneous lateral arm flap: anatomy and clinical applications. *Microsurgery.* 2003;23(2):87–95.

Hage JJ, Woerdeman LA, Smeulders MJ. The truly distal lateral arm flap: rationale and risk factors of a microsurgical workhorse in 30 patients. *Ann Plast Surg.* 2005;54(2):153–159.

Hamdi M, Coessens BC. Distally planned lateral arm flap. *Microsurgery.* 1996;17(7):375–379.

Harpf C, Papp C, Ninkovic M, et al.. The lateral arm flap: review of 72 cases and technical refinements. *J Reconstr Microsurg.* 1998;14(1):39–48.

Hou SM, Liu TK. Vascularized tendon graft using lateral arm flap. 5 microsurgery cases. *Acta Orthop Scand.* 1993;64(3):373–376.

Hennerbichler A, Etzer C, Gruber S, et al. Lateral arm flap: analysis of its anatomy and modification using a vascularized fragment of the distal humerus. *Clin Anat.* 2003;16(3):204–214.

Karamursel S, Bagdatly D, Markal N, et al.Versatility of the lateral arm free flap in various anatomic defect reconstructions. *J Reconstr Microsurg.* 2005;21(2):107–112.

Katsaros J, Schusterman M, Beppu M, et al. The lateral upper arm flap: anatomy and clinical applications. *Ann Plast Surg.* 1984;12(6):489–500.

Kuek LB. The extended lateral arm flap: a detailed anatomical study. *Ann Acad Med Singapore.* 1992;21(2):169–175.

Lai CS, Tsai CC, Liao KB, et al. The reverse lateral arm adipofascial flap for elbow coverage. *Ann Plast Surg.* 1997;39(2):196–200.

Mooshammer HE, Hellbom BA, Schwarzl FX, et al. Reconstruction of a complex defect of the foot with an osteotendofasciocutaneous lateral arm free flap. *Scand J Plast Reconstr Hand Surg.* 1997;31:271–273.

Morrison WA, Cavallo AV. Revascularization of an ischemic replanted thumb using a lateral arm free fascial flap. *Ann Plast Surg.* 1993;31(5):467–470.

Moser VL, Gohritz A, van Schoonhoven J, et al.. The free lateral arm flap in reconstructive hand surgery. *Eur J Plast Surg.* 2004;27:81–85.

Ninkovic M, Harpf C, Schwabegger AH, et al. The lateral arm flap. *Clin Plast Surg.* 2001;28(2):367–374.

Scheker LR, Kleinert HE, Hanel DP. Lateral arm composite tissue transfer to ipsilateral hand defects. *J Hand Surg Am.* 1987;12(5 Pt 1):665–672.

Scheker LR, Lister GD, Wolff TW. The lateral arm free flap in releasing severe contracture of the first web space. *J Hand Surg Br.* 1988;13(2):146–150.

Shenaq SM. Pretransfer expansion of a sensate lateral arm free flap. *Ann Plast Surg.* 1987;19(6):558–562.

Shenaq SM, Dinh TA. Total penile and urethral reconstruction with an expanded sensate lateral arm flap: case report. *J Reconstr Microsurg.* 1989;5(3):245–248.

Song R, Song Y, Yu Y, et al. The upper arm free flap. *Clin Plast Surg.* 1982;9:27–35.

Summers AN, Matloub HS, Sanger JR. Salvage of ischemic digits using a lateral arm fascial flap. *Plast Reconstr Surg.* 2001;107(2):398–407.

Summers AN, Sanger JR, Matloub HS. Lateral arm fascial flap: microarterial anatomy and potential clinical applications. *J Reconstr Microsurg.* 2000;16(4):279–286.

Teoh LC, Khoo DB, Lim BH, et al. Osteocutaneous lateral arm flap in hand reconstruction. *Ann Acad Med Singapore.* 1995;24(4 suppl):15–20.

Tung TC, Wang KC, Fang CM, et al. Reverse pedicled lateral arm flap for reconstruction of posterior soft-tissue defects of the elbow. *Ann Plast Surg.* 1997;38(6):635–641.

Upton J, Mutimer KL, Loughlin K, et al. Penile reconstruction using the lateral arm flap. *J R Coll Surg Edinb.* 1987;32(2):97–101.

Waterhouse N, Healy C. The versatility of the lateral arm flap. *Br J Plast Surg.* 1990;43(4):398–402.

Yousif NJ, Warren R, Matloub HS, et al. The lateral arm fascial free flap: its anatomy and use in reconstruction. *Plast Reconstr Surg.* 1990;86(6):1138-1145; discussion 1146–1147.

16 Posterior Interosseous Artery Island Flap for Dorsal Hand Coverage

Eduardo A. Zancolli

The posterior interosseous flap is an island pedicled fasciocutaneous flap from the dorsal aspect of the forearm supplied by the cutaneous branches of the posterior interosseous artery. The posterior interosseous artery is located in the septum between the extensor carpi ulnaris and the extensor indicis propius. This flap has proven to be an excellent coverage option for the dorsum of the hand and the first interdigital web. The dorsal cutaneous area of the forearm supplied by the posterior interosseous artery was initially described by Manchot in 1889 (8) and later by Salmon in 1936 (12).

The vascular anatomy of the flap was described along with 20 initial cases (17 cases to cover the first web and three cases to cover the dorsum of the hand). The dorsal cutaneous area of the forearm irrigated by the posterior interosseous artery was initially described by Manchot in 1889 (8) and later by Salmon in 1936 (12).

This island flap was presented for the first time by the author at the VIth European Hand Surgery Course in Ümea (Sweden) (13). In this opportunity the vascular anatomy of the flap and an experience on 20 initial cases were presented (17 cases to cover the first web and three cases to cover the dorsum of the hand). Hand outs distributed during the course were published by the author in 1993 (18). The procedure was also presented in the same year in the XI Congress of the Argentine Society for Surgery of the Hand (awarded with the "J. Goyena Prize"), in November 1985, Buenos Aires, Argentina (14). Other papers on the procedure were published by us in 1986 (15,16), 1988 (17) and 1993 (1,18). The vascular anatomy of the posterior interosseous island flap was presented by Penteado et al in 1986 (11), and other studies on the posterior interosseous flap have been published by Masquelet et al (9), Costa et al (3,4), Gilbert et al (7), Buchler et al (2), Dap et al (5), Mazzer et al (10), and Goubier et al (6). These studies have further supported the efficacy of the this flap.

INDICATIONS/CONTRAINDICATIONS

The posterior interosseous artery island flap is capable of transporting the skin of the distal two-thirds of the forearm. The flap's pedicle length determines its coverage possibilities.

It is particularly useful for covering extensive defects on the back of the hand as far distally as the dorsal aspect of the proximal phalanges of the fingers and for obtaining a complete coverage of the first web after the release of severe adduction contractures of the thumb. Buchler et al (2) noted that the flap could reach the dorsum of the proximal interphalangeal joints. It can be indicated in different types of pathologies such as burn sequelae, wounds on the dorsum of the hand, tumors, and congenital deformities.

Contraindications for flap use include any injury to the posterior interosseous artery or deep laceration or crush wounds to the posterior forearm in the area of the flap pedicle. The flap is not recommended in patients with diabetes, in whom small vessels may be diseased. The flap has been used successfully in smokers, but smoking certainly carries a higher risk of flap complications.

PREOPERATIVE PLANNING

Successful flap harvest is predicated on a thorough knowledge of the flap anatomy. Normally the anterior and posterior interosseous arteries in their course through the forearm are united through two main anastomoses, one proximal, at the level of the distal border of the supinator muscle, and one distal at the most distal part of the interosseous space (2 cm proximally of the distal radioulnar joint) (Fig. 16-1). The island posterior interosseous island flap is supplied by the reverse arterial blood flow through the distal anastomosis once the proximal anastomosis has been ligated. Venous drainage is produced by the venae comitantes of the posterior interosseous artery.

The angiosomal territory of the posterior interosseous artery was studied in a series of 80 cadaveric forearms in 1993 (1). Ink injections performed through catheter placed in the distal part of the anterior interosseous artery stained the distal two-thirds of the posterior forearm skin through the reverse flow through the distal anastomosis. The proximal third of the forearm skin remained unstained even when larger amounts of ink were injected (see Fig. 16-5). Ink injections through the catheter placed in the proximal part of the posterior interosseous artery stained the proximal two-thirds of the posterior forearm through the direct flow through the proximal cutaneous branch (1).

Other anatomic conclusions from this study can be summarized as follows: the posterior interosseous artery usually branches from the common interosseous artery in the proximal third of the forearm in 90% of cases, it can however be a direct branch of the ulnar artery in 10% of cases (1). It pierces the interosseous membrane about 6 cm distal to the lateral epicondyle of the humerus (14–18) forming its origin or proximal anastomosis between the anterior and posterior interosseous arteries. It enters into the posterior compartment of the forearm below the distal edge of the supinator muscle, located at the union of the proximal with the distal two-thirds of the dorsal aspect of the forearm (60 mm distal to the lateral epicondyle). At its entrance into the posterior compartment of the forearm, the posterior interosseous artery gives off branches to the recurrent interosseous artery that anastomoses at the elbow with a descending branch from the superior profunda, with the posterior ulnar recurrent and the anastomotica magna. In its ascending course the artery runs between the lateral condyle and the olecranon (Figs. 16-1 and 16-2).

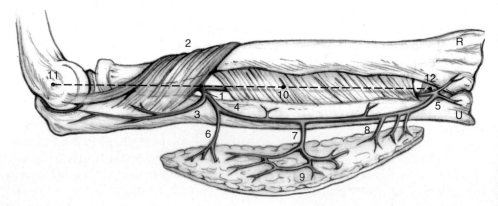

FIGURE 16-1

Anatomy of the posterior interosseous artery. (*1*) Proximal end of the posterior interosseous artery at the distal border of the supinator muscle. (*2*) The artery is emerging as a division of the common interosseous artery. (*3*) Recurrent interosseous artery. (*4*) Posterior interosseous artery following the longitudinal line X-X', between the lateral epycondile (*11*) and the distal radio-ulnar joint (*12*). (*5*) Distal anastomosis between both interosseous arteries (2 cm proximal to the distal radio-ulnar joint). Cutaneous branches from the posterior intererosseous artery that irrigte the two distal thirds of the posterior skin of the forearm. Proximal (*9*), middle (*7*), and distal (*8*) branches. (*10*) Middle of the forearm where the middle cutaneous branch is located 1–2 cm distal to this point.

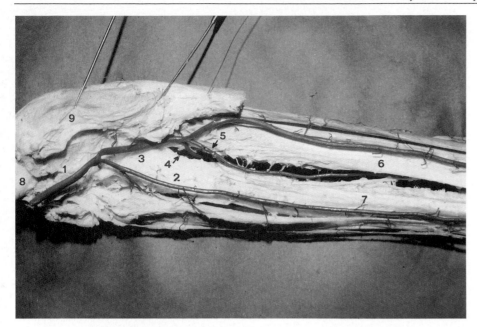

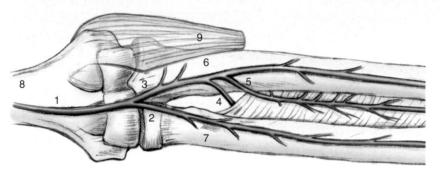

FIGURE 16-2

Cadaver specimen dissected to show the proximal origin of the posterior interosseous artery. Volar view of the proximal part of the forearm and the elbow. (*1*) Brachial artery. (*2*) Radial artery. (*3*) Ulnar artery showing the separated origin of the posterior interosseous artery (*4*) and the anterior interosseous artery (*5*). (*6*) Ulna. (*7*) Radius. (*8*) Humerus. (*9*) Medial epicondyle muscles.

From the proximal anastomosis, the posterior interosseous artery follows a line between the lateral epicondyle and the distal radio-ulnar joint. In its course it can be divided into three parts: proximal, middle, and distal (17).

In the proximal part, the artery runs deep to the abductor pollicis longus muscle and is covered by the extensor digiti minimi and the extensor carpi ulnaris muscles and in close relation with the posterior interosseous nerve and a large venous plexus. In the middle part, it becomes superficial, just beneath the superficial antebrachial fascia in the middle third of the forearm, running between the extensor digiti minimi and the extensor carpi ulnaris muscles. In this part, the artery reduces its diameter in 90% of the cases and is usually found to be between 0.3 and 0.6 mm in diameter (1) (see Fig. 16-4).

In the distal part, the posterior interosseous artery joins with the distal end of the anterior interosseous artery, forming the distal anastomosis between the two vessels (13,15). This anastomosis is located 2 cm proximal to the distal radio-ulnar joint and very close to the periosteum of the ulnar metaphysis (Figs. 16-1 and 16-3). This anastomosis has been present in all our cadaver specimens and operative cases and represents the point of rotation of the vascular pedicle of the posterior interosseous flap. At the distal anastomosis the posterior interosseous artery enlarges between 0.9 and 1.1 mm (1).

During its course, the posterior interosseous artery gives four to six cutaneous branches which run through the septum between the extensor digiti minimi and the extensor carpi ulnaris muscles to reach the dorsal skin of the forearm, of these the principal cutaneous branches are the proximal and middle branches.

The proximal cutaneous branch emerges from the proximal part of the artery, forming a large branch that irrigates the skin over the upper third of the dorsal aspect of the forearm. It is consistently present but it has a variable origin. Of our 80 specimens, it was found as a branch of the recurrent interosseous artery in 28, a branch of the common interosseous artery in 22, and as a branch of the posterior interosseous artery in 30. This variation indicates that the proximal cutaneous branch cannot be preserved to supply the flap in all cases.

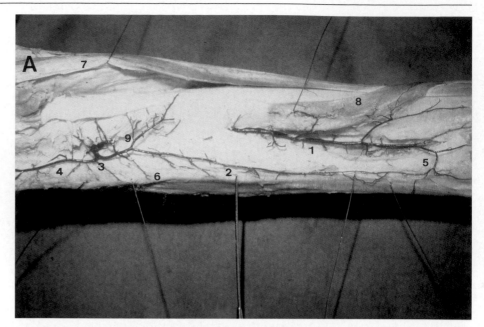

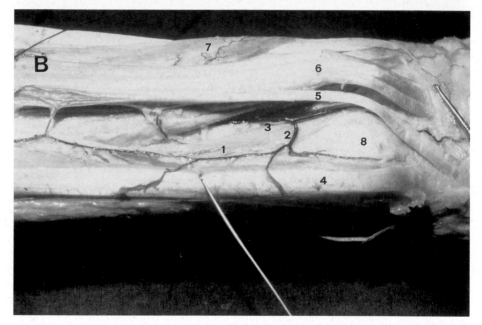

FIGURE 16-3

A: Cadaver specimen injected with latex (right forearm). Dissection of both interosseous arteries. (*1*) Anterior interosseous artery. (*2*) Posterior interosseous artery piercing the interosseous membrane (*3*) and showing the emergence of the recurrent interosseous artery (*4*). The cutaneous branches have been eliminated. (*7*) Distal anastomosis between both interosseous arteries located very close to the periostum of the distal metaphysis of the ulna. (*8*) Extensor carpi ulnaris. (*9*) Extensor carpi radialis brevis muscle. (*10*) Extensor pollicis brevis and abductor pollicis longus muscles. (*11*) Large branch of the posterior interosseous artery to irrigate common extensor muscle. **B:** Posterior interosseous artery showing its proximal anastomosis (*2*) with the anterior interosseous artery (*3*). Right forearm. Several branches to the dorsal muscles of the forearm are seen. (*4*) Extensor carpi ulnaris tendon. (*5*) Extensor digiti quinti tendon. (*6*) Extensor communis digitorum tendons. (*7*) Extensor pollicis brevis and abductor pollicis longus muscles. (*8*) Distal head of the ulna.

The middle cutaneous branch originates in the middle third of the forearm where the posterior interosseous artery becomes superficial. It represents a large branch located at 1 to 2 cm distal to the middle of the forearm. It was consistently present in our cadaveric investigations and clinical cases.

No cutaneous branches were found between the described proximal and middle branches. In our cadaveric observations, one or two large interconnecting venous perforators were consistently found running together with the middle cutaneous arterial branch, uniting the superficial to the deep venous system (the venae comitants of the posterior interosseous artery) (1).

At the distal third of the posterior forearm, the posterior interosseous artery may also contribute six to eight cutaneous branches to the skin of variable diameter (1).

The posterior interosseous artery also gives several branches to the muscles of the posterior compartment of the forearm (see Fig. 16-10E) and contributes some blood supply to the periosteum of the radius and ulna.

In only two cases the continuity of the posterior interosseous artery was absent at the level of the middle of the forearm: one in an anatomic specimen and one in a clinical case. This uncommon anatomic finding is in accordance with other reports in the medical literature. Thus, Penteado et al. (11) found absence of the posterior interosseous artery in the forearm in 4 of 70 specimens. In their same series, the distal anastomosis was absent in only one case. Buchler and Frey (2) found the posterior interosseous artery missing at the middle of the forearm in 2 of 36 cases. Despite this, angiograms and Doppler examination are not part of our standard preoperative protocol.

SURGERY

The surgical procedure is performed under general anesthesia. Pneumatic tourniquet is employed. Exsanguination is obtained by simple elevation of the upper limb for 30 seconds. Loop magnification (4×) permits a better identification of the vascular pedicles and their cutaneous branches. The patient is placed in the supine position with the forearm placed in pronation over the inferior-lateral thoracic wall with the elbow flexed in 90 degrees (Fig. 16-6). This position facilitates flap preparation and raising. The tourniquet is insufflated (250 mmHg) after the flap has been designed. The operation consists into two main steps: flap design and flap elevation.

Flap Design

Flap design (Fig. 16-7A) is strictly related to the shape and size of the recipient area. A longitudinal line (X-X') is drawn from the lateral humeral epicondyle to the distal radioulnar joint. This line represents the course of the posterior interosseous artery in the posterior forearm. A point *A* is marked 1 cm distal to the middle of line. This point corresponds to the emergence of the middle cutaneous branch of the posterior interosseous artery and to the medial interconnecting venous perforator. The

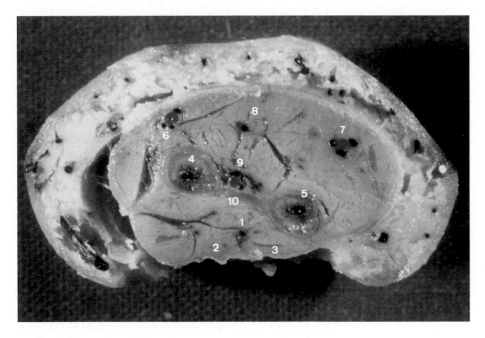

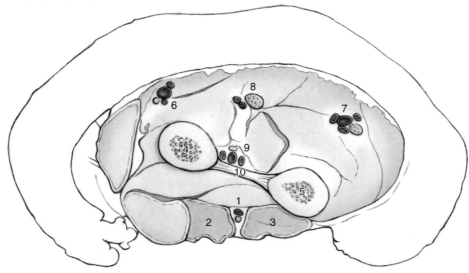

FIGURE 16-4

Transverse section of the forearm at its middle third. (*1*) Posterior interosseous artery—in its proximal course—running deep between the extensor digiti quinti (*2*) and the extensor carpi ulnaris (*3*) muscles. (*4*) Radius. (*5*) Ulna. Radial artery (*6*) and ulnar artery (*7*) both with their venae. Median nerve and median nerve artery (*8*). Anterior interosseous artery and its venae (*9*). Interosseous membrane (*10*).

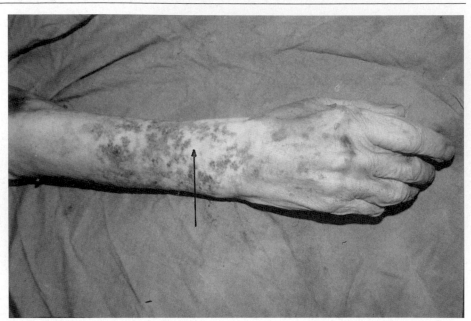

FIGURE 16-5

Fresh cadaver injected with 20 mL of black ink through a catheter placed in the distal anterior interosseous artery. The distal and middle thirds of the dorsal forearm are stained.

flap is planned to be irrigated by this middle cutaneous pedicle, so the point A must be always included in the flap. A second point *B* is marked at the distal end of the line X-X', 2 cm proximal to the distal radio-ulnar joint. This point corresponds to the distal anastomosis between both interosseous arteries and is the point of rotation of the pedicle flap.

The proximal limit of the flap can be safely placed to a point 6 cm distal to the lateral epicondyle (point *C*). The flap may be extended distally up to the wrist joint. In this case distal cutaneous branches can be included. It should be remarked that the medial vascular cutaneous pedicle is capable of irrigating a flap as large as the complete width of the posterior forearm. The center of the flap always corresponds to the line X-X'.

It was observed in our clinical cases that there is no venous insufficiency in the posterior interosseous reverse forearm flap if it is raised with the large middle venous interconnecting perforator. It ensures sufficient drainage of the subcutaneous tissue and skin into the venae comitants of the posterior interosseous artery (1).

A flap of approximately 3 to 4 cm in width will allow for direct closure of the donor area of the forearm leaving an inconspicuous scar (14–16) (Figs. 16-8 and 16-10). Wider flaps will need free skin graft to cover the dorsum of the forearm and may lead to a poorer aesthetic result (Fig. 16-9).

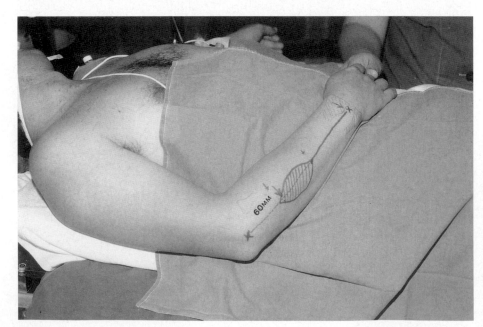

FIGURE 16-6

Position of the upper limb during surgery. In this patient a posterior interosseous artery island flap 4 cm wide has been designed to cover the first interdigital web. The flap is located at the level of the middle cutaneous branch of the posterior interosseous artery. Details on the flap design are completed in Figure 16-7.

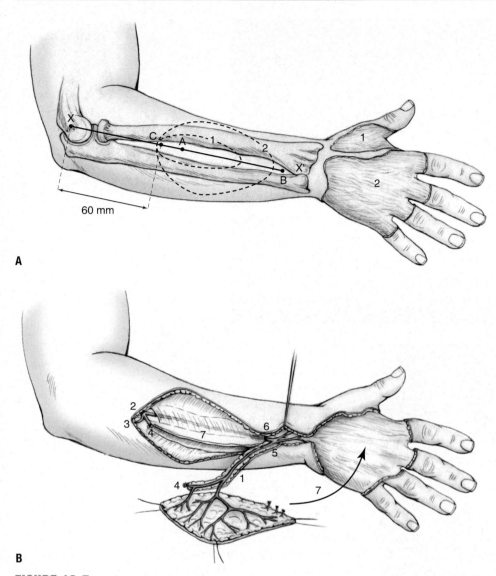

A

B

FIGURE 16-7

A: Design of the flap. The location of the island flap is in the line X-X', between the lateral epicondyle (X) and the distal radio-ulnar joint (X'). Three points are marked in the skin. Point *A* corresponds to the location of the middle cutaneous branch of the posterior interosseous artery. Point *B* is located 2 cm proximal to the distal radio-ulnar point and corresponds with the location of the distal anastomosis; and point *C* is located at the distal edge of the supinator muscle where the posterior interosseous artery pierces the interosseous membrane. This point is 60 mm distal to the lateral epicondyle. The width, length, and shape of the island flap is in accordance with the defect to be covered: *1* is representing the shape, size, and location of a flap to cover the first interdigital web, and *2* represents a flap to cover the dorsal aspect of the hand. **B:** Raising of the island flap. The flap has been raised with the posterior interosseous artery and its venae comitantes (*1*). In this case the middle and the proximal cutaneous branches are irrigating the flap. The intermuscular septum and a strip of fascia are raised with the posterior interosseous artery. (*2*) Common interosseous artery. (*3*) Recurrent interosseous artery. (*4*) The posterior interosseous artery has been ligated at its emergence (proximal anastomosis between both interosseous arteries). (*5*) Distal anastomosis is preserved (point of rotation of the flap). (*6*) Anterior interosseous artery. (*7*) In this case the flap is rotated to cover the dorsum of the hand. The donor area is covered with a free skin graft (see Figs. 16-8 and 16-9).

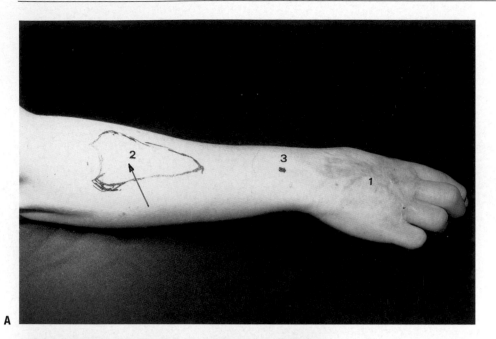

A

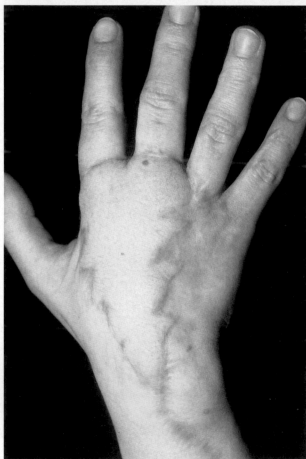

B

FIGURE 16-8

A: Sequela of an injury in a 16-year-old girl on the dorsum of the hand (*1*) with laceration of the long extensor tendons of the index and middle fingers and stiffness of their metacarpophalangeal joints. A posterior interosseous artery island flap was designed (*2*) with the shape of the area to be covered on the hand. Middle and proximal pedicles were preserved to irrigate the flap. Excision of the injured extensor tendons and metacarpophalangeal capsulectomies were indicated simultaneously with the island flap. The fingers were immobilized in flexion during the postoperative period. Location of the distal anastomosis (*3*). **B:** Finger extension obtained after a secondary surgical stage with Z plasties at the borders of the flap and tendon transfer from the flexor superficialis tendon of the ring finger, divided into two strips, to the base of the middle and index fingers proximal phalanges. The interdigital webs were reconstructed with the flap. *(Continued)*

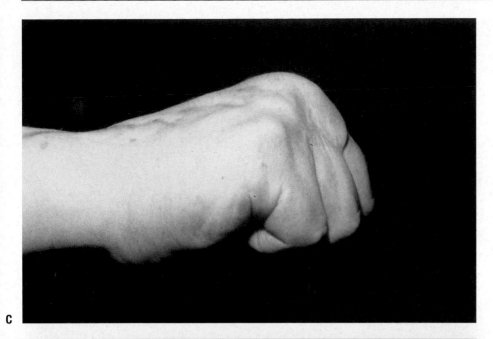

C

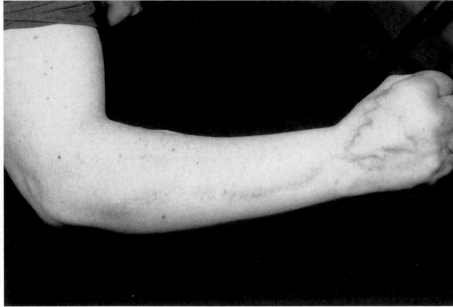

D

FIGURE 16-8

Continued **C:** Digital flexion obtained. **D:** The donor area of the forearm was initially closed.

Flap Elevation

Flap elevation (see Fig. 16-7B) begins at its radial side. The dissection is carried out between the subcutaneous tissue and the superficial fascia. The incision is continued in the direction of the wrist, and the proximal and medial cutaneous branches are easily identified. The interconnecting venous perforator that accompanies the medial cutaneous branch is clearly visualized. The proximal cutaneous branch can be coagulated. Our clinical cases have shown that the flap can be safely raised with the middle cutaneous branch. The posterior interosseous artery is sectioned at its proximal origin proximal to the medial cutaneous branch. The posterior interosseous artery with its venae comitants are raised with the intermuscular septum located between the extensor carpi ulnaris and the extensor indicis propius and a very thin strip of fascia covering the muscles. Elevation is completed after sectioning the skin at the ulnar side of the flap. Finally, the flap is turned through 180 degrees to cover the recipient area: to the dorsum of the hand, or to a released first web space, or to both. Now the pneumatic tourniquet is released to observe flap circulation.

At the end of the procedure, the hand is immobilized in a neutral position of the wrist or with some dorsiflexion. In the case of coverage of the back of the hand, where the extensor tendons have been

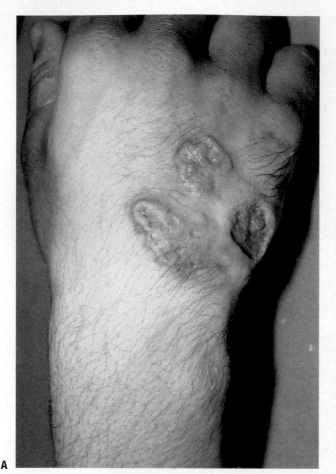

A

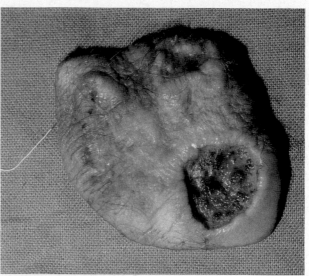

C

FIGURE 16-9

A: An epitheloid sarcoma with invasion of skin on the dorsal aspect of the forearm in a 20-year-old man. **B:** An ample excision of the affected skin, including the extensor tendons of the two last fingers, was indicated. **C:** Piece of the lesion. *(Continued)*

B

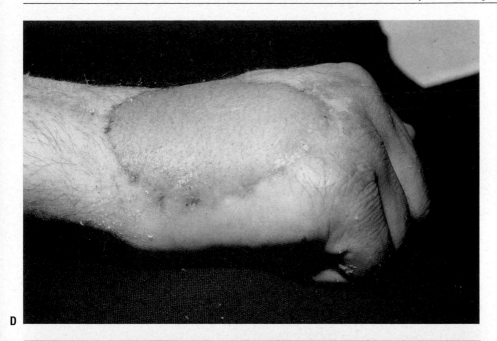

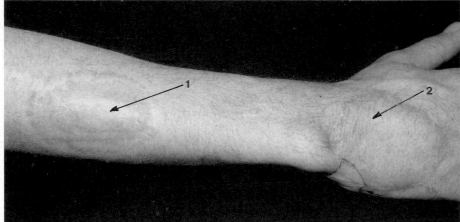

FIGURE 16-9

Continued **D:** Immediate postoperative period after a posterior interosseous artery island flap. In a secondary surgical stage, the extensor tendons were reconstructed. **E:** Result after 2 years following the initial operation showing the free skin graft in the donor area (*1*) and the posterior interosseous artery island flap in the recipient area (*2*). Complete function of the fingers was obtained.

excised and a metacarpophalangeal capsulotomy has been performed, the fingers are immobilized in flexion to prevent the recurrence of metacarpophalangeal stiffness in extension. In these cases tendon grafts can be indicated during a second surgical stage (see Figs. 16-8 and 16-9).

POSTOPERATIVE MANAGEMENT

The hand and wrist are immobilized in a long plaster splint for 2 weeks following the surgery. A large window is left in the dressing to monitor the flap for signs of ischemia or venous congestion. No blood thinning agents are used during the postoperative period. Following removal of the splint, the sutures are removed and the patient may begin postoperative therapy.

RESULTS

Our series of 80 cases (47 males and 33 females) was published in 1993 (1). In this series, 22 flaps were indicated for the coverage of skin defects in the dorsum of the hand, 37 for the reconstruction of the first interdigital web, 5 to cover the dorsum of the hand and first web space, 15 for the volar wrist, and 4 for the palm of the hand. In three cases extensor tendon grafts to extend the fingers were indicated in a second surgical stage. Seventy-six flaps were successful and four were lost. Two of these were clearly due to twisting of the pedicle. The flap provides a large amount of skin for hand reconstruction without interfering with lymphatic drainage, venous drainage, or the integrity of the

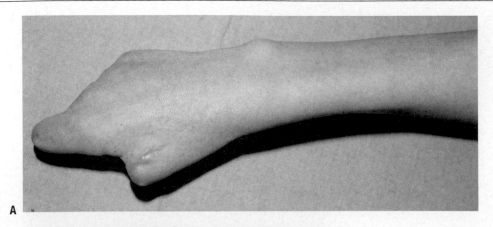

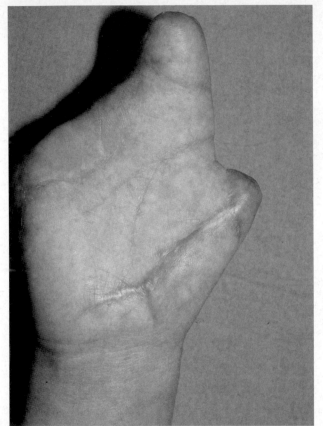

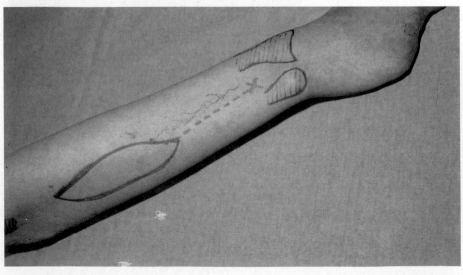

FIGURE 16-10

A,B: Sequela of a trauma with amputation of the digits and adduction contracture of the first intermetacarpal space in a 18-year-old man. **C:** Design of the posterior interosseous artery island flap of 3 cm width. The middle cutaneous branch was preserved to nourish the island flap. *(Continued)*

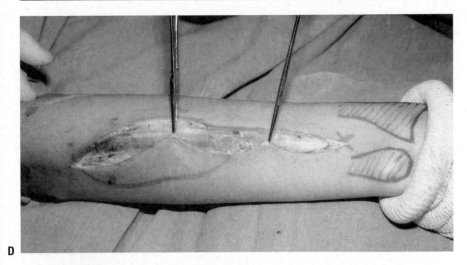

D

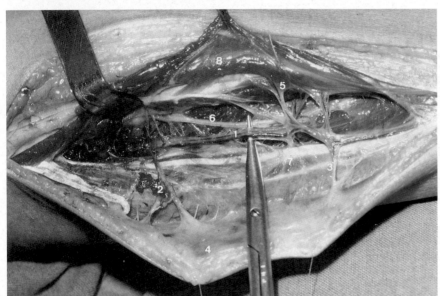

E

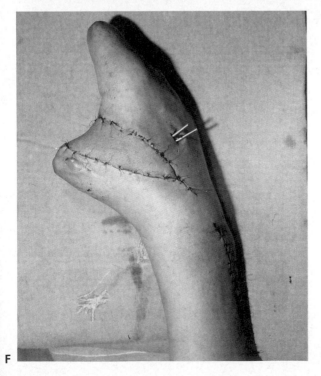

F

FIGURE 16-10

Continued **D:** The initial skin incision is shown. The radial side of the flap is initially elevated from its radial side. **E:** Anatomy of the dissected posterior interosseous artery (*1*) with its middle (*2*) and distal (*3*) cutaneous branches to the dorsal skin of the forearm (*4*). Several arterial branches to the dorsal muscles of the forearm (*5*) and the posterior interosseous nerve (*6*) are shown. The extensor carpi ulnaris muscle (*7*) and the extensor muscles to the fingers (*8*) are separated. The hand is at the right of the picture. **F:** A few days after the release of the first intermetacarpal space and the transport of the island flap. Two KW are maintaining the separation of the first two metacarpals. *(Continued)*

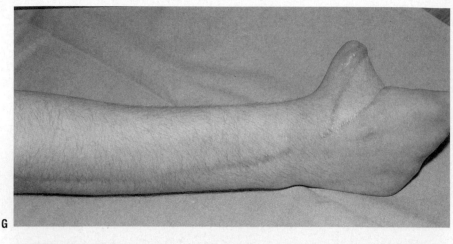

G

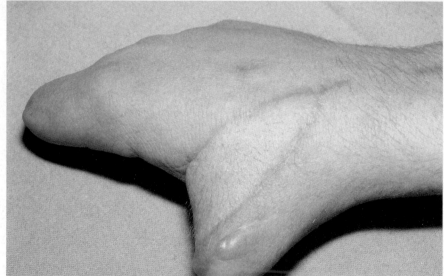

H

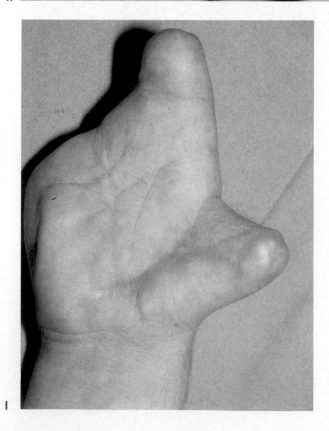

I

FIGURE 16-10

Continued **G:** Direct closure of the donor area. **H,I:** Result obtained.

principal vessels of the volar side of the forearm. It furnishes good-quality skin to permit secondary surgical reconstructions of tendons or the skeleton of the hand.

COMPLICATIONS

As mentioned previously, flap loss is the most serious complication; this is most commonly due to inadvertent twisting of the pedicle or injury to the veins during dissection resulting in flap congestion. Injury to the radial nerve has also been reported with temporary paralysis to the extensor carpi ulnaris and extensor digiti minimi muscles following flap harvest. Such occurrences are rare.

REFERENCES

1. Angrigiani C, Grilli D, Dominikow D, et al. Posterior interosseous reverse forearm flap: experience with 80 consecutive cases. *Plast Reconst Surg.* 1993;92(2):285–293.
2. Buchler U, Frey HP. Retrograde posterior interosseous flap. *J Hand Surg.* 1991;16A(2):283–292.
3. Costa H, Soutar DS. The distally based island posterior interosseous flap. *Br J Plast Surg.* 1988;41:221–227.
4. Costa H, Smith R, McGrouther DA. Thumb reconstruction by the posterior interosseous flap. *Br J Plast Surg.* 1988;41:228–233.
5. Dap F, Dantel G, Voche P, et al. The posterior interosseous flap in primary repair of hand injuries. *J Hand Surg.* 1993;18-B(4):437–445.
6. Goubier JN, Romaña C, Masquelet AC. Le Lambeaux interosseoux posterieur chez l'enfant. *Chirurgie de la Main.* 2002;21:102–106.
7. Gilbert A, Masquelet AC, Hentz VR. Pedicle flaps of the upper limb. In: Dunitz M, ed. *Vascular anatomy: surgical technique and current indications.* 1992.
8. Manchot C. *The cutaneous arteries of the human body* (translation of Hautarterien des menslischen Korpers. 1889.) New York: Springer; 1983.
9. Masquelet AC, Penteado CV. Le Iambeau interosseoux posterieur. *Ann Chir Main.* 1987;6:131–139.
10. Mazzer N, Barbieri CH, Cortez M. The posterior interosseous forearm island flap for skin defects in the hand and elbow. A prospective study of 51 cases. *J Hand Surg.* 1996;21B:237–243.
11. Penteado CV, Masquelet AC, Chevrel JP. The anatomic basis of the fascio-cutaneous flap of the posterior interosseous artery. *Surg Radiol Anat.* 1986,8.209–215.
12. Salmon M. Les arteres de la peau. Etude anatomique et chirurgicale. Paris: Masson and Companie; 1936.
13. Zancolli EA. Posterior interosseous island forearm flap. *Vascular anatomy.* VIth European Hand Surgery Course. June 6th, 1985. Ümea, Sweden (handouts published in 1993).
14. Zancolli EA, Angrigiani C, Lopez Carlone H. *Contractura severa en aducción de la primera comisura de la mano.* Colgajo dorsal del antebrazo. November 29-30, 1985. XI Congress of the Argentine Society for Surgery of the Hand (Paper awarded with the "Jorge Goyena Prize," 1985). Buenos Aires, Argentina (not published).
15. Zancolli EA, Angrigiani C. Colgajo dorsal del antebrazo (en "isla)(Pedículo de vasos interoseos posteriores). *Revista de la Asociación Argentina de Ortopedia y Traumatología.* 1986;51(2):161–168.
16. Zancolli EA, Angrigiani C. Dorsal forearm island flap. *Posterior interosseous vessels pedicle.* 3rd Congress of the International Federation of Societies for Surgery of the Hand, Tokyo, 1986 (abst).
17. Zancolli EA, Angrigiani C. Posterior interosseous island flap. *J Hand Surg.* 1988;13-B(2):130–135.
18. Zancolli EA, Cozzi E. *Atlas de Anatomía Quirúrgica de la Mano.* Ed. Medica Panamericana. Madrid, 1993:93.

17 Fillet Flaps in Cases of Mutilating Trauma

Bradley Medling and Michael W. Neumeister

Fillet flaps can be a very important reconstructive option in many cases of hand and lower limb trauma. Fillet flaps are, by definition, axial flaps that may provide skin, muscle, fascia, and bone. They can be harvested either as a pedicled flap or as a free flap. Careful a planning and execution of the flaps can allow for reconstruction of local defects with a flap of a similar tissue type. This technique takes advantage of spare parts that would otherwise be discarded, avoiding associated morbidity of a separate flap harvest.

Fillet flaps are most commonly employed after mutilating trauma to the hand. The concept of spare parts surgery should be broadly applied to include any tissue that would otherwise be discarded; these flaps may include bone, nerve, tendon, joints, or the whole digit. Segments of the injured part can be harvested with their blood supply intact, and thereby be used as a vascularized tissue graft or flap.

Frequently, a traumatized extremity is left without soft tissue coverage, leaving exposed vital structures such as bone, joint, tendon, or neurovascular bundles. Vascularized coverage can be salvaged from attached parts of the mangled hand that are otherwise rendered dysfunctional or from amputated parts where a flap is designed over a preserved vascular bundle.

The key component to the safe harvest of a fillet flap is an understanding of the vascular supply to tissue. Since the entire upper extremity and lower extremity can be used in a fillet fashion, the blood supply to the arm and leg must be understood. In the upper extremity, the axillary artery terminates at the lateral border of the pectoralis minor muscle becoming a brachial artery to a point just distal to the antecubital fossa. The brachial artery runs in the medial upper arm in relative proximity to the ulnar and median nerve. At the level of the elbow, the brachial artery is lateral to the median nerve. The brachial artery bifurcates into the radial and ulnar arteries, respectively, under the superficial flexor muscles of the forearm. The radial artery travels under the flexor carpi radialis muscle exiting more superficial in the forearm just lateral to the tendon of the flexor carpi radialis. The ulnar artery travels with the ulnar nerve under the muscle belly of the flexor carpi ulnaris becoming more superficial in the distal forearm. The ulnar artery travels through Guyon's canal and bifurcates into a superficial and deep branch, each of which communicates with the radial artery component of the superficial and deep palmar arches. The radial artery bifurcates at the wrist into a superficial palmar and deep dorsal branch. The superficial palmar branch courses around the base of the thenar eminence, and the larger deep branch travels under the abductor pollicis longus, extensor pollicis brevis, and the extensor pollicis longus, through the anatomical snuffbox. It then courses between the first and second metacarpals, through the adductor space to form the radial component of the superficial and deep palmar arches. The common digital vessels arise from the superficial palmar arch and travel to the level of the metacarpophalangeal joint, where these vessels now bifurcate to become the digital vessels proper (Fig. 17-1).

In the lower extremity, the superficial femoral and the profunda femoral vessels may be used as arterial inflow for fillet flaps of the thigh. The superficial femoral vessels continue distally to form the

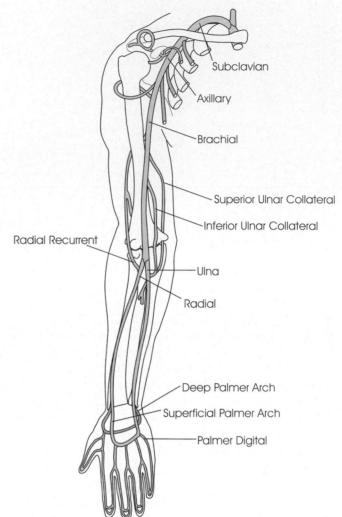

FIGURE 17-1

Upper extremity vascular anatomy. Axial pattern flaps can be designed from known vasculature and their smaller branches.

popliteal artery, which bifurcates in the popliteal fossa to the anterior tibial and posterior tibial arteries. The posterior tibial artery subsequently bifurcates to become the posterior tibial artery and the peroneal artery. The anterior tibial artery travels in the anterior compartment above the interosseous membrane, becoming more superficial as it approaches the extensor retinaculum of the ankle. At this point, this vessel becomes the dorsalis pedis artery, which travels between the first and second metatarsal to the foot. The superficial arcuate branch provides arterial inflow to the dorsum of the foot, while the deep branch pierces between the first and second metatarsal to form the plantar vascular arch. The common digital vessels arise from this arch, and bifurcate at the metatarsal-phalangeal joints to become the digital vessels to the toes. The peroneal artery travels beside the medial aspect of the fibula and terminates as the lateral calcaneal artery behind the lateral malleolus. The poster tibial artery travels in the poster compartment of the lower leg and exits superficial behind the medial malleolus and subsequently bifurcates into the medial and lateral plantar vessels (Fig. 17-2).

INDICATIONS/CONTRAINDICATIONS

Before harvesting a fillet flap for soft tissue coverage, the surgeon should identify the ultimate goal of the immediate and delayed reconstructive procedures. Decisions may be less complex for some lower extremity trauma, where discarding the mutilating limb may be in the best interest of the patient from a functional point of view. Prostheses may be much more functional than attempts at salvage where stability and sensation are compromised. Conversely, mangled hands can have significant function if pinch and grasp can be restored. Reconstructive efforts may be turned toward

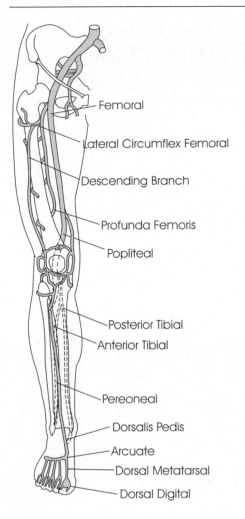

- Femoral
- Lateral Circumflex Femoral
- Descending Branch
- Profunda Femoris
- Popliteal
- Posterior Tibial
- Anterior Tibial
- Pereoneal
- Dorsalis Pedis
- Arcuate
- Dorsal Metatarsal
- Dorsal Digital

FIGURE 17-2

Lower extremity vascular anatomy.

salvaging fingers or the thumb, rather than using their tissue as spare parts for soft tissue coverage for the remaining injured hand. The ability to restore some sensate function is a key component of the hand's role in activities of daily living. This separates the overall treatment protocols and goals of upper extremity reconstruction from that of lower extremity reconstruction (Fig. 17-3). The reconstruction process is dictated by the complexity and level of injury. Nerve regeneration, tendon and bone reconstruction, and secondary toe to hand procedures are alternatives to amputation of digits or hands and permit acceptable restoration of function. In both upper and lower extremity, however, there are opportunities that arise to use tissue that would otherwise be discarded, for definitive soft tissue closure.

The availability of adequate tissue often depends on the mechanism of injury to a limb. Clean guillotine lacerations or amputations, with minimal tissue loss, offer the best results at restoration of function. Fortunately, most of these injuries do not mandate that need of spare parts or fillet flaps due to the lack of soft tissue deficits. More traumatic injuries, such as crush and avulsion injuries, or electrical burns, require greater debridement and have more tissue loss. Consequently, these injuries frequently take advantage of spare parts and fillet flap surgery for coverage.

Pedicle or free tissue fillet flaps can be used for proximal amputations that require stable coverage to better preserve function, such as elbow flexion or knee mobility. This technique is usually indicated for amputations with significant proximal tissue loss and where there is a contraindication for replantation. The remaining distal tissue is filleted, based on one neurovascular bundle, and transferred to cover the proximal exposed structures as a free tissue transfer. If there is an intact neurovascular bundle, but with segmental intervening loss of tissue in the limb, the fillet flap can be harvested as a pedicle flap, leaving the vessels and nerves intact. Indications for fillet flaps are included in Table 17-1.

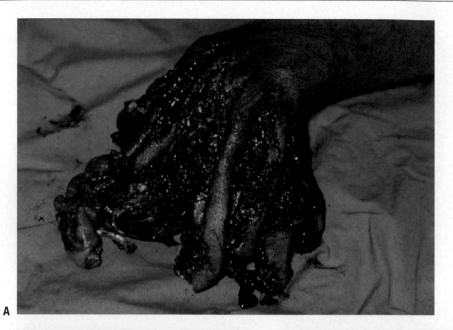

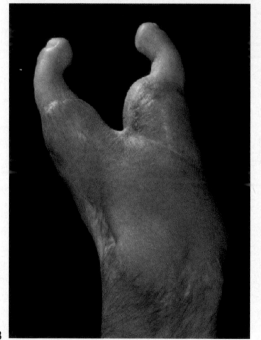

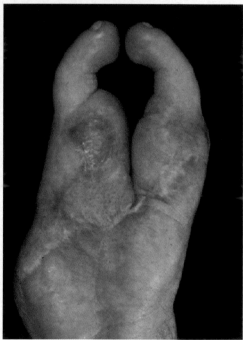

FIGURE 17-3

A: Mutilated hand from corn picker injury with complete loss of all fingers. **B,C:** Restoration of pinch from two toe-to-hand transfers.

TABLE 17-1.   Indications for Fillet Flap

Nonreplantable extremity with adjacent tissue loss from trauma	Availability of tissue from discarded, amputated, or nonfunctioning limb or digit
Nonsalvageable digit with proximal or adjacent digit/hand defect	Segmental loss tumor extirpation or trauma

PREOPERATIVE PLANNING

The preoperative planning should take into consideration patient stability, premorbid health, a history of smoking, limb function (i.e., preservation of elbow flexion), available local tissue, prostheses application, and patient occupation. Patient selection is very important when contemplating the use of fillet flaps for soft tissue coverage of limb or trunk defects. In acute, mutilating trauma, the patient must be stabilized initially as survival should be the first goal. Following the full advanced trauma life support (ATLS) workup, with primary and secondary surveys, limb salvage is planned to optimize function.

The initial surgery should entail an aggressive debridement and irrigation to make sure all tissue is viable. Many times, a second and third surgery are required to allow tissue to demarcate and to avoid infection. Before using fillet tissues, the surgeon should plan to transfer based on the blood supply to the spare tissue. The fillet flaps can either be transferred as a free flap or a pedicle flap. Digital fillet flaps are neurovascular flaps usually based on the digital arterial and nerve supply to the finger (Fig. 17-4). The surgeon will plan to use the digit that has been, in part, rendered dysfunctional as a result of the proximal trauma but where viability is still present distally through an

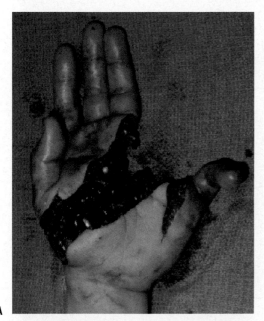

A

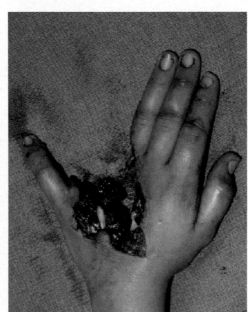

B

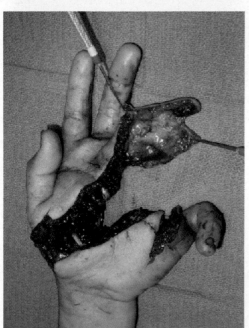

C

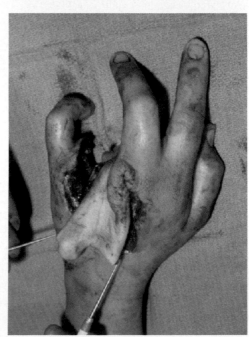

D

FIGURE 17-4

A–D: Tablesaw to the right hand with intrusion through the web space between the small and ring finger in an ulnar to radial direction. Complex repair of flexor/extensor tendons, neurovascular repair of the arch and common digital vessels was undertaken. The ring finger is filleted based on its radial neurovascular bundle. Resection of the head of the fourth metacarpal was performed secondary to the level of comminution. Long-term follow-up reveals good prehension. *(Continued)*

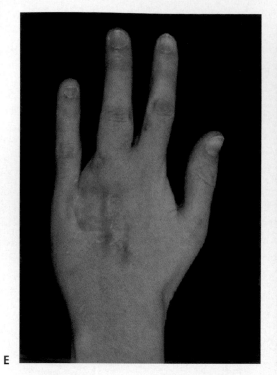

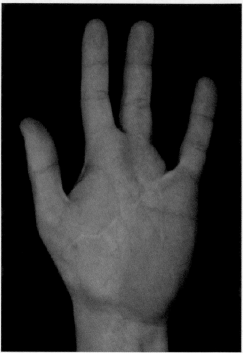

FIGURE 17-4

Continued **E–G:** Tablesaw to the right hand with intrusion through the web space between the small and ring finger in an ulnar to radial direction. Complex repair of flexor/extensor tendons, neurovascular repair of the arch and common digital vessels was undertaken. The ring finger is filleted based on its radial neurovascular bundle. Resection of the head of the fourth metacarpal was performed secondary to the level of comminution. Long-term follow-up reveals good prehension.

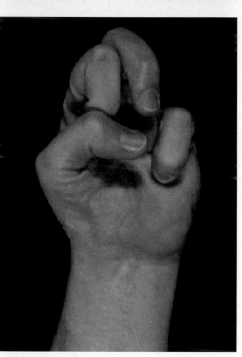

intact neurovascular bundle. In the elective cases, angiography may help to identify intact vascular anatomy before transfer. Angiography is rarely indicated in the acute traumatic case as the surgeon can visualize the vessels and observe the vascularity (bleeding) of the distal tissues.

SURGERY

Patient Positioning

The patient should be positioned appropriately to allow dissection of any digit, arm, or leg based on the blood supply of that part. The patient is usually in the supine position for most upper extremity and lower extremity flaps. An exception to this is the use of a fillet flap for recurrent, recalcitrant pressure sores on the ischial and para-sacral areas, for which the patient should be placed in the prone position.

Technique

The assessment of vascular integrity should be performed before inflation of the tourniquet. Although a pulse-lavage system can be employed, a simple spray bottle allows adequate force to propel smaller particulate debris from the wound (Fig. 17-5). Larger debris should be mechanically debrided with sharp dissection. The preservation of questionable tissue is acceptable if further assessment is planned in 24 to 48 hours for further debridements. Temporary coverage with dressings, xenograft, or allograft can be used in the interim to prevent desiccation in the interim (Fig. 17-6).

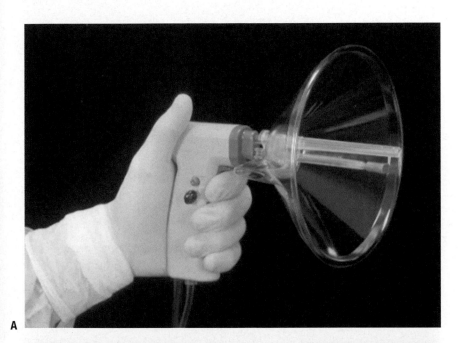

A

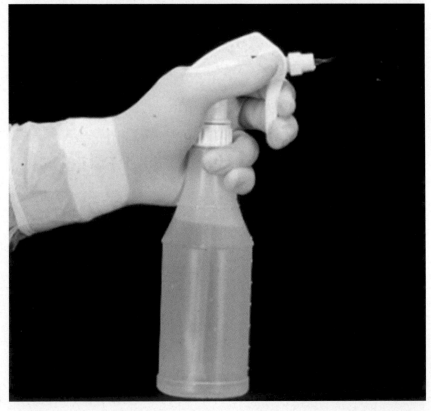

B

FIGURE 17-5

A: Pulse lavage system. **B:** Simple spray bottle.

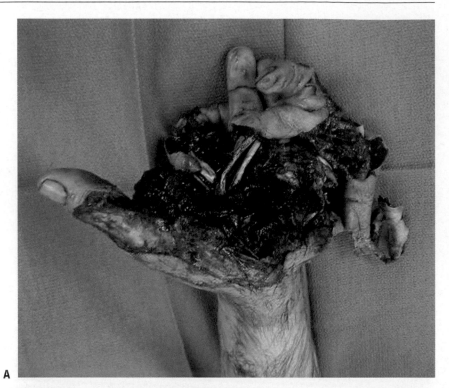

A

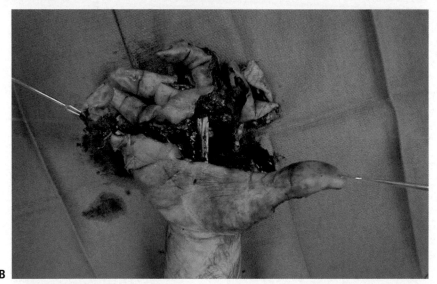

B

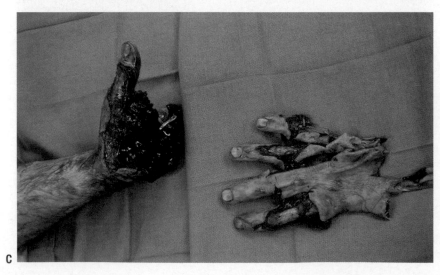

FIGURE 17-6

A–C: Mutilating injury necessitating temporary coverage with allograft secondary to the size of the wound, and possible need for further debridement. *(Continued)*

C

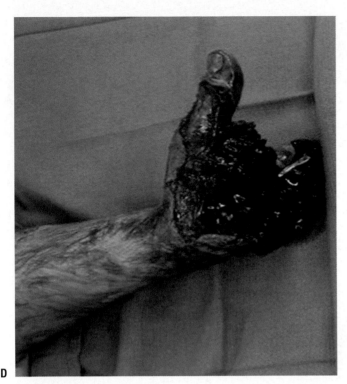

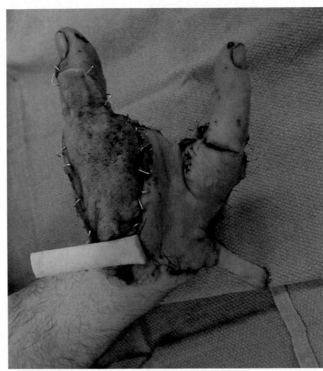

D

E

FIGURE 17-6

Continued **D–E:** Mutilating injury necessitating temporary coverage with allograft secondary to the size of the wound, and possible need for further debridement.

Digital Fillet Flaps of the Hand   The hand provides an ideal setting for the use of fillet flaps for soft tissue coverage of mutilating injuries. A single finger can provide all the components required for composite reconstruction of the hand. Digital fillet flaps can be designed to cover both palmar and dorsal hand defects (Fig. 17-7). The use of adjacent digits that are rendered dysfunctional from the injury can provide coverage with glaborous skin and normal sensibility (Fig. 17-8). Similarly, microsurgical techniques can be used to move the filleted digit to an area of the hand not immediately adjacent to the flap. Idler describes the use of a filleted digit as a free flap to transfer to cover proximal hand wounds. An osteocutaneous fillet flap was described by Gainor in which the index finger with the bone intact was transferred to reconstruct the thumb. A composite, neurovascular island flap can be used in a similar fashion incorporating the distal phalanx, nail bed, and skin for sensate reconstruction of a hemi-thumb defect (Fig. 17-9).

The vascularity of the digit to be a fillet is determined by gross inspection and the use of a handheld Doppler. The arc of rotation depends on the fillet flap's vascular pedicle. The fillet flap must reach the primary defect based on the pivot point of a pedicle. Al-Qattan described lengthening a fillet finger flap by incising the skin at the finger. He then recommends basing the flap on either the radial or ulnar vessel, which will allow one to unfold of the flap and increase its functional pedicle length. Preoperative planning using a surgical sponge to measure the arc of rotation and the subsequent length of the flap required is a helpful tool in determining the utility of the proposed flap. Incomplete filling of the defect will result in the need for skin grafting some other form of soft tissue coverage. Split or full thickness skin grafts can be harvested from remaining spare parts. Excess tissue within the fillet flap can be used to fill in contour defects. In such cases, the distal portion of the fillet flap can be de-epithelialized and folded beneath the remaining flap to augment soft tissue bulk.

Fillet Flaps of the Legs and Arms   Fillet flaps of the legs and arms are used to cover proximal amputation stumps to prevent further shortening of the limb or to add length around the elbow or shoulder. In upper extremity trauma, these fillet flaps are based on the radial or ulnar arteries. The flap is usually a free tissue transfer because there is often an intervening defect in the vessels. The brachial artery and venae commitantes act as the recipient vessels around the elbow. In lower extremity trauma, the fillet flap can be based on either the anterior tibial or the posterior tibial vessels. Incisions in the distal amputated part are made on the opposite side of the limb from where the blood

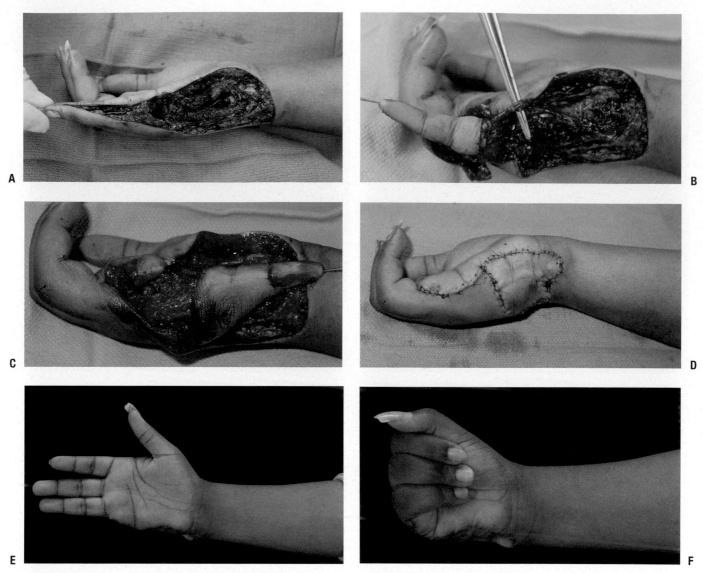

FIGURE 17-7

Fourteen-year-old patient with hypothenar defect. **A–D:** The small finger is filleted based on its radial neurovascular bundle for coverage. This technique provides stable, sensate closure of the defect. **E,F:** Three-month follow-up reveals stable coverage and good hand function.

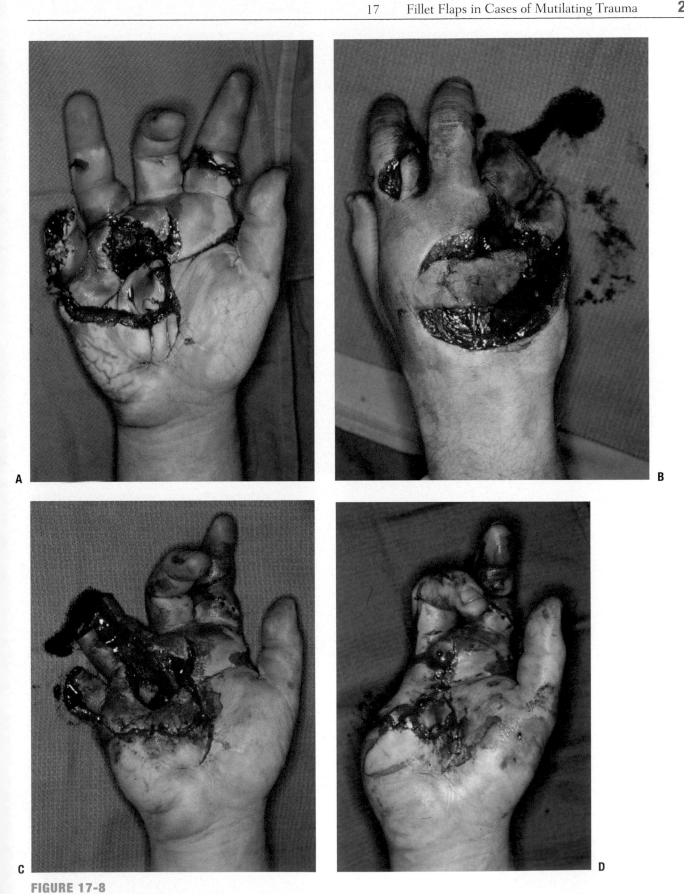

FIGURE 17-8

A–D: Punch press injury to ulnar aspect of left hand. Ring and small fingers filleted for coverage. A small skin graft is placed dorsally beyond the reach of the tip of the flap. Long-term postoperative follow-up reveals stable coverage. *(Continued)*

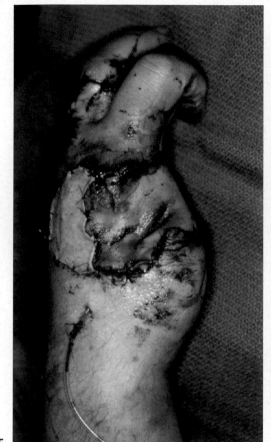

E

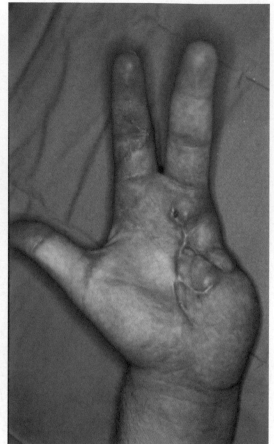

F

G

FIGURE 17-8

Continued **E–G:** Punch press injury to ulnar aspect of left hand. Ring and small fingers filleted for coverage. A small skin graft is placed dorsally beyond the reach of the tip of the flap. Long-term postoperative follow-up reveals stable coverage.

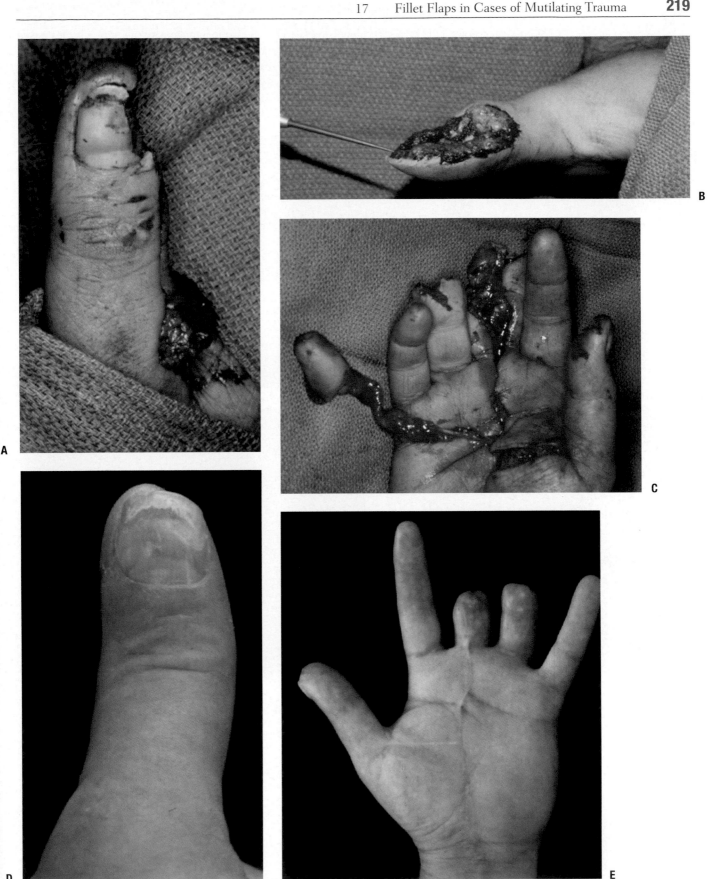

FIGURE 17-9

A,B: Table saw injury to ulnar aspect of a thumb. **C–E:** Additional injury to the middle and ring fingers. Neurovascular island flap harvested from the middle finger transferred for composite coverage of the thumb.

supply is present. This keeps the blood supply to the skin, subcutaneous tissue, and muscles based axially with the medial and lateral tissue equal distances from the primary vessels. Care must be taken during the removal of the bony and muscular components of the flap not to injure the neurovascular bundles. The flap is trimmed appropriately to fit the recipient defect. The fillet flaps can be harvested as a pedicle flap or as a free tissue transfer (Fig. 17-10).

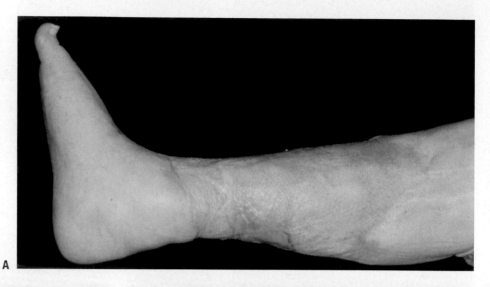

A

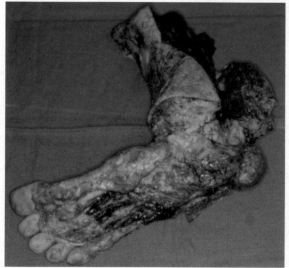

B

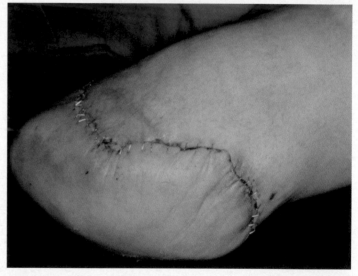

C

FIGURE 17-10

Lower extremity reconstruction after amputation. The sole of the foot is filleted and transferred proximally to cover the proximal stump after amputation.

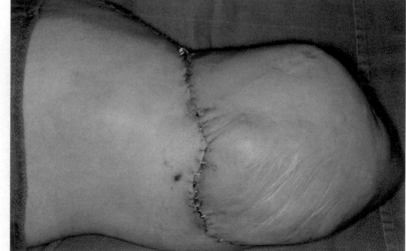

D

POSTOPERATIVE CARE

Postoperative care depends on the area reconstructed. For upper extremity defects, bulky noncompressive dressings are used to protect lacerated or damaged digits. A window is left within the dressing to monitor the vascular status of the fillet flap. If the spare part has been transferred as a free flap, then flap monitoring is performed hourly for the first 24 to 48 hours to ensure there are no signs of arterial ischemia or venous congestion. Signs of either problem will necessitate anastomotic re-exploration to prevent flap failure.

If extensive skin grafting has been performed, motion within the digit or extremity is usually delayed for 5 to 7 days to allow for skin graft take. If a bolster dressing has been placed or if skin grafts have been secured with the use of vacuum-assisted-closure (VAC), motion may be initiated sooner.

Lower extremity wounds are also treated initially with bulky noncompressive dressings and immobilization with the application of a posterior splint. Leg elevation is essential to limit swelling and minimize the risk of venous congestion within the flap. At 1 week postoperatively, compressive wraps may be initiated to the flap and reconstructive area to help with the resolution of postoperative edema. Compressive wrapping may also aid in long-term flap contours.

RESULTS/COMPLICATIONS

Flap loss is obviously the most devastating complication following fillet flap reconstruction. In such cases, alternative means of wound coverage will be necessary to cover resultant defects. Kuntscher et al. present their results from pedicle fillet flaps of fingers for dorsal, palmer, and adjacent digit defects secondary to trauma, burn wounds, Dupuytren's disease, malignant tumor resection, and diabetic gangrene. In their series of 30 patients, the fillet flap provided a stable coverage option with normal sensibility compared to the unaffected digits. The overall complication rate was 18%, with a flap loss, revision surgery, and infection rate of 7.5%.

RECOMMENDED READING

al Qattan MM. Lengthening of the finger fillet flap to cover dorsal wrist defects. *J Hand Surg*. 1997;22:550.

Cave EF, Rowe CR. Utilization of skin from deformed and useless fingers to cover defects in the hand. *Ann Surg*. 1947;125;126.

Chan SW, LaStayo P. Hand therapy management following mutilating hand injuries. *Hand Clin*. 2003; 9(1):133-148.

Goitz RJ, Westkaemper JG, Tomaino MM, et al. Soft-tissue defects of the digits. Coverage considerations. *Hand Clin*. 1997;13:189.

Hammond DC, Matloub HS, Kadz BB, et al. The free-fillet flap for reconstruction of the upper extremity. *Plast Reconstr Surg*. 1994;94:507.

Idler RS, Mih AD. Soft tissue coverage of the hand with a free digital fillet flap. *Microsurgery*. 1990;11:215.

Küntscher MV, Erdmann D, Homann HH, et al. The concept of fillet flaps: classification, indications, and analysis of their clinical value. *Plast Reconstr Surg*. 2001;108:885.

Russell RC, Vitale V, Zook EC. Extremity reconstruction using the fillet of sole flap. *Ann Plast Surg*. 1986;17:65.

Singer DI, Morrison WA, McCann JJ, et al. The fillet foot for end weight-bearing cover of below knee amputations. *Aust N Z J Surg*. 1988;58:817.

18 The Use of Free Flaps in Upper Extremity Reconstruction/ Anterolateral Thigh Flap

Lawrence Lin, Samir Mardini, and Steven L. Moran

INDICATIONS/CONTRAINDICATIONS

Soft tissue deficiencies within the upper extremity are common following trauma, burns, infection, and tumor extirpation. The coverage of such defects can usually be accomplished with the use of pedicled flaps or local rotational flaps. However, when defects are very large or encompass multiple structures including nerve, bone, or muscle, the use of composite free tissue transfer provides a reliable and single stage means of reconstructing complex defects.

The benefits of free tissue transfer within the upper extremity include the transfer of additional vascularized tissue to the injured area, the ability to carry vascularized nerve, bone, skin, and muscle to the injured area in one procedure, and the avoidance of any additional functional deficits to the injured limb which may be incurred with the use of a local or pedicled flap. Free flaps are not tethered at one end, as is the cases for pedicled flaps, and this allows for more freedom in flap positioning and insetting. More recent fasciocutaneous and perforator flaps also allow for primary closure of donor sites with minimal sacrifice of donor site muscle. With current microsurgical techniques, free flap loss rates are between 1% and 4% for cases requiring elective free tissue reconstruction. Finally, the upper extremity is particularly suited for free tissue transfer as the majority of recipient blood vessels utilized for anastomosis are located close to the skin, and are of relatively large caliber.

Major indications for free tissue transfer are: (a) primary coverage of large traumatic wounds with exposed bone, joint, and tendons or hardware, (b) coverage of complex composite defects requiring bone and soft tissue replacement, (c) coverage of soft tissue deficits resulting from release of contractures or scarring from previous trauma, and (d) significant burns.

There are few absolute contraindications for free flap transfer and in many cases free tissue transfer may be the only option for upper limb salvage following significant soft tissue loss. Despite this, relative contraindications to free tissue transfer include a history of a hypercoagulable state, history of recent upper extremity DVT, and evidence of ongoing infection with the traumatic defect. Other contraindications would include inadequate recipient vessels for flap anastomosis. Disregarding technical error, the status of the recipient vessel used for flap anastomosis may play the greatest role in flap failure; recipient vessels within the zone of injury are prone to postoperative and intraoperative thrombosis. Recipient vessels for microvascular transfer should ideally be located out of the zone of injury, radiation, or infection. In rare cases, arterial venous fistulas may be created proximally within the upper extremity or axilla using the cephalic or saphenous vein. These fistulas can be brought into the zone of injury and divided to provide adequate inflow and outflow for free tissue transfer.

Specific Indication for the Anterolateral Thigh Flap

There are many choices for free flap coverage of the upper extremity. The scapular, parascapular, latissimus dorsi myocutaneous, and lateral arm flap have long been favorites of surgeons for reconstruction of traumatic upper extremity injuries. Many of these flaps will be described in later chapters of this text. If joints are to be crossed, fasciocutaneous flaps are much preferred as muscle flaps can undergo atrophy and restrict flexion and extension across joints or fingers (Fig. 18-1).

Classic cutaneous free flaps, such as the radial forearm flap, lateral arm flap, and scapular flap, have limitations in size, donor site morbidity, and overall thickness. Musculocutaneous flaps such as the latissimus dorsi and rectus abdominus flaps result in functional loss and donor site morbidity including, particularly in the abdomen, potential hernia formation. In addition, in coverage of joint surfaces, muscle flaps tend to undergo fibrosis and atrophy over time, which may limit muscle excursion, particularly when placed over the elbow or dorsum of the hand. Muscle is still indicated for those circumstances involving osteomyelitis or significant soft tissue contamination. More recently, chimeric flaps have been harvested to include both muscle and a large component of skin, providing the ideal coverage for many complex defects in the upper extremity.

FIGURE 18-1

A: An extensive iv infiltrate to back of hand and forearm resulted in full thickness skin loss over the majority of the hand and forearm in this 56 year old woman. **B:** Soft tissue coverage was obtained with the use of a rectus abdominus free flap. **C,D:** Despite successful soft tissue coverage, atrophy and fibrosis within the muscle over time has lead to limitations in wrist motion resulting in decreased wrist flexion.

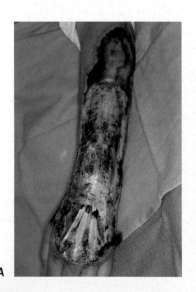
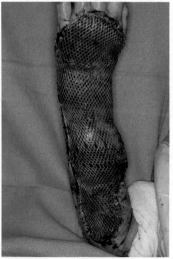
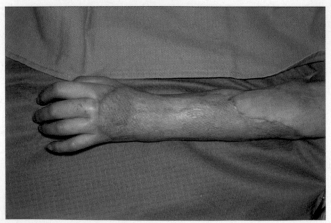
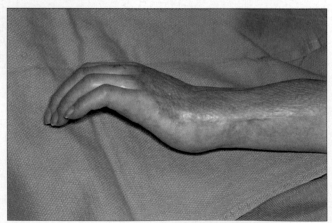

In recent years, the anterolateral thigh flap has become the major flap in reconstructive microsurgery, including head and neck defects and extremity wounds. It has replaced many other flaps. The skin overlying the anterior thigh region has relatively constant anatomy with the descending branch of the lateral femoral circumflex artery (LFCA), giving rise to either pure muscular (musculocutaneous) or subcutaneous (septocutaneous) perforators that supply the area. Based on their experience with over 1,500 anterolateral thigh flaps for various anatomic defects including the upper extremity, Chen et al determined that 12% were based on direct septocutaneous perforators, and 88% were based on musculocutaneous perforators. Variations in perforator anatomy can exist, which include absence of skin perforator, perforators which are too small for elevation, a perforator artery which does not run with the vein, and perforator arteries that have no accompanying vein. These anatomical variations are rare, accounting for 2% of cases, however they need to be noted by the surgeon. As proposed by Chen, an algorithm for managing anatomical variations begins with attempting to identify a more proximal perforator in the upper thigh, usually arising from the transverse branch of the LFCA, and harvesting the flap based on this perforator. Alternatively, an anteromedial thigh flap may be raised or the vastus lateralis may be taken as a musculocutaneous flap. Finally, exploration can be performed on the contralateral side as the anatomy may be different.

The anterolateral thigh flap serves as the ideal flap for upper extremity coverage due to its many considerable advantages. The flap provides a long pedicle (up to 16 cm) with suitable vessel diameters; the arterial pedicle can measure up to 2.5 mm and the two venae comitantes can measure up to 3 mm in diameter. It is also a versatile flap with the ability to incorporate different tissue components with large amounts of skin, as the flap can be harvested as a cutaneous, fasciocutaneous, or musculocutaneous flap with vastus lateralis. In addition, based on the supply of the LFCA system, a chimeric flap incorporating the rectus femoris or tensor fascia lata can be raised to cover extensive, complex defects. The flap may be harvested as a sensate flap by including the lateral femoral cutaneous nerve or as a flow-through flap in cases of significant arterial trauma. Inclusion of thigh fascia with the flap allows its use as an interposition graft for tendon reconstruction. The thickness of the flap may be debulked primarily, optimizing the match of donor tissue for the upper extremity. Ordinary skin flaps can sometimes produce bulkiness with poor aesthetics. Thick skin paddles, such as with parascapular flaps, may interfere with motor function and flexion of the metacarpal phalangeal joints or inter-phalangeal joints. Flaps as thin as 3 mm to 5 mm have been harvested for tendon coverage. The donor site results in minimal morbidity with most sites able to be closed primarily, resulting in a linear scar and absence of any long term leg dysfunction. Lastly, its anatomic location allows for a two-team approach for flap elevation and recipient site preparation, saving considerable operative time.

ANTEROLATERAL THIGH FLAP FOR UPPER EXTREMITY RECONSTRUCTION

Preoperative Planning

Preoperative requirements for flap consideration begin with the preparation of a clean wound bed. Radical debridement of all necrotic tissue is the most important component of a successful reconstruction. Tissue considered to be of marginal viability should be debrided early rather than performing multiple dressing changes or utilizing vacuum-assisted therapy in the hopes of rescuing traumatized tissue; such measures can lead to delayed definitive surgical reconstruction, perpetuate the inflammatory component of wound healing, perpetuate distal edema, and result in hand and limb stiffness. If the surgeon can guarantee a clean wound bed, free of any necrotic material, immediate flap coverage may be attempted in cases of acute trauma. We have found that most high energy traumatic injuries and agricultural accidents require at least one to two surgical debridements prior to definitive wound closure. Wound debridements in these cases are performed in conjunction with wound cultures for bacteria and fungal species. The ideal timing for upper limb free tissue reconstruction has been debated within the literature but should be within 72 to 96 hours of injury.

The upper extremity is evaluated for any evidence of concomitant bony or neurovascular injury. A careful vascular evaluation is also performed and if there is any question as to the status of the inflow vessels, an angiogram or a CT angiogram may be obtained to verify inflow. Our preference is to perform the majority of arterial anastomosis in end-to-side fashion, while the veins are anastomosed in an end-to-end fashion. If consideration is being given to performing an arterial anastomosis in end-to-end fashion to either the radial or ulnar artery, the surgeon must verify a patent palmar arch with an Allen's test or Doppler examination prior to surgery. The donor leg for the anterior lateral thigh flap should be free of concomitant soft tissue trauma. If the patient has a history of lower extremity arterial atherosclerotic disease or diabetes, examination of the lower extremity is warranted, to verify that there is an intact profundus femoral artery which gives rise to the lateral femoral circumflex system.

Patient positioning

The patient is positioned in the supine position for harvest of the anterior lateral thigh flap. The injured arm is positioned on a standard hand table. Recipient site preparation is aided with the use of an upper extremity tourniquet.

Flap harvest is usually performed under general anesthesia, though spinal/epidural block for flap elevation and axillary block of the affected extremity can be undertaken when general anesthesia is contraindicated.

Flap Elevation Surgery

General principles and steps in elevation for perforator flap include:

1. Doppler mapping of the perforator,
2. Design of the flap for operation,
3. Identification of the perforators leading to the main pedicle,
4. Intra-muscular dissection of the perforator with preservation of the nerves,
5. Elevation of the flap,
6. Thinning of the flap, and
7. Transfer of the flap to cover the defect.

The anterolateral thigh flap is based on the lateral femoral circumflex vessel, particularly the descending branch, which courses inferiorly along the intermuscular septum giving rise to subcutaneous and/or intramuscular perforators that penetrate the fascia to supply the skin and subcutaneous tissue overlying the anterolateral thigh. A preoperative Doppler examination of the lower leg is performed to identify these perforators. A line is drawn from the anterior superior iliac spine to the lateral margin of the patella. At the midpoint of this line is a reliable perforator identifiable in almost 90% of cases (Fig. 18-2). An additional perforator can be identified in 80% of cases within the upper third of the line, again using a hand held Doppler. The skin paddle, incorporating both perforators if possible, is designed in an elliptical fashion based on the dimensions of the defect in the upper extremity.

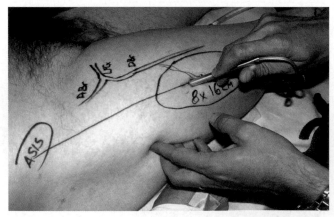
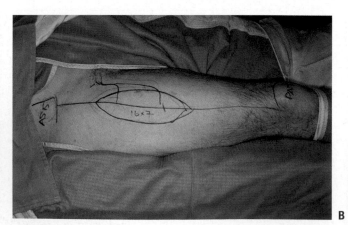

A   **B**

FIGURE 18-2

Prior to flap elevation the arterial perforators to the ALT flap are identified on the leg. A line is drawn from the anterior superior iliac spine (ASIS) to the lateral margin of the patella. In 90% of cases a major perforator can be identified within 3 cm of the middle portion of this line. A second major perforator is usually identified at the upper third of this line. **A:** The sites for the perforators are confirmed with a handheld Doppler probe and marked with a skin scribe. **B:** The flap is then designed around the perforators in an elliptical fashion.

Dissection begins medially by dissecting down to the rectus femoris fascia. The fascia of the rectus femoris muscle is divided and dissection proceeds in a lateral direction until the intermuscular septum separating the rectus femoris and vastus lateralis muscles is encountered. Medial retraction of the rectus femoris muscle exposes the entire septum, allowing for visualization of the descending branch of the lateral femoral circumflex artery in addition to its branch going to the rectus femoris itself (Fig. 18-3). At this point there may be 1–3 major perforators exiting from the descending branch and passing through the muscle of the vastus lateralis as musculocutaneous perforators or passing directly through the septum as septocutaneous perforators to the skin. Usually, one large perforator is sufficient to supply a large skin island, and allows for easy thinning of the flap. However, more perforators may be included if the skin island is very large, and flaps as large as 15 x 35 cm

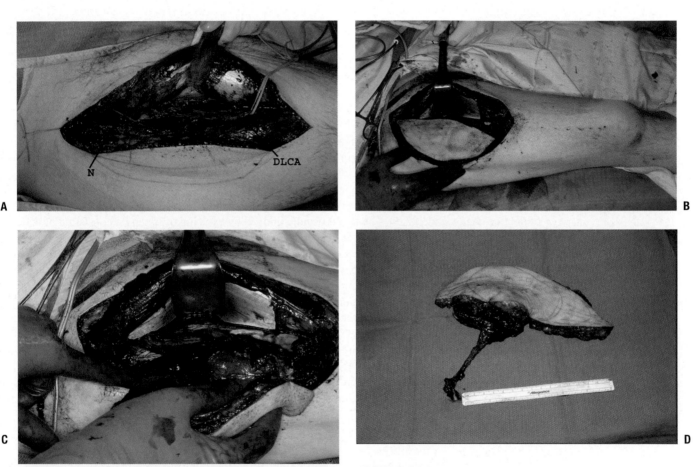

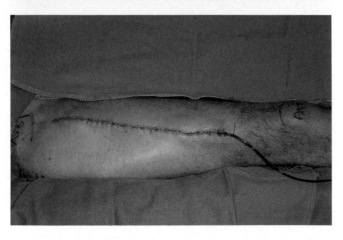

FIGURE 18-3

A: After the flap has been marked the medial incision is made first and the rectus femoris muscle is identified. The rectus femoris (RF) muscle is retracted medially to reveal the descending branch of the lateral femoral circumflex vessels (DCLA). A branch of the lateral femoral cutaneous nerve (n) can usually be identified running superior to the vastus lateralis muscle **B:** Once the flap perforators are identified, dissection may begin at the lateral margin of the flap. **C:** In this photograph 2 perforators of the lateral femoral circumflex vessels are seen passing into the vastus lateralis. These vessels may be dissected through the muscle into the fascia of the overlying skin flap or a small cuff of muscle may be preserved around the vessels. **D:** The flap is now ready for transfer to the arm. The muscle cuff can be seen beneath the skin paddle. The pedicle length and large diameter allow for easy insetting and microvascular anastomosis. **E:** The donor site may be closed primarily over a closed suction drain.

have been reported. If septocutaneous perforators are present, one may simply proceed to the posterior incision, including the portion of the tensor fascia lata, and elevate the flap. If intramuscular perforators are encountered then dissection must proceed as one would for a true perforator flap, in which case the artery needs to be carefully dissected free from the surrounding muscle. A cuff of muscle may be included in the flap should the upper extremity wound require additional bulk or if the wound contains exposed bone or significant dead space (see Figure 18-3D).

Dissection proceeds along the descending branch of the LFCA separating venae comitantes from the artery. The pedicle can be dissected back to the main trunk of the lateral femoral circumflex artery, or divided at the descending branch. If one traces the vessels back to the origin, the motor nerve to the vastus lateralis will need to be dissected free from the arterial pedicle. This may be a tedious dissection as the nerve may pass through and around the venous pedicle. Dissection of the vessels back to the origin results in very large caliber vessels of up to 3 mm in some cases.

Preparation of the arterial recipient site is then performed. If the radial artery is going to be used, a Henry approach is usually carried out. For approach to the brachial artery a curved lazy-S incision is performed over the antecubital fossa and exposure of the brachial artery at the level of the medial forearm is performed. The flap is then transferred to the upper extremity. The tourniquet is then released in order to verify adequate arterial inflow. Once adequate arterial inflow has been verified, the anterolateral thigh flap may be divided from the lower extremity and transferred to the upper extremity. The anastomosis is then performed in end-to-side fashion using 8-0 nylon. Venous coupling may also be used to expedite the microsurgical procedure (Fig. 18-4).

The donor site is approximated primarily over closed suction drainage when flap width is less than 8 cm, or a skin graft may be used for larger width flaps. For cases involving intramuscular perforator dissection, the muscle edges are reapproximated to preserve maximal quadriceps function.

In certain cases, such as coverage of the hand, a thin flap may be required and primary defatting of the flap can be undertaken. The flap is usually thinned by excising the deep fat consisting of wide, flat fat lobules up to the junction of the superficial fat, made up of smaller, round lobules. Defatting before ligation of the pedicle allows for monitoring of flap perfusion during the thinning process. The flap may be thinned up to 3 mm without compromise to the blood supply. A more conservative approach towards primary flap thinning should be undertaken until adequate experience is gained as flap debulking can be performed safely and easily as a secondary procedure (Fig. 18-5). Innervated flaps can be achieved by including the lateral femoral cutaneous nerve in the proximal portion of the flap. The nerve arises from the deep fascia approximately 10 cm caudad to the anterior superior iliac spine and divides into two or three branches. As previously mentioned, when added bulk is required to cover a complex wound, the anterolateral thigh flap can be harvested as a chimeric flap along with the vastus lateralis or rectus femoris muscles, the tensor fascia lata, or other skin flaps in the thigh based on the supply of lateral femoral circumflex system.

Postoperative Management

Monitoring   Flap monitoring is of paramount importance following microvascular surgery. Postoperative thrombosis of either the artery or vein can be salvaged in greater than 50% of patients if detected early. Intraoperatively, a stitch is placed over the perforator on the skin paddle to facilitate postoperative monitoring with a Doppler probe. Alternatively, an implantable Doppler probe can be placed around the vein or artery intraoperatively to allow for continuous monitoring of the anastomosis. The Doppler signal over the marked skin paddle is checked hourly with the use of a hand held Doppler while the patient remains in the Intensive Care Unit. The highest incidence of postoperative arterial thrombosis is within the first 24 hours, with the incidence of venous thrombosis occurring most frequently within the first three days. Donor site drain output is recorded and drains are kept in place until daily output is less than 30 cc. The patient is allowed to ambulate on postoperative day 2. Postoperative complications include partial to total flap loss, temporary weakness in the lower extremity which usually resolves within the first two weeks, and sensory deficit at the donor site if there has been any stretching or injury to the lateral femoral cutaneous nerve. In cases of venous congestion, exploration of the anastomosis is necessary. If prolonged venous thrombosis is experienced, the use of either TPA or leeches can sometimes be used to salvage the flap.

The use of postoperative anticoagulation is debated. Our patients are given one baby aspirin per day, and are continued on subcutaneous heparin while they are in the hospital. Formal anticoagulation with heparin is discouraged and has been linked to an increase risk of hematoma formation and

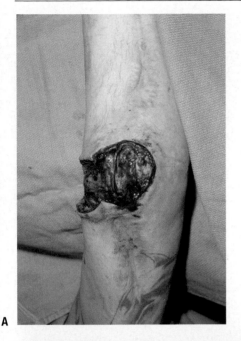

FIGURE 18-4

A: 34 year old male, status post liver transplantation, with a chronic left posterior elbow wound. The multiple posterior scares are evidence of previous attempts to close this defect. **B:** The skin incision for an ipsilateral ALT flap is marked on the thigh after identification of the underlying perforators. **C:** The flap is separated from surrounding tissue. **D:** The lateral femoral circumflex vessels can be seen above the surgeon's index finger entering the flap. **E:** In preparation for flap transfer the brachial artery is exposed at the level of the elbow. *(Continued)*

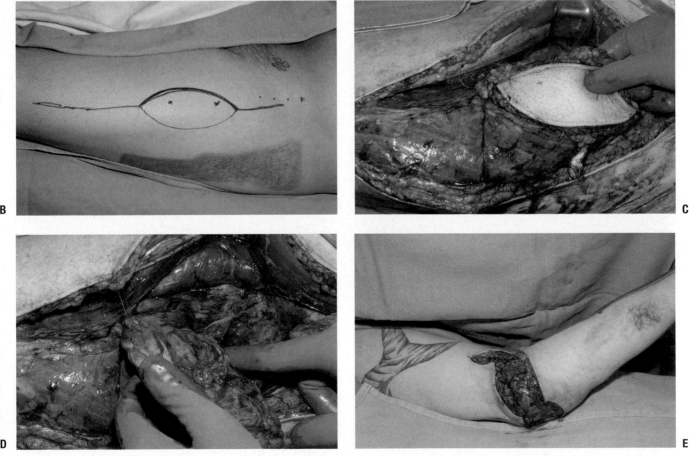

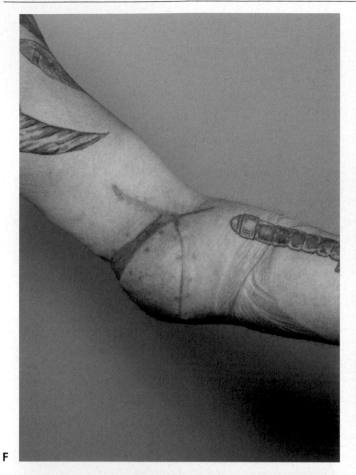

F

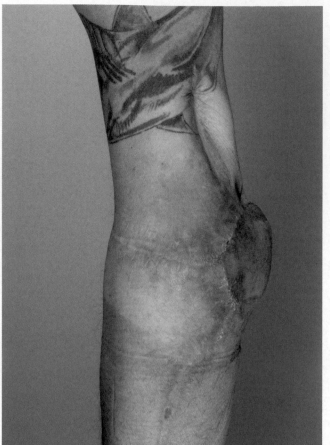

G

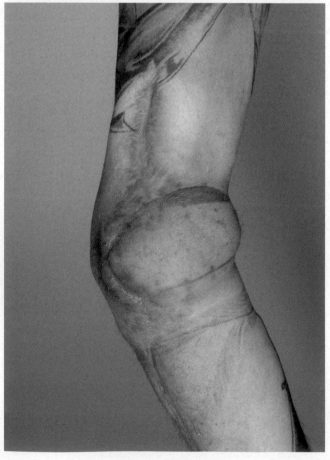

H

FIGURE 18-4

Continued **F–H:** The result at 3 months postop with well healed wound, with good contour and no signs of infection.

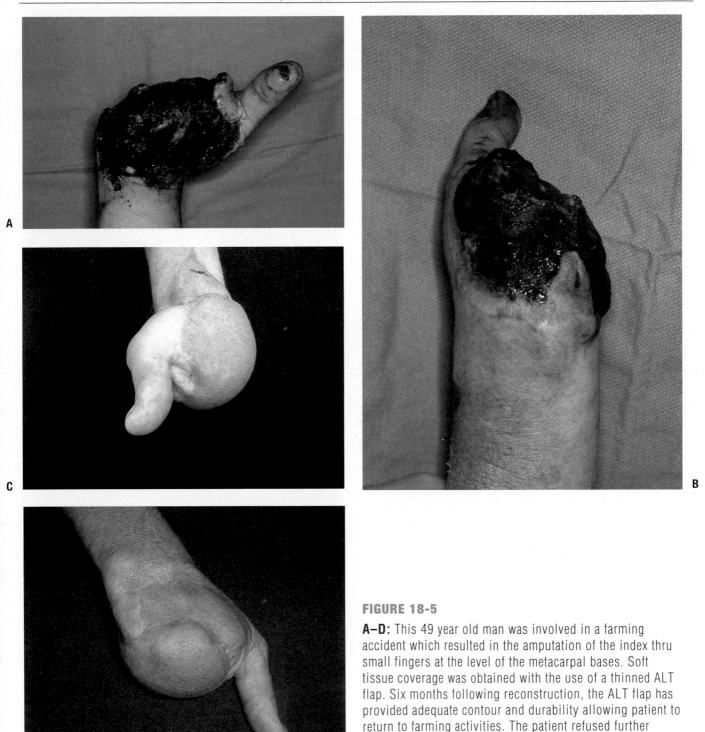

FIGURE 18-5

A–D: This 49 year old man was involved in a farming accident which resulted in the amputation of the index thru small fingers at the level of the metacarpal bases. Soft tissue coverage was obtained with the use of a thinned ALT flap. Six months following reconstruction, the ALT flap has provided adequate contour and durability allowing patient to return to farming activities. The patient refused further surgery for finger reconstuction **(C,D)**.

flap loss. For those situations where arterial inflow has been difficult to establish, dextran at 25 mL/hour may be used in adults.

Rehabilitation   Underlying injuries usually dictate when motion may begin. We usually wait 5 days for the anastomosis to mature and for the postoperative swelling to subside. At this point if the underlying bone injury is stabilized, early mobilization is initiated. A light ace wrap is applied to the flap beginning on day five to help aid in resolution of post-operative swelling. Re-elevation of the flap for additional bone grafting or tendon grafting can be done as soon as 4 to 6 weeks. Defatting or thinning of the flap is usually delayed for 6 to 9 months after the original surgery.

Complications

The greatest complication of free flap surgery is flap loss due to arterial or venous thrombosis. The best means of preventing these problems is adequate preoperative planning. Repairs within the zone of injury, technical errors including inadequate visualization of vessels, and tension or kinking at the anastomosis site can all lead to flap failure. Ongoing infection can also result in partial flap loss. For the anterolateral thigh flap, twisting of the pedicle can occur easily due to the absence of muscle to keep its proper orientation. Marking the anterior wall of the pedicle and lifting of the flap in the air to allow the pedicle to lie in its natural orientation prior to final inset may prevent pedicle twisting. It is also important to avoid compression of the flap.

Results

Good success has been reported with the use of anterolateral thigh flaps in the upper extremity. Flap failure rates have been noted to be as low as 2%. Additional thinning procedures may be required in patients with continued bulk. Microvascular surgery and free tissue transfer within the upper extremity is facilitated by large recipient vessels, and a relatively shallow operating field.

CONCLUSION

With proper planning, the anterolateral thigh flap is capable of managing many complex injuries within the upper extremity. It is now often our first choice for coverage of upper extremity defects. The advantages of the ALT flap are: relatively consistent anatomy; ease in dissection; long pedicle length; ability to achieve a thin, pliable flap; ability to provide sensate coverage through the lateral femoral cutaneous nerve; no sacrifice of major artery of the lower limb; and versatility in flap construct which allows one to harvest not only muscle, but also functional muscle such as the rectus femoris. The donor site can be closed primarily.

RECOMMENDED READING

Breidenbach WC. Emergency free tissue transfer for reconstruction of acute upper extremity wounds. *Clin Plast Surg.* 1989;16:505–514.

Celik N, Wei FC, et al. Technique and strategy in anteriorlateral thigh perforator flap surgery, based on an analysis of 15 complete and partial failures in 439 cases. *Plast Reconstr Surg.* 2002;109:2211–2216.

Chen HC, Tang YB, et al. Reconstruction of the hand and upper limb with free flaps based on musculocutaneous perforators. *Microsurgery.* 2004.

Chen SH, Wei FC, et al. Emergency free-flap transfer for reconstruction of acute complex extremity wounds. *Plast Reconstr Surg.* 1992;89:882–888.

Derderian CA, Olivier WA, et al. Microvascular free-tissue transfer for traumatic defects of the upper-extremity: a 25 year experience. *J Reconstr Microsurg.* 2003;19:455–462.

Godina M. Early microsurgical reconstruction of complex trauma of the extremities. *Plast Reconstr Surg.* 1986;78:285–292.

Hamdi M, Van Landuyt K, et al. A clinical experience with perforator flaps in the coverage of extensive defects of the upper extremity. *Plast Reconstr Surg.* 2004;113: 1175–1183.

Hong JP, Shin HW, et al. The use of the anterolateral thigh perforator flaps in chronic osteomyelitis of the lower extremity. *Plast Reconstr Surg.* 2005;115(142–148).

Kimata Y, Uchiyama K, et al. Anterolateral thigh flap donor-site complications and morbidity. *Plast Reconstr Surg.* 2000;106:584.

Koschnick M., Bruener S, et al. Free tissue transfer: An advanced strategy for postinfection soft-tissue defects in the upper extremity. *Ann Plast Surg.* 2003;51:147–154.

Kuo YR, Jeng SF, et al. Free anterolateral thigh flap for extremity reconstruction: clinical experience and functional assessment of donor site. *Plast Reconstr Surg.* 2001;107:1766.

Lin CH, Mardini S, et al. Sixty-five clinical cases of free tissue transfer using long arteriovenous fistulas or vein grafts. *J Trauma.* 2004;56:1107–1117.

Wei FC, Jain V, et al. Have we found an ideal soft tissue flap? An experience with 672 anterolateral thigh flaps. *Plast Reconstr Surg.* 2002;109:2019–2226.

19 Groin Flap Coverage of the Hand and Wrist

Jeffrey B. Friedrich and Nicholas B. Vedder

INDICATIONS/CONTRAINDICATIONS

The pedicled groin flap is an extremely versatile and reliable flap that was initially described in 1972 by MacGregor and Jackson. It enjoys a revered place in the field of reconstructive surgery because it was one of the first axial-pattern flaps to be described and applied in humans. After several decades, many surgical techniques, including pedicled flaps, have been supplanted by new methods. However, despite the advent of microsurgery, the pedicled groin flap continues to be a venerable technique with a variety of applications.

The groin flap has been used most commonly for upper extremity reconstruction, and is indicated for soft tissue defects in which there is destruction or devitalization of soft tissue on the hand, wrist, and distal forearm. The groin flap is not designed to supplant skin-grafting on wounds that will accept a graft; rather, it is to be used when the injury or resection leaves exposed structures that will not accept a skin graft, such as tendon or bone. It has been described for soft tissue reconstruction of a number of traumatic etiologies including crush injuries, avulsions, gunshots, blast wounds, and burns. Additionally, the flap is warranted for soft tissue defects following elective resection such as contractures, hypertrophic scarring, or tumor, and has even been described as soft tissue coverage following recurrent carpal tunnel syndrome.

In the setting of trauma, the groin flap is most often used for delayed primary coverage of upper extremity wounds. Several groups have employed the flap for very early coverage (within 24–48 hours from injury); however, the complication rate has been found to be high. Therefore, unless a clean and healthy wound bed can be ensured initially, it is generally prudent to thoroughly debride the wound, observe it for a few days, and then apply the groin flap only after a clean, healthy wound surface is ensured.

As noted above, the groin flap will provide reliable soft tissue coverage to practically any portion of the hand as well as the distal forearm. It is particularly well-suited to the dorsal surface of the hand. The flap can certainly be used to provide coverage for the palmar surface of the hand; however, the flap can be bulky, and does not at all approximate the native, adherent, glabrous skin of the palm. This can leave the palm with a bulky flap that is prone to shearing motion when weight is borne on the palmar surface of the hand, such as seen with pushing, gripping, tool use, or twisting motions. For this reason, it is wise to consider other thinner flaps such as the reversed radial forearm flap or free fasciocutaneous flaps such as the anterolateral thigh flap for most palmar reconstructions.

A brief mention must be made of the groin flap for use as a free tissue transfer. The free groin flap was the first free flap described and can be used for many of the same indications for which other free flaps are currently used. Its reliability is somewhat limited because of the variable arterial pedicle and the short length of the pedicle. Furthermore, even in experienced hands, the free groin flap failure rate is notably higher than it is for other free flaps, thus limiting its utility.

The authors gratefully acknowledge the assistance of Douglas P. Hanel, MD in preparation of the figures for this chapter.

Another chief indication for use of the groin flap is in the setting of thumb reconstruction. Often with total or near-total thumb loss, it is necessary to use free digit transfers such as the great or second toe. Unfortunately, traumatic thumb amputations can leave the patient with insufficient soft tissue of the thenar region. In these cases, the groin flap is an excellent choice to provide a soft-tissue "base" on to which the digit transfer can be placed at a later date.

The contraindications for the use of the pedicled groin flap are few. In general, the flap should not be implemented in patients who are deemed to be uncooperative, or who would otherwise not be able to tolerate a 2- or 3-week interval in which their affected hand is immobilized and attached to the groin. In the past, it was felt that elderly patients were not good candidates for this flap because of the risk of shoulder and elbow stiffness. However, a recent study has shown that elderly patients are able to tolerate the procedure with no more complications (including upper extremity stiffness) than the average young patient.

As with any flap, active tobacco use is a concern with the groin flap. Specifically, the flap can be subject to marginal necrosis in active smokers. The surgeon must balance the need for complex reconstruction with the potential morbidity that may be incurred by patients who smoke.

Previous groin surgery may or may not be a contraindication to the use of this flap. In general, inguinal hernia repair does not preclude the use of the groin flap, nor do other scars in the general vicinity such as abdominoplasty or Pfannenstiel incisions. However, a previous inguinal lymph node dissection would render this flap tenuous, or outright unsafe. The potential disruption of superficial vessels in the groin is too high to risk use of a flap based on these vessels. Additionally, patients who have had groin lymph node dissections have quite often had external beam radiation to the same region, further rendering flap dissection in this area a dangerous proposition.

PREOPERATIVE PLANNING

When using the groin flap in the acute posttraumatic setting, wound preparation is of paramount importance. The surgeon must perform any hand or forearm repairs that are necessary in the acute phase. This includes fracture reduction and fixation, as well as tendon, vessel, and nerve repair. Wound debridement must also be complete so as to minimize the infection risk once the site is covered with a flap. Wound debridement and cleansing may need to be done several times in the operating room prior to flap coverage, and several days of dressing changes may be necessary to ensure that the wound bed is as healthy as possible. This is especially true with crush and avulsion injuries.

In the posttraumatic setting, timing of coverage with a groin flap has become an important issue. In general, most published reports advocate use of the flap in a delayed-primary fashion, specifically between 48 hours and 7 days following injury. Others have attempted to employ the flap in a more acute setting (24–48 hours following injury); however, the consensus seems to be that early timing leads to an unacceptably high rate of infection and dehiscence, and is thus not advocated. In the end, timing of flap implementation should be based on the surgeon's best clinical judgment about the mechanism of injury, and the status of the wound bed.

In the elective setting, the preoperative preparation for a groin flap is somewhat less crucial. The patient must understand that the interval between flap elevation and flap division will entail a moderate amount of disability, and will require a significant amount of diligence in regard to their self-care. Additionally, it is a good idea for the patient to make prior arrangements to have a friend or family member at home who will be able to assist them with various activities of daily living.

SURGERY

The groin flap coverage surgery must be done with a general anesthetic. Additionally, it is recommended that a bladder catheter be placed as the operation can be in excess of 3 hours. If the patient is not already being administered intravenous antibiotics for prophylaxis of a traumatic wound, one dose of antibiotics should be administered 30 minutes before skin incision.

Patient Positioning

Once anesthetized, care should be taken with patient positioning. Although an ipsilateral groin flap is most commonly used, a contralateral flap is sometimes acceptable if the ipsilateral side is for some reason unavailable. Regardless of which side is chosen, a small towel roll or "bump" should be placed under the hip of the side that will undergo groin flap dissection to allow extension of the flap dissection back to the flank. The upper extremity to be reconstructed should be placed on a hand table for initial wound preparation. Additionally, one should leave enough room on the side of the operating table to be able to comfortably lay the upper extremity beside the torso during groin flap inset. The other necessary step before initiating the operation is placement of a pneumatic tourniquet on the upper extremity to be reconstructed.

Technique

The operation is begun by preparation of the recipient bed. If the flap is being employed for traumatic wound coverage, a final thorough debridement is done at this time. If it is being done for scarring or other elective soft tissue coverage, the creation of the recipient wound to be covered is done in its entirety before moving to the groin.

In preparation for flap elevation, measurements are taken to determine the required dimensions of the groin flap. This can be done in several ways. One can simply use a ruler to determine the largest dimensions of the wound, or a template can be fashioned. The paper wrapper from surgical glove packaging makes a nice template material and is readily available. This can be pressed onto the wound so that the wound fluid makes an imprint in the paper. Then the template can be made simply by cutting around the outline of the defect. Alternatively, one can use a piece of the elastic wrap used to exsanguinate the hand (Fig. 19-1). The template is then transferred to the groin. In general, the more ulnar aspects of the wound will be covered by the distal end of the flap.

When designing the flap, one must keep in mind the arterial anatomy of the flap. Specifically, the flap is supplied by the superficial circumflex iliac artery and vein (Fig. 19-2). Numerous studies have shown the artery to consistently extend to the level of the anterior superior iliac spine (ASIS) before any significant caliber diminishment. In other words, the flap is an axial pattern flap medial to the ASIS, and a random-pattern flap lateral to this point. The area lateral to the ASIS can be used as part of the flap design; however, its effectiveness is limited by its random nature. Therefore, the operator should generally design a flap that, at the portion lateral to the ASIS, has a width:length ratio between 1:1 to 1:1.5 (although the medial portion needs only be wide enough to include the axial vessels). It is possible to design a flap whose distal extent is more posterior than this limit, but a delay procedure should then be employed for the flap. A delay procedure involves incision, but not eleva-

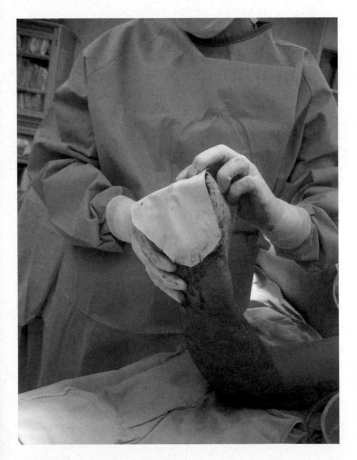

FIGURE 19-1

Use of a piece of the elastic exsanguination wrap to create a template of the defect to be covered with a groin flap.

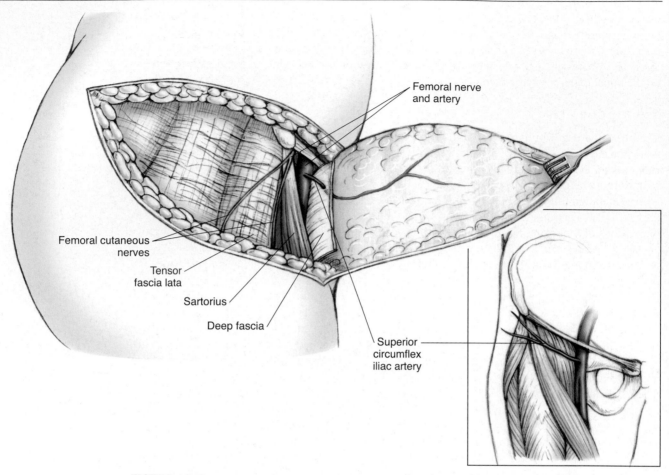

FIGURE 19-2

Detail of groin flap anatomy (right-sided), showing the pedicle (superficial circumflex iliac artery), inclusion of the superficial sartorius fascia with the flap, and the location of the lateral femoral cutaneous nerve branches as they emerge from under the inguinal ligament. (Adapted from Brown EZ Jr, Pederson WC. Skin grafts and skin flaps. In: *Green's operative hand surgery*. 5th ed. Philadelphia: Elsevier/Churchill Livingstone; 2005:1692-1702, with permission.)

tion of the desired flap. The incised flap is then left in situ for a week so that the circulation at the distal end of the flap can be augmented during that time. Following that interval, the flap can then be elevated and inset in the upper extremity wound.

When beginning the overall design of the flap, it is best to keep in mind the recommendations of Chuang, who published a set of groin flap design rules based on experience amassed via the use of over 200 groin flaps. The mainstay of these guidelines is the "two fingerbreadths" rule (the two fingerbreadths being at the level of the index and long finger distal interphalangeal joint of the operator) (Fig. 19-3). The first step is to estimate the location of the superficial circumflex iliac artery, done by marking a point two fingerbreadths below the junction between the inguinal ligament (which runs along a line between the anterior superior iliac spine and the pubic tubercle) and the femoral artery. Once that artery location is estimated, its true path should be verified by Doppler ultrasound. The upper flap border is marked two fingerbreadths above the inguinal ligament (parallel to the artery), while the lower flap border is a line two fingerbreadths below and parallel to the artery. Also, as will be further discussed following, the superficial branch of the superficial circumflex iliac artery (SCIA) emerges from the deep fascia two fingerbreadths medial to the ASIS, then continues laterally in a subcutaneous plane.

It should be noted that if using the two fingerbreadths rule for flap design, a relatively slender flap will result medially. In reality, when the flap is centered over the SCIA, the cephalad-caudad width of the flap lateral to the ASIS can be quite substantial. However, most authors agree that flap widths up to 10 cm enable primary closure of the groin wound site, while those that are wider stand a good

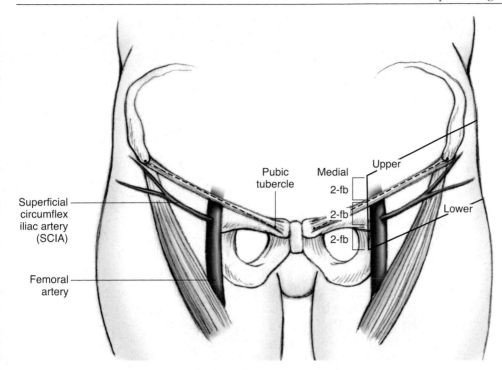

FIGURE 19-3

Drawing of the application of the two-fingerbreadth rule. The *dashed line* on the left of the patient is the location of the inguinal ligament. The *solid line* immediately below that is the location of the superficial circumflex iliac artery. Note that the upper border of the flap is two fingerbreadths above the inguinal ligament, and the lower border is two fingerbreadths below the vascular pedicle (SCIA). (Adapted from Chuang DC, Colony LH, Chen HC, Wei FC. Groin flap design and versatility. *Plast Reconstr Surg.* 1989;84(1):100–107, with permission.)

chance of requiring closure with a split-thickness skin graft because of inability to achieve primary closure. It is usually possible to determine how wide a flap can safely be harvested and closed primarily by pinching the skin and subcutaneous tissue together. Flexing the operating table at the hip to relieve some of the tension can facilitate closure.

Once the marks are drawn, the incisions of the flap are made. The incision is carried down to the level of the external oblique fascia on the abdomen, and the muscle fascia on the leg. Then the flap dissection is begun at the lateral end in the plane between the subcutaneous fat and the muscle fascia of the thigh (below the inguinal ligament); and between the subcutaneous fat and the external oblique muscle fascia (above the inguinal ligament). The flap is most easily and safely raised with curved Metzenbaum scissors, although low-powered electrocautery can be used as well. The dissection proceeds in this fashion until reaching the lateral border of the sartorius muscle. On reaching the sartorius, the fascia over this muscle is incised at its lateral border. The sartorius fascia is then elevated from the muscle. Above the inguinal ligament, the dissection plane remains immediately superficial to the external oblique fascia. At the medial border of the sartorius muscle, the SCIA divides into a superficial and a deep branch. By elevating the sartorius fascia, the superficial branch (which supplies the lateral extent of the groin flap) is preserved with the flap. When the medial sartorius fascia is reached, and the deep branch of the SCIA encountered, it is divided and ligated with either vascular clips or sutures. This deep branch of the SCIA is not necessary for flap survival, and it will only serve to tether the flap if more flap length is desired (Fig. 19-4).

During the flap dissection, one must remain cognizant of the lateral femoral cutaneous nerve and its course in the vicinity of the flap. The nerve emerges from under the inguinal ligament at the medial edge of the sartorius muscle (see Fig. 19-2). The nerve branches run deep to the SCIA; therefore, care should be taken to preserve the nerve branches in this area. If nerve branches are found in the sartorius muscle fascia, efforts must be made to dissect free and preserve them. Despite attempts to preserve the nerve branches, patients should be told before the procedure that nerve damage (both transient and permanent) is possible and can lead to numbness of the lateral thigh.

The endpoint of flap dissection is generally determined by the acquisition of enough flap length to be easily inset in the defect of the hand or forearm. Some references caution against proceeding more medially than the lateral border of the sartorius muscle; however, we have found that a longer flap can be raised if proper precautions are taken. That said, the absolute anatomic endpoint of flap dissection is at the lateral border of the femoral artery.

While this chapter chiefly concentrates on the use of the pedicled groin flap, a brief mention of the free groin flap will be made. The dissection of the flap proceeds in an identical manner to that described previously. However, one of the over-arching goals of free flap harvest is to obtain donor

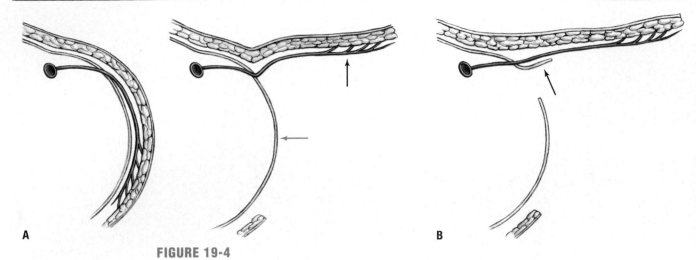

FIGURE 19-4

A: Schematic representation of vascular kinking that is possible if the sartorius fascia is not elevated with the groin flap. The illustration shows an axial view of the lower extremity. The *black arrow* points to the superficial circumflex iliac artery (SCIA); the π points to the fascia of the sartorius muscle. **B:** Schematic representation of the relatively straight course of the superficial branch of the SCIA following elevation of the sartorius fascia with the groin flap. The *black arrow* points to the now-released sartorius fascia. (Adapted from Brown EZ Jr, Pederson WC. Skin grafts and skin flaps. In: *Green's operative hand surgery.* 5th ed. Philadelphia: Elsevier/Churchill Livingstone; 2005:1692–1702, with permission.)

vessels that are as long as safely possible. With the free groin flap, this involves dividing the SCIA very close to the femoral artery, and dividing the donor vein very close to the femoral vein. This must be done carefully as vascular clips or sutures placed too close to the femoral vessels can serve to narrow the lumen of the vessel. When harvesting the groin flap for free tissue transfer, one anatomic caveat must be kept in mind: in a minority of persons (estimated at 30%), the SCIA emerges from a common vessel that bifurcates into the SCIA and the superficial inferior epigastric artery (SEIA). When this is found to be the case, the common trunk is dissected back to the femoral artery and used as the arterial donor. Both the SCIA and SEIA will reliably supply the groin skin; so when they emerge separately, the larger of the two vessels is chosen as the arterial donor. Usually, the larger vessel is the SCIA.

Several steps must be taken before inset of the flap into the upper extremity. First, one must close the donor defect, because closure will be much more difficult if it is done after flap inset. This closure should optimally be a three-layered one, with 0-0 or 2-0 braided absorbable suture in the superficial fascia (Scarpa's fascia on the abdominal wall to superficial fascia on the lower extremity), 2-0 or 3-0 braided absorbable suture in the dermis, and 3-0 or 4-0 nonabsorbable monofilament or staples in the skin. This closure is done over a suction drain, usually brought out through a separate stab incision. The closure is facilitated by flexion of the operating table at the hip, and use of towel clips or staples to temporarily approximate the skin while the sutures are being placed (Fig. 19-5). It is also important for the patient's bed to remain flexed at the hip in the immediate postoperative period to minimize tension on the suture line.

Next, the flap base should be "tubed" before inset. Tubing of the flap diminishes the amount of exposed flap undersurface, thereby helping with postoperative wound care. The tubing is done simply by suturing the upper and lower sides of the flap together such that it forms a cylinder (Fig. 19-6). The closure of the tube can be done with a single layer of nonabsorbable monofilament sutures. One must be cautious about tubing the flap, as this can cause vascular compromise. A simple way to deal with a congested flap is to release a few sutures at the base (since this is the thickest part of the flap). In a seminal article on groin flap design, Schlenker illustrates another method to increase the circumference of the tube while simultaneously positioning the flap for inset depending on whether the hand defect is dorsal or volar. This is done by incising either the cephalad or caudad side of the flap longer than the other, then performing either a clockwise or counterclockwise closure of the donor defect. This then positions the portion of the flap that will be inset into a more optimal orientation for coverage (Fig. 19-7).

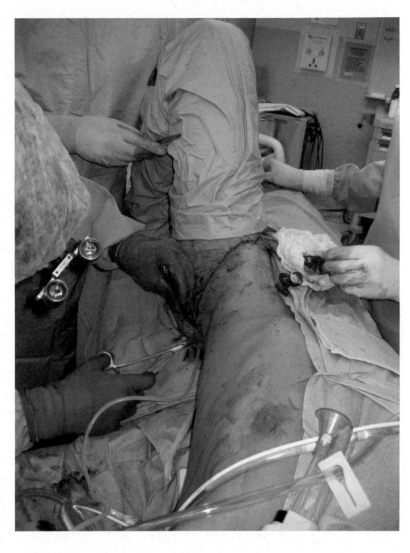

FIGURE 19-5

Flexion of the hip to facilitate groin flap donor site closure.

The other task to be done before flap inset is to thin the distal part of the flap that was originally lateral to the ASIS. This is most easily performed with curved Mayo or Metzenbaum scissors, trimming the fat down to the subdermal level. This will facilitate flap inset, and will reduce the amount of defatting that needs to be done in the secondary setting.

Once elevated, the inset of the groin flap is relatively simple. The affected hand is moved into the groin, and the flap is then inset into the recipient site, usually over a closed-suction drain. This is typically performed with a two-layered closure, specifically 3-0 or 4-0 braided absorbable suture in the dermis, and 3-0 or 4-0 nonabsorbable monofilament suture in the skin (Fig. 19-8).

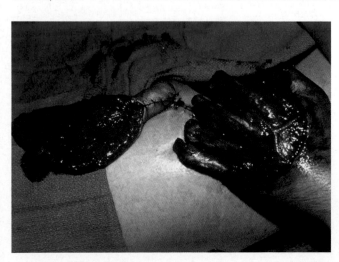

FIGURE 19-6

Groin flap following "tubing" of the proximal portion of the flap.

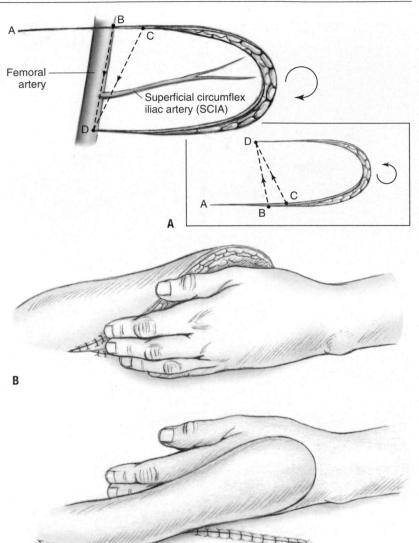

FIGURE 19-7

A: Schlenker's modification of the groin flap incisions. By making the top incision longer, and closing points B and C to point D, clockwise rotation is facilitated. Similarly, by making the lower incision longer, counterclockwise rotation is facilitated. **B:** By creating a flap that is rotated clockwise, and therefore facing downward, closure of a palmar defect is made easier. **C:** Similarly, counterclockwise rotation of the flap causes the raw surface to face upward, allowing easier closure of a dorsal hand defect. (Adapted from Schlenker JD. Important considerations in the design and construction of groin flaps. *Ann Plast Surg.* 1980;5(5):353–357, with permission.)

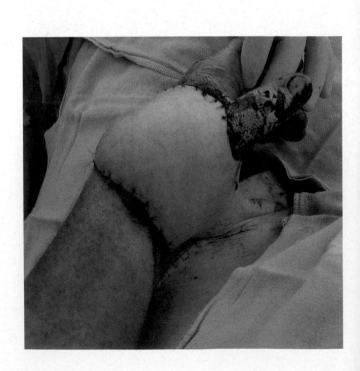

FIGURE 19-8

Completion of groin flap inset on the hand.

Care must be taken with postoperative dressings and positioning. The wounds on the hand can simply be covered with antibiotic ointment. We find that it is best to cover the small exposed portions of the flap (at the base) with antibiotic (bismuth)-impregnated gauze. The closed groin wound can be dressed with a gauze dressing or covered with antibiotic ointment. Cast padding or soft towels should be placed in the affected axilla and under the hand as these areas will become moist with the arm at the side. A pillow should be placed underneath the elbow to give the arm support, and to ensure that the flap itself is just the slightest bit extended anterior and lateral to the body. It is important to avoid kinking of the flap since this will easily cause venous congestion. Finally, the donor-side leg should have a pillow placed under the knee to relieve tension on the groin flap closure. Once the patient is awake, it is important to educate them in positioning of the flap to avoid kinking.

Flap Division and Final Inset

In general, the pedicle of the groin flap is divided between 2 and 3 weeks after flap elevation. Wei's group and others have done numerous studies using ischemic preconditioning of the flap to allow flap division at an earlier time (7–10 days). However, we have found that, with proper patient selection, the groin flap will be tolerated for 3 weeks just as easily as it would be tolerated for 1 week. Furthermore, we have not found any complications associated with the longer attachment times.

Flap division proceeds as follows: one should test the vascularity of the flap by firmly occluding the tubed pedicle with thumb and forefinger or by using a penrose drain clamped around the pedicle, then observing capillary refill of the flap. If there is *any* question about the perfusion of the flap, the flap division should be delayed. A hand table should be set up before the start of the case. An arm tourniquet is not necessary for this procedure, and in fact, it is discouraged because the vascularity of the flap needs to be assessed during this operation. The arm is prepared from at least the elbow down, and the entire groin area is prepared simultaneously. The flap is marked where it is thought that it will cover the remaining wound, taking care to make this marking generous. The flap is then incised with a scalpel and carried through with electrocautery. The arm is then placed on the hand table. Sometimes, there is a residual flap "stump," which is excised to the point that the remaining groin wound can be easily closed without a large dog-ear deformity. If the stump of the SCIA is large, this should be ligated with a suture or vascular clips. The remaining groin wound is closed in a fashion similar to that of the original groin wound closure.

Finally, the remainder of the groin flap is inset to the hand. Some very judicious defatting of the open end of the flap can be undertaken at this time. This can be done with scissors, but it should not be overly aggressive. Both the donor and recipient sites should be well debrided and cleansed before closure. The closure should be loose to allow drainage, as these will be contaminated wounds. The wound is sutured with 4-0 nylon in the skin (Fig. 19-9). A soft dressing should then be applied to the

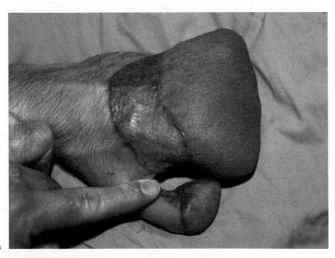
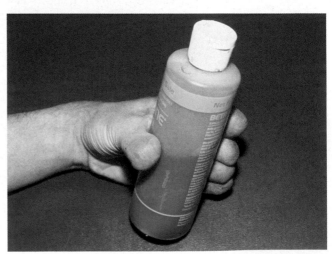

A   B

FIGURE 19-9

A: Photograph of same patient in Figure 19-6 after division of groin flap pedicle. The hand has a "mitten" appearance after covering the finger stumps with the groin flap. **B:** Long-term results seen in patient from Figures 19-5 and 19-8B. The groin flap has been divided into individual flaps for each finger, and they have each been further contoured.

hand, usually with moist gauze in the layer next to the skin as this will encourage drainage from these contaminated wounds. We find it helpful to take advantage of the general anesthesia by manipulating the patient's elbow and shoulder before his or her awakening.

POSTOPERATIVE MANAGEMENT

After the first stage of the groin flap procedure, most patients will need a significant amount of assistance from physical and/or occupational/hand therapists. The involvement of the therapist is essential to help with the transition to home life for the interval in which the hand is attached to the groin. For the purposes of practicality and cost of care, it is beneficial to send the patient home a few days after the initial stage of the procedure, rather than keeping the patient in an inpatient setting for 2 to 3 weeks. The therapist will assist the patient with normal self-care activities such as dressing (including any modifications of clothing made necessary by the attachment of the hand to the groin), hygiene, and other daily activities.

The chief purpose of the hand therapist is to ensure joint mobility to the degree that it is possible during the pedicled stage of the flap. This includes range of motion exercises with the involved shoulder and elbow, as well as the affected hand. In our experience, the groin flap is most often used to cover hand and wrist defects. Therefore, if the patients' other hand injuries permit, we encourage them to work on range of motion exercises with the hand, most commonly in the interphalangeal and metacarpophalangeal joints.

Postoperative wound care is relatively simple after the first stage of the surgery. The chief aim is to keep any flap surfaces that are exposed (i.e., any raw surfaces that are not covered by tubing of the flap) moist and clean. The application of antibiotic (bismuth)-impregnated gauze or antibiotic ointment serves this purpose quite well. Patients are encouraged to wash the wounds daily with soap and water and even to shower. Suture removal depends on the surgeon's preference: they can be removed in 10 to 14 days, or this can be done at the time of flap division 2 to 3 weeks after the initial procedure.

After the conclusion of the flap division procedure 2 to 3 weeks after flap elevation, physiotherapy continues to be an important part of the patients' care. Range of motion exercises should be continued, especially in the affected elbow and shoulder. These joints can become quite stiff between the two procedures; however, this stiffness is most often transient if physical therapy is maintained. Finally, aggressive rehabilitation of the injured hand is a long-term endeavor.

Much later during the patient's care, debulking, revision, and functional improvement of the reconstruction can be taken into consideration. In many patients, the groin flap can be relatively bulky, potentially giving the reconstructed hand a "loaf of bread" appearance. Once the flap has completely healed, this problem is relatively easily treated by partial opening of the flap followed by direct lipectomy in the subcutaneous plane, or by using suction lipectomy with a small (3 mm) suction cannula.

COMPLICATIONS

In the intraoperative setting, a potential complication is construction of a flap that is too wide in the cephalocaudal dimension, thereby preventing primary closure of the donor site. This is not a grave complication, but it does require closure of the donor site with a split-thickness skin graft, which obviously creates another donor site. Additionally, the appearance of the groin wound covered by a skin graft is less desirable than that of a groin wound that has been closed primarily.

The most dreaded complication of the use of the groin flap is flap loss, either partial or total. Fortunately, the pedicled groin flap is quite hardy, making flap loss unusual if care is taken with flap design and tubing. Most series have found flap loss rates in pedicled groin flaps around 1%, and these are most often partial, rather than total flap losses. Not surprisingly, the rate of flap loss when using the groin flap as a free tissue transfer is higher than that of pedicled groin flaps. This can be attributed to the relatively increased difficulty of free groin flap dissection, and to the nature of free flaps in general. Cooper analyzed a series of 130 patients who had undergone free groin flaps for a variety of indications. The series had seven partial and nine total flap losses, and a total flap failure rate of 8.5%. This is slightly higher than most published series of free tissue transfers, where the general free flap failure rate is around 5%. Cooper's series corroborates these numbers in that they experienced an overall free tissue transfer failure rate (using flaps other than the free groin flap) of 4.2%, which is less than half of the failure rate of the free groin flap in their hands.

A complication that is of low morbidity, but can be somewhat distressing to the patient is lateral thigh numbness due to lateral femoral cutaneous nerve injury. Many of these injuries are transient, and sensation will return within several weeks. More distressing to the patient is permanent numbness of the lateral thigh. The true incidence of permanent nerve injury is difficult to gauge due to the variable amount reported in the literature (1%–50%). This can be prevented by careful dissection around the area of the ASIS during flap elevation, taking care to identify and protect the adjacent cutaneous nerves.

Joint stiffness of the elbow and shoulder, though usually transient, is almost a guarantee with the use of the pedicled groin flap. Joint stiffness was thought to be more pronounced and problematic in elderly (over 55 years) patients; however, Buchman published a small series of elderly patients who underwent groin flaps in which they contend that the severity of joint stiffness in this population is not any worse than that of a younger population. As mentioned in the previous section, aggressive physiotherapy is crucial to ensure that any joint stiffness is merely transient.

As with any procedure that involves a period of immobilization, deep venous thrombosis is a concern when dealing with patients who have undergone a groin flap reconstruction. Because groin flap patients are at least initially confined to bed, it is recommended that these patients all be administered low-dose subcutaneous heparin or low-molecular-weight heparin as prophylaxis against deep venous thromboses.

Finally, there are a number of complications that are possible with just about every flap surgery, including the groin flap. Some groups have reported significant seromas in the groin donor site, but these are usually adequately treated with needle aspiration or the opening of a small part of the donor incision. Infection is certainly a possibility, especially with raw wound surfaces for a number of days. However, these are surprisingly uncommon, and are usually sufficiently treated with intravenous or oral antibiotics, along with limited wound opening.

RECOMMENDED READING

Arner M, Moller K. Morbidity of the pedicled groin flap. A retrospective study of 44 cases. *Scand J Plast Reconstr Surg Hand Surg.* 1994;28(2).143–146.

Barillo DJ, Arabitg R, Cancio LC, et al. Distant pedicle flaps for soft tissue coverage of severely burned hands: an old idea revisited. *Burns.* 2001;27(6):613–619.

Buchman SJ, Eglseder WA Jr, Robertson BC. Pedicled groin flaps for upper-extremity reconstruction in the elderly: a report of 4 cases. *Arch Phys Med Rehabil.* 2002;83(6):850–854.

Cheng MH, Chen HC, Wei FC, et al. Combined ischemic preconditioning and laser Doppler measurement for early division of pedicled groin flap. *J Trauma.* 1999;47(1):89–95.

Cheng MH, Chen HC, Wei FC, et al. Devices for ischemic preconditioning of the pedicled groin flap. *J Trauma.* 2000;48(3):552–557.

Chow JA, Bilos ZJ, Hui P, et al.. The groin flap in reparative surgery of the hand. *Plast Reconstr Surg.* 1986;77(3):421–426.

Chuang DC, Colony LH, Chen HC, et al. Groin flap design and versatility. *Plast Reconstr Surg.* 1989;84(1):100–107.

Chuang DC, Jeng SF, Chen HT, et al.. Experience of 73 free groin flaps. *Br J Plast Surg.* 1992;45(2):81–85.

Clodius L, Smith PJ, Bruna J, et al.. The lymphatics of the groin flap. *Ann Plast Surg.* 1982;9(6):447–458.

Cooper TM, Lewis N, Baldwin MA. Free groin flap revisited. *Plast Reconstr Surg.* 1999;103(3):918–924.

Dahlin LB, Lekholm C, Kardum P, et al. Coverage of the median nerve with free and pedicled flaps for the treatment of recurrent severe carpal tunnel syndrome. *Scand J Plast Reconstr Surg Hand Surg.* 2002;36(3):172–176.

DeHaan MR, Hammond DC, Mann RJ. Controlled tissue expansion of a groin flap for upper extremity reconstruction. *Plast Reconstr Surg.* 1990;86(5):979–982.

Dvir E. The groin flap for immediate reconstruction. *Plast Reconstr Surg.* 1987;79(3):505.

Graf P, Biemer E. Morbidity of the groin flap transfer: are we getting something for nothing? *Br J Plast Surg.* 1992;45(2):86–88.

Hanumadass M, Kagan R, Matsuda T. Early coverage of deep hand burns with groin flaps. *J Trauma.* 1987;27(2):109–114.

Harii K, Ohmori K, Torii S, et al. Microvascular free skin flap transfer. *Clin Plast Surg.* 1978;5(2):239–263.

Heath PM, Jackson IT, Cooney WP III, et al. Simultaneous bilateral staged groin flaps for coverage of mutilating injuries of the hand. *Ann Plast Surg.* 1983;11(6):462–468.

Ikuta Y, Kimori K. Flap reconstruction in the upper limb. *Ann Acad Med Singapore.* 1995;24(4 Suppl):124–130.

Isenberg JS, Nguyen H, Salomon J. Bilateral simultaneous groin flaps in the salvage of a pediatric blast-injured hand. *Ann Plast Surg.* 1994;33(4):415–417.

Jones NF, Lister GD. Free skin and composite flaps. In: Green DP, Hotchkiss RN, Pederson WC, ed. *Operative hand surgery.* 4th ed. New York: Churchill Livingstone;1993:1159–1200.

Li YY, Wang JL, Lu Y, et al. Resurfacing deep wound of upper extremities with pedicled groin flaps. *Burns.* 2000;26(3):283–288.

McGregor IA, McGregor AD. Hand surgery. In: McGregor IA, McGregor AD, ed. *Fundamental techniques of plastic surgery.* 9th ed: New York: Churchill Livingstone;1995:183–213.

McGregor IA. The groin flap. *Br J Plast Surg.* 1972;25:3–9.

Mih AD. Pedicle flaps for coverage of the wrist and hand. *Hand Clin.* 1997;13(2):217–229.

Murakami R, Fujii T, Itoh T, et al. Versatility of the thin groin flap. *Microsurgery.* 1996;17(1):41–47.

Nuchtern JG, Engrav LH, Nakamura DY, et al. Treatment of fourth-degree hand burns. *J Burn Care Rehabil.* 1995;16(1):36–42.

O'Brien BM, MacLeod AM, Hayhurst JW, et al. Successful transfer of a large island flap from the groin to the foot by microvascular anastomoses. *Plast Reconstr Surg*. 1973;52(3):271–278.

Parmaksizoglu F, Beyzadeoglu T. Composite osteocutaneous groin flap combined with neurovascular island flap for thumb reconstruction. *J Hand Surg [Br]*. 2003;28(5):399–404.

Rasheed T, Hill C, Riaz M. Innovations in flap design: modified groin flap for closure of multiple finger defects. *Burns*. 2000;26(2):186–189.

Reinisch JF, Winters R, Puckett CL. The use of the osteocutaneous groin flap in gunshot wounds of the hand. *J Hand Surg [Am]*. 1984;9A(1):12–17.

Schlenker JD. Important considerations in the design and construction of groin flaps. *Ann Plast Surg*. 1980;5(5):353–357.

Swartz WM. Immediate reconstruction of the wrist and dorsum of the hand with a free osteocutaneous groin flap. *J Hand Surg [Am]*. 1984;9A(1):18–21.

Trumble TT, Vedder NB. Tissue transfer: pedicle and free tissue flaps. In: Trumble TT, ed. *Principles of hand surgery and therapy*. Philadelphia: WB Saunders; 2000:499–528.

Van Wingerden JJ. The groin flap revisited—what the textbooks do not tell. *S Afr J Surg*. 1999;37(1):21–23.

Watumull D, Orenstein HH. Soft tissue coverage for the upper extremity. *Orthopedics*. 1993;16(4):459–465.

Williams G, Baek SM, Gilbert MS, et al. The groin flap: report of a case of complications in the donor site. *Mt Sinai J Med*. 1981;48(1):63–65.

Winspur I. Distant flaps. *Hand Clin*. 1985;1(4):729–739.

Wray RC, Wise DM, Young VL, et al. The groin flap in severe hand injuries. *Ann Plast Surg*. 1982;9(6):459–462.

PART IV

SOFT TISSUE COVERAGE OF THE FINGERS FOLLOWING TRAUMA

20 Cross-Finger Flaps for Digital Soft Tissue Reconstruction

Bassem T. Elhassan and Alexander Y. Shin

Injuries of the fingertips are very common occurrences secondary to both domestic and industrial accidents and are among the most common hand injuries encountered in the emergency room and the hand practice. To function properly, the fingertip requires adequate padding with durable, sensate skin coverage. As such, any reconstructive procedure of the fingertip must include the provision of durable skin coverage, preservation of adequate sensation, maintenance of finger length, prevention of proximal joint stiffness, and restoration of cosmesis when possible.

Several techniques have been described to address tissue loss of the fingertips. These techniques include direct wound approximation, healing by secondary intention (i.e., allowing the wound to granulate), split and full thickness skin grafting, cross-finger and reverse cross (deepithelialized) finger flaps, adipofascial turnover flaps, revision amputation, volar V-Y advancement flap, Kutler's bilateral V-Y advancement, vascularized island flaps (homodigital flaps), and partial toe transfers (1–6). Each technique has its own indications and contraindications depending on the size of soft tissue loss and the concomitant injuries (exposed bone, tendon, nerve, or vessels).

Cross-finger flaps are local flaps that can reliably provide padding and durable cover for fingertip injuries and have been in use for over 50 years (7,8). The anatomy, indications and contraindications, technique, and results of treatment of the cross-finger flap and the reverse (deepithelized) cross-finger flap for coverage of fingertip injuries will be described.

ANATOMY

Cross-Finger Flap

The cross-finger flap is a random local (regional) flap that is usually raised from the dorsum of the donor finger at the level of the proximal or middle phalanx. The blood supply of this flap is from the many small vessels of the subdermal and subcutaneous plexus. These plexi are fed by two major blood supplies. The first is the dorsal digital arteries that originate from the dorsal metacarpal arteries, which in turn originate from the dorsal carpal arterial arch. These branches mostly feed the plexus covering the skin and subcutaneous tissues of the dorsum of the proximal phalanx. The second blood supply is the proper digital arteries, which feed the plexus of vessels covering the skin and subcutaneous of the dorsum of the middle and distal phalanges.

When used as an innervated flap, the cross-finger flap derives its innervation from the sensory innervation of the dorsum of the hand (9,10). The superficial branch of the radial nerve and the dorsal sensory branch of the ulnar nerve innervate the dorsum of the hand up to the level of the proximal one-third of the dorsal skin of the proximal phalanx. Distal to this point, most of the innervation comes from the proper digital nerves through dorsal and distal branches (Figs. 20-1 and 20-2).

Reverse Cross-Finger Flap

The flap used for reverse cross-finger flap consists of the same tissues used for the standard cross-finger flap but without the covering skin, and thus has also been called a deepithelialized cross-fin-

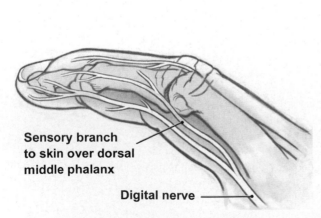

FIGURE 20-1

Innervation to the dorsum of the middle and distal phalanges from the proper digital nerves through dorsal and distal branches. (Reproduced with permission of the Mayo Foundation, 2005.)

Sensory branch to skin over dorsal middle phalanx

Digital nerve

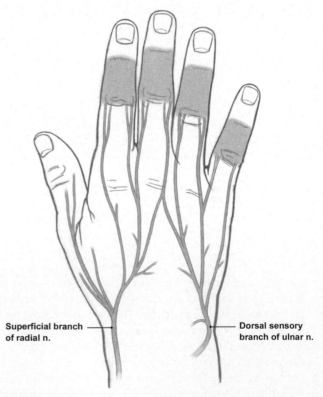

FIGURE 20-2

Innervation to the dorsum of the hand and dorsum of the proximal fingers from branches of the radial and ulnar nerves. (Reproduced with permission of the Mayo Foundation, 2005.)

Superficial branch of radial n.

Dorsal sensory branch of ulnar n.

ger flap. The subdermal plexus becomes the main blood supply to this flap, fed by branches of the dorsal digital arteries and the proper digital arteries as previously described.

INDICATIONS/CONTRAINDICATIONS

Cross-Finger Flap

A cross-finger flap can be used any age group. In the pediatric patient, its use is reported to be successful as early as the first year of life (11). Some authors have recommended alternative tissue coverage in patients older than 50 years because of the risk of development of persistent postoperative stiffness at the proximal interphalangeal (IP) joint (12,13).

The main indication for this flap coverage is a volar fingertip wound with a major loss of skin and subcutaneous tissue with exposed bones and/or tendons. It can also be used for volar defects of the middle phalanx.

As a random flap, the base is longer than the limbs of the flap. Thus, the entire dorsal skin of the finger can be raised and used. However, if the flap includes skin from the dorsal creases of the IP joints, the resultant dorsal scar may lead to stiffness and possible flexion contracture. It is recommended that the flap be raised between the IP creases. The flap's size therefore varies from patient to patient and depends on the size of the finger.

Contraindications include (14–16):

- Multiple injuries to the hand involving the potential donor finger
- Vasospastic conditions such as Raynaud disease and Berger disease
- Preexisting disabling problem such as Dupuytren contracture

Advanced age, diabetes mellitus, and rheumatoid arthritis are considered relative contraindications.

Reverse Cross-Finger Flap

A reverse cross-finger flap is indicated in adults with defects on the dorsum of the finger with major loss of skin and subcutaneous tissue and exposed bones and tendons or a nail bed defect that cannot be covered by other techniques (17).

The best donor site is the dorsum of the middle and proximal phalanges. The skin over the distal interphalangeal (DIP) and proximal interphalangeal (PIP) joints should be avoided because the subcutaneous tissue over these areas is thin and there is higher risk of developing contractures.

The size and contraindications of this flap are similar to those of the cross-finger flap.

SURGERY

Cross-Finger Flap

The donor finger is adjacent to the injured finger. Typically, the donor finger is chosen based on how the injured finger approximates to the middle phalanx of the donor finger. A majority of these flaps can be performed as outpatient surgery under regional anesthesia. Preoperative radiographs of the injured hand should be evaluated for concomitant injuries, which should be treated prior to commencement of the cross-finger flap procedure. Prophylactic antibiotic is given per the discretion of the surgeon.

Under brachial or digital tourniquet control, the injured digit is debrided and irrigated and the skin edges freshened (Fig. 20-3).

The donor and recipient fingers are placed in a position of comfort, before planning the location and the shape of the donor area. To ensure adequate soft tissue coverage, the size of the defect can be outlined on a piece of glove paper allowing 20% excess for the flap pedicle (Fig. 20-4). The outlined site is drawn on the dorsum of the adjacent donor digit. The three sides of the flap are raised as a full thickness graft on the donor finger down to but not including the paratenon (Fig. 20-5A). It is essential that the paratenon layer not be violated, as the full thickness skin graft, which is placed over the donor area, may not adhere. Meticulous hemostasis is obtained. If mobility of the raised flap is limited, or if there is kinking of the flap when the recipient site is covered, further dissection of the flap is performed by incising carefully Cleland's ligament, while protecting the neurovascular bundle that lies volar. Once elevated, the tourniquet is deflated and the vascularity of the flap and the paratenon is evaluated. The donor defect is covered with a full thickness skin graft obtained form

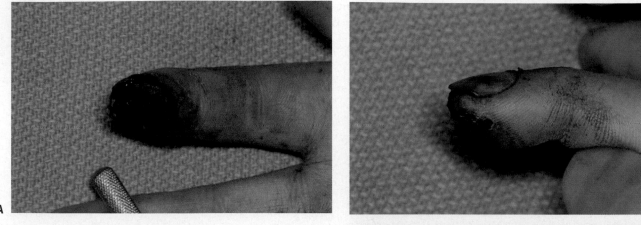

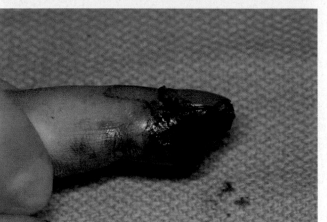

FIGURE 20-3

A-C: Front and side views of an oblique volar fingertip amputation.

the anticubital fossa, upper brachium, or groin (Fig. 20-5B). The flap is sutured in place on the finger defect with nonabsorbable 5-0 suture in adults or absorbable suture in children (Figs. 20-6 through 20-9). A compressive dressing of the surgeon's choice is applied over the skin graft, followed by a bulky hand dressing with appropriate splints. The wound is kept elevated, with encouragement of movement of the uninjured digits. The dressing can be lightened at 1 week postoperatively, whereas the sutures are removed between 10 and 14 days. Between 2 and 3 weeks postoperatively, the patient is returned to the operating room, where the flap is divided, contoured, and inset (Figs. 20-10 through 20-12).

Reverse Cross-Finger Flap

The reverse cross-finger flap is useful for dorsal tissue loss, unlike the standard cross-finger flap, which is indicated for volar wounds. The preparations for this flap are similar to those of the standard cross-finger flap. The differences include the hinge of the flap and the donor tissue. A thin full thickness skin flap is raised from the dorsum of the donor finger at the level of the middle phalanx, preserving the subcutaneous layer.

The hinge of the skin flap is opposite to the primary defect. This is in contradistinction to the standard cross-finger flap, where the hinge is adjacent to the site of the defect (Figs. 20-13 and 20-14). Attention should be paid to keep the dissection at the level of the dermis, below the hair follicles, and above the layer of subcutaneous veins (Fig. 20-15). The subcutaneous tissue is raised, keeping the paratenon intact, with the hinge of the subcutaneous tissue adjacent to the defect. The subcutaneous flap is inset into the defect and the skin is placed back over the donor site (Fig. 20-16). A thin full thickness skin graft is harvested and set on the flap (Fig. 20-17). Division of the flap occurs between 2 and 3 weeks postoperatively (Fig. 20-18). A clinical example of a reverse cross-finger flap is illustrated in Figure 20-19.

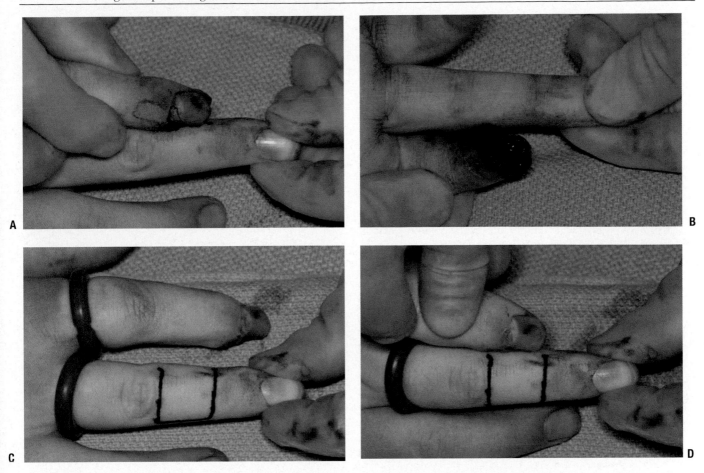

FIGURE 20-4

A-D: Intraoperative pictures showing the steps of preparation for cross-finger flap coverage of a ring fingertip defect. The injured finger is placed at the level of the planned flap from the dorsum of the middle finger at the level of the middle phalanx. The flap should be 20% larger than the actual defect to minimize tension at the time of closure.

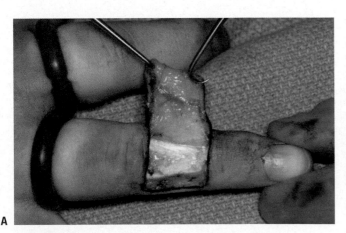
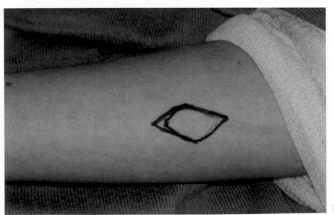

FIGURE 20-5

A: Elevation of the cross-finger flap, keeping the paratenon intact. **B:** Drawing the site for the full-thickness skin graft harvesting from the forearm of the involved finger. (Reproduced with permission of the Mayo Foundation, 2005.)

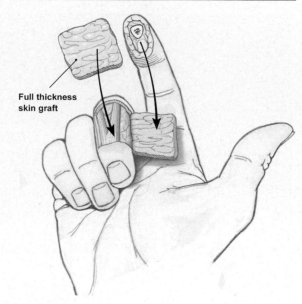

FIGURE 20-6

Illustration demonstrating where the cross-finger flap from the dorsum of the middle finger is to be inset onto the amputated index tip. The full thickness graft is placed to cover the defect over the dorsum of the donor area. (Reproduced with permission of the Mayo Foundation, 2005.)

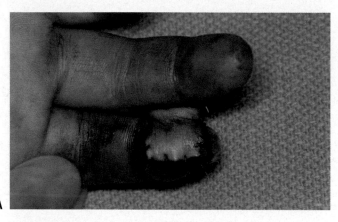

A

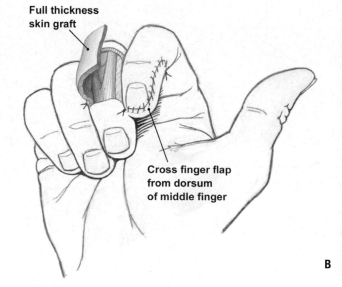

B

FIGURE 20-7

A: A clinical example of a cross-finger flap taken from the dorsum of the middle finger to cover the ring finger. **B:** Illustration demonstrating insetting of the flap. (Reproduced with permission of the Mayo Foundation, 2005.)

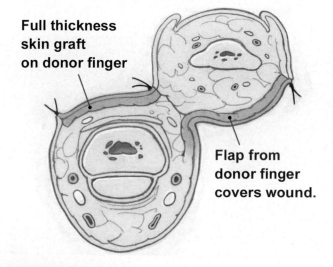

Full thickness skin graft on donor finger

Flap from donor finger covers wound.

FIGURE 20-8

Illustration demonstrating cross section through donor and recipient sites. (Reproduced with permission of the Mayo Foundation, 2005.)

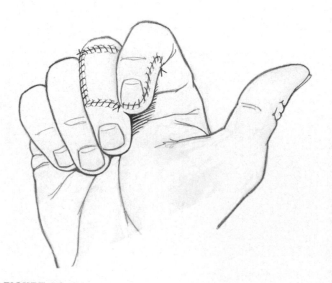

FIGURE 20-9

Illustration of the position of the finger after insetting of flap and skin grafting of donor defect. (Reproduced with permission of the Mayo Foundation, 2005.)

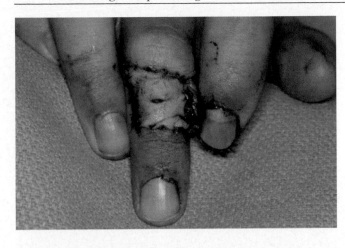

FIGURE 20-10

A full thickness graft from the forearm is used to cover the defect over the donor site.

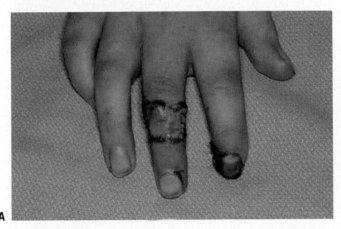

A

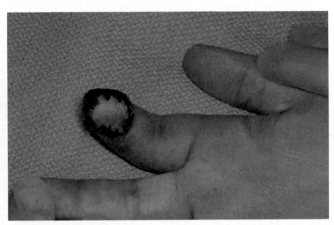

B

FIGURE 20-11

A,B: Division of the flap at 3 weeks postoperatively, with contouring and insetting of the flap.

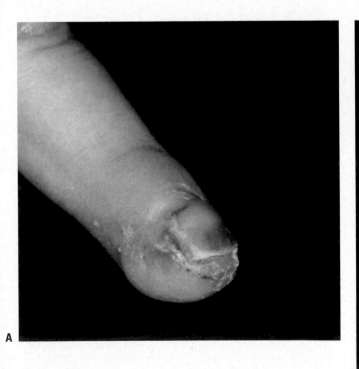

A

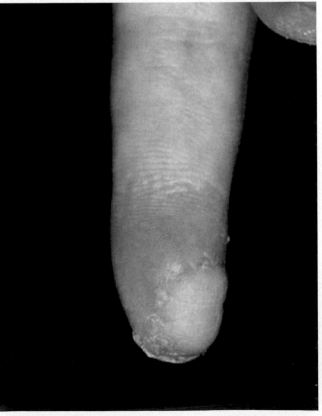

B

FIGURE 20-12

A,B: The appearance of the finger 3 months after surgery.

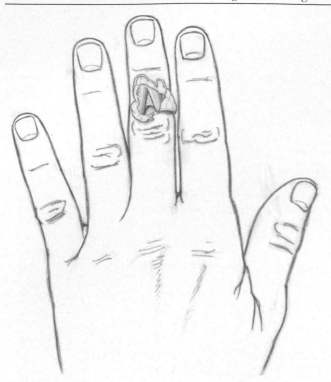

FIGURE 20-13

A defect on the dorsum of middle finger at the level of the middle phalanx with exposure of the extensor tendon denuded of its paratenon is an ideal indication for a reverse cross-finger flap. (Reproduced with permission of the Mayo Foundation, 2005.)

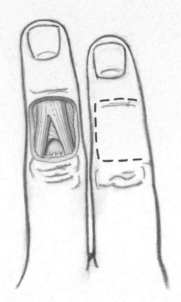

FIGURE 20-14

After the wound is debrided to fresh edges, the reverse cross-finger flap can be designed. (Reproduced with permission of the Mayo Foundation, 2005.)

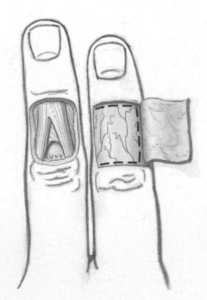

FIGURE 20-15

A thin full thickness skin flap is raised from the dorsum of the donor finger at the level of the middle phalanx, keeping the subcutaneous fat flap intact. The *dotted dashed lines* indicate the site of the planned reverse cross-finger flap, which is divided to the level of the paratenon. (Reproduced with permission of the Mayo Foundation, 2005.)

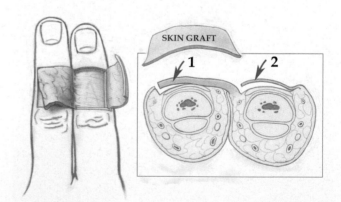

FIGURE 20-16

The hinge of the skin flap is opposite to the primary defect. The drawing shows how the reversed fat flap covers the dorsal finger skin defect (*arrow 1*). The raised thin thickness skin graft is re-placed again into its native site (*arrow 2*). Then, a thin thickness skin graft is placed over the reversed cross-finger flap. (Reproduced with permission of the Mayo Foundation, 2005.)

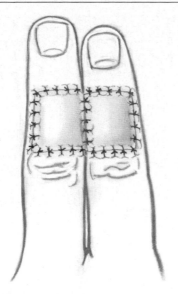

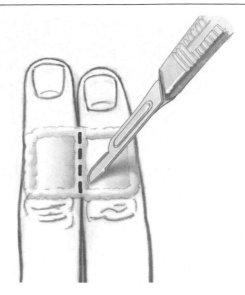

FIGURE 20-17

A drawing showing the appearance of the fingers after the after insetting of the reverse flap and placement of the skin graft. (Reproduced with permission of the Mayo Foundation 2005).

FIGURE 20-18

Division of the reverse cross-finger flap 2–3 weeks after the procedure. (Reproduced with permission of the Mayo Foundation 2005).

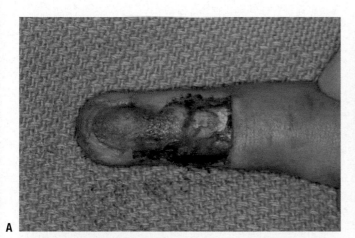

A

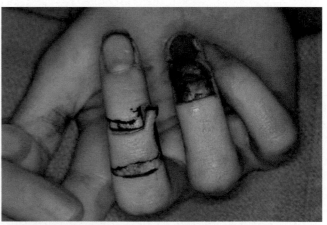

B

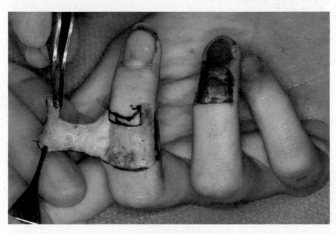

C

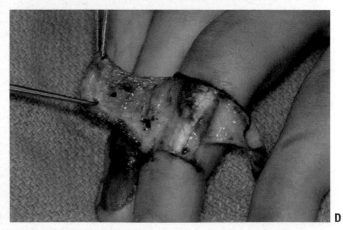

D

FIGURE 20-19

A-G: Clinical example of a reverse cross-finger flap, illustrating flap harvest and insetting. *(Continued)*

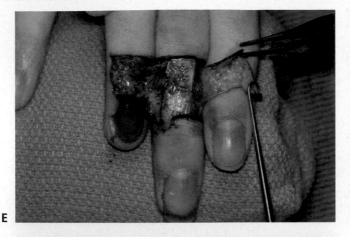

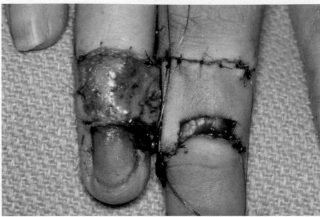

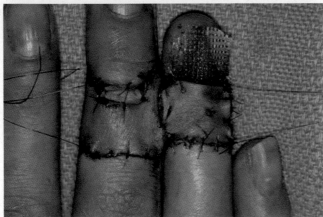

FIGURE 20-19 *Continued*

POSTOPERATIVE MANAGEMENT AND RESULTS

After flap division, supervised finger range of motion commences, which includes combined active motion and passive stretching to eliminate stiffness and regain lost motion (see Fig. 20-9).

Postoperative infection, wound problems, and loss of flap are unusual (15).

The appearance of the skin graft and defect over the donor site are minimized or eliminated with the use of full thickness skin graft. Color mismatch between the dorsum and the pulp of the fingers is minimal, except in individuals with dark-colored skin.

The most common complications encountered with the reverse cross-finger flap include cold sensitivity and decreased sensation in the new transferred skin. In one report reviewing several follow-up studies of finger pulp loss coverage, 30% to 50% of patients developed cold sensitivity and 30% developed altered sensation regardless of the technique used (18). In another study of 54 patients followed over a 5-year period, 92% of the patients were satisfied with the result. However, 53% suffered cold sensitivity. All fingers developed protective sensation, but none had normal sensation or normal sweating (19). The altered sensory recovery varies by age. More than 90% of patients younger than 12 years had 6 mm or less two-point discrimination, compared to 40% of patients older than 40 years (20).

Atasoy (17) reported on four patients who had this reverse cross-finger flap done for nail bed defects (2 patients) with dorsal digital skin avulsions and/or extensor tendon injuries (2 patients). All patients had satisfactory results at the time of final follow-up. The patients with nail bed injury had satisfactory nail growth, and all patients had satisfactory extensor tendon function and good coverage of the defect. A potential complication of the reverse cross-finger flap is creation of an epithelial cyst. Atasoy recommended not grafting the reverse flap in case of large nail bed defect with an intact germinal matrix, in order not to preclude the nail from growing. However, if the there is a complete avulsion of the germinal matrix, nail bed, and skin, with exposure of bone and tendon and little possibility for the nail to return, the reversed flap should be skin grafted.

In another study, Al-Qattan compared the results of deepithelialized cross-finger flap reconstruction (31 patients) versus adipofascial turnover flaps (42 patients) for reconstruction of small complex dorsal digital defects (21). All flaps survived with no infection or hematoma. Patients who underwent reverse cross-finger flap had the following complications: flap dehiscence in one patient, stiffness of the donor finger in five patients, inclusion cyst in one patient, and significant skin graft loss in two patients.

Six patients who underwent adipofascial turnover flaps developed epidermolysis of the donor site, which resolved spontaneously. Al-Qattan recommended using the latter flap in children to avoid using of general anesthesia during flap division, and in older patients to avoid stiffness, and in multiple defects of adjacent border digits.

CONCLUSIONS

The cross-finger and reverse cross-finger flaps are reliable and dependable methods to cover volar and dorsal fingertip soft tissue defects. If carefully performed in properly selected patients, they are versatile flaps that provide a superior means of reconstruction for the injured finger with loss of significant tissue. The cross-finger flap has been used in a wide variety of patients of all ages with rewarding overall patient satisfaction.

REFERENCES

1. Atasoy E, Iokimidis E, Kasdan ML, et al. Reconstruction of the amputated finger tip with a triangular volar flap. *J Bone Joint Surg.* 1970;52-A:921–926.
2. Fisher RH. The Kutler method of repair of finger tip amputation. *J Bone Joint Surg.* 1967;49-A: 317–321.
3. Fox JW, Golden GT, Rodeheaver G, et al. Non-operative management of finger-tip pulp amputation by occlusive dressings. *Am J Surg.* 1977;133:255–256
4. Frandsen PA. VY Plasty as treatment of finger tip amputation. *Acta Orthop Scand.* 1978;49:255–259.
5. Koshima I, Inagawa K, Urushibara K, et al. Fingertip reconstructions using partial-toe transfers. *Plast Reconstr Surg.* 200;105(5):1666–1674.
6. Ma GFY, Cheng CJY, Chan KT, et al. Finger tip injuries—a prospective study on seven methods of treatment on 200 cases. *Ann Acad Med Singapore.* 1982;11(2):207–213.
7. Cronin TD. The cross finger flap, a new method of repair. *Am Surg.* 1951;17:419–425.
8. Gurdin M, Pangman WJ. Repair of surface defects of fingers by transdigital flaps. *Plast Reconstr Surg.* 1950;5:308–371.
9. Cohen BE, Cronin ED. An innervated cross-finger flap for fingertip reconstruction. Review. *Plast Reconstr Surg.* 1983;72(5):688–697.
10. Hasting H II. Dual innervated index to thumb cross finger or island flap reconstruction. *Microsurgery.* 1987;8(3):168–172.
11. Thomson HG, Sorokolit WT. The cross-finger flap in children: a follow-up study. *Plast Reconstr Surg.* 1967;39(5):482–487.
12. Barclay TL. The late results of finger-tip injuries. *Brit J Plat Surg.* 1955;8:38–42.
13. Porter RW. Functional assessment of transplanted skin in volar defects of the digits. *J Bone Joint Surg.* 1968;50A:955–963.
14. Horn JS. The use of full thickness hand skin flaps in the reconstruction of injured fingers. *J Plast Reconstr Surg.* 1951;78:463.
15. Kappel DA, Burech JG. The cross-finger flap. An established reconstructive procedure. *Hand Clin.* 1985;1(4):677–683.
16. Smith JR, Bom AF. An evaluation of fingertip reconstruction by cross-finger and palmar pedicle flap. *J Plast Reconstr Surg.* 1965;35:409–418.
17. Atasoy E. Reversed cross-finger subcutaneous flap. *J Hand Surg [Am].* 1982;7(5):481–483.
18. Louis DS, Jebson PJL, Graham TJ. Amputations. In: Green DP, Hotchkiss RN, Pederson WC, eds. *Green's operative hand surgery.* 4th ed., vol 1. Philadelphia: Churchill Livingstone; 1999:48–94.
19. Nishikawa H, Smith PJ. The recovery of sensation and function after cross-finger flaps for fingertip injury. *J Hand Surg [Br].* 1992;17(1):102–107.
20. Kleinert HE, McAlister CG, MacDonald CJ, et al. A critical evaluation of cross finger flaps. *J Trauma.* 1974;14:756–763.
21. Al-Qattan MM. De-epithelialized cross-finger flaps versus adipofascial turnover flaps for the reconstruction of small complex dorsal digital defects: a comparative analysis. *J Hand Surg.* 2005;30(3):549–557.

21 Heterodigital Arterialized Flap

Shian Chao Tay and Lam Chuan Teoh

INDICATIONS/CONTRAINDICATIONS

Hand trauma that results in exposed bone, tendon, joint, or neurovascular structures requires some type of flap coverage. Defects located around joints and web spaces may also require flap coverage to avoid contractures that could occur following split thickness grafting. The location and size of these defects can often preclude the use of small rotation or advancement flaps. Free flap coverage is an option, but the presence of surrounding infection or a wide zone of trauma may make the recipient vessels' dissection difficult. In such situations, a heterodigital arterialized (HTA) flap may be the best option.

The HTA flap is raised from the lateral side of a donor finger together with the digital artery and a dorsal digital vein. Unlike Littler's neurovascular island flap, or Hueston's extended neurovascular island flap, the heterodigital arterialized flap's main function is to provide non-sensory reconstruction of skin defects in the hand or fingers. Thus, this flap is never harvested with the finger pulp or the digital nerve of the donor finger. This is an important feature that serves to reduce morbidity to the donor finger. The inclusion of the digital dorsal vein into the flap improves venous drainage of the flap and reduces the incidence of venous congestion, which is a well-documented complication of the classic Littler flap,.

The heterodigital arterialized flap is a thin flap. In this aspect it is ideal for reconstruction in the hand and fingers as it provides near like-to-like reconstruction. The other advantages of this flap is that being regional, it obviates the need to prepare a separate surgical site and allows for almost immediate motion of the reconstructed finger. The reconstruction can be performed as a single-stage procedure (as compared to the cross-finger flap or groin flap).

In our experience, the heterodigital arterialized flap has been used to reconstruct volar, lateral, or dorsal defects in the fingers proximal to the distal interphalangeal joint, web spaces, palm, dorsum of the hand, and the thumb. The average flap dimensions are 4.1 cm (range, 1.5 to 5.5 cm) in the longitudinal axis and 2.1 cm (range, 1.0 to 3.5 cm) in the transverse axis. The HTA flap is thus a useful option to consider when faced with the problem of a relatively large defect in the hand or finger that requires non-sensory flap reconstruction. The HTA flap has been used for reconstruction of defects following infection, trauma, post-replantation of digits, electrical burns, chemical burns, and high-pressure injection injuries.

In terms of flap mobility, the reach of the heterodigital arterialized flap is limited to coverage of defects in the adjacent fingers or thumb or adjacent parts of the hand. This is principally due to the combined limitations in the reach of the dorsal vein and the digital artery of the flap. In situations where a greater reach is required, it is possible to divide the dorsal vein of the flap over the dorsum of the hand and reanastomose it in a region of healthy tissue after flap transfer. With this maneuver, the flap should have the ability to reach defects two to three fingers away, much like the traditional reach of Littler's neurovascular island flap, when pivoting at the common digital artery's offshoot at the superficial palmer arterial arch.

The HTA flap is absolutely contraindicated if there is only one functioning digital artery in the donor finger and when the vascular viability of any other adjacent fingers is threatened by flap harvesting. It is also relatively contraindicated if the functional prognosis of the finger to be reconstructed is judged to be so poor that it might be better to amputate it. However, we recognize that social or cultural practices may still dictate reconstruction for the purpose of cosmesis or the maintenance of the "whole" self. Conversely, if there is a rare situation wherein a need to perform a digital amputation exists in a hand containing a defect requiring flap reconstruction, the HTA flap can be used as a fillet flap from the amputated finger for defect reconstruction. In such a situation, the HTA flap is very useful in spare parts surgery as there is no concern for donor finger morbidity. If the defect occurs beyond the reach of the flap or in the contralateral hand, a free fillet HTA flap can be created from the finger to be amputated provided the conditions at the recipient finger allows for a free flap.

PREOPERATIVE PLANNING

All practical options available for reconstruction should be considered by the surgeon before deciding on the HTA flap. Risks of heterodigital donor finger morbidity should be carefully weighed against benefits of reconstruction. Often, the location, size, and nature of the defect will preclude other reconstructive options, leaving the HTA flap as the most viable option with the highest flap survival rate.

The choice of donor finger is often dictated by the location of the defect and is often an adjacent finger. The outside borders of the index and little fingers are not used as donor sites to preserve hand cosmesis and to maintain native skin for protection and sensation. This requirement is not absolute; however, we prefer the use of the middle finger, ring finger, and the ulnar border of the index finger. Theoretically, the radial border of the little finger can be used as a donor site but this is rare as the little finger is small, providing little skin, and the remaining ulnar digital artery is often absent or vestigial.

A digital Allen's test must be performed on the intended donor finger to ensure that both digital arteries are sufficiently patent. In addition, the Allen's test should also be performed on the finger that is adjacent to the donor site as this would dictate if the digital artery mobilization can proceed proximal to the point of bifurcation of the common digital artery. More often than not, a longer reach is required and ligation and division of the neighboring branch of the digital artery to the adjacent finger would need to be performed to create an arterial pedicle of sufficient length.

If the donor site is just next to the defect in the adjacent finger, also known as the contiguous or near side of the adjacent finger (e.g., defect on ulnar side of index finger with donor site on radial side of middle finger), the pivot point can be at the bifurcation of the common digital artery, as a short pedicle would be sufficient. This pivot point can be approximately landmarked in the intermetacarpal space at the level of the distal palmer crease. The distance from this pivot point to the proximal edge of the defect can then be measured to determine the reach needed by the flap and hence the location of the proximal margin of the flap. If the flap is not coming from the contiguous side of the adjacent finger, it is likely that a more proximal pivot point would be required to ensure sufficient reach of the flap. The most proximal point would be the superficial palmer arterial arch, which can be approximated to the level of the proximal palmar crease in the relevant intermetacarpal space. In such situations, as mentioned previously, it will be necessary to ligate and divide the neighboring digital artery of the common digital artery that supplies the adjacent finger to maximize the reach of the flap.

Experience has shown that the reach of the flap increases by 10% once the digital artery is adequately mobilized. However, in the interests of safety and ensuring minimum tension in the pedicle, a 1:1 ratio should still be maintained for the length of the arterial pedicle during preoperative planning of flap surgery.

The timing for reconstruction depends on the pathology. As far as possible, early reconstruction (within 1 week) is preferred as it minimizes overall hand stiffness from prolonged disuse. For traumatic conditions, the reconstruction is ideally performed within 1 week. For post-replantation surgery with residual skin defects, the resurfacing is performed within 10 to 15 days when re-endothelialization of the vascular anastomoses is completed. Infection cases are ideally resurfaced within 4 to 7 days when the surrounding cellulitis and edema have subsided. In order to achieve this time line in infective cases, infection reversal should be achieved within one to two formal definitive excisional debridement surgeries in conjunction with appropriate intravenous antibiotics.

The surgery can be performed under general or regional anesthesia with sedation. The patient's general condition and coagulation profile should be optimized as per any reconstructive surgery. The patient should be consented and counseled as to the surgery, the postoperative course, and the duration of stay following surgery.

SURGERY

Patient Positioning

The patient should be in the supine position, and care should be taken to protect bony prominences with suitable pressure-relieving bolsters. The upper limb with the hand requiring reconstruction should be abducted to not more than 80 degrees at the shoulder to prevent excessive stretch to the nerves in the axilla. The elbow should be flexed slightly so that the forearm can be placed transversely on a stable hand table. A pneumatic tourniquet should be applied to the most proximal part of the upper arm, and the upper limb should be cleaned and draped as far proximal until the distal edge of the tourniquet. If the surgery is expected to last more than 2 hours, urinary catheterization should be considered.

Technique

The surgery is performed under tourniquet control, which should be inflated with the upper limb elevated but not exsanguinated. This is to facilitate identification and mobilization of the digital artery and the digital dorsal vein. The defect should be thoroughly debrided and irrigated. A template of the defect is made. At this point, the digital Allen's test can be repeated to confirm the adequacy of both digital arteries in the donor finger, and also in the adjacent finger if the flap is not taken from the contiguous side of the finger adjacent to the defect.

Using the template created, the appropriate dimension of the flap is then transferred onto the donor site. The flap should be centered on the lateral or dorsolateral side of the finger, depending on the width of flap required, to ensure the inclusion of the digital artery and a dominant digital dorsal vein. The maximum width of the flap should not exceed the mid-palmer line and the mid-dorsal line (a width of approximately 3 cm). The maximum length of the flap is from the base of the finger to the distal interphalangeal joint crease (usually 4 to 5 cm depending on the size of the finger). If necessary, the flap length may be extended 0.5 cm distal to the distal interphalangeal joint crease. Next, a palmar Z incision is drawn, biased to the respective side of the finger to access the proximal part of the digital artery. This incision is carried into the palm to the level of the common digital artery. The location of the dominant dorsal digital vein is then verified and marked to ensure that it will drain the flap. Once this is completed, the flap is ready to be harvested.

Heterodigital arterialized flap harvesting is performed with the aid of loupe magnification. The flap is first raised from its palmar margin (Fig. 21-1). If the palmar margin of the flap crosses any digital palmer flexion creases, a mini-z cut can be made at these creases, to break up the resultant scar line. Superficial palmer veins can be carefully cauterized with bipolar electrocautery and divided. As one proceeds deeper, the dissection follows the digital artery from proximal to distal starting from the bifurcation of the common digital artery. The angle of dissection toward the neurovascular bundle is an oblique plane skiving dorsal to the digital nerve, which is more central and superficial compared to the digital artery. As far as possible, the nerve should be left undisturbed in its bed with a collar of fat kept around it. Besides ensuring that the nerve is not traumatized, the collar of fat also provides additional cushioning and enhances the take of the full-thickness skin graft at the donor site. Ideally, a collar of fat or soft tissue should also be kept around the digital artery to preserve the venae comitantes. Fortunately, in the HTA flap, this is not as critical, as the dorsal vein would provide the main conduit for venous drainage.

At this point, an intraoperative occlusion test can be performed using non-traumatic microsurgical vascular clamps to determine the integrity of the contralateral digital artery in the donor finger. If mobilization of the digital artery to the level of the superficial palmer arch is necessary, a similar occlusion test should be performed on the bifurcated digital artery supplying the adjacent non-donor finger to ensure that it also has a healthy contralateral digital artery.

As mobilization of the digital artery progresses, the transverse palmer arches of the digital artery will be encountered. These are rather large and short. Sufficient room is developed and the arches can be carefully cauterized with bipolar electrocautery before division. Care should be taken to ensure that the bipolar electrocautery is applied at least 2 mm from the parent artery to prevent compromising flow in the main digital artery.

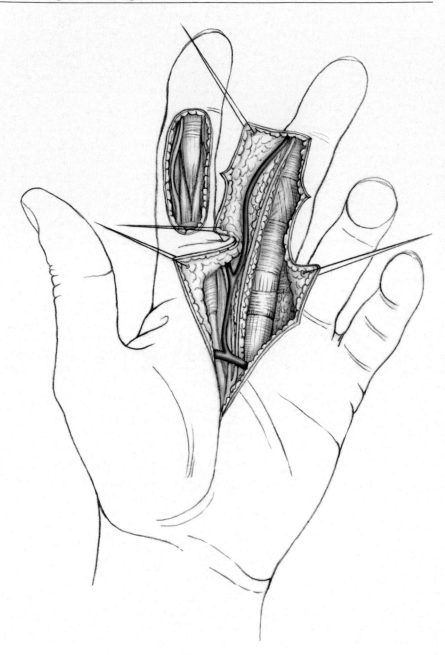

FIGURE 21-1

Completed palmar dissection of the HTA flap with the digital nerve left undisturbed in its bed with a collar of fat around it. Proximal dissection of the arterial pedicle is facilitated by a palmar Z incision into the palm.

Dorsal dissection is performed next with proximal to distal dissection and mobilization of the dominant dorsal digital vein to ensure inclusion of the vein in the flap. The flap is dissected free from the extensor tendons in the plane superficial to the paratenon. Care should be taken not to damage the dorsal skin branches of the digital artery supplying the flap. At the distal margin of the flap, the distal end of the dominant dorsal vein is ligated and divided, and the same is performed for the digital artery on the palmer side.

At this stage, the flap should be detached from distal to proximal. The adherent fibrous septa and Cleland's ligaments are divided. At the base of the digit, some dissection may be necessary to complete the division of subcutaneous tissues attached to the flap. The natatory ligament at the web space may also be divided to prevent kinking of the dorsal vein and lengthen the reach of the flap.

A generous subcutaneous tunnel is created between the donor and the recipient site. Tunneling is performed from the proximal edge of the recipient site into the palm to reach the pivot point of the flap. A hemostat forceps is used to gently enlarge the tunnel for easy flap delivery. The distal end of the flap is carefully grasped and gently maneuvered into the tunnel. A recommended method of flap delivery is to completely wrap the flap with tulle gras dressing and deliver the flap by grasping only

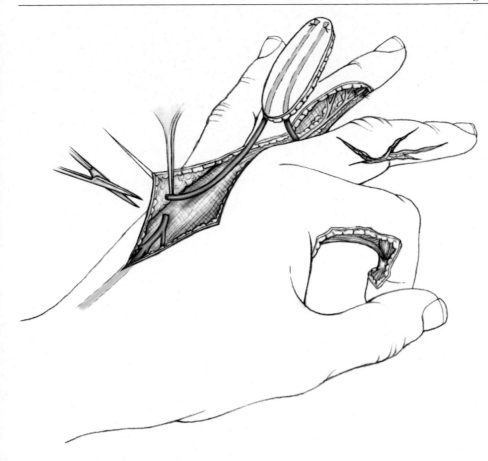

FIGURE 21-2

Completed dorsal and palmar dissection of the HTA flap with the flap completely islanded from the donor ring finger. The flap is now to be transferred. In this case, the defect requiring resurfacing is on the volar side of the index finger. The middle finger has a significant injury and is not suitable as a donor. The bi-pedicled nature of the flap will obstruct the transfer through the palmar subcutaneous tunnel. Thus, the venous pedicle of the flap has been divided over the dorsum of the hand to partially free the flap and convert it into a mono-pedicled flap.

on the tulle gras. This serves to prevent direct grasping of the flap and also protects the flap and pedicles from being avulsed if the delivery in the tunnel is inadvertently rough or jerky. As the flap traverses the tunnel, care is taken to ensure that the digital artery and the dorsal vein do not become twisted or kinked. The flap should not be rotated more than a half turn. If there is any uncertainty, the flap should be re-delivered to ensure its correct orientation.

When a longer reach of the flap is required, and the bipedicled nature of the flap is restricting the transfer, the dominant dorsal vein may be divided before the transfer (Fig. 21-2) and anastomosed to the original vein or another vein over the dorsum of the hand in an area free of adversity, after the flap has been transferred (Fig. 21-3). When this procedure is performed, it is called the "partially free HTA flap."

After flap transfer, the flap is provisionally held in place with a few fine sutures. The tourniquet is then deflated to check for flap perfusion and to secure hemostasis. If flap perfusion does not return after 5 minutes or if there is flap congestion, some sutures may have to be removed. If this fails to improve flap color, kinks in the vascular pedicle may have to be located and relieved. If the vascular pedicle suffered mild inadvertent trauma during surgery, appropriate flap resuscitation measures such as warming the patient, warm saline soaks to the artery, and immersion of the arterial pedicle in 2% lidocaine or papavrine may have to be performed before adequate flap perfusion is restored.

Once adequate flap perfusion is restored, the flap is then fully inset with fine sutures, usually non-absorbable monofilament 5-0 sutures, spaced not less than 3 to 5 mm apart. Care should be taken during the insetting to ensure that both the dorsal vein and the digital artery are not compressed or traumatized. The donor defect is resurfaced with a full-thickness skin graft. This can be taken from the medial proximal forearm, the anterior elbow, or groin if necessary. As early postoperative active rehabilitation is required, it is highly recommended to secure the skin graft with a cotton wool bolster and a meticulous tie-over dressing to prevent skin graft loss during therapy. The rest of the surgical wounds are closed with fine sutures with or without non-suction drains. A bulky, non-constrictive dressing is applied with a window left open for flap monitoring. Healthy flap perfusion should be confirmed before leaving the operating room.

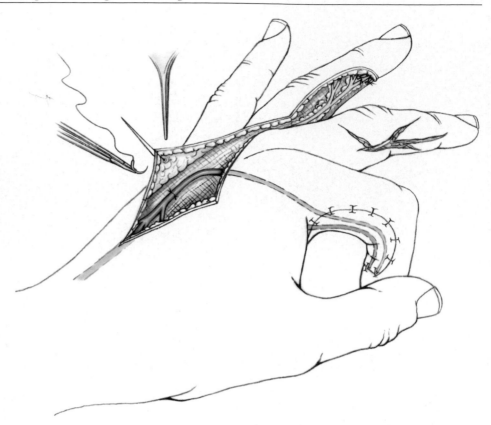

FIGURE 21-3

The partially free HTA flap after successful transfer to the defect site on the index finger. The venous pedicle of the flap has been tunnelled back for microsurgical repair to the original draining vein over the dorsum of the hand.

RESULTS

A total of 40 HTA flaps were performed between 1991 and 2001. Thirteen of these flaps involved division and repair of the dominant dorsal digital vein to extend the reach of the flap. Total active range of motion of the donor finger was excellent in 82.5%, good in 15%, and fair in 2.5% (1 patient) according to Strickland and Glogovac's criteria for flexor tendon surgery (see Figs. 21-4, 21-5, and 21-12). The fair result was due to the development of reflex sympathetic dystrophy and associated flexion contracture. Donor finger two-point discrimination was 3 to 5 mm, except in one case (6 mm). None of the donor fingers had hypersensitivity, symptomatic neuromas, or suffered from cold intolerance.

Flap survival was 100% with no cases of flap congestion or ischaemia documented. All flaps healed primarily and provided supple coverage of the defects. Full-thickness skin graft take was similarly successful at 100% in the donor fingers. Although a contour concavity is present at the time of removal of the cotton wool bolus on the fifth postoperative day, the concavity usually fills out within

FIGURE 21-4

A sizeable defect (5 ×2 cm) over the volar-ulnar aspect of the right index finger exposing bare flexor tendons and the neurovascular bundles following trauma. The HTA flap would come from the radial side of the middle finger. Thus, it would be a contiguous transfer of the HTA flap. There is no need to divide the venous pedicle to partially free the HTA flap in such a situation. (From Teoh LC, Tay SC, Yong FC, Tan SH, Khoo DBA. Heterodigital arterialized flaps for large finger wounds: results and indications. *Plast Reconstr Surg.* 2003;111(6):1905–1913. With permission.)

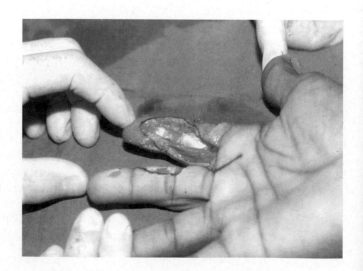

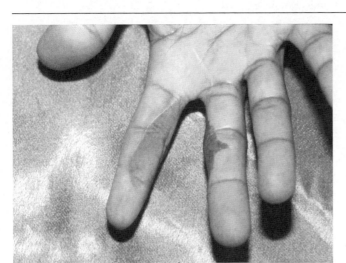

FIGURE 21-5
Cosmetic result in this dark-skinned individual at 3 months postoperatively. Patient has full extension of the donor middle finger and has excellent primary healing of the HTA flap on his index finger. (From Teoh LC, Tay SC, Yong FC, Tan SH, Khoo DBA. Heterodigital arterialized flaps for large finger wounds: results and indications. *Plast Reconstr Surg.* 2003;111(6):1905–1913. With permission.)

3 months after surgery. None of the cases required any further surgery to the flap such as insetting or defatting.

We evaluated the total active motion in 22 fingers which had undergone reconstruction with the HTA flap. According to Strickland and Glogovac's criteria, 45.4% achieved excellent and good results, with the remainder achieving fair to poor results. It should be noted that the poorer outcomes in the reconstructed fingers are due to severe insults resulting in multiple tissue involvement with concomitant damage to joints, tendons, and/or ligaments and not due to contractures of the HTA flap.

POSTOPERATIVE MANAGEMENT

The first 24 hours are the most critical for the flap. The flap should be monitored frequently with the hand nursed in an elevated position during this time and the patient kept nil per oral (NPO). The ambient temperature can be raised to a level appropriate for the season at least for the first night depending on the surgeon's preference. Drains, if used, should be removed within the first 24 to 48 hours. Rehabilitation should commence on the second postoperative day but can be delayed if circumstances dictate. An early and active rehabilitation program is crucial in minimizing heterodigital donor finger morbidity. Active and passive range of motion exercises are instituted for both the recipient and donor digits. Regional anesthesia in the form of infusion blocks can be maintained during the postoperative period to assist with pain control during rehabilitation. The use of a cotton bolster ensures that the full-thickness skin graft is firmly secured so as to allow progressive hand therapy within the first week. Interval splinting of the donor digit between exercises may be necessary to prevent flexion contractures.

COMPLICATIONS

Heterodigital donor finger morbidity is the main concern. As mentioned previously, the preservation of the digital nerve and the finger pulp on the donor finger is critical toward preserving sensory function in the donor finger. In addition, the meticulous dissection of the digital artery away from the digital nerve is crucial in minimizing inadvertent trauma to the digital nerve, which can affect sensory function in the finger pulp and produce sensitive mini-neuromas along the digital nerve. Together with careful resurfacing of the donor site using full-thickness skin grafting and institution of early active finger mobilization, stiffness of the donor and reconstructed finger can be significantly reduced.

Mild loss of total active motion can be expected in about 10% to 15% of cases. Reflex sympathetic dystrophy with flexion contracture is another serious complication that can occur. Flap failure, either partial or complete, is always a potential complication, but it has not occurred in our series. In the five cases of free HTA flap, we did not experience any vascular complications and all the free flaps survived completely. In dark-skinned races, the darker dorsal skin may be a poor cosmetic match for defects on the volar side of the hand (Fig. 21-5).

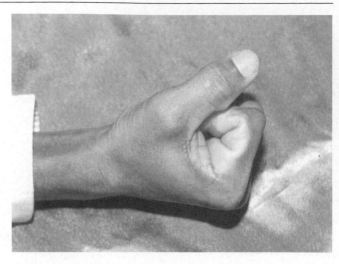

FIGURE 21-6

Excellent result and hand function with full finger flexion in both donor and reconstructed fingers. (From Teoh LC, Tay SC, Yong FC, Tan SH, Khoo DBA. Heterodigital arterialized flaps for large finger wounds: results and indications. *Plast Reconstr Surg.* 2003;111(6): 1905–1913.

VARIANTS OF THE HETERODIGITAL ARTERIALIZED FLAP

Besides the free fillet flap, other variants of the HTA flap include the cross-finger HTA flap, which is particularly suited for coverage of dorsal defects distal to the proximal interphalangeal joint which cannot be reached by the reverse dorsal intermetacarpal flap or the Quaba flap. Another indication for the cross-finger HTA flap is in situations where proximal dissection of the digital artery in the hand is not advisable due to previous trauma or infection. The cross-finger HTA flap only requires dissection of the venous and arterial pedicle up to the level of the base of the finger and will allow transfer to any surface on the adjacent finger (Fig. 21-6). This is accessed via mid-lateral incisions raising small dorsal and volar soft tissue flaps proximal to the donor site. Care should be taken not to extend these incisions into the web space or the lateral walls of the web commissure. A similar mid-lateral incision is performed proximal to the defect on the injured finger. The flap is directly transferred across the interdigital space and onto the defect (Fig. 21-7). This avoids the need to tunnel the pedicles and flap through the distal part of the hand and also allows the flap to reach a defect on any surface of the finger distal to the proximal interphalangeal joint. The dorsal and volar soft tissue flaps of the mid-lateral incisions are then sutured together to create a soft tissue pouch that will protect the flap pedicle and prevent separation of the digits. Division of the cross-finger

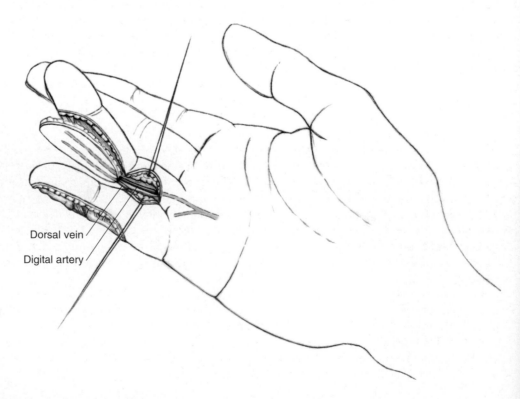

Dorsal vein
Digital artery

FIGURE 21-7

Cross-finger HTA flap from the ulnar side of the ring finger for transfer to a defect on the ulnar side of the distal little finger. Note that minimal pedicle length is required for this direct cross-finger transfer and there is no need to perform any pedicle dissection in the palm.

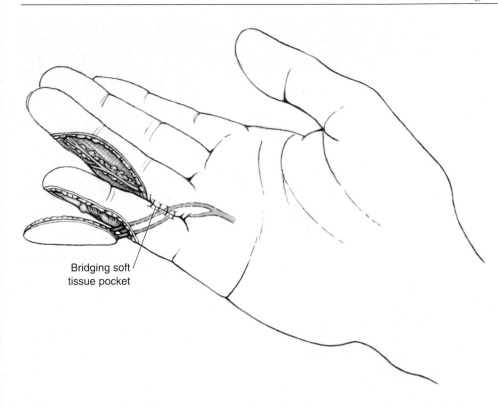

Bridging soft
tissue pocket

FIGURE 21-8

Cross-finger HTA flap after transfer to the defect site. The flap has been tunnelled through volar tissue of the little finger. The vascular pedicles of the flap are now protected by a soft tissue skin bridge that has been created between the base of the ring and little finger. A full-thickness skin graft with a cotton wool bolus with tie over will be applied to the donor site. The soft tissue skin bridge, together with the HTA flap vascular pedicles, will be divided at 3 weeks postoperatively when the cross-finger HTA flap has established its own vascular supply in the reconstructed little finger.

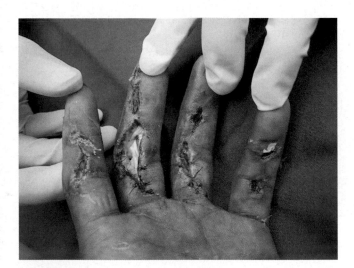

FIGURE 21-9

A patient referred from another hospital with a sizeable chronic non-healing defect on his left middle finger with concomitant injuries to all the other fingers.

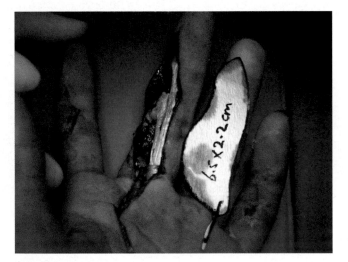

FIGURE 21-10

After debridement, the true defect size is apparent (6.5 × 2.2 cm) with exposed bare flexor tendons. The patient will be undergoing free HTA flap procedure with the flap being harvested from the ulnar side of the right middle finger.

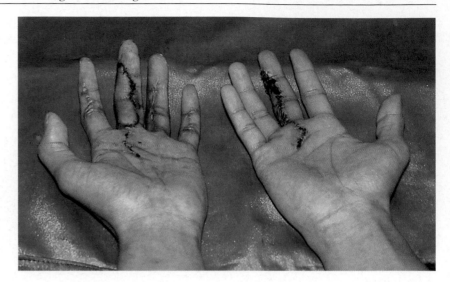

FIGURE 21-11

Two weeks post free HTA flap with 100% survival of the free HTA flap with excellent primary healing in the reconstructed left middle finger. The full-thickness skin graft is also healing well on the donor site (ulnar side of the right middle finger).

version of the HTA flap is performed at 3 weeks. In the interim, active rehabilitation of the joined fingers should be started to prevent finger stiffness.

The final variant is the free HTA flap. This free flap should only be used by hand microsurgeons already well experienced with the HTA flap. In occasional situations, a sizeable defect exists in a hand in which there is concomitant or prior injuries to the other fingers, rendering them unsuitable as donors of the HTA flap. In such situations, if the defect is amenable for a free flap procedure and other free flaps are not available, the HTA flap may be harvested as a completely free flap from the uninjured contralateral hand. In such situations, the free HTA flap is taken from the ulnar side of the middle finger. The indication for the free HTA flap is certainly unique and rare. First performed in 1991, we have since found cause to only have performed five such flaps. In one case, it was used to electively resurface a sizeable defect on the small finger following a successful four-finger replantation. In another case, it was used to resurface a non-healing chronic defect on the middle finger following an injury which also involved the other three fingers (Figs. 21-8 and 21-9). In two cases, there were acute concomitant injuries to the other fingers. In the last case, the free HTA flap was used as a free flow-through arterial flap, not only to reconstruct the skin defect, but also to reconstruct a digital artery segment defect in a finger that had arterial insufficiency following an injury that also involved all the fingers. The excellent size matching of the digital arteries certainly contributed significantly to the success of the procedure. In all five cases, except for the mild cosmetic defect of the full thickness skin graft at the donor site, all the donor fingers retained full and complete range of active motion and preservation of normal pulp sensation (Figs. 21-10 and 21-11). An important reason why the free HTA flap might have such an excellent result in the donor fingers might be due to the fact that there were no other injuries in the donor hand, which greatly facilitated active rehabilitation.

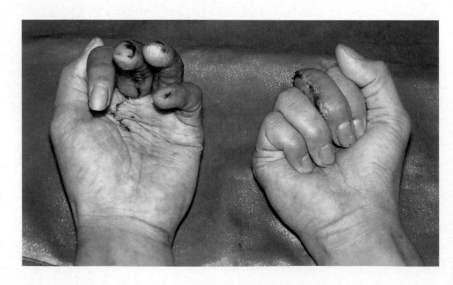

FIGURE 21-12

Full flexion of the right middle donor finger demonstrated. The stiffness that is apparent in the left hand is due to prolonged immobilization and disuse as a result of the chronic non-healing wound. With successful and robust coverage of the defect in the left hand with excellent primary healing, aggressive rehabilitation of the hand can be started to alleviate the stiffness.

RECOMMENDED READING

Adani R, Squarzina PB, Castagnetti C, Lagana A, Pancaldi G, Caroli A. A comparative study of the heterodigital neurovascular island flap in thumb reconstruction with and without nerve reconnection. *J Hand Surg.* 1994;19B:552–559.

Brunelli F, Mathoulin C. Digital island flaps. In: Gilbert A, Masquelet AC, Hentz VR, eds. *Pedicle flaps of the upper limb: vascular anatomy, surgical technique, and current indications.* London: Martin Dunitz; 1992:169–176.

Buchler U. The dorsal middle phalangeal finger flap. *Handchir Mikrochir Plast Chir.* 1988;20:239–243.

Caffee HH, Ward D. Bipolar coagulation in microvascular surgery. *Plast Reconstr Surg.* 1986;78:374–377.

Chow SP, Zhu JK, So YC. Effect of bipolar coagulation and occlusion clamping on the patency rate in microvascular anastomosis. *J Reconstr Microsurg.* 1986;2(2):111–115.

Eaton RG. The digital neurovascular bundle. A microanatomic study of its contents. *Clin Orthop.* 1968;61:176–185.

Edwards EA. Organization of the small arteries of the hand and digits. *Am J Surg.* 1960;99:837–846.

Endo T, Kojima T, Hirase Y. Vascular anatomy of the finger dorsum and a new idea for coverage of the finger pulp defect that restores sensation. *J Hand Surg.* 1992;17A:927–932.

Foucher G, Braun FM, Merle M, Michon J. La technique du "débranchement-rebranchment" due lambeau en ilot pédiculé. *Ann Chir.* 1981;35:303.

Hirase Y, Kojima T, Matsuura S. A versatile one-stage neurovascular flap for fingertip reconstruction: The dorsal middle phalangeal finger flap. *Plast Reconstr Surg.* 1992;90(6):1009–1015.

Hood JM, Lubahn JD. Bipolar coagulation at different energy levels: effect on patency. *Microsurgery.* 1994;15:594–597.

Hueston J. The extended neurovascular island flap. *Br J Plast Surg.* 1965;18:304–305.

Isogai N, Kamiishi H, Chichibu S. Re-endothelialization stages at the microvascular anastomosis. *Microsurgery.* 1988;9(2):87–94.

Henderson HP, Reid DA. Long term follow up of neurovascular island flaps. *Hand.* 1980;12(3):113–122.

Kumta SM, Yip KMH, Pannozzo A, Fong SL, Leung PC. Resurfacing of thumb-pulp loss with a heterodigital neurovascular island flap using a nerve disconnection/reconnection technique. *J Reconstr Microsurg.* 1997;13(2):117–122.

Kurokawa M, Ishikawa K, Nishimura Y. A neurovascular island flap including a vein for the treatment of an acquired ring constriction. *Br J Plast Surg.* 1995;48(6).401-404.

Lee YL, Teoh LC, Seah WT. Extending the reach of the heterodigital arterialised flap by cross finger transfer. *Plast Reconstr Surg.* In press.

Leupin P, Weil J, Buchler U. The dorsal middle phalangeal finger flap. Mid-term results of 43 cases. *J Hand Surg Br.* 1997;22(3):362-371.

Littler JW. Neurovascular pedicle method of digital transposition for reconstruction of the thumb. *Plast Reconstr Surg.* 1953;12:303–319.

Lucas GL. The pattern of venous drainage of the digits. *J Hand Surg.* 1984;9A:448–450.

Moss SH, Schwartz KS, von Drasek-Ascher G, Ogden LL, Wheeler CS, Lister GD et al. Digital venous anatomy. *J Hand Surg.* 1985;10A:473–482.

Murray JF, Ord JVR, Gavelin GE. The neurovascular island flap : an assessment of late results in sixteen cases. *J Bone Joint Surg.* 1967;49A:1285–1297.

Paterson P, Titley OG, Nancarrow JD. Donor finger morbidity in cross-finger flaps. *Injury.* 2000;31:215–218.

Quaba AA, Davison PM. The distally based dorsal hand flap. *Br J Plast Surg.* 1990;43(1):28–39.

Riordan DC, Kaplan EB. Surface anatomy of the hand and wrist. In: Spinner M, ed. *Kaplan's functional and surgical anatomy of the hand.* 3rd ed. Philadelphia: Lippincott Williams and Wilkins; 1984:353.

Rose EH. Local arterialized island flap coverage of difficult defects preserving donor digit sensibility. *Plast Reconstr Surg.* 1983;72:848–858.

Roth JH, Urbaniak JR, Boswick JM. Comparison of suture ligation, bipolar cauterization, and hemoclip ligation in the management of small branching vessels in a rat model. *J Reconstr Microsurg.* 1984;1:7–9.

Strauch B, de Moura W. Arterial system of the fingers. *J Hand Surg.* 1990;15A:148–154.

Strickland JW, Glogovac SV. Digital function following flexor tendon repair in Zone II: a comparison of immobilization and controlled passive motion techniques. *J Hand Surg.* 1980;5A:537–543.

Tay SC, Teoh LC, Tan SH, Yong FC. Extending the reach of the heterodigital arterialized flap by vein division and repair. *Plast Reconstr Surg.* 2004;114(6):1450–1456.

Tay SC, Teoh LC. The heterodigital arterialized flap—discussion. *Plast Reconstr Surg.* 2005. In press.

Teoh LC, Tay SC, Yong FC, Tan SH, Khoo DBA. Heterodigital arterialized flaps for large finger wounds: results and indications. *Plast Reconstr Surg.* 2003;111(6):1905–1913.

Tubiana R, Duparc J. Restoration of sensibility in the hand by neurovascular skin island transfer. *J Bone Joint Surg.* 1961;43B:474.

Tubiana R, Duparc J. O'peration palliative pour paralysie sensitive a la main. *Mem Acad Chir.* 1959;85:66–70.

Weeks PM. Discussion. Local arterialized island flap coverage of difficult hand defects preserving donor digit sensibility. *Plast Reconstr Surg.* 1983;72:858.

22 Homodigital Island Flap

Bradon J. Wilhelmi and Damon Cooney

Single-stage reconstruction of the finger pulp has become possible with a better understanding of hand anatomy and the advent of new surgical techniques. Single-stage reconstruction eliminates the risk of a stiff finger resulting from immobilization and the necessity of a second operation that is required with traditional regional flap reconstruction. The options for one-stage reconstruction of pulp defects include heterodigital and homodigital neurovascular island flaps. The heterodigital neurovascular island flap has the disadvantage of late or no development of sensory reorientation and paresthesia in the donor finger. Harvesting the flap from the injured finger, as is the case in a homodigital island flap, avoids unnecessary surgery to an adjacent uninjured finger as well as potentially enhancing rehabilitation by minimizing additional hand trauma. Many homodigital neurovascular flaps based on one or two volar digital pedicles have been described which can provide the fingertip with sensate coverage. The palmar advancement flap based on bilateral neurovascular pedicles has been used for reconstruction of the thumb and fingers. The interphalangeal (IP) joint is usually needed to be kept in flexion to obtain adequate advancement of the flap, which increases the complication risk for flexion contracture of the distal joint with these advancement flaps. Also, the use of the advancement flap increases the risk for dorsal skin necrosis if the dorsal branches from the proper digital artery are severed for distal advancement of the flap. The volar V-Y flap is still a suitable flap for small fingertip defects less than 1 cm when there is sufficient skin distal to the distal interphalangeal (DIP) crease to base the flap.

INDICATIONS/CONTRAINDICATIONS

The homodigital neurovascular flap has been described with elevation of the dorsal finger skin to repair pulp deficits which cannot be closed with the volar V-Y advancement flap. Anatomic studies have demonstrated that a dorsal arterial branch from the proper digital artery exists over the middle phalanx which runs obliquely, dorsally, and distally over the distal interphalangeal crease. The dorsal branch at the middle phalanx collateralizes with the dorsal blood supply of the finger from another dorsal branch from the proper digital artery at the level of the distal phalanx, forming a dorsal arterial arcade over the DIP joint. Also, a dorsal nerve branch can be found leaving the proper digital nerve to innervate the dorsal finger skin proximal to the nail fold. The dorsal homodigital neurovascular island flap can be based on one or both of these arteries and this dorsal nerve. When the flap is harvested on the distal-most branches, it can be called the distal dorsal homodigital artery (DDHDA) flap. This DDHDA flap can be used to close defects of 2 × 2.5 cm just proximal to the tip and hyponychium (Fig. 22-1). Larger defects in this region can be reconstructed by a flap based on the dorsal branch at the middle phalanx, called the middle dorsal homodigital neurovascular island flap, or MDHDA flap. This MDHDA flap can be used to close defect 2 × 4 cm in size (Fig. 22-2). Alternatively, when the loss is very distal and an antegrade homodigital neurovascular island flap will not reach the defect, a reverse homodigital island flap (RHDA flap) can be used. The RHDA flap is harvested from the lateral base of the finger and based on proximal dorsal branches of the proper digital artery (Fig. 22-3). Dorsal branches of the proper digital nerve can be used to innervate this skin paddle, coapting this nerve to the transected nerve at the tip. These homodigital flaps are contraindicated when there is significant injury involving the pedicle or the skin on which the flap is based over the dorsum of the finger. Moreover, these homodigital flaps should not be used when

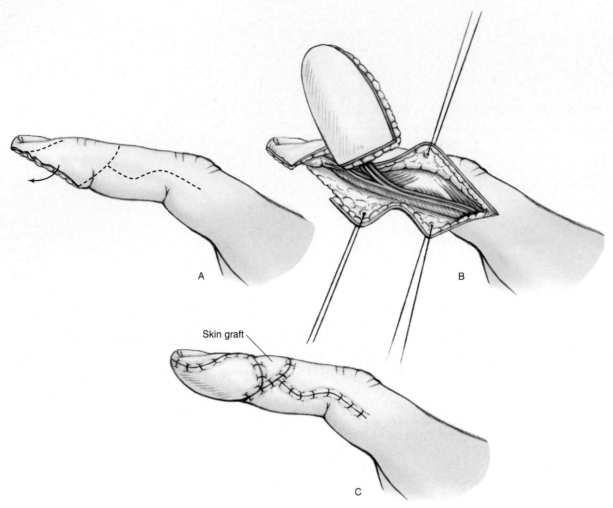

FIGURE 22-1

A: The design of the incision and distal dorsal homodigital neurovascular island (DDHD) flap. The axis of the flap curves obliquely and dorsally toward the contralateral side. **B:** The flap is elevated with its neurovascular pedicle and transposed obliquely into the defect and the typical wound suitable for a DDHDA flap with an intact tip and hypochium. **C:** The flap inset and grafted donor defect.

a skin bridge cannot be preserved for venous drainage to the distal finger. If the harvest of the flap would result in the exposure of already injured extensor tendon, devoid of paratenon, then the flap should be avoided. Crush and electrical injuries to the dorsal finger are also relative contraindications for the homodigital flap.

PREOPERATIVE PLANNING

The reconstruction of fingertip defects with homodigital island flaps should be performed in the operating room. The flap should be harvested with the use of a tourniquet to facilitate identification of anatomic structures. A microscope should be available should the digital artery be injured and require repair, or if the nerve has to be coapted. Amputated remnants should be saved. These amputated parts can be used as a source for a skin graft for the tip defect if the flap cannot be used or even as the donor defect of the flap. The risks of the procedure should be explained to the patient and family. Patients need to understand that if the flap fails, they may require an amputation, as well as other risks such as loss of extension, cold intolerance, swelling, and loss of some sensation.

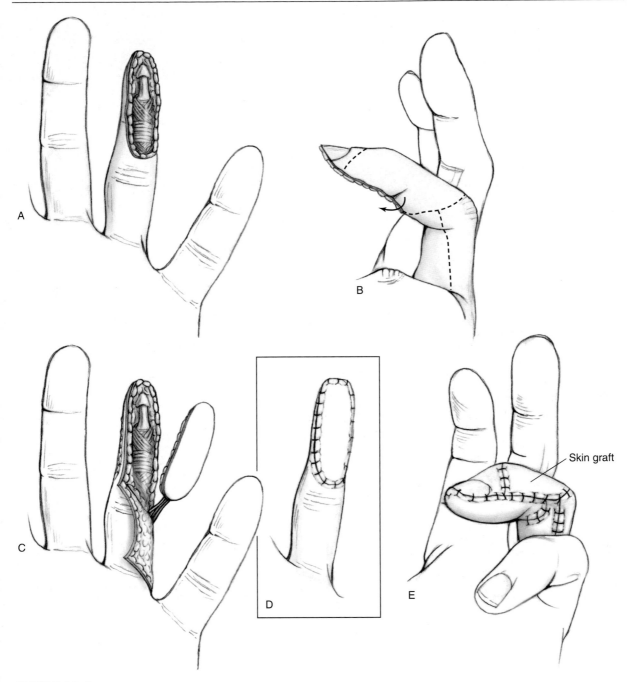

FIGURE 22-2

A,B: The rectangular flap design for the middle dorsal homodigital neurovascular island flap. **C:** The proximal pedicle dissection. **D,E:** The insetting of the flap and the grafted donor.

SURGERY

Patient Positioning

The homodigital flap reconstruction of a finger defect can be performed in the operating room with the patient in the supine position with the involved hand on an arm board and an upper arm tourniquet. The arm is prepared up to the tourniquet. The procedure can be performed with a regional block, such as a bier block or axillary block, or under general anesthesia.

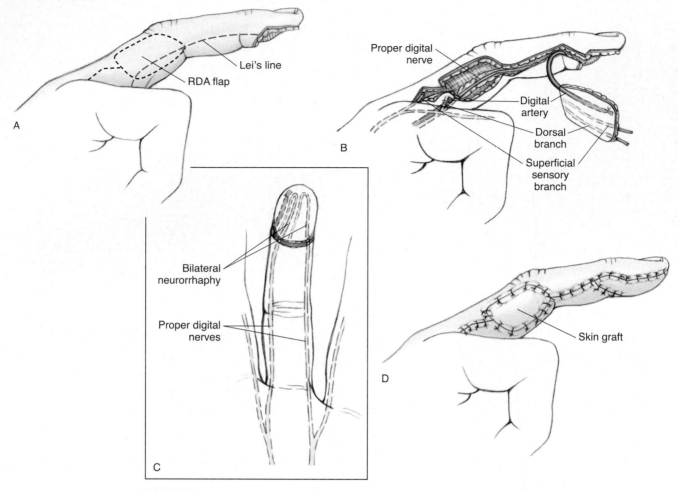

FIGURE 22-3

The required size of RDHDA flap is marked on the dorsolateral aspect of the involved proximal phalanx. **A:** The flap is based on the digital artery which topographically courses under the dorsoventral skin junction line. **B:** The vascular pedicle is ligated at its proximal end. Both the dorsal branch from the proper digital nerve and the superficial sensory branch from the corresponding radial or ulnar nerve are sectioned proximally, leaving 1 cm nerve tails attached to the flap. **C:** The flap is transposed to the recipient wound. The attached sensory nerves of the flap are microanastomosed with both ulnar and radial digital nerves at the recipient wound. **D:** The flap donor site is resurfaced with full thickness skin graft. The pivot area of the vascular pedicle is also covered with a piece of skin to eliminate the pressure completely. (From *Br J Plast Surg.* 1990;46B:484. With permission.)

Technique for Distal Dorsal Homodigital Artery (DDHDA) Flap

A template of the defect is made and is used to design the skin paddle of the flap. The flap is outlined on either the ulnar-dorsal side or the radial-dorsal side of the involved digit, depending on the wound location. When either digital artery can be used, the non-opposition side of the digit is preferred. The flap design is based either over the distal phalanx and DIP joint (defect <2.5 cm) or the middle and distal phalanx, depending on the size of the defect. The distal margin of the flap should be maintained 4 mm proximal to the nail fold to avoid germinal matrix and resultant nail abnormality. Based on the width of the pulp defect, the DDHDA flap proximal incision line is marked obliquely from the volar edge of the pulp defect toward the DIP crease, reaching proximally to the dorsum of the middle phalanx of the finger. The flap may include a portion of volar tissue of the terminal phalanx if any residual pulp tissue remains intact. The extension for the distal and proximal incision lines on the dorsum of the digit is determined by the length of the designed flap. The length of the flap should be longer than the defect to ensure adequate coverage of the flap pedicle (see Fig. 22-1). The neurovascular bundle is approached first via a zig-zag midlateral incision extending at least into the proximal interphalangeal crease. The digital pedicle is dissected proximal to distal with inclusion of surrounding fatty tissue to preserve the venae commitante with the proper digital artery to ensure venous drainage of the flap. This dissection should be performed with loupe magnification. In the proximal edge of the flap, particular attention is paid to include sufficient soft tissue between the pedicle and the flap to ensure adequate blood supply to the flap because the dorsal feeder arteries coming off the proper digital artery in the middle phalanx of the finger are usually divided during dissection. The flap is elevated in the plane above the paratenon from the dorsum of the finger toward the pedicle, then to the volar edge (see Fig. 22-1). Once the flap elevation is complete, the flap is advanced obliquely to fill the pulp defect. The donor site on the dorsum of the finger is covered with a full thickness graft taken from the hypothenar eminence or upper forearm.

Technique Middle Homodigital Neurovascular Island (MDHDA) Flap

When a larger skin paddle (>2.5 cm and extending into the middle phalanx) is needed, the MDHDA flap is preferred. The MDHDA flap is designed as a rectangular island, with the axis of the flap parallel to the length of the volar skin defect. The rest of the procedure proceeds as described previously, except the proximal incision line is extended obliquely toward the proximal interphalangeal crease, and the dorsal digital branches at the middle phalanx are included (see Fig. 22-2).

Technique for Reverse Digital Island Flap

For very distal level injuries, when the arc of pedicle length might not reach for the DDHDA and MDHDA flaps, the reverse homodigital island flap can be used. The reverse digital island flap is designed on the dorsolateral side of the involved proximal phalanx according to the size and shape of the pulp defect (Fig. 22-3). The dissection begins proximally at the proximal digital neurovascular bundle at the base of the finger (Fig. 22-4). The dorsal nerve and artery branches from the proper digital nerve and artery are identified while preserving a thick tuft of soft tissue from the proper digital artery to the skin paddle. The skin paddle is elevated in the dorsal to volar direction. The skin over the neurovascular bundle is incised in zig-zag fashion. The proper neurovascular bundle is dissected in the proximal to distal direction, preserving the soft tissue around the proper digital artery to include the venae comitante to avoid venous insufficiency of the flap. Ideally, the proper digital nerve to the finger is preserved. Collateral flow from the contralateral digital artery to the pedicle proper digital artery should be preserved. The flap is inset and the dorsal nerve branch is coapted to

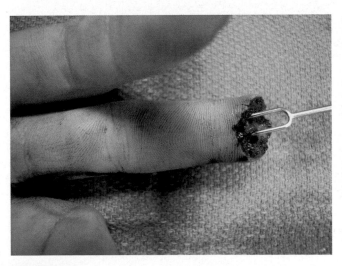 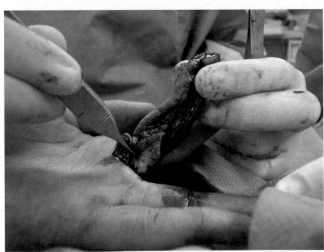

A   B

FIGURE 22-4

A: Distal tip amputation of the long finger with exposure of underlying bone. In such a case, further shortening of the finger to allow for primary coverage would lead to a loss of the profundus tendon insertion and decrease finger function. **B:** A reverse homodigital island flap is designed on the ulnar aspect of the long finger. *(Continued)*

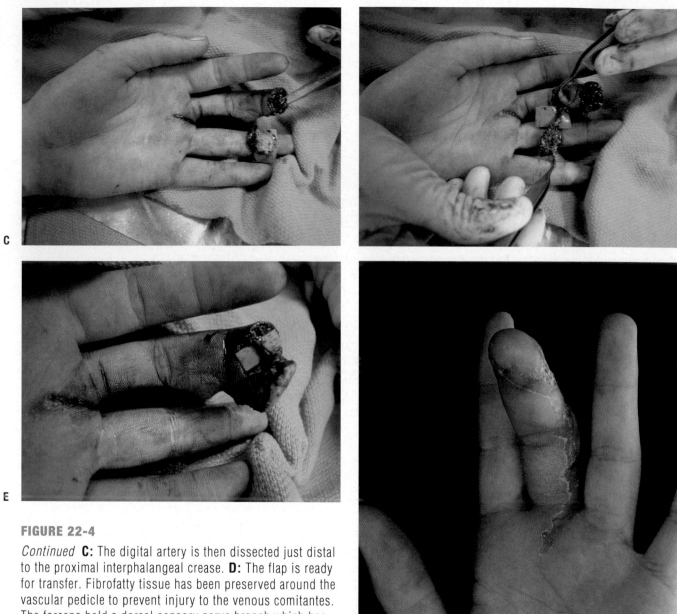

FIGURE 22-4

Continued **C:** The digital artery is then dissected just distal to the proximal interphalangeal crease. **D:** The flap is ready for transfer. Fibrofatty tissue has been preserved around the vascular pedicle to prevent injury to the venous comitantes. The forceps hold a dorsal sensory nerve branch which has been included in the flap. **E:** The flap is rotated 180 degrees allowing the dorsal sensory nerve to be coapted to the injured radial digital nerve. **F:** The early postoperative appearance with excellent contour and well-healed donor site.

the digital nerve in the defect. Alternatively, the proper digital nerve can be included with the pedicle and repaired to the contralateral digital nerve in the defect. However, this sacrifice of the proper digital nerve renders the finger insensate on the pedicle side, which can be avoided by using a dorsal nerve branch. The donor site at the base of the finger can usually be closed primarily, if a full thickness graft is not preferred.

RESULTS

Several reports with these flaps have demonstrated that the flaps have reliable arterial and venous flow. Moreover, these studies have shown good return of sensation in the 5–9 mm range of 2-point discrimination. Some of the reviews have demonstrated a mild loss of extension complicating the skin grafted donor site on the dorsum of the injured fingers.

POSTOPERATIVE MANAGEMENT

After the homodigital island artery flap, splint immobilization is unnecessary. Early mobilization can be encouraged which will lower the risk for a stiff finger postoperatively. If the RDHDA flap is used, usually the donor can be closed primarily. If a skin graft is required at the base of the finger, a splint is used postoperatively for 1 week.

COMPLICATIONS

Postoperative complications from the homodigital flap include loss of extension, loss of sensation, cold intolerance, and flap loss, most likely from venous compromise. The risk of loss of extension can be minimized with early motion. Fingers that have been reconstructed with innervated homodigital flaps can achieve 5 mm 2-point discrimination, but the grafted donor site can be less sensate. There is no increased risk for cold intolerance in patients reconstructed with homodigital flaps over other options. The risk for venous compromise can be lessened by harvesting the pedicle to include soft tissue and venae comitante with the digital artery.

RECOMMENDED READING

Atasoy E, Ioakimidis E, Kasdan ML, et al. Reconstruction of the amputated finger tip with a triangular volar flap: a new surgical procedure. *J Bone Joint Surg.* 1970;52A:921–926.

Flint MH, Harrison SH. A local neurovascular flap to repair loss of the digital pulp. *Br J Plast Surg.* 1965;18:156–163.

Foucher G, Smith D, Pempinello C, et al. Homodigital neurovascular island flaps for digital pulp loss. *J Hand Surg.* 1989;14B:204–208.

Joshi BB. A local dorsolateral island flap for restoration of sensation after avulsion injury of fingertip pulp. *Plast Recontr Surg.* 1974;54:175–182.

Lai CS, Lin SD, Chou CK, et al. Innervated reverse digital artery flap through bilateral neurorrhaphy for pulp defects. *Br J Plast Surg.* 1993;46:483–488.

Lucas GL. The pattern of venous drainage of the digits. *J Hand Surg.* 1984;9A:448–450.

Mober E. Aspects of sensation in reconstructive surgery of the upper extremity. *J Bone Joint Surg.* 1964;46A;817–825.

O'Brien B. Neurovascular island pedicle flaps for terminal amputations and digital scars. *Br J Plast Surg.* 1968;21:258–261.

Posner MA, Smith RJ. The advancement pedicle flap for thumb injuries. *J Bone Joint Surg.*1971;53A:168. 10. Shaw WH. Neurovascular island pedicle flaps for terminal digital scars—a hazard. *Br J Plast Surg.* 1971;24:161–165.

Strauch B, de Moura W. Arterial system of the fingers. *J Hand Surg.* 1990;15A:148–154.

Tsai TM, Yuen JC.A neurovascular island flap for volar oblique finger tip amputations. *J Hand Surg.* 1996;21B:94–98.

Weeks PM. Local arterialized island flap coverage of difficult hand defects preserving donor digit sensibility. *Plast Reconstr Surg* 1983;72:858.

23 First Dorsal Metacarpal Artery Island Flap

Günter Germann and Katrin Palm-Bröking

Soft tissue defects in the hand, and particularly in the thumb, frequently present difficult reconstructive problems because of the restricted availability of local tissue. Although local skin flaps have been employed and time-proven over decades, the philosophy of immediate wound closure of complex defects with exposure of tendon, bone, or joints has stimulated interest in anatomic research and the development of refined reconstructive techniques (10).

Traditional flaps have many disadvantages such as two-stage operations (i.e., cross-finger flap [17,24]), tedious dissections with considerable donor-site morbidity and loss of discriminative power (i.e., Littler flap [27,28]), or limited arc of rotation and mobility (i.e., transposition flaps [7] and the Moberg flap [1,8]). On the other hand, more recent microsurgical reconstructions such as the free pulp flap (7) require a significant amount of time and a familiarity with microsurgical technique. The first dorsal metacarpal artery island flap overcomes the disadvantages of traditional hand flaps and can provide a moderate-sized skin paddle on a long consistent vascular leash, allowing one-stage reconstruction for thumb and dorsal hand wounds without the need for microsurgical anastomosis.

The first dorsal metacarpal artery island flap was originally described by Hilgenfeldt in 1950 (16) and subsequently refined by Paneva-Holevic in 1968 and finally described as a pure island flap ("kite flap") by Foucher and Braun in 1979 (8). Many variations of the flap have since been described and established in daily clinical use based on the consistent anatomy of the dorsal metacarpal arterial arcade (3–5,6,7,9,10–12,19–20). The majority of the flaps in recently published reports are raised from the dorsal aspect of the hand with only a few being found on the palmar surface (2,13,14).

The dorsum of the hand is supplied by the network of dorsal metacarpal arteries which are fed from the main forearm vessels: the radial, ulnar, and interosseus arteries. The first dorsal metacarpal artery (FDMA) consistently arises from the radial artery or the princeps pollicis artery and runs distally to the fascia of the interosseus muscle, frequently embedded in a fascial pocket. In most cases the first dorsal metacarpal artery divides in the middle of the second metacarpal into three terminal branches (18,22,24,30). The radial branch of the first dorsal metacarpal artery goes to the thumb, while the intermediate branch runs to the first web space. Distally the ulnar branch usually terminates at the level of the metacarpo-phalangeal joint and then arborizes into the dorsal skin of the index finger after giving off a perforating branch at the level of the metacarpal neck.

The exact location of the artery with respect to the first dorsal interosseous muscle may vary. Kuhlmann and de Frenne found the artery to run superficial to the muscle in 75% of specimens, while the FDMA was found within the muscle in 15% of specimens; in 10% of specimens the artery ran within and on top of the muscle during its course. Dautel and Merle identified a superficial course of the FDMA in 36% of specimens, a supra-fascial course in 23% of specimens, and a deep, intramuscular course in 56%. Despite its exact location all authors agree on the consistency of a FDMA (11,13,18,22,24,30) (Fig. 23-1).

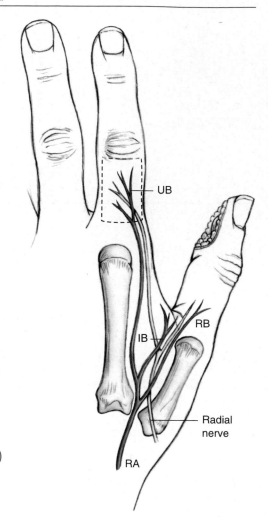

FIGURE 23-1

The three branches of the radial artery (*RA*). The radial branch of the first dorsal metacarpal artery (*RB*) goes to the thumb, the intermediate branch (*IB*) to the first web space, and the ulnar branch (*UB*) of the first dorsal metacarpal artery runs to the index finger.

Overall, the flap provides excellent sensibility, pliability, and stability for a variety of hand defects. We feel the first dorsal metacarpal island flap is one of the workhorses for reconstructive hand surgery (22,24–27).

INDICATIONS/CONTRAINDICATIONS

Indications

Indications for the first dorsal metacarpal artery flap ("kite flap") are based on the following criteria:

- Etiology, location, size, and condition of the defect
- Availability of the flap (i.e., previous injuries that may compromise the vascular pedicle)
- Suitability of the flap for the defect (e.g., size, arc of rotation)
- Inclusion of other tissue components (i.e., tendon, bony segment)
- Patient's wishes (donor site morbidity, aesthetic appearance)
- Surgeon's familiarity with the technique

Based on these decision-making criteria, the flap is indicated for primary or secondary reconstructions of:

- The dorsal aspect of the thumb
- Restoration of sensibility with pulp reconstruction in the thumb
- Skin defects at the dorsal aspect of the hand within the arc of rotation of the antegrade kite flap
- Palmar defects of the index finger
- Defects of the web space

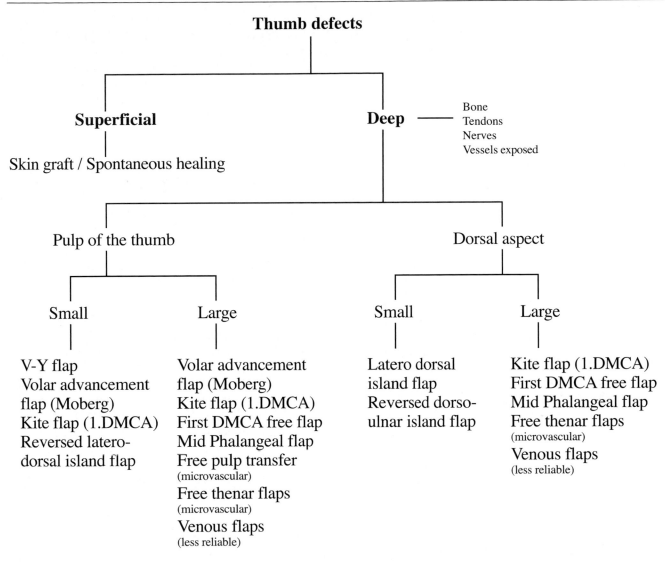

FIGURE 23-2

Decision-making algorithm for flap selection in treatment of thumb defects.

- Defects around the wrist
- Defects at the base of the thumb or the middle finger ("retrograde kite flap")
- Complex flaps including various tissue components
- Microvascular flap transfer based on the vascular pedicle in the snuff box

The list of indications demonstrates the versatility of the flap: however, reconstruction of the thumb takes precedence as the main indication in most centers.

Following the pioneer work of Tränkle et al, the flap has replaced other sensate neurovascular island flaps for restoration of sensibility in the thumb (10,13,26,29) due to the dissection technique, the discriminative power that can be achieved, and the acceptable donor site morbidity. Based on this study, the flap is now widely used for this indication (Fig. 23-2).

Contraindications

Contraindications for flap use include acute trauma or a history of significant trauma to the donor site (15). In addition, injury mechanisms such as crush avulsions, wringer injuries, high-energy trauma (e.g., blast injuries or gun shot wounds) may limit the reliability of this flap if they have disrupted the course of the FDMA (10,13). If the tissue viability of the donor site cannot be estimated properly in the first hours of the trauma, wound closure should be delayed or a different flap should be used for wound coverage.

Burn injuries of the dorsum of the hand do not present a contraindication for the use of a first dorsal metacarpal artery flap in all cases. The dorsal metacarpal artery system is not damaged by deep partial-thickness burns that are excised and grafted. In 80% of patients with full-thickness burns, the dorsal metacarpal artery system is still intact. The potential for elevating a first dorsal metacarpal artery flap is therefore preserved after burn excision and grafting (11). Nevertheless, preoperative Doppler ultrasound examination is recommended before flap elevation.

PREOPERATIVE PLANNING

As in any surgical procedure, careful preoperative assessment and planning are key factors to success and the avoidance of complications or failure. Decision making follows an algorithmic approach in which the defect must be assessed for:

- Size
- Etiology
- Characteristics

The decision for flap selection is based on the criteria outlined previously (see indications). The patient should be thoroughly informed about the therapeutic options, and his or her expectations and wishes should also be discussed. Special attention should be paid to donor site morbidity including numbness over the radial aspect of the dorsum of the hand and the implications of a full-thickness skin graft to the donor site. The postoperative management and potential complications such as flap failure or impaired mobility of the fingers, impaired sensibility, and other possible undesirable results should be discussed with the patient. Donor-site morbidity is an important issue that should also be discussed with the patient before surgery. The functional and aesthetic morbidity of the donor site is an issue often neglected in the choice of a flap, and it must be borne in mind that the donor area of a first dorsal metacarpal artery island flap is in a very exposed position.

Clinical examination should exclude prior injuries in the area of the vascular pedicle. In most cases the artery is palpable, but Doppler ultrasound examination before flap elevation is mandatory (13) since the course of the artery is variable (see previous discussion). The course of the artery should be marked on the skin preoperatively after Doppler examination (13,19,26,27).

SURGERY

The defect size is templated to the dorsum of the index finger. The course of the artery is marked on the dorsum of the hand with the aid of a hand-held Doppler ultrasound device. Surgery is performed using either an axillary bloc, or general or regional anesthesia. The use of a pneumatic tourniquet and loupe magnification are necessary for the dissection. The flap is harvested from the dorsum of the index finger and includes the first dorsal metacarpal artery, a branch of the superficial radial nerve, and at least one subcutaneous vein (Figure 23-3).

Dissection is performed starting with the vascular pedicle including a large subcutaneous vein which has first to be identified and mobilized. Elevation of the flap starts radially by incising the interosseus fascia at the most radial edge of the muscle. The fascia is then peeled off the muscle towards the second metacarpal. Thereby, a wide pedicle including the subcutaneous vein, a branch of the superficial radial nerve, and the vascular pedicle is created (24). A vessel loop is used to mark this pedicle. The pedicle is traced back to its origin in the snuff-box. There is no need to isolate the vascular pedicle from the interosseus fascia, since this may injure the delicate vessels. Transillumination will verify the inclusion of the artery and the small accompanying veins in the pedicle.

Dissection now proceeds from the distal border of the flap. The flap is incised and dissected off of the paratenon of the extensor apparatus toward the proximal border of the flap. Care must be taken to preserve the paratenon in order to secure graft-take at the donor site. A critical point in the dissection is the radial aspect of the extensor hood of the metaphalangeal joint where the vessels enter the subcutaneous network of the flap. It is recommended to include a small strip of extensor hood to secure the vessel entrance. This area can be easily repaired without any functional deficit by a 4.0 polydioxanone (PDS) suture.

Once the flap is raised, the tourniquet is deflated to assess the blood supply of the flap. Occasionally, the flap may first appear pale but usually begins to turn pink within a few minutes (26,27). The flap may be passed through a subcutaneous tunnel into the defect (21,24,27). If the skin is too

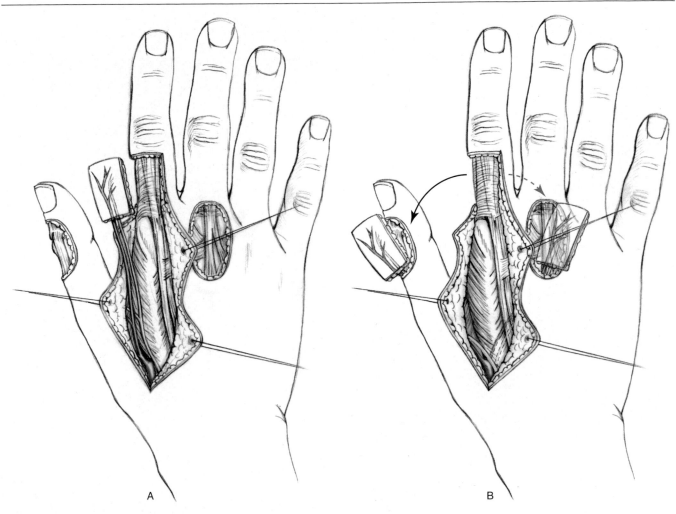

FIGURE 23-3

Schematic drawing of the dissected **(A)** first dorsal metacarpal artery flap and the first dorsal metacarpal artery flap with its pedicle passed distally under the skin tunnel **(B)**. (From Germann G, et al. *Decision-making in reconstructive surgery—upper extremity.* Berlin: Springer-Verlag; 2000. With permission.)

tight, the tunnel is opened and the pedicle is skin grafted. As a sensory island flap, the first dorsal metacarpal artery island flap allows a wide arc of rotation due to its pedicle length of up to 7 cm (24).

The donor defect of the index finger is covered with a full-thickness skin graft (19). A split-thickness skin graft may also be used; however a full-thickness skin graft will provide a better color match (23). Full-thickness grafting will provide an aesthetically acceptable appearance at the donor site within a shorter period of time, although the long-term results using a split–thickness graft are comparable (19) (Figs. 23-4 and 23-5).

Extensive experience with this flap has lead to some refinements. To avoid any tension on the pedicle, the subcutaneous tunnel has to be opened frequently. We now raise the flap constantly with a "cutaneous tail" extending from the proximal border of the flap to the radial aspect of the second metacarpal. This extension allows opening of the tunnel and direct skin-skin closure after flap transfer. This technique does not only provide a more stable skin closure, but also a better aesthetic appearance (see Fig. 23-4C,F). In addition, segments of the second metacarpal or the extensor indicis proprius tendon can be included in the flap for more complex reconstruction.

The first dorsal metacarpal artery flap can also be raised as a microvascular free flap (10,12,13). The flap is harvested using the same technique as the pedicled first dorsal metacarpal artery flap described previously. Dissection of the FDMA back to its origin from the radial artery provides an artery of adequate diameter for microvascular anastomosis. A long pedicle length facilitates mi-

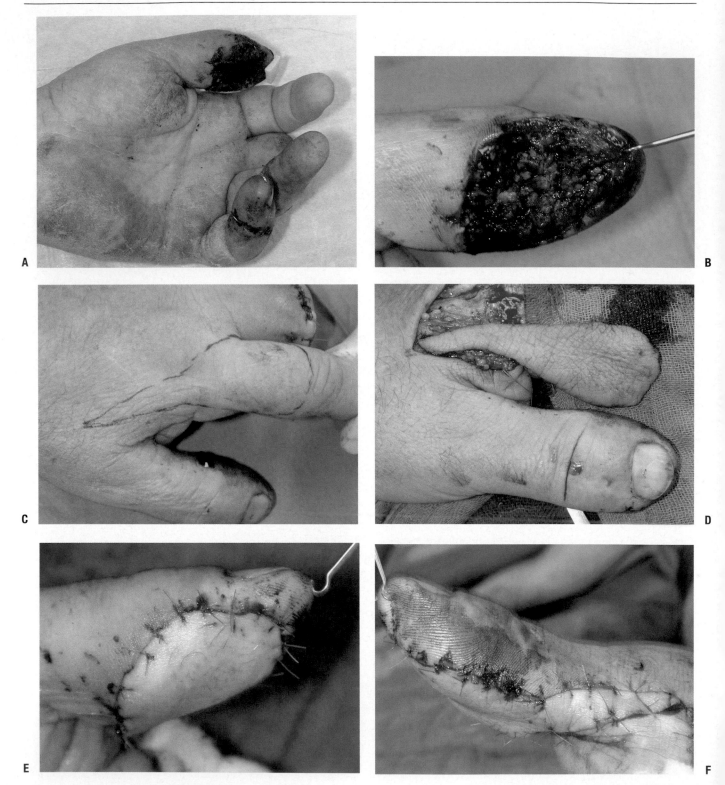

FIGURE 23-4

A: A 63-year-old man sustained a mutilating saw injury of the hand with avulsion of the palmar aspect of the distal phalanx of the left thumb (additional injuries in the middle and small fingers). Six days after the injury: complete necrosis of the pulp of the thumb. **B:** Intraoperative view after radical debridement. **C:** Flap design: the first dorsal metacarpal artery island flap is outlined over the dorsal aspect of the proximal phalanx of the index finger. **D:** The first dorsal metacarpal artery island flap is elevated. Note the "cutaneous tail" of the flap that allows primary skin-skin closure. **E,F:** After tunneling the flap into the defect, primary skin-skin closure is achieved. *(Continued)*

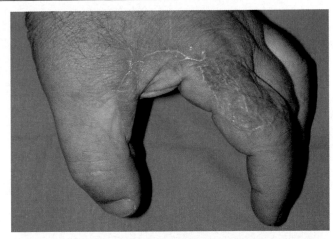

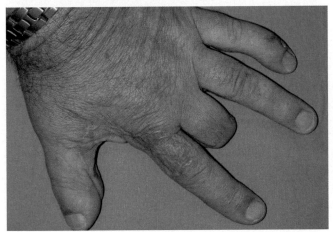

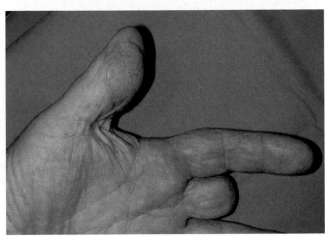

FIGURE 23-4

Continued **E,F:** After tunneling the flap into the defect, primary skin-skin closure is achieved. **G:** Reconstruction of the donor site with skin graft. **H–J:** Aesthetic and functional outcome 2 years postoperatively. Full extension of thumb and index finger. The patient describes cold intolerance of the donor site. Two PD of the flap: 6.5 mm; 2 PD of the donor site: 6 mm.

crovascular reconstruction outside the area of trauma; inclusion of the cutaneous nerve permits reconstruction of sensibility. We believe that dissection of this flap is easier and faster than a toe and first web-space flap (19) (Fig. 23-6).

POSTOPERATIVE MANAGEMENT

The hand may be immobilized in a bulky dressing following surgery. A palmar plaster splint may be used to immobilize any concomitant fractures. A window is left in the dressing for evaluation of the flap. Care is taken not to apply the dressing too tight for fear of causing arterial or venous compromise. Forty-eight to 72 hours after surgery, the flap's vascularity is ensured, and (13) physical therapy may be initiated if underlying fracture fixation is stabile. The index finger metacarpalphalangeal joint is usually immobilized for 5 to 7 days to ensure take of the skin graft over the donor site, but the proximal and distal interphalangeal joints may be mobilized as soon as possible to avoid postoperative stiffness. Occupational therapy is also initiated for sensory re-education of the flap. Initially, sensation in the flap will be perceived as coming from the dorsum of the index finger, or a dual sensation phenomenon may result. Cortical reorientation of sensation is possible with a structured sensory re-education program. The first dorsal metacarpal artery island flap allows immediate restoration of sensibility even in older patients, among whom neuronal co-adaptation of a pedicled or a free flap yields poorer results than in younger people (26,27).

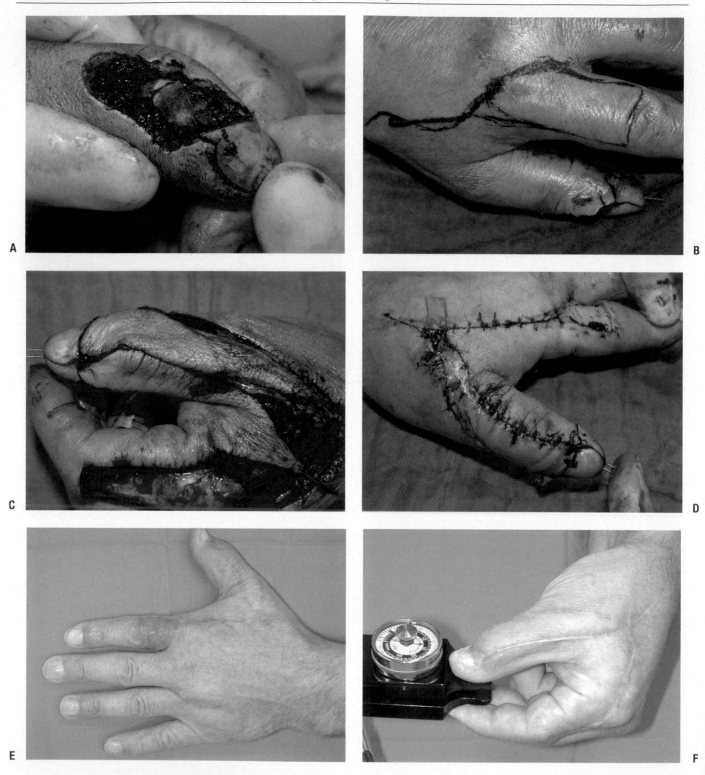

FIGURE 23-5

A: A 44-year-old man suffered a work-related accident with a chain saw, resulting in a skin defect including a defect of the extensor pollicis longus tendon at its insertion and exposure of the interphalangeal joint. **B:** Design of the first dorsal metacarpal artery island flap on the dorsal of the index finger. **C:** The first dorsal metacarpal artery island flap prior to insertion into the defect. **D:** Result after insetting of the first dorsal metacarpal island flap. The flap shows perfect capillary refill. The donor site has been diminished in size by mobilization of the surrounding skin. Aesthetic **(E)** and functional **(F)** outcome 2 years postoperatively. Excellent hand function and aesthetic appearance have been achieved. The patient returned to his previous employment without limitations.

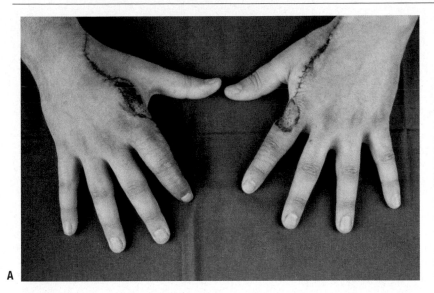
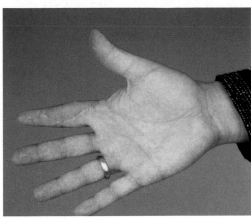

A   B

FIGURE 23-6

A 22-year-old carpenter sustained an occupational high pressure-injection injury of the palmar aspect of the proximal interphalangeal joint of the index finger of the non-dominant right hand. A soft-tissue defect resulted, which included a large portion of the palmar aspect of the finger and exposure of both flexor tendons and neurovascular bundles. This was successfully reconstructed with a free kite flap **(A)**. The flap healed uneventfully with excellent aesthetic and functional result. Follow-up after 40 months **(B)** demonstrated a static two-point discrimination of 15 mm. Grip strength values were excellent. Time off work was 11 weeks.

COMPLICATIONS

Although the first dorsal metacarpal artery island flap has proven to be very reliable, various complications can occur. These complications include planning errors, complications during the operation, and postoperative difficulties. To avoid an inadequate arc of rotation or an inadequate flap size, the surgeon can add 10% to 15% more length to the pedicle, and the flap can be planned and harvested 10% to 15% larger in size (10,13).

Care should be taken to exert only gentle traction when passing the flap through the subcutaneous tunnel to close the thumb pulp defect. Excessive tension can cause a partial compression of the vessels, and marginal necrosis could result. Whereas vascular insufficiency on the arterial side is frequently the result of tunnelling, a short pedicle or tight wound closure can compromise the venous outflow. In case of postoperative vascular insufficiency, sutures can be released and leech therapy may be employed.

Donor-site morbidity of dorsal metacarpal artery island flaps is low compared with axial homodigital island flaps. Neuromas are rare, and the patients report less hypersensitivity than in homodigital island flaps (13). However, one of the most important donor-site problems of the first dorsal metacarpal artery island flap is a diminished protective sensation over the transplanted skin graft, and patients may complain of cold intolerance. Hypertrophic scars present a minor donor-site problem. Functional limitation because of the donor site is negligible, and the range of motion of the donor finger reaches approximately 95% of the opposite index finger (26,27).

RECOMMENDED READING

Adani R, Busa R, Castagnetti C, Bathia A, Caroli A. Homodigital neurovascular island flaps with "direct flow" vascularization. *Ann Plast Surg.* 1997;38(1):36–40.

Adani R, Squarzina PB, Castagnetti C, Lagana A, Pancaldi G, Caroli A. A comparative study of the heterodigital neurovascular island flap in thumb reconstruction, with and without nerve reconnection. *J Hand Surg.* 1994;19(5):552–559.

Dellon AL. Sensory recovery in replanted digits and transplanted toes. *J Reconstr Microsurg.* 1986;2:123.

Early MJ, Milner RH. Dorsal metacarpal flaps. *Br J Plast Surg.* 1987;40:333–341.

Gebhard B, Meissl G. An extended first dorsal metacarpal artery neurovascular island flap. *J Hand Surg.* 1995;20(4):529–531.

Grossman JAI, Robotti EB. The use of split-thickness hypothenar grafts for coverage of fingertips and other defects of the hand. *Ann Chir Main (Ann Hand Surg).* 1995;14:239–243.

Holevich J. A new method of restoring sensibility to the thumb. *J Bone Joint Surg.* 1963;45B:496–502.

Inoue G, Maeda N, Suzudi K. Resurfacing of skin defects of the hand using the arterial venous flap. *Br J Plast Surg.* 1990;43(2):135–139.

Krag C, Rasmussen KB. The neurovascular island flap for defective sensibility of the thumb. *J Bone Joint Surg [Br].* 1975;57(4):495–499.

Lister G. Local flaps to the hand. *Hand Clin.* 1995;1(4):621–640.

Masquelet AC, Gilbert A. *An atlas of flaps in limb reconstruction.* London: Martin Duniz; 1995.

Oka Y. Sensory function of the neurovascular island flap in thumb reconstruction: comparison of original and modified procedures. *J Hand Surg.* 2000;25(4):637–643.

Pfeiffer KM. Kombinierte Verletzungen des Daumenstrahls: Eine Übersicht über die Behandlungsmöglichkeiten. *Mikrochir Plast Surg.* 1993;25:80–84.

Prakash V, Chawla S. First dorsal metacarpal artery adipofascial flap for a dorsal defect of the thumb. *Plast Reconstr Surg.* 2004;114(5):1353–1355.

Ratcliff RJ, Regan PJ, Scerri GV. First dorsal metacarpal artery flap cover for extensive pulp defects in the normal length thumb. *Br J Plast Surg.* 1992;45:544–546.

Rose EH. Local arterialized island flap coverage of difficult hand defects preserving donor digit sensibility. *Plast Reconstr Surg.* 1983;72(6):848-858.

Rose EH. Small flap coverage of hand and digit defects. *Clin Plast Surg.* 1989;16(3):427–442.

trauch B, Greenstein B. Neurovascular flaps to the hand. *Hand Clin.* 1995;1(2):327–333.

Voche P, Merle M. Vascular suply of the palmar subcutaneous tissue of fingers. *Br J Plast Surg.* 1996;49(5):315–318.

Williams RL, Nanchahal J, Sykes PJ, O'Shaughenessy M. The provision of innervated skin cover for the injured thumb using the first dorsal metacarpal artery island flap. *J Hand Surg.* 1995;20B:231–236.

REFERENCES

1. Baumeister S, Menke H, Wittemann M, Germann G. Functional outcome after the moberg advancement flap in the thumb. *J Hand Surg.* 2002;27A:105–114.

2. Bertelli JA, Catarina S. Neurocutaneous island flaps in upper limb Coverage: experience with 44 clinical cases. *J Hand Surg.* 1997;22(3): 515–526.

3. Chang SC, Chen SL, Chen TM, Chuang CJ, Cheng TY, Wang HJ. Sensate first dorsal metacarpal artery flap for resurfacing extensive pulp defects of the thumb. *Ann Plast Surg.* 2004;53(5):449–454.

4. Chen C, Wie F. Lateral-dorsal neurovascular island flaps for pulp reconstruction. *Ann Plast Surg.* 2000;45:616–622.

5. Dautel G, Merle M. Dorsal metacarpal reverse flaps. *Br J Hand Surg.* 1991;16B: 400–405.

6. Ege A, Tuncay I, Ercetin O. Foucher's first dorsal metacarpal artery flap for thumb reconstruction: evaluation of 21 cases. *Isr Med Assoc J.* 2002;4(6):421–433.

7. El-Khatib HA. Clinical experiences with the extended first dorsal metacarpal artery island flap for thumb reconstruction. *J Hand Surg.* 1998;23A:647–652.

8. Elliot H. Small flap coverage of hand and digit defects. *Clin Plast Surg.* 1989;16:427-442.

9. Foucher G, Braun JB. A new Island flap transfer from the dorsum of the index to the thumb. *Plast Reconstr Surg.* 1979;63:344–349.

10. Germann G. Principles of flap design for surgery of the Hand. *Atlas Hand Clin.* 1998;3:33–57.

11. Germann G, Funk H, Bickert B. The fate of the dorsal metacarpal arterial system following thermal injury to the dorsal hand: a doppler sonographic study. *J Hand Surg.* 2000;25(5):962–967.

12. Germann G, Hornung R, Raff T. Two new applications for the first dorsal metacarpal artery pedicle in the treatment of severe hand injuries. *J Hand Surg [Br].* 1995;20(4):525–528.

13. Germann G, Levin LS. Intrinsic flaps in the hand: new concepts in skin coverage. *Techniques in Hand and Upper Extremity Surgery.* 1997;1(1):48–61.

14. Germann G, Raff T, Schepler H, Wittemann M. Salvage of an avascular thumb by arteriovenous flow reversal and a microvascular "kite" flap: case report. *J Reconstr Microsurg.* 1997;13:167–291.

15. Giessler G, Erdmann D, Germann G. Soft tissue coverage in devastating hand injuries. *Hand Clin.* 2003;19:63–71.

16. Hilgenfeld O. *Operativer daumenersatz.* 1st ed. Stuttgart: Enke Verlag; 1950.

17. Lassner F, Becker M, Berger A, Pallua N. Sensory reconstruction of the fingertip using the bilaterally innervated sensory cross-finger flap. *Plast Reconstr Surg.* 2002;109(3):988–993.

18. Marx, A, Preisser P, Peek A, Partecke BD. Anatomy of the dorsal mid-handarteries-anatomic study and review of the literature. *Handchir Mikrochir Plast Chir.* 2001;33(2):77–82.

19. Pelzer M, Sauerbier M, Germann G, Tränkle M. Free "kite" flap: a new flap for reconstruction of small hand defects. *J Reconstr Microsurg.* 2004;20(5):367–372.

20. Preisser P, Marx A, Klinzig S, Partecke BD. Covering defects of the basal finger area by pedicled flaps anastomosed to the dorsal metacarpal arteries. *Handchir Mikrochir Plast Chir.* 2001;33(2):83–88.

21. Quaba AA, Davison PM. The distally based dorsal metacarpal artery flap. *Br J Plast Surg.* 1990;43:28–32.

22. Sherif MM. First dorsal metacarpal artery flap in hand reconstruction. I. Anatomical study. *J Hand Surg.* 1994;19A:26–38.

23. Sherif MM. First dorsal metacarpal artery flap in hand reconstruction. II. Clinical application. *J Hand Surg.* 1994;19(1):32–38.
24. Shun-Cheng CH, Shao-Liang CH, Tim Mo Chen, Chuang CH, Cheng T, Wang H. Sensate first dorsal metacarpal artery flap for resurfacing extensive pulp defects in the thumb. *Ann Plast Surg.* 2004;53:449–454.
25. Small JO, Brennen MD. The first dorsal metacarpal artery neurovascular island flap. *J Hand Surg.* 1988;15:145–148.
26. Tränkle M, Germann G, Heitmann C, Sauerbier M. Defect coverage and reconstruction of thumb sensibility with the first dorsal metacarpal artery Island flap. *Chirurg.* 2004;75:996–1002.
27. Tränkle M, Sauerbier M, Heitmann C, Germann G. Restoration of the thumb sensibility with the innervated first dorsal metacarpal artery island flap. *J Hand Surg.* 2003;28A(5):758–766.
28. Vlastou C, Earle AS, Blanchard JM. A palmar cross-finger flap for coverage of thumb defects. *J Hand Surg.* 1985;10(4):566–569.
29. Wilhelm K, Putz R, Hierner R, Giunta RE. *Lappenplastiken in der Handchirurgie-Angewandte Anatomie, Operationstechniken, Differentialtherapie.* München: Urban and Schwarzenberg; 1997.
30. Yang D, Morris SF. Vascular basis of dorsal digital and metacarpal skin flaps. *J Hand Surg.* 2001;26(1):142–146.

24 Thumb Coverage

David Elliot

The primary goals of thumb reconstruction are to restore length and sensation. A thumb should be of adequate length to allow for pinch to the index and middle fingertips and to participate in span grasp with all five digital tips. Adequate length is also essential for developing power grip. The surgeon aims to provide adequate coverage of the deeper, vital structures with soft tissue and skin of good quality. Sensibility of the tip is of particular importance, being crucial to fine pinch. A thumb "post" with no or little movement distal to the basal joint, and/or poor tip shape and sensation, can still work to aid in hand function but will not allow for finesse of function.

In attempting to obtain optimum reconstruction one should avoid shortening the thumb unless absolutely necessary. We encourage distal replantation or composite graft replacement, and also look to homodigital flap reconstruction whenever possible. Care should be spent in nail bed preservation and repair. Any nail greater in length than one third of its normal length should be retained, at least at primary surgery. Reconstruction of the thumb defects with the use of skin grafts from elsewhere on the body can create patches of dissimilar color, texture, and thickness and a noticeably poor cosmetic result. Finally, with respect to mobility and rehabilitation, the time-honored plastic surgical techniques of skin cross-finger, thenar, groin, and cross-arm flaps should be avoided, if possible, as they tether the injured thumb to another part of the body, thus preventing adequate therapy, which may promote edema and stiffness.

HOMODIGITAL FLAP RECONSTRUCTION

Homodigital flap reconstruction involves rearrangement of the soft tissues of the injured digit to achieve healing without seeking tissue for reconstruction from outside that digit. This concept of reconstruction has definite advantages for thumb reconstruction. In particular, it reconstructs "like with like" and avoids the creation of further scarring and morbidity elsewhere on the hand or body. While homodigital reconstruction is advantageous in these respects, the availability of donor tissues within the thumb is obviously limited.

Perhaps the single most important surgical pearl to remember when using homodigital reconstruction is that the thumb and fingers have an astonishing ability to close skin defects of considerable size by a combination of wound contraction and re-epithelialization (Fig. 24-1). Thus, if a portion of the wound can heal under moist antiseptic dressings through secondary intention, the surgeon may use the homodigital flaps to cover only those portions of the wound which contain exposed vital structures or to improve soft tissue coverage over bone. The flap does not have to cover the entire defect, only the essential components of the defect.

Preoperative Planning

Preoperative planning should include AP and lateral radiographs in addition to a thorough hand exam. Concomitant arterial and nerve injuries can often be identified prior to exploration within the operating room. Many thumb injuries will occur in conjunction with other hand injuries and revascularization of injured digits takes precedence over coverage issues. Wounds should be debrided of all necrotic tissue and free of infection before embarking on soft tissue coverage.

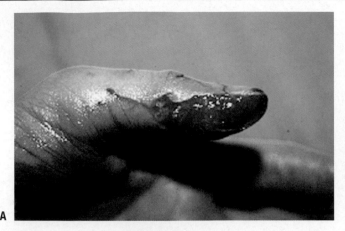
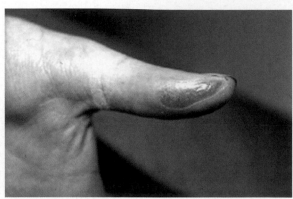

FIGURE 24-1

A: Industrial scalpel wound of the thumb tip. **B:** Same digital surface after healing by re-epithelialization under moist antiseptic dressings for 3 weeks. (Reproduced from Elliot D. Specific flaps for the thumb. *Tech Hand Up Extrem Surg.* 2004;8(4):198–211, with permission.)

Patient Positioning

Patients are positioned supine on the operating room table. General or regional anaesthesia may be used during the surgical procedures. In some cases, thumb or wrist blocks may be used when performing smaller flaps or for debridement procedures. An upper arm tourniquet is placed prior to prepping and draping the patient. Surgery is always performed under tourniquet control to aid in visualization of vital structures.

The following sections present our preferred techniques for thumb reconstruction based on location of the original defect.

Palmar Defects

Neurovascular Tranquilli-Leali or Atasoy-Kleinert Flap

INDICATIONS/CONTRAINDICATIONS   Historically, the original Tranquilli-Leali or Atasoy-Kleinert flap has been described to cover partial amputation defects of the distal phalanx; however, these flaps do not work well on the thumb because of the inflexibility of the subcutaneous soft tissues. Laterally based single pedicle flaps, vascularized in the same way by the small vessels beyond the trifurcations of the digital arteries, also move poorly. The *neurovascular* Tranquilli-Leali *or* Atasoy-Kleinert flap is designed to be much larger and is islanded on both neurovascular pedicles bilaterally (Fig. 24-2). The flap is designed to extend to, or across, the IP joint crease proximally. This flap works well for minor transverse or oblique injuries of the distal phalanx with exposure of bone.

This flap can be used for stump reconstruction of any length of amputated thumb and is more useful than the original Tranquilli-Leali flap; however, it moves less freely than on a finger, partly because of the fibrous nature of the subcutaneous tissues of the thumb and partly because of what has been described as the "vertical dimension" of the thumb, that is its palmar-dorsal width at the tip (1). On fingers, it can be used to reconstruct defects with a palmar slope of up to 30 degrees; on the thumb it can only reconstruct defects with bone exposure which are dorsally facing, transverse, or palmar facing with less than 10 degrees of slope (Fig. 24-3).

SURGICAL TECHNIQUE   The incisions of the V cross the interphalangeal joint crease at an angle and thus do not cause contractures (see Figs. 24-2 and 24-3). When designing the flap, one takes the V incisions out almost to the lateral nail folds distally. Having made the flap wide, the leading edge of the flap after advancement is wider than the original thumb tip. Unless the lateral corners of the flap are excised, this results in a spatulate end to the digit. Cutting off the lateral corners and allowing the resulting raw edges and tip to epithelialize not only narrows the digital tip but also rounds it to achieve a good appearance. The flap is designed as a "V" at its proximal extremity and was conceived to close proximally as a "Y" after the flap has moved distally. Mostly, the proximal donor defect is left open to close under dressings as primary closure of the vertical limb of the "Y" tightens

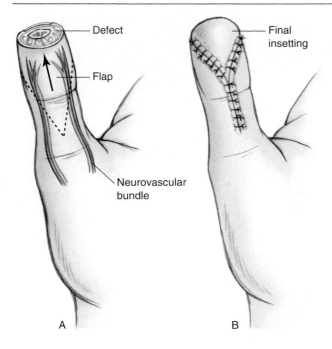

A   B

FIGURE 24-2

A,B: Illustration of the neurovascular Tranquilli-Leali flap. The flap extends proximally beyond the IP crease and includes both the neurovascular bundles.

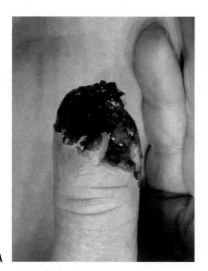

A

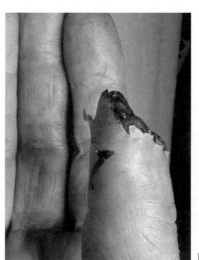

B

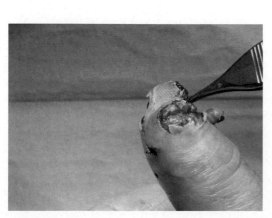

C

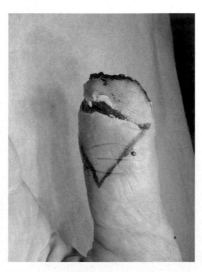

D

FIGURE 24-3

A,B: Dorsal sloping crush amputation of the right thumb tip of a 70-year-old man. **C:** Simple folding back of the palmar tissues after excision of the nail germinal   matrix to suture the skin to the proximal nail fold is not possible because of the bulk of the pulp tissue. **D:** A neurovascular Tranquilli-Leali flap designed to allow easier folding back of the palmar tissues and shaping of the thumb tip. The transverse skin split just beyond the "V" was part of the injury, but only skin deep, so not affecting the vascularity of the tissues distal to it. *(Continued)*

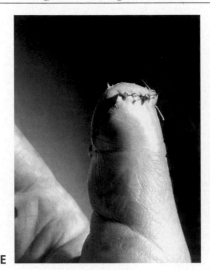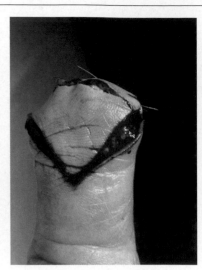

FIGURE 24-3

Continued **E,F:** The reconstructed shape after trimming the lateral points of the advanced flap to round the thumb tip. (Reproduced from Elliot D. Specific flaps for the thumb. *Tech Hand Up Extrem Surg.* 2004;8(4):198–211, with permission.)

E

F

the thumb too much proximally over the vascular pedicles of the flaps and compromises vascular inflow into the flap.

Moberg Flaps

INDICATIONS/CONTRAINDICATIONS   With greater losses of palmar thumb tissue, more sloping palmar oblique injuries, and when the whole distal pulp of the thumb has been avulsed, the neurovascular Tranquilli-Leali flap is too small and cannot advance sufficiently. For larger thumb defects confined to the distal phalanx we favor the use of a modified Moberg flap. The Moberg flap, as described by Moberg in 1964, is an advancement flap based on both neurovascular bundles of the thumb (2). The advantages of this flap are that it returns sensation and glabrous skin to the defect site. The downside to the original flap design was the IP joint flexion contracture necessary to achieve suture of the flap distally to the nail. Our preferred modification of the Moberg flap avoids the IP joint flexion necessary with the original to advance the flap to the tip of the digit. This is, essentially, O'Brien's modification of the Moberg flap, but uses a "V" tail proximally instead of a skin graft at the base of the thumb (Fig. 24-4) (3). This **V-Y Moberg flap** achieves the same excellent results as the original Moberg flap in terms of sensibility of the thumb tip, but without the restrictions of interphalangeal joint movement associated with the original flap or the need for skin graft of the O'Brien modification.

There is no danger of dorsal skin loss in raising Moberg-type flaps on the thumb, as the dorsal skin of the thumb has a separate blood supply. Because of the safety of the V-Y Moberg flap, the speed and ease with which it can be dissected, and the excellent sensibility of the thumb tip which can be achieved with it, this technique remains our favorite thumb tip reconstruction if the defect is limited to the distal phalangeal segment of the thumb.

TECHNIQUE   The flap is created laterally along the mid-lateral lines on each side of the thumb and with the tip of the proximal "V" well back on the thenar eminence, at least as far proximally as a line drawn proximally from the ulnar border of the middle finger. This creates a large flap which incorporates the more lax subcutaneous tissues of the thenar eminence. Smaller flaps with the proximal "V" at the base of the thumb move less easily and less far distally. The wider and longer flap avoids any need for addition of techniques to accommodate tightness at the base of the thumb. The use of this flap is considerably extended in reconstructing palmar oblique defects if the pulp distally which is denuded of skin cover remains as the leading edge of the flap, with suture of subcutaneous tissue, not skin, to the nail distally then epithelialization under dressings (Fig. 24-4).

Other Flaps   Other flaps have an infrequent use in reconstruction of the tip and palmar surface of the thumb but can be useful.

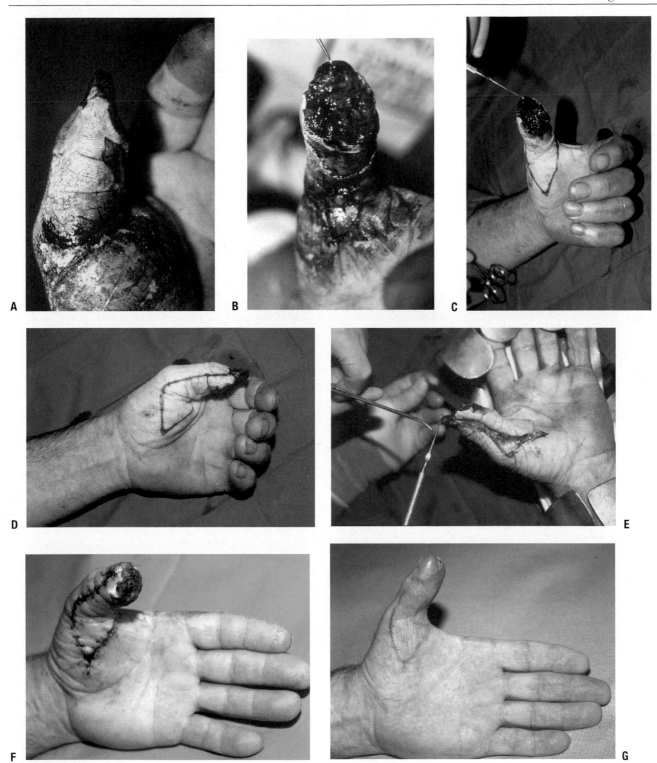

FIGURE 24-4

A,B: Preoperative views of the thumb of a 47-year-old man with a typical crush avulsion of the distal pulp. **C,D:** Markings of a V-Y modification of the Moberg flap shown preoperatively. **E:** Intra-operative view of the fully mobilized flap. **F:** Immediate postoperative view with the flap advanced to provide pulp cover of the distal bone. **G:** Final result after epithelialization of the tip under moist antiseptic dressings. (Reproduced from Elliot D, Yii NW. Homodigital reconstruction of the digits—the perspective of one unit. *Handchir Mikrochir Plast Chir.* 2001;33(1):7–19, with permission.)

LATERAL PULP FLAP   We devised the Lateral Pulp Flap for losses of the radial border of the tip of the index finger with exposure of bone but it is also useful on either border of the thumb tip (Fig. 24-5). This flap exploits the excess of pulp in the digital tip.

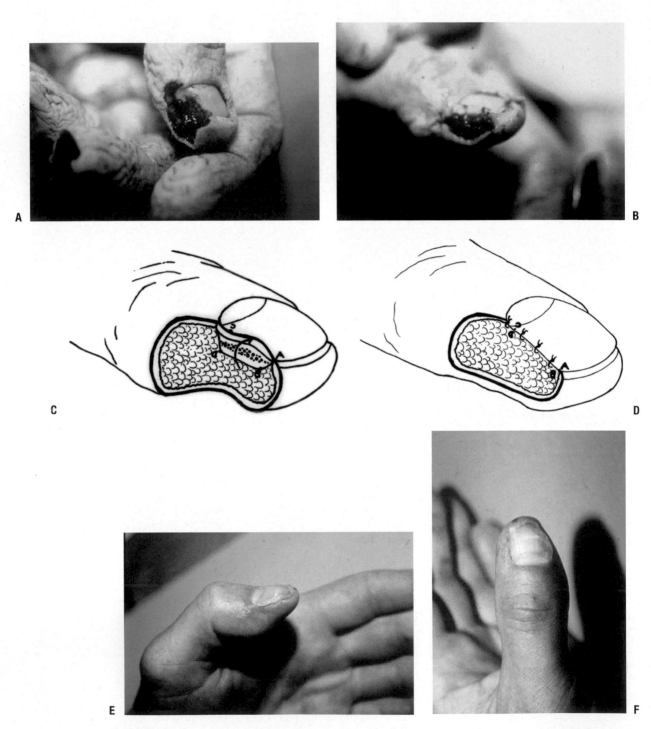

FIGURE 24-5

A: A slicing defect with loss of the radial lateral pulp, lateral nail fold, and lateral one-third of the nail of the thumb in a 50-year-old man. **B:** Lateral pulp transposed to cover the distal phalanx. **C,D:** Diagrams to show the original injury and transposition of the pulp to cover the bone of the distal phalanx. **E,F:** Late views of the reconstruction, 1 year after the injury. (Parts C and D reproduced from Elliot D, Jigjinni VS. The lateral pulp flap. *J Hand Surg Br.* 1993;18(4):423–426, with permission.)

The flap is raised by opening the tip of the digit with a fish mouth incision close to the distal nailbed and freeing the pulp attachments to the bone. The pulp then moves laterally and is lifted over the bone and sutured to the edge of the nail. The deep edge of the pulp—not the superficial edge—is brought up to the nailbed to cover the bone. The pulp is then epithelialized under moist antiseptic dressings. This reconstruction creates a digital tip which is sensate but has no lateral nail fold. This seems to cause no functional problems and is less obvious than most lateral nail fold reconstructions, as these are usually too bulky.

SIDE-TO-SIDE HOMODIGITAL SWITCH FLAPS Side-to-side homodigital switch flaps, which reconstruct or re-innervate one side of a digital tip at the expense of the other side, can be useful to resurface areas of pulp sensibility in the hand which are critical for pinch activity after localized loss of tissue or irrevocable digital nerve injury. Replacement of the radial side of the index or middle fingertips by a vascularized composite transfer from the ulnar side of the same digit is well established, both as a simple transposition and as an island flap. Use of the radial pulp of the thumb tip to reconstruct and/or reinnervate the ulnar side is logical, as the ulnar portion of the thumb tip is most involved in majority of gross and fine pinch (Fig. 24-6).

LITTLER FLAPS

Indications/Contraindications The classic Littler flap, as described by Littler in 1956, was designed for thumb tip and palmar thumb resurfacing. Unlike the flaps described above, the Littler flap is a heterodigital flap, which means a donor site defect will be created on the middle or ring finger. The flap utilizes tissue from either the ulnar border of the ring or middle finger; this tissue is transferred on its neurovascular bundle, thus allowing for the return of sensation to the thumb (Fig. 24-7). This differs from the heterodigital flaps described elsewhere in this text, which are designed to spare the digital nerves. This flap is easy to dissect and transfer. However, the flap can considerably downgrade the donor finger function and restoration of adequate two-point sensation after transfer has been a problem and suffers problems of achieving "thumb-tip" sensibility. To improve thumb-tip sensation, and avoid patient's perception of the thumb-tip as still coming from the donor finger, division of the donor finger nerves and reconnection of the nerves in the flap to those of the recipient thumb has been recommended. Nerve disconnection and reconnection extends its usefulness in younger patients but, like all neurorrhaphies, gives less satisfactory tip innervation in the middle-aged and elderly patients.

Direct contraindications for this flap include injury to the neurovascular pedicle to the donor finger. Laceration of the superficial arterial arch or common vascular bundle to the donor finger could potentially lead to compromise of the flap or donor finger following transfer. Very distal tip injuries may also be difficult to cover with this flap.

Complications Specific complications to be noted with the use of the Littler flap include the risk of venous congestion, specifically if the nerve is dissected or divided in preparation for neurorrhaphy at the level of the thumb. In such cases leech therapy may be required for resolution of venous congestion. Poor return of thumb sensation may also occur or the inability of the patient to recorticate, in which case the sensation within the flap is always perceived by the patient as coming from the donor finger donor site. Either sensory problem may necessitate a secondary nerve graft or nerve repair, but two-point discrimination may well remain >12 mm within the flap.

Reconstruction of the Dorsal Surface of the Thumb

The Hatchet Flaps

INDICATIONS/CONTRAINDICATIONS For the more common, smaller defects of the dorsum of the thumb, homodigital techniques are very useful. They are generally simpler and quicker to execute and avoid injury of adjacent fingers. For these small defects the **Hatchet Flap** provides an easy reconstructive option. **Hatchet Flaps** are also very useful in replantation, as they allow one to advance the dorsal veins of the proximal part of the thumb to the replant and achieve direct vein anastomoses under good skin cover without recourse to either vein grafts or a separate skin cover procedure. These flaps can be used as far distally as the proximal nail fold (Fig. 24-8).

SURGICAL TECHNIQUE The flap is designed as a random dorsal cutaneous flap (Fig. 24-8). A curvilinear incision is made over the radial (Fig. 24-9) or ulnar (Fig. 24-8) aspect of the thumb. A broad base is preserved on the opposite side of the digit. As on the palmar surface when utilizing a Moberg flap, a V-Y tail can be added to these flaps to avoid the need to skin graft the donor site proximally (Fig. 24-9)

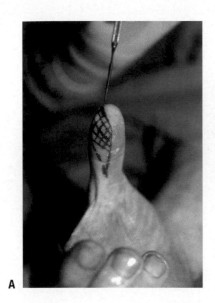
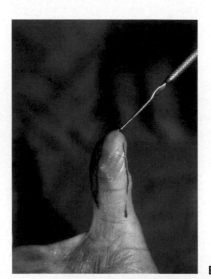
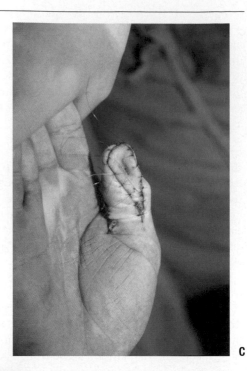

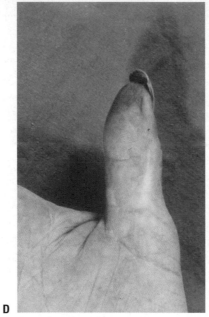
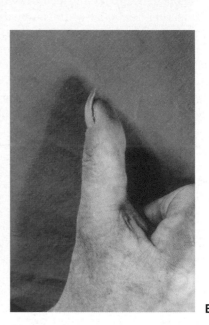

FIGURE 24-6

A: Thumb of a patient with irreparable damage to the ulnar digital nerve. A triangle of the denervated ulnar digital nerve territory is shaded, prior to excision down to bone. **B:** The same thumb showing the pre-operative marking of the radial switch flap. **C:** The thumb at surgery, after transposition of the flap and with the graft applied to the donor defect. **D:** Late view of the grafted donor site. **E:** Late view of the switch flap. (Reproduced from Elliot D, Southgate CM, Staiano JJ. A homodigital switch flap to restore sensation to the ulnar border of the thumb tip. *J Hand Surg Br.* 2003; 28(5):409–413, with permission)

(4). On this surface of the digits, it is necessary to close the proximal V as a Y to protect the extensor paratenon from desiccation.

RESULTS   In a review of 1,077 dorsal wounds of all digits, which we treated over a 6-year period, 154 digits required flap reconstruction (5). The dorsal V-Y flap accounted for 42% of the flaps used and was the most common skin flap used on this surface of the digits, reflecting the relative incidence of defects of this size and shape.

Brunelli Flap

SURGICAL TECHNIQUE   This homodigital flap is a useful adjunct for reconstructing smaller defects of the dorsum of the thumb. In 1993, Brunelli and his colleagues in Paris described a very easily and quickly raised flap based on the dorsoulnar artery of the thumb which is useful for reconstruction of dorsal defects of the tip of the thumb involving all or parts of the nail complex (Fig. 24-10) (6). The artery may be verified preoperatively with a handheld Doppler probe, but is very consistent running on the ulnar aspect of the extensor tendons. The flap is raised with a skin tail to reduce the risk of com-

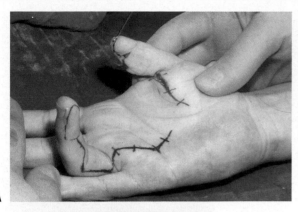

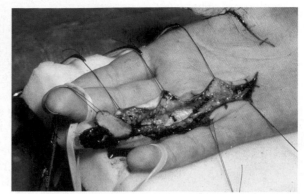

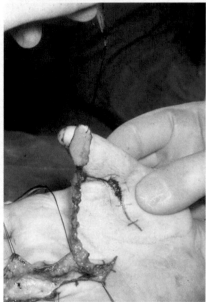

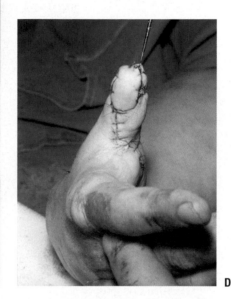

FIGURE 24-7

A: Intra-operative view showing dissection of damaged and denervated skin on the ulnar aspect of the thumb tip and the markings of a Littler flap on the ulnar side of the ring finger.
B: Dissection of the pedicle of the flap.
C: Demonstration of the transfer.
D: Final view of the flap after tunnelling across the palm and insetting.

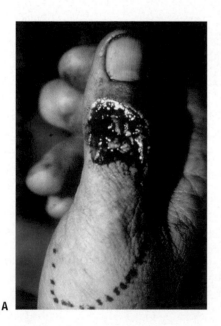

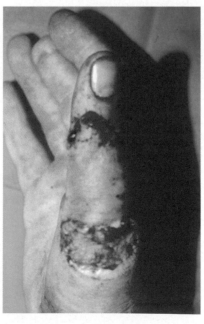

FIGURE 24-8

A: Preoperative view of a typical "small" skin defect on the dorsum of the thumb. A simple dorsal hatchet flap is marked.
B: Closure of the defect with this flap, with split skin graft reconstruction of the donor defect. (Reproduced from Elliot D. Specific flaps for the thumb. *Tech Hand Up Extrem Surg.* 2004;8(4):198–211, with permission.)

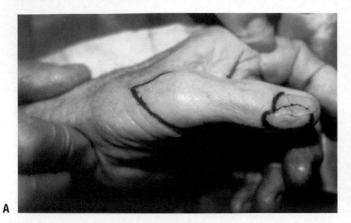

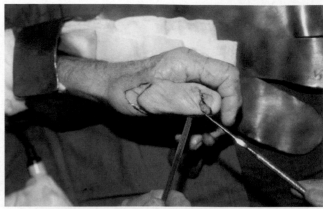

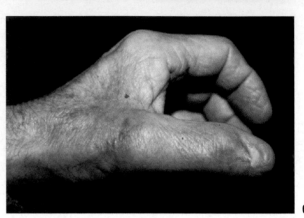

FIGURE 24-9

A: Preoperative view of the thumb of a 73-year-old man with a squamous cell carcinoma of the radial lateral fold of the nail. The thumb is marked with a dorsal V-Y hatchet flap for reconstruction. **B:** Intra-operative view of the flap being advanced. **C:** Late postoperative view. (Reproduced from Elliot D. Specific flaps for the thumb. *Tech Hand Up Extrem Surg.* 2004;8(4):198–211, with permission.)

pression of the pedicle just proximal and lateral to the nail fold, which is the tightest part of its course. The flap may be safely elevated to the proximal margin of the interphalangeal joint skin crease. The donor site may be closed with a skin graft or advancement flap from the dorsum of the hand (Fig. 24-10).

This flap can be innervated for reconstruction of the thumb tip but, like the other flaps of dorsal origin, carries skin with poor innervation. It has more recently been redescribed carrying a segment of vascularized bone from the first metacarpal with it and may prove a very useful means of placing vascularized bone at the tip of the thumb without microsurgical transfer from the foot (7).

RECONSTRUCTION OF LARGE DORSAL DEFECTS

A very few techniques of reconstruction suffice to cover almost all full-thickness soft tissue losses on the dorsum of the thumb. Complete loss of the dorsal surface cover can be replaced using the first dorsal metacarpal artery or with a reverse posterior interosseous artery flap; both flaps are described in detail elsewhere in the text. The latter is particularly useful if the adjacent dorsal tissues of the hand have been injured and are not available as a donor site. It can also carry vascularized bone (and tendon) to the thumb.

The posterior interosseous vessel is small and the dissection relatively difficult, requiring microsurgical instrumentation and expertise. However, this flap is mostly safe and does not involve sacrifice of a major blood vessel of the forearm. For this reason, it is preferred to the use of the radial forearm flap for larger defects of the dorsum of the thumb, although the latter is useful for complete wrap-around of the first ray. When used to reconstruct the dorsum of the thumb, the reverse posterior interosseous artery flap donor site can almost always be closed primarily and then heals with a fine, narrow scar which may be almost invisible in the hair of a male forearm.

Postoperative Management

We remove all dressings and splints from reconstructed hand injuries on the day after surgery to allow washing and dressing of the raw wounds and verification of flap viability. Although this some-

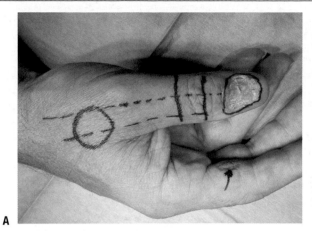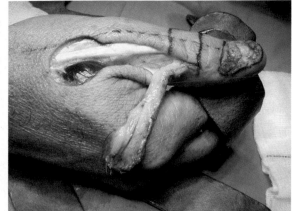

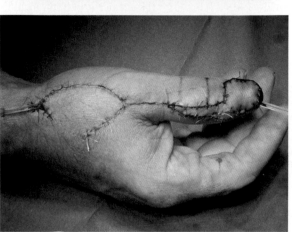

FIGURE 24-10

A: A thumb with a badly damaged nail before excision for biopsy. The Brunelli flap and its pedicle have been marked. **B:** The flap has been raised and shows the artery on which it is based on its undersurface. **C:** The flap inset after total excision of the nail complex. The flap has been taken with a "tail" to ease pressure on the pedicle beyond its turning point. The donor site has been closed with a dorsal V-Y hatchet flap. (Reproduced with permission from Elliot D. Homodigital reconstruction of the digits: The perspective of one unit. *Indian J Plast Surg.* 2003;36:106–119.)

times has to be done with care to avoid tension on flap pedicles, it allows the hand to be bathed in warm water. This both helps general cleaning and debridement of the wounds and is a comfortable environment in which to encourage very early hand mobilization. The wounds are dressed as lightly as possible while maintaining a moist antiseptic presence around any areas without skin which will heal through secondary intention. Suture lines that are not oozing are not covered. Sometimes homodigital and more distant reconstructions require that one or more joints be prevented from moving in a certain direction to take tension off the pedicle. For example, with all of the advancement flaps on the palmar surface, full extension will pull on the flap pedicles, so the thumb is splinted in slight flexion. Conversely, a slightly extended wrist position will ease tension on the pedicle of reverse posterior interosseous artery flaps. Protection of pedicles and flaps is continued during bathing and dressing changes by appropriate positioning and guarding with the other hand and between dressing changes by use of thermoplastic splints. Bathing and dressing changes are carried out twice a day with the patients learning to do this themselves as soon as possible.

Rehabilitation

The use of homodigital flaps allows for early mobilization of the reconstructed thumb. Motion will be restricted by concomitant tendon, nerve, and bony injuries; however with stable skeletal fixation, most thumbs can be mobilized using limited motion and passive motion protocols under the supervision of a hand therapist within the first 72 hours following surgery. Whenever possible, we avoid techniques of bandaging, splinting, and skeletal fixation which will completely immobilize the reconstructed thumb. Over and above the early mobilization under water during dressing changes, mobilization of as much of the thumb and the rest of the hand as possible is continued from this early stage by exercises three or four times daily with the splint in place, albeit sometimes with loosening of some straps if this is possible without loss of the protection of flap pedicles. The splint provides a solid resting position for the thumb at night and gives the patient confidence that their thumb will not suffer from jarring by unexpected contact with external forces. Splints are generally used for 1 to 2 weeks. However, this period may lengthen to 4 or 5 weeks, if required to protect structures repaired under the flap. Between activities, the hand is elevated. This regimen of elevation and enthusiastic exercising is intended to eliminate edema from the hand as quickly as possible to minimize fibrin restriction of joint and extensor tendon movements.

Complications

Major complications include flap loss, partial flap loss, infection, and iatrogenic injury to the digital arteries or nerves. Partial flap loss is often best managed by allowing the wound to heal through secondary intention. Total flap loss, while infrequent with these homodigital flaps, will necessitate the use of a heterodigital island flap such as the first dorsal metacarpal artery island flap, or a larger pedicled forearm flap, such as the posterior interosseous flap or radial forearm flap. Obviously such flaps will create further injury to the arm but are reliable means of providing soft tissue coverage. An additional downside to the use of heterodigital flaps is that they are often insensate or require a neurorrhaphy to re-establish sensation. Return of sensation in these situations may be dependent on the age of the patient. In addition, heterodigital flaps will create an injury to another digit, which may further compromise hand function.

RESULTS

The techniques described here have proved adequate to reconstruct most of the thumb defects we have seen in our practice over the last 12 years. The principle used in the smaller cases, particularly in reconstructing the tip of the thumb, has been to capitalize on the enormous healing capacity of digital skin and assist this, when necessary, by simple local flap reconstructions. These provide the best sensation possible and the best cosmetic profile to the thumb tip. For larger defects we prefer to use homodigital techniques whenever possible, although there are upper limits to the size of defects which can be reconstructed by these. For any defect, our choice of flaps is, in part, determined by the site, size, and shape of the defect and, in part, by flap reliability and ease of use. The homodigital flaps described above have proved particularly versatile and reliable in the hands of surgeons of varying levels of experience within our unit, although requiring some familiarity with microsurgical technique and instrumentation. They are quick to perform, which can be an advantage following lengthy bony or soft tissue reconstructions. They allow early and independent mobilization of the thumb and the use of local tissue respects the cosmetic principle of reconstruction of "like with like." Donor site morbidity is also limited to the already injured part. When used for fingertip reconstruction, advancement homodigital flaps cannot achieve the sensibility of the original, but are durable and intrinsically more likely to restore good sensory function in the digital tips than most of the reconstructive alternatives. For larger defects, the Littler transfer, the dorsum of the index ray, and, more recently, the reverse posterior interosseous artery flap are our local work horses and are discussed in detail in subsequent chapters.

REFERENCES

1. Gaul JS. A palmar-hinged flap for reconstruction of traumatic thumb defects. *J Hand Surg Am.* 1987;12:415–421.
2. Moberg E. Aspects of sensation in reconstructive surgery of the upper extremity. *J Bone Joint Surg Am.* 1964;46:817–825.
3. O'Brien B. Neurovascular island pedicle flaps for terminal amputations and digital scars. *Br J Plast Surg.* 1968;21:258–261.
4. Yii NW, Elliot D. Dorsal V-Y advancement flaps in digital reconstruction. *J Hand Surg Br.* 1994;19:91–97.
5. Yii NW, Elliot D. Bipedicle strap flaps in reconstruction of longitudinal dorsal skin defects of the digits. *Plast Reconstr Surg.* 1999;103:1205–1211.
6. Brunelli F, Vigasio A, Valenti P, et al. Arterial anatomy and clinical application of the dorsoulnar flap of the thumb. *J Hand Surg Am.* 1999;24:803–811.
7. Pelissier P, Pistre V, Casoli V, et al. Dorso-ulnar osteocutaneous reverse flow flap of the thumb. Anatomy and clinical application. *J Hand Surg Br.* 2003;26:207–211.

RECOMMENDED READING

Allen MJ. Conservative management of finger tip injuries. *Hand.* 1980;12:257–265.
Bang H-H, Kojima T, Hayashi H. Palmar advancement flap with V-Y closure for thumb tip injuries. *J Hand Surg Am.* 1992;17:933–934.
Baumeister S, Menke H, Wittemann M, et al. Functional outcome after the Moberg advancement flap in the thumb. *J Hand Surg Am.* 2002;27:105–114.

Elliot D, Jigjinni VS. The lateral pulp flap. *J Hand Surg Br.* 1993;18:423–426.

Elliot D, Moiemen NS, Jigjinni VS. The neurovascular Tranquilli-Leali flap. *J Hand Surg Br.* 1995;20B:815–823.

Elliot D, Southgate CM, Staino JJ. A homodigital switch flap to restore sensation to the ulnar border of the thumb tip. *J Hand Surg Br.* 2003;28:409–413.

Elliot D, Wilson Y. V-Y advancement of the entire volar soft tissue of the thumb in distal reconstruction. *J Hand Surg Br.* 1993;18:399–402.

Foucher G, Smith D, Pempinello C, et al. Homodigital neurovascular island flaps for digital pulp loss. *J Hand Surg Br.* 1989;14:204–208.

Henderson HP, Reid DAC. Long term follow up of neurovascular island flaps. *Hand.* 1980;2:113–122.

Lee LP, Lau PY, Chan CW. A simple and efficient treatment for fingertip injuries. *J Hand Surg Br.* 1995;20B:63–71.

Littler JW. Neurovascular pedicle transfer of tissue in reconstructive surgery of the hand. *J Bone Joint Surg Am.* 1956;38:917.

Markley JM. The preservation of close two-point discrimination in the interdigital transfer of neurovascular island flaps. *Plast Reconstr Surg.* 1977;59:812–816.

Oka Y. Sensory function of the neurovascular island flap in thumb reconstruction: comparison of original and modified procedures. *J Hand Surg Am.* 2000;25:637–643.

Omer GE, Day DJ, Ratliff H, et al. Neurovascular cutaneous island pedicles for deficient median-nerve sensibility. New technique and results of serial functional tests. *J Bone Joint Surg Am.* 1970;52:1181–1192.

PART V

MANAGEMENT OF THE SOFT TISSUES OF THE LOWER EXTREMITY

25 Soft Tissue Management Following Traumatic Injury to the Femur

Thomas F. Higgins

Open injuries of the femur and thigh are common. The need for major soft tissue coverage in this area in the setting of trauma is uncommon due to the generous surrounding muscular envelope. Soft tissue coverage of the femur can be a concern in certain situations such as power takeoff injuries or pedestrians struck by motor vehicles; however, the majority of these defects may be covered with skin grafts, and the need for vascularized free tissue transfer is unusual. Despite this, there are several components to soft tissue management in this area which may be used during exposure to the proximal and distal portions of the femur. Simple alterations in established techniques can lead to improved postoperative contour, improved soft tissue coverage of hardware, and decreased rates of postoperative infection and stiffness following elective and emergent surgical procedures.

This chapter covers four major areas of concern with regard to soft tissue management in the thigh:

- The approach to the proximal femoral shaft and intertochanteric zone
- The approach for the repair of supracondylar and intra-articular distal femur fractures
- Exposure for the treatment of open femur fractures
- The management of post-traumatic arthrofibrosis of the knee with the use of a Judet quadricepsplasty

APPROACH TO THE LATERAL PROXIMAL FEMUR

Indications/Contraindications

Fractures of the proximal femur, whether femoral neck or intertrochanteric, constitute the majority of all femur fractures (9). The soft tissue management issues in this portion of the proximal femur are the relative dearth of coverage over the greater trochanter and the area of the femur just distal to the vastus lateralis. Frequently, plate and screw implants and laterally based orthopaedic constructs will be prominent and symptomatic, particularly in thin patients. An approach that maximizes soft tissue coverage over the lateral aspect of the proximal femur and restores the most normal anatomy will be described. Rather than a direct lateral approach cutting through the vastus lateralis, which has been frequently advocated for this operation, a simple modification provides a more anatomic dissection and a friendlier soft tissue reconstruction.

Patient Positioning

The patient is positioned as desired for ultimate reduction and fixation goals.

Surgery

A direct lateral approach begins 1 cm proximal to the vastus ridge and extends as far distally as necessary for osteosynthesis. On the coronal plane, the incision should be 1 cm posterior to the mid-coronal point of the femur (Fig. 25-1). Dissection is taken down to the iliotibial band, and this is divided in line with its fibers (Figs. 25-2 and 25-3).

A gentle sweeping motion with a sponge will clear trochanteric bursa or areolar soft tissue that lies in this layer. Particularly fibrotic bursal tissue may need to be excised with scissors (Fig. 25-4). This will reveal quite clearly the proximal extent of the vastus lateralis and its insertion at the vastus ridge and the confluence with the distal extent of the vastus medialis tendon. Rather than directly incising the vastus lateralis in the midcoronal point of the femur, a J-shaped incision is performed. Leaving several millimeters of the vastus lateralis tendon still attached to the vastus ridge, the tendon is incised from its anterior extent posteriorly until connecting with the lateral intermuscular septum (Figs. 25-5 and 25-6). The dissection is then taken through the most posterior fibers of the vastus lateralis extending from proximal to distal, just anterior to the lateral intermuscular septum. The

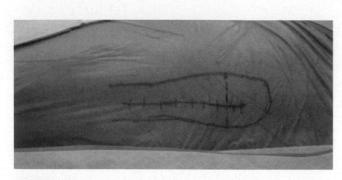

FIGURE 25-1

Incision drawn over the greater trochanter. *Dotted transverse line* represents the vastus ridge.

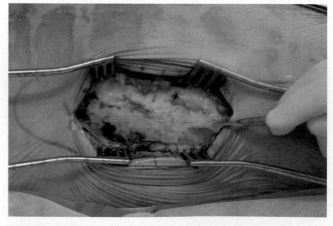

FIGURE 25-2

Iliotibial band is incised in line with its fibers.

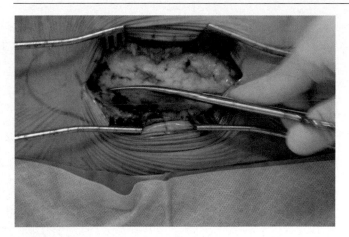

FIGURE 25-3

Iliotibial band is divided proximal to distal with curved Mayo scissors.

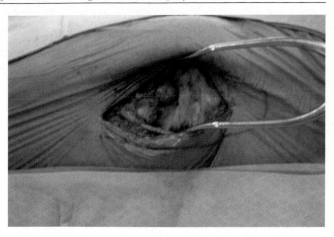

FIGURE 25-4

Fibrotic trochanteric bursa may need to be excised.

vastus tendon is tagged with a heavy braided nonabsorbable suture before being detached from the vastus ridge (see Fig. 25-5). As the dissection extends greater than 5 cm distal to the vastus ridge, the first perforating branch off the profunda femoris will be encountered penetrating the lateral intermuscular septum. These perforators should be ligated or cauterized. A gentle sweeping motion with an elevator from posterior to anterior along the proximal femur will allow reflection of the vastus lateralis in an anterior direction (Fig. 25-7). The periosteum and deepest soft tissues should not be stripped off the femur. For ideal visualization at this point, a Bennett retractor is placed anterior to the femur, and an assistant holds this forward (Fig. 25-8). Osteosynthesis proceeds as planned.

The Bennett retractors make for easy retraction and permit reduction and fixation. At the conclusion of the procedure, Bennett retractors are simply removed, and gravity allows the vastus to fall back into place, padding and directly covering the implant (Fig. 25-9). The most proximal origin of the vastus lateralis is then repaired back to its tendinous origin with a heavy braided nonabsorbable suture (Figs. 25-10 and 25-11). The posterior aspect of the vastus lateralis does not need to be repaired. The iliotibial band is repaired with interrupted nonabsorable suture, and the skin may be closed according to surgeon preference (Figs. 25-12 and 25-13).

This approach is most helpful for the placement of a dynamic hip screw, blade plate, or locking proximal femoral plate. It offers less scarring, as the muscle belly has not been interrupted. This should also be a more functional repair, as less damage presumably has been done to the vastus origin by dividing it and repairing it, rather than by directly insulting it with a midgastric approach.

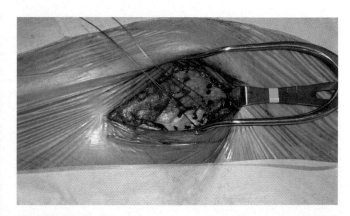

FIGURE 25-5

Proximal tendon of vastus lateralis is to be incised in a posteriorly based "J."

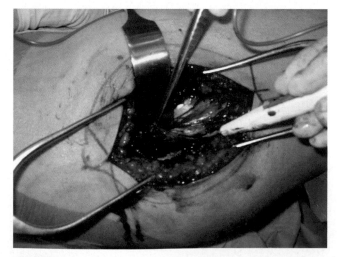

FIGURE 25-6

Vastus lateralis origin is elevated in along the "J."

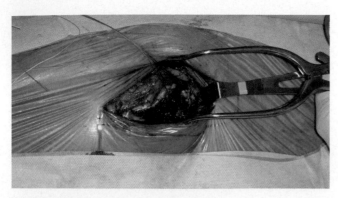

FIGURE 25-7
Lateralis is retracted anteriorly with tagging sutures.

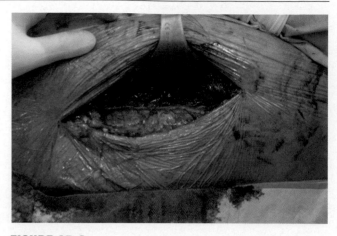

FIGURE 25-8
Bennett retractor is used to reflect the vastus anteriorly.

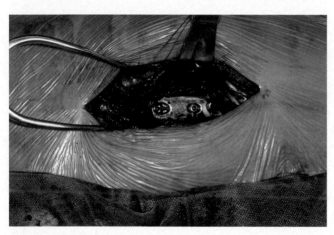

FIGURE 25-9
Osteosynthesis hardware, after placement, is covered by vastus.

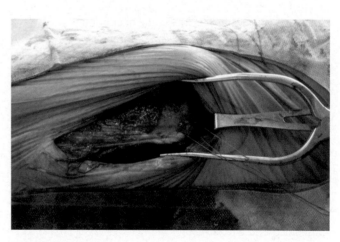

FIGURE 25-10
Vastus lateralis pulled back to its origin at the vastus ridge.

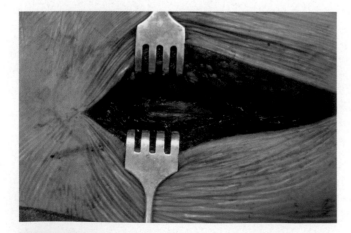

FIGURE 25-11
Through the closing iliotibial band, repair of the vastus origin may be visualized.

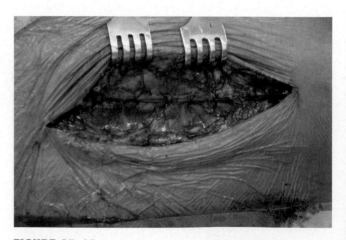

FIGURE 25-12
Iliotibial band is repaired with interrupted nonabsorbable suture.

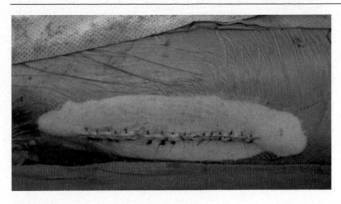

FIGURE 25-13
Skin closure at completion of intertrochanteric fracture osteosynthesis.

Postoperative Management

In the elderly population with intertrochanteric hip fractures, patients are generally allowed to bear weight as tolerated to facilitate mobilization (8). The first 2 weeks postoperatively focus on range of motion of the hip and knee, and gait training with assistive devices as necessary. At 2 weeks postoperatively, strengthening of the abductors, hip flexors, and quadriceps is added to the regimen.

In younger patients, or fractures with a subtrochanteric component, weight bearing may be protected initially, and advanced as desirable by the treating surgeon.

Complications

Complications of operations through this approach are generally related to the osteosynthesis, and these may be avoided somewhat with careful attention to achieving reduction and adherence to correct placement of implants.

APPROACH TO THE DISTAL FEMUR AND KNEE

Indications/Contraindications

Multiple variations on parapatellar and lateral parapatellar approaches have been described. Similar to the muscle sparing approach described for the proximal femur, the "swashbuckler" approach described by Starr et al at Parkland Hospital (14) offers excellent visualization of the joint for anatomic fixation of interarticular fracture while preserving the vastus and quadriceps with no intramuscular dissection.

This approach offers the advantage of not interfering with or dividing the extensor mechanism while gaining adequate visualization of the joint space. With proximal and distal retraction, the intervening metaphyseal soft tissues may be largely undisturbed to enhance healing of comminuted metaphyseal bone.

Surgery

Patient Positioning   The patient is positioned supine. The lower extremity is prepared and draped free. A bump may be used under the knee to facilitate exposure and/or reduction.

Technique   The skin incision starts at the insertion of the patellar ligament and extends directly cephalad to the apex of the patella. It then extends lateral and proximal toward the lateral intermuscular septum (Fig. 25-14). A full thickness skin flap is elevated off the extensor fascia. The lateral margin of the patella and patellar ligament are identified distally. Proximally, the lateral margin of the vastus lateralis is identified.

The knee capsule is incised immediately along the lateral aspect of the patellar ligament (Fig. 25-15). Care must be taken not to cut the anterior horn of the lateral meniscus. Dissection is taken directly along the lateral margin of the patella, leaving a small cuff of tissue for eventual repair. At the superolateral shoulder of the patella, the deep dissection extends laterally toward the lateral intermuscular septum. The vastus lateralis is thus spared and is elevated anteriorly off the lateral intermuscular septum. As dissection nears the femur, perforating branches of the profunda femoris artery must be identified and ligated. These will be located every 3 to 4 cm approximately 1 cm lateral to the femoral cortex.

Right angle retractors may be placed at the level of the quadriceps tendon for medial excursion of the quadriceps and patella (Fig. 25-16). Bennett retractors may be placed over the femoral diaphysis. These

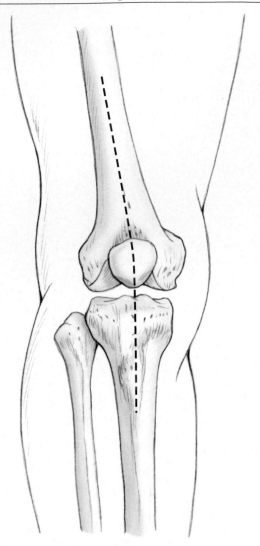

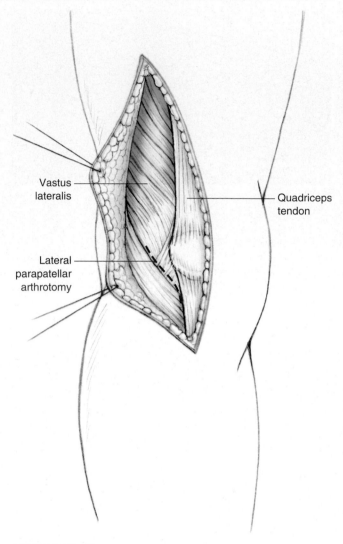

FIGURE 25-14

The skin incision for the "swashbuckler" approach to the distal femur. (Redrawn from Starr AJ, Jones AL, Reinert CM. The "swashbuckler": a modified anterior approach for fractures of the distal femur. *J Orthop Trauma.* 1999;13(2):138–140. With permission.)

FIGURE 25-15

The lateral parapatellar arthrotomy extends to the lateral margin of the vastus lateralis. (Redrawn from Starr AJ, Jones AL, Reinert CM. The "swashbuckler": a modified anterior approach for fractures of the distal femur. *J Orthop Trauma.* 1999;13(2):138–140. With permission.)

retractors in combination will allow adequate visualization of the femur for reconstruction. If possible, no retractors at all should be placed medially at the level of the metaphysis, as most techniques demand preservation of the medial soft tissues so as to not interfere with healing of metaphyseal comminution. Adequate visualization may easily be achieved with retractors placed proximal and distal to this area.

For full visualization of the femoral condyles, the patella may be everted. This may be facilitated by elevating a small proximal portion of the most lateral insertion of the patellar ligament off the tibia. Osteosynthesis is then performed.

Closure is achieved with repair of the lateral parapatellar retinaculum and capsule lateral to the patellar ligament. A drain may be placed in the knee and run along the lateral intermuscular septum, exiting the skin proximally. Subcutaneous tissue and skin are repaired according to surgeon preference.

Postoperative Management

Assuming stable osteosynthesis has been achieved, immediate range of motion is initiated. A physical therapist may perform passive supervised range of motion, 0 to 90 degrees, with no strengthening and no active quadriceps. Alternatively, a continuous passive motion machine may be used. Quadriceps strengthening begins at 6 weeks postoperatively, and weight bearing is advanced according to surgeon judgment.

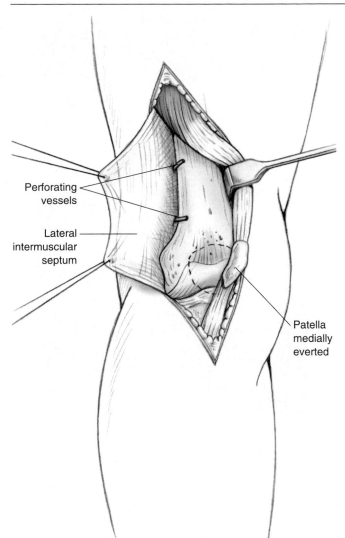

Perforating
vessels

Lateral
intermuscular
septum

Patella
medially
everted

FIGURE 25-16

With quad retracted and patella everted, visualization of the distal femur is excellent. Starr AJ, Jones AL, Reinert CM. The "swashbuckler": a modified anterior approach for fractures of the distal femur. *J Orthop Trauma.* 1999;13(2):138–140. With permission.)

Complications

Potential complications of complex distal femur fractures include infection, nonunion, and arthrofibrosis. Judet quadricepsplasty for loss of knee motion will be addressed later in this chapter.

SURGICAL EXPOSURE OF OPEN FEMORAL FRACTURES

Indications/Contraindications

Given the wide girth of soft tissues around the femur, an open fracture by definition implies a high-energy injury. There are compelling data to support early irrigation and debridement of open fractures for the prevention of infection (3,4). Small lacerations or puncture wounds are often the tell-tail signs of an open fracture and should not be overlooked; these relatively small surface injuries often disguise a significant deeper soft tissue insult (13). Open fractures of the distal femur in particular will present with a very small opening of the skin where the femoral shaft has pistoned distally to penetrate the vastus medialis obliquus or the vastus lateralis and the skin (Figs. 25-17 and 25-18).

Frequently, the treatment of open intra-articular distal femur fractures will necessitate an aggressive irrigation and debridement at the time of presentation and transarticular spanning external fixation for definitive stabilization. Even in the hemodynamically unstable trauma patient, early stabilization of the femur is mandatory. Prolonged maintenance of a patient in Hare traction is not advisable given the attendant complications of skin breakdown and sciatic nerve palsy, and so spanning external fixation is recommended over prolonged traction.

The initial management of these fractures should not include the placement of a pulsatile irrigation catheter through the small traumatic wound. This may succeed only in further embedding de-

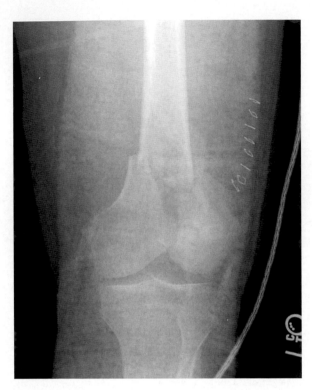

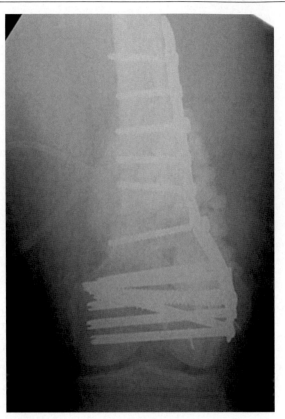

FIGURE 25-17

Skin staples demonstrate the length of the inadequate incision used to debride this open intracondylar distal femur fracture.

FIGURE 25-18

This inadequate index debridement leads to a long and complicated course of treatment, including a deep infection and the placement of antibiotic beads.

bris in an open fracture site and will certainly not provide an adequate debridement of the injured soft tissues that would ultimately be responsible for the development of a deep infection. Adequate debridement of an open femoral fracture demands wound extension (5).

Preoperative Planning

Initial debridement entails some insight by the initially treating surgeon into the definitive fixation plan. Frequently, the entire approach for the eventual repair of an open femur fracture may be performed at the time of debridement, particularly if this will include plating of a distal femur fracture. Open fractures of the femoral diaphysis may still be treated quite successfully with intramedullary nailing after wound extension and debridement (13). Regardless of eventual fixation plan, proximal and distal extension of soft tissue wounds is always necessary.

Surgery

Extension of the skin laceration is performed both proximally and distally down to the investing fascia of the thigh, which is always torn due to the pre-existing trauma. Fracture exposure will often require intramuscular dissection. Specific landmarks or structures to avoid will vary depending on location of the open wounds. Extensive dissection through muscle may be required, but most of this muscle has been traumatized and may not be viable. It is exactly this tissue that must be removed for the adequate debridement of the open femoral fracture and the prevention of a potential deep infection.

If, following aggressive irrigation and debridement, it is determined that a transarticular spanning external fixation is going to be used for definitive or temporary stabilization, consideration must be given to the underlying soft tissues. In applying joint spanning external fixation, one should be careful to place the femoral pins proximal enough that the eventual internal fixation is not communicating with the pin sites if at all possible. Femoral pins may be introduced directly anterior through the quadriceps, anterolateral, or directly lateral. Tibial pins are generally introduced anteromedially. Spanning external fixation may be maintained for several weeks while waiting for physiologic or soft tissue stabilization. Nowotarski et al. demonstrated in non-spanning external fixation that patients could safely undergo one-stage conversion to internal fixation without significant infectious problems (11). However, waiting much longer than 3 weeks may create problems in having to take down interval callus formation and makes the articular reconstruction more difficult.

Postoperative Management

In an effort to stabilize the soft tissue envelope, initiation of range of motion may be delayed after open fracture of the distal femur. If an open distal femur fracture has been spanned with an external fixator, subsequent debridements may be necessary, and the exact timing of definitive internal fixation is at the surgeon's discretion.

If a thorough debridement and immediate intramedullary nailing of an open diaphyseal fracture has been completed, range of motion and weight bearing may be initiated right away.

Complications

The prompt and aggressive debridement of open fractures is an attempt to avoid the most obvious complication, osteomyelitis. Further complications from open fractures include knee stiffness and non-union. In cases with a segmental bone loss, or a high degree of metaphyseal comminution, patients may be informed at the time of definitive fixation that an elective bone grafting procedure will be performed 4 to 6 weeks later. The author prefers to use proximal tibial cancellous autograft, as it is biologically active, is a low morbidity harvest site when compared to iliac crest, and limits the affected area of the patient to a zone already involved in the injury. For large segmental defects, a cement spacer may be placed at the time of index fixation, with the plan to exploit the "biologic membrane" formed around this spacer to promote healing at the time of subsequent bone grafting (12).

JUDET QUADRICEPSPLASTY

Indications/Contraindications

Frequently, patients who have suffered comminuted intra-articular injuries of the distal femur or supracondylar femur will suffer from poor range of motion secondary to post-traumatic scarring and contracture. Various methods have been proposed for the treatment of this loss of flexion at the knee. Arthroscopic lysis, closed manipulation, and quadriceps tendon lengthening have all been advocated (15). For particularly stubborn cases of post-traumatic arthrofibrosis and quadriceps contracture leading to loss of knee flexion, the author finds the Judet quadricepsplasty to be the most effective way to regain functional motion of the knee (1,2,6,7,10,16).

This approach recognizes that, in addition to the skeletal injury apparent on the radiographs, there was great soft tissue damage sustained at the time of distal femoral fracture. It is this damage to the rectus and vastus musculature that is at least in part responsible for the subsequent loss of range of motion. Arthrofibrosis and capsular contracture also contribute to post-traumatic stiffness and are addressed by this operation.

Judet attributed the stiffness of the knee to four principle anatomic reasons. First was adhesion of the subquadricipital pouch with tethering of the patella. Second was retraction of the parapatellar fibrous elements and intra-articular adhesions. Third was adherence of the vastus intermedius muscle of the femur. Fourth was degenerative fibrosis of the quadriceps. The surgical procedure is based on a sequential release of these various parts of the contracture. Range of motion is to be assessed after each stage, and the operation proceeds until the desired results are achieved or maximum range of motion is achieved after completion of all steps.

Preoperative Planning

An epidural catheter is placed preoperatively. General and epidural anesthetic are used intraoperatively, but the regional anesthesia will help with patient compliance and tolerance with postoperative continuous passive motion.

Surgery

Range of motion is assessed on administration of the general anesthetic (Fig. 25-19). Two incisions are generally used (Fig. 25-20). The first is a medial parapatellar approach. This allows access to the medial aspect of the patellar tendon, the suprapatellar pouch medially, and the medial gutter. The medial retinaculum is released, and adhesions of the medial joint and suprapatellar pouch are excised.

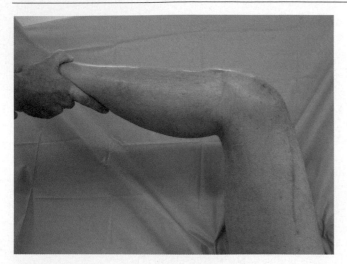

FIGURE 25-19
Range of motion is assessed preoperatively.

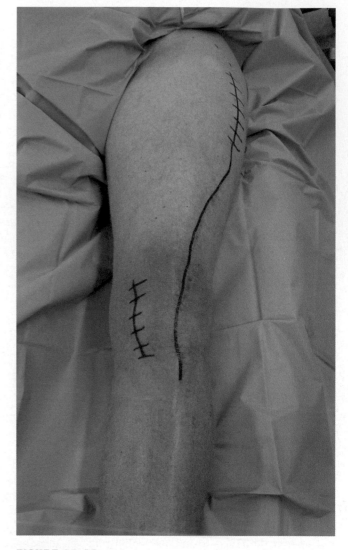

FIGURE 25-20
Two incisions planned preoperatively for Judet quadricepsplasty.

The second incision often follows the incision made from the operative repair of the fracture (Fig. 25-21). This will usually follow the lateral aspect of the patella ligament through the lateral patellar retinaculum and proximal up along the lateral intramuscular septum to the level of the greater trochanter. In the distal segment the parapatellar and lateral retinacular tissues are released and intra-articular adhesions are excised. The patella is freed until it may be easily lifted off the femoral condyles (Fig. 25-22). Scar tissue along the medial and lateral aspects of the patellar ligament, particularly distally, would likewise need to be excised. At this point, range of motion is checked, and the quadriceps may be manipulated at each subsequent step. The vastus lateralis is elevated from the linea aspera, and perforating vessels are ligated as they are encountered. The vastus intermedius is then lifted extraperiosteally from the front and side of the femur (Fig. 25-23). Much of the intermedius will be replaced by scar and fibrotic tissue, and much of this may be excised without significant functional impact (Fig. 25-24). Frequently, one will find heterotopic bone formation within the muscle bellies, and this may be excised along with fibrotic muscle tissue in an effort to regain length. Once again, the knee is manipulated and range assessed.

Next, the vastus lateralis is released from its femoral origin superolaterally, and the rectus femoris may be released from its origin on the anterior capsule (Figs. 25-25 and 25-26). This allows distal excursion of much of the quadriceps mechanism in an effort to regain range of motion at the knee. The knee is manipulated for a final time and final range of motion is measured (Fig. 25-27). Only the skin is closed, and a drain is used (Fig. 25-28). Given the somewhat sanguinous nature of the dissection along the well-perfused margins of scar tissue, postoperative hematoma must be guarded against, and drain use is encouraged.

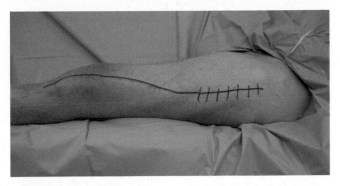

FIGURE 25-21

Lateral incision planned as extension (*dotted line*) off existing scar (*solid line*).

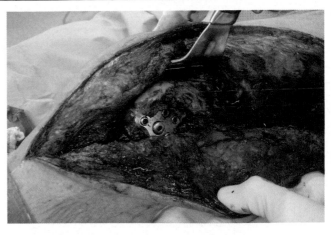

FIGURE 25-22

Supracondylar zone shows dense fibrotic scar tissue.

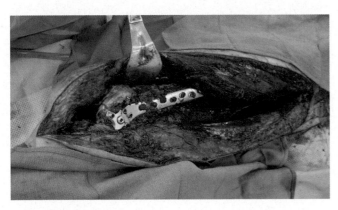

FIGURE 25-23

Scar tissue release mobilizes the extensor mechanism off the anterior femur.

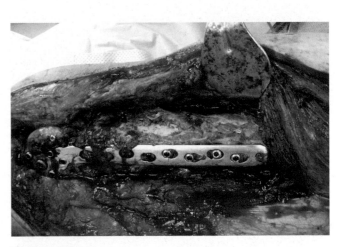

FIGURE 25-24

Heterotopic bone may scar the quadriceps to the femur and must be excised.

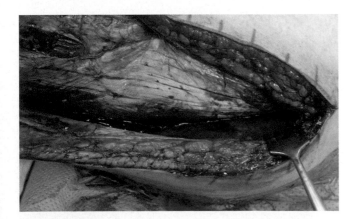

FIGURE 25-25

Disection may be extended up to the level of the vastus lateralis origin and the rectus origin anteriorly.

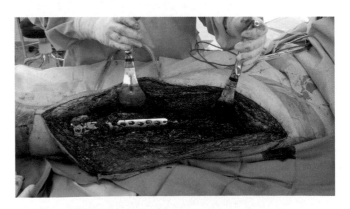

FIGURE 25-26

With release of the rectus proximally, ultimate excursion of the extensor mechanism may be achieved.

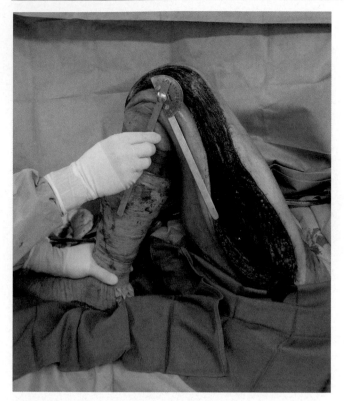

FIGURE 25-27

Ultimate range of motion should be assessed before and after closure.

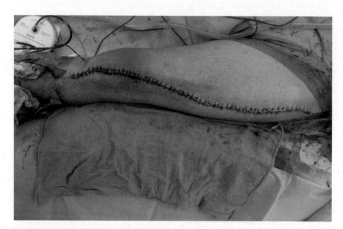

FIGURE 25-28

Final skin closure of the lateral incision.

Postoperative Management

The knee may be immobilized in a position of flexion so that, on awakening from anesthetic, the patient may have some idea of what the range of motion may be achieved (Fig. 25-29). Epidural anesthetic is generally used, and continuous passive motion is initiated after the recovery room. The drain is removed in approximately 48 hours. Due to the bleeding which may be encountered in dissection of scar and muscle, we have found that blood transfusion may be necessary before discharge.

No postoperative immobilization is typically used at the time of discharge, and patients may need crutches for ambulation, as they frequently will have a functional extensor lag postoperatively. This extensor lag resolves over time.

Complications/Results

The most common immediate complication following this procedure is hematoma formation. This complication can be minimized with intraoperative hemostasis and with the routine use of closed

FIGURE 25-29

Knee is immobilized in flexion postoperatively, and continuous passive motion is initiated after the recovery room.

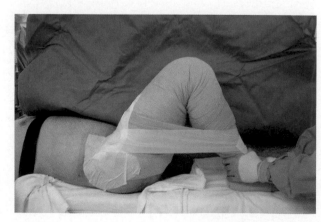

suction drains in all patients. Secondary complications include extensor lag, which will resolve in most cases with postoperative therapy. Recurrent stiffness and arthrofibrosis can also complicate postoperative results; however, the results of this operation in the literature have been encouraging (1,2,6,7,10,16), with total gains in range of motion between 55 to 69 degrees in the two largest series.

SUMMARY

The soft tissue around the femur and thigh segment is adequate enough to sustain extensive trauma without requiring free tissue transfer. Some of the techniques listed in this chapter may facilitate the correct handling of the soft tissues, help to prevent infection in the setting of open fracture, or help patients to regain motion after a comminuted supracondylar injury.

REFERENCES

1. Ali AM, Villafuerte J, Hashmi M, Saleh M. Judet's quadricepsplasty, surgical technique, and results in limb reconstruction. *Clin Orthop Relat Res.* 2003;(415):214–220.
2. Bellemans J, Steenwerckx A, Brabants K, Victor J, Lammens J, Fabry G. The Judet quadricepsplasty: a retrospective analysis of 16 cases. *Acta Orthop Belg.* 1996;62(2):79–82.
3. Gustilo RB, Anderson JT. Prevention of infection in the treatment of one thousand and twenty-five open fractures of long bones: retrospective and prospective analyses. *J Bone Joint Surg Am.* 1976;58(4):453–458.
4. Gustilo RB, Merkow RL, Templeman D. The management of open fractures. *J Bone Joint Surg Am.* 1990;72(2):299–304.
5. Giannoudis PV, Papakostidis C, Roberts C. A review of the management of open fractures of the tibia and femur. *J Bone Joint Surg Br.* 2006;88(3):281–289.
6. Daoud H, O'Farrell T, Cruess RL. Quadricepsplasty. The Judet technique and results of six cases. *J Bone Joint Surg Br.* 1982;64(2):194–197.
7. Judet R. Mobilisation of the stiff knee. *J Bone Joint Surg Br.* 1959;41B:856–857.
8. Koval KJ, Sala DA, Kummer FJ, Zuckerman JD. Postoperative weight-bearing after a fracture of the femoral neck or an intertrochanteric fracture. *J Bone Joint Surg Am.* 1998;80(3):352–356.
9. Martinet O, Cordey J, Harder Y, Maier A, Buhler M, Barraud GE. The epidemiology of fractures of the distal femur. *Injury.* 2000;31(suppl 3):C62–63.
10. Merchan EC, Myong C. Quadricepsplasty: the Judet technique and results of 21 posttraumatic cases. *Orthopedics.* 1992;15(9):1081–1085.
11. Nowotarski PJ, Turen CH, Brumback RJ, Scarboro JM. Conversion of external fixation to intramedullary nailing for fractures of the shaft of the femur in multiply injured patients. *J Bone Joint Surg Am.* 2000;82(6):781–788.
12. Pelissier P, Masquelet AC, Bareille R, Pelissier SM, Amedee J. Induced membranes secrete growth factors including vascular and osteoinductive factors and could stimulate bone regeneration. *J Orthop Res.* 2004;22(1):73–79.
13. Starr A, Bucholz R. *Fractures of the shaft of the femur.* Philadelphia: Lippincott Williams & Williams; 2001.
14. Starr AJ, Jones AL, Reinert CM. The "swashbuckler": a modified anterior approach for fractures of the distal femur. *J Orthop Trauma.* 1999;13(2):138–140.
15. Wang JH, Zhao JZ, He YH. A new treatment strategy for severe arthrofibrosis of the knee. A review of twenty-two cases. *J Bone Joint Surg Am.* 2006;88(6):1245–1250.
16. Warner JJ. The Judet quadricepsplasty for management of severe posttraumatic extension contracture of the knee. A report of a bilateral case and review of the literature. *Clin Orthop Relat Res.* 1990;(256):169–173.

26 Management of Soft Tissue Defects Surrounding the Knee and Tibia: The Gastrocnemius Muscle Flap

Steven Myerthall, David J. Jacofsky, and Steven L. Moran

Defects surrounding the knee and patellar region are common and may result from trauma, tumor, or infection. One of the most important goals in the management of open wounds surrounding the knee is stable soft tissue coverage. Soft tissue coverage with muscle can seal the joint and bone from ongoing contamination and help to revascularize underlying structures, while preventing the development of late infection and nonunion. Options for soft tissue coverage are determined by the size of the wound, location, and surrounding zone of injury. The gastrocnemius muscle flap has historically been used to cover defects surrounding the knee, lower thigh, and patellar region. Its consistent vascular anatomy and superficial location have made it a workhorse for coverage of defects in this area.

The gastrocnemius is the most superficial muscle of the posterior calf. The muscle has two heads arising from the medial and lateral condyles at the femur, and the adjacent capsule of the knee; these muscles then insert into the calcaneal tendon (Fig. 26-1). The two muscle heads, medial and lateral, unite at the level of the fibular head. Proceeding distally the muscles join with the tendon of the soleus at the mid-leg to form the Achilles tendon. The medial sural artery is the dominant vascular pedicle for the medial gastrocnemius muscle, whereas the lateral sural artery supplies the lateral head. The origin of the arteries is approximately 4 cm above the head of the fibula and both originate from the popliteal artery. Innervation to the muscles originates from the tibial nerve and lies posterior to the vascular pedicle as it enters the muscle.

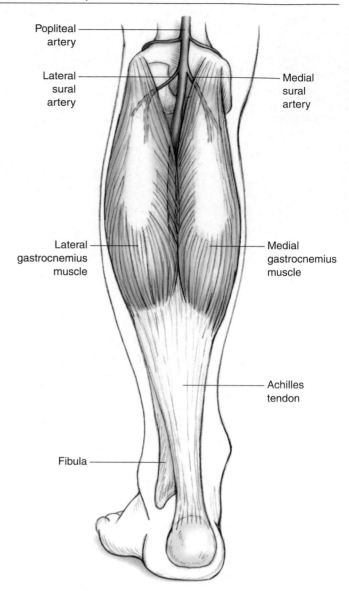

FIGURE 26-1

The medial and lateral gastrocnemius muscles as seen from the posterior approach.

INDICATIONS/CONTRAINDICATIONS

Both the medial and lateral gastrocnemius muscles may be used independently or in conjunction with each other. The medial gastrocnemius will cover the inferior thigh, knee, and proximal tibia. The medial head of the muscle is used most frequently as a proximally based flap due to its larger size in comparison to the lateral head of the muscle. The lateral head may also be used alone or in combination with the medial head for coverage of large tibial defects or for lateral distal thigh wounds. For defects at the level of the mid-portion of the tibia, the gastrocnemius muscle may not provide adequate coverage and the soleus muscle is preferred for coverage of middle third defects. For defects involving the distal third of the tibia and ankle, free tissue transfer is usually required. The tendinous inferior margin of the gastrocnemius muscle may be used to augment the repair of an injured suprapatellar tendon.

Contraindications to the use of the gastrocnemius muscle flap include active infection and/or significant disruption of the soft tissue and/or vascular pedicle. Additional contraindications for flap use include any procedure or injury which may have traumatized or injured the sural artery, such as a previous repair of a popliteal arterial laceration or repair of popliteal aneurysm. Occasionally, severe compartment syndromes may render the muscle fibrotic and useable for transfer, but due to its superficial location and high take off of the sural artery, this is unusual. Direct trauma to the posterior calf may result in muscle destruction and should be ruled out prior to proceeding with flap elevation. Radiation to the knee following tumor extirpation may also compromise the vascular pedicle, increasing the chance of total or partial muscle necrosis following transfer. The muscle should not be used if the soleus and contralateral gastrocnemius muscle are no longer functional, as this will create postoperative difficulty with plantar flexion. A history of a recent deep venous thrombosis within the involved extremity is a relative contraindication for the use of the flap, although we have used the flap successfully in such situations.

Distally based gastrocnemius muscle flaps have been described for coverage of middle third and lower leg defects. Vascular supply to the muscle in these cases is supplied through crossing anastomotic arterial connections between the medial and lateral gastrocnemius muscle bellies extending across the midline raphe. Use of the flap in this manner is not common, as more reliable methods of middle third and lower leg coverage are available and include the soleus muscle flap, the sural artery flap, and free flap coverage.

PREOPERATIVE PLANNING

The preoperative management of severe open fractures involves stabilization of the patient, tetanus prophylaxis, and broad-spectrum antibiotics. Trauma often compromises the availability of the skin and soft tissue surrounding the knee. Nonviable tissue requires aggressive debridement. Serial debridements may be needed if tissue viability is uncertain. Once the wound bed is clean, flap coverage may proceed, ideally within 72 to 96 hours following initial injury. Preoperative physical examination should focus on determining the function of the remaining muscles of the lower leg to determine if sacrifice of the gastrocnemius could result in a significant loss of plantar flexor following muscle transfer. A vascular examination should also be performed to assess for the patency of the popliteal artery. In those patients with a history of peripheral vascular disease or a history of popliteal arterial trauma, an angiogram can confirm patency of the sural artery prior to surgery.

SURGERY

Patient Positioning

Operating room setup is standard for lower extremity coverage. A leg tourniquet may facilitate dissection, especially in cases of lateral gastrocnemius harvest where the perineal nerve must be identified and protected during flap elevation.

The muscle may be harvested with the patient in prone or supine position. If the patient is prone, a stockinette or mid-posterior S-shaped incision is made and significantly facilitates exposure of the muscle's origin posteriorly over the femoral condyle. The posterior approach is made with an incision starting 5 cm above the popliteal crease and extending down to the distal end of the muscle belly. More commonly, however, for anterior traumatic defects surrounding the patellar and tibial region, the patient is positioned in the supine position with the leg internally or externally rotated to facilitate exposure of the medial or lateral heads, respectively. Lateral decubitus positioning is also an option for lateral gastrocnemius muscle elevation.

The patient may receive either general or spinal anesthesia. In additional, depending on associated injuries, the ipsilateral or contralateral thigh should be prepared for a skin graft donor site. After sterile preparation, the entire extremity is draped and fully exposed. Appropriate preoperative antibiotics should be given 30 to 60 minutes prior to incision.

Technique

Medial Gastrocnemius Muscle Flap   A longitudinal incision is made where the separation of the bellies of the gastrocnemius and soleus muscle can be palpated. This should parallel the medial border of the tibia and can be curved proximally in a posterior direction to facilitate exposure and dissection of the proximal portion of the muscle. The incision should extend from the level of the tibial plateau to 10 cm above the medial malleolus. If the flap is to be tunneled into position on the anteromedial aspect of the leg, a skin bridge of at least 7 cm must be maintained to prevent skin necrosis. For more anterior defects, or preexisting peripatellar defects, a curved incision can be extended both proximally and distally from the defect site to a line 4 cm medial to the edge of the tibia (Fig. 26-2A,B).

During initial subcutaneous dissection, the saphenous vein is identified and preserved (Fig. 26-2C). The underlying deep investing fascia of the leg is then opened to expose the plane between the

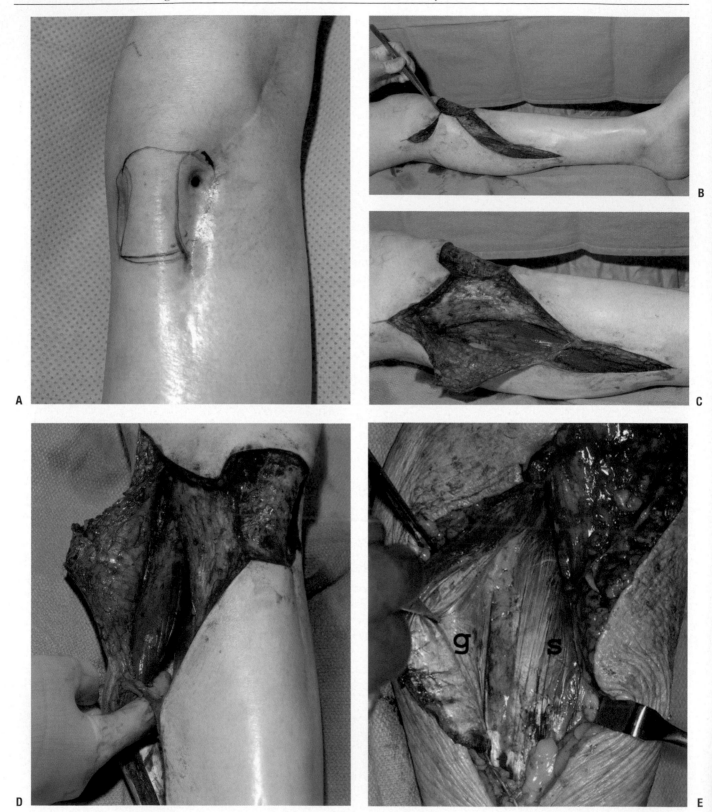

FIGURE 26-2

A: A 53-year-old patient with longstanding osteomyelitis of the tibia requiring debridement and soft tissue coverage. **B:** The skin surrounding the defect is excised. The bone is debrided and filled with antibiotic beads. The skin defect is incorporated into the skin incision for exposure of the gastrocnemius muscle. The skin incision is curved posterior approximately 4 cm beyond the medial border of the tibia. **C:** This incision gives excellent exposure of the posterior compartment. Note that the saphenous vein has been preserved at the inferior extent of the skin incision. **D,E:** The deep investing fascia of the leg is divided and the plane between the gastrocnemius and the soleus muscle may be identified using finger dissection. *(Continued)*

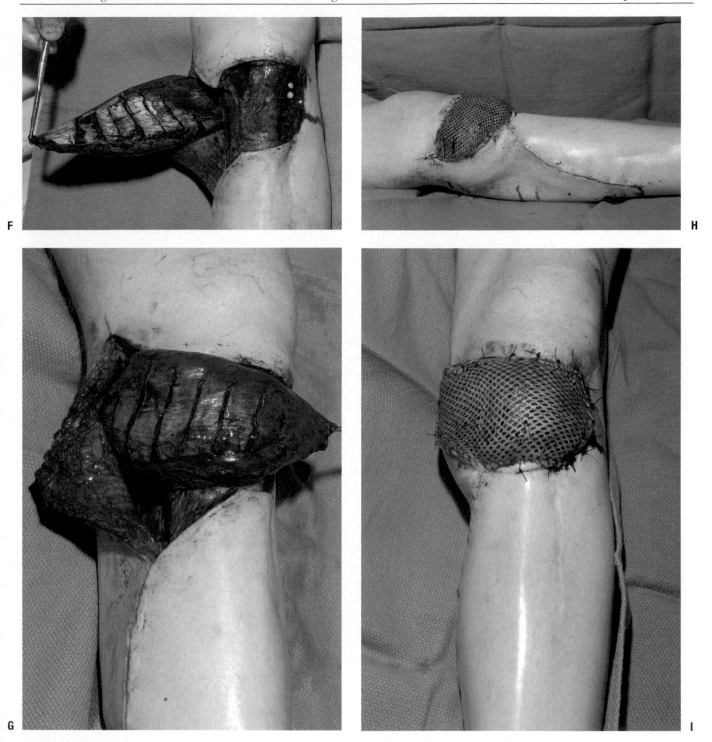

FIGURE 26-2

Continued **F,G:** Once the muscle is mobilized, the anterior and posterior fascia may be transversely scored to allow for easier insetting. **H,I:** Once the muscle is inset, it is covered with a split thickness skin graft. The leg incision is closed over a suction drain. g, gastrocnemius; s, soleus.

gastrocnemius and soleus muscles (Fig. 26-2D,E). In most patients, the plantaris tendon is located in this interval and should be left intact. This plane is easily opened with blunt finger dissection. The plane between the external fascia of the muscle and the overlying skin should also be opened using blunt dissection. Large, perforating vessel can be identified running from the muscle to the overlying skin. These vessels serve as the main blood supply to the skin paddle of a gastrocnemius fasciocutaneous flap. These vessels should be ligated in the gastrocnemius muscle flap dissection. The sural nerve and lesser saphenous vein can be identified running between the medial and lateral heads of the gastrocnemius muscle and should be preserved.

Dissection is then continued medially between the plane of the gastrocnemius and the soleus until the midline raphe of the gastrocnemius muscle is identified. Often this raphe will be identified by decasations of the muscle fibers distally. More proximally, the two heads may be more easily separated and identified if the raphe is not clearly visualized distally. Once the limits of the medial muscle have been clearly identified, the inferior margin of the muscle is divided from the Achilles tendon with a 2-cm cuff of tendon, which facilitates insetting of the muscle. This cuff of tendon is also very valuable for reconstruction of the terminal extensor mechanism of the quadriceps muscle.

The sural nerve will be identified within the gastrocnemius raphe and should be preserved. Using cautery, the raphe can be divided and the gastrocnemius can be separated from the Achilles tendon. At this point, the muscle may be pedicled and mobilized for coverage of the upper one-third of the lower leg. If the knee or distal thigh requires coverage, the origin of the muscle will require release. For release from the femoral condyle, posterior extension of the skin incision significantly facilitates visualization of the muscle's vascular pedicle. Skeletonization of the sural vessels from the deep surface of the muscle will also allow further mobilization of the muscle. The muscle can be transferred with either its deep or superficial surfaces exposed. Cross-hatching or removal of the fascia will allow for further mobility and advancement of the muscle without impairing blood supply (Fig. 26-2F,G).

The fascia is then inset into the defect using horizontal mattress sutures, pulling the muscle beneath the overlying skin on the far side of the defect. If there is excessive tension, sutures may be mattressed through the skin and tied over bolster dressings. Prior to inset, a 10-mm flat or round drain can be placed under the flap; a second drain should be placed at the donor site prior to closure.

A meshed skin graft should then be obtained and placed on the transposed muscle flap, followed by a bolster dressing. This dressing should include a nonadherent layer followed by a bolster with gentle compression maintained on the graft. A VAC sponge may also be applied to facilitate skin graft take to the underlying muscle (Fig. 26-2H,I). The remainder of the wound should be covered with sterile dressings and the leg placed in a knee immobilizer for support. The skin graft donor site may be dressed with a single-layer transparent dressing.

Lateral Gastrocnemius Muscle   The lateral gastrocnemius muscle will cover the inferior thigh, knee, and proximal tibia. For harvesting of the lateral gastrocnemius the skin incision is made at the posterior midline of the lower calf extending to the lateral popliteal fossa. The proximal mark is placed 2 or 3 cm posterior to the fibula. Once again, an adequate skin bridge must be maintained between the traumatic defect and the incision to avoid skin bridge necrosis. Alternatively, the existing skin defect may be extended proximally and distally over the posterior margin of the fibula to allow for exposure of the muscle (Fig. 26-3).

Dissection begins 5 to 6 fingerbreadths below the fibular head so as not to encounter the peroneal nerve. Once the plane between the soleus and gastrocnemius is clearly identified, superficial dissection can begin between the gastrocnemius and the investing fascia of the lower leg. The common peroneal nerve must be identified at the level of the neck of the fibula and protected throughout the rest of the dissection. Since the common peroneal nerve passes between the lateral head of the gastrocnemius and the tendon of the biceps femoris, particular attention should be paid to identify the nerve during this portion of the dissection. The muscle is then separated as described for the medial gastrocnemius muscle flap, and may then be pedicled into the overlying defect site (Fig. 26-4).

The flap is inset, and the donor site closed as previously described for the medial gastrocnemius flap.

POSTOPERATIVE MANAGEMENT

The patient should be maintained on bed rest for 5 to 7 days. The bolster dressing may be removed on postoperative day 5 to ensure adequate skin graft "take." Following skin graft take, Xeroform dressing changes are performed once to twice a day until the skin graft has matured, at which point the patient is encouraged to keep the skin graft lubricated with a petroleum-based lotion to prevent desiccation of the newly grafted skin. If immediate postoperative motion is essential, the origin of the gastrocnemius muscle should be divided to minimize forces across the flap in the early postoperative period. A VAC sponge may also aid in securing skin grafts if immediate motion is essential.

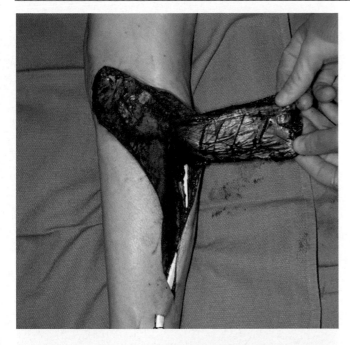

FIGURE 26-3

The incision for exposure of the lateral gastrocnemius muscle flap is made 2–3 cm posterior to the fibula.

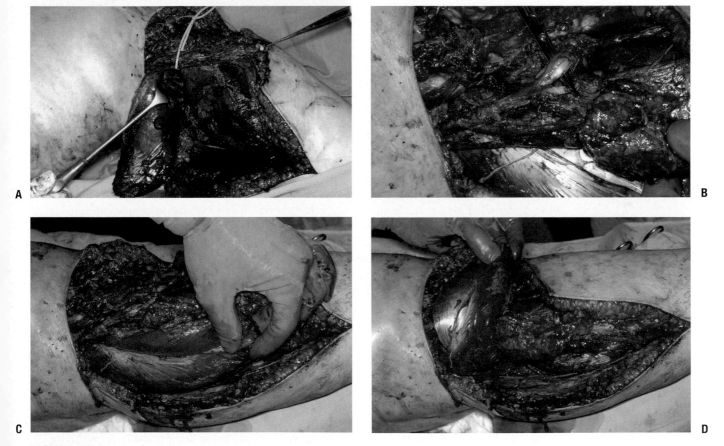

FIGURE 26-4

A: A traumatic lateral tibial and patellar defect in 28-year-old woman. The lateral gastrocnemius muscle has been harvested with a posterior and inferior incision extended from the original defect site. Note that the common perineal nerve has been identified and marked with blue vessel loop. The soleus muscle belly (*s*) can be seen below the gastrocnemius muscle (*g*). **B:** The common perineal nerve (seen here running above the scissors) must be identified prior to pedicling the flap into the defect site to ensure it is not inadvertently compressed or injured during flap insetting. **C,D:** Once the lateral gastrocnemius muscle is isolated from midline raphe, it can easily reach the lateral aspect of the peri-patellar region.

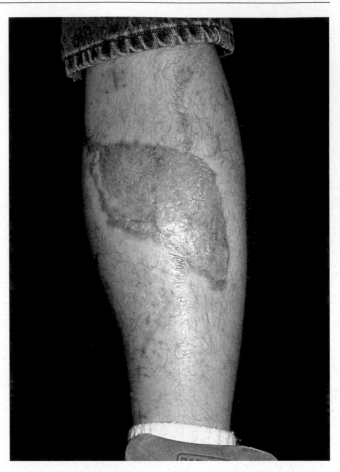

FIGURE 26-5

A 2-year follow-up of a 35-year-old man who underwent medial gastrocnemius muscle coverage for exposed tibia following a motor vehicle accident. Significant improvement in contour is obtained with long-term use of a compression wrap or compression stocking.

The drains are removed once drainage is less than 30 mL/day. Gentle range of motion should then begin at 10 to 14 days, increasing the motion by 5 or 10 degrees per day. Ambulation can begin on the postoperative day 10, with knee flexion limited with the use of a knee immobilizer. If the flap is inset under tension or if the healing environment is less than ideal, the knee immobilizer can be maintained for an additional week to prevent undo tension on the margins of the muscle flap.

Postoperative swelling is minimized with the use of elastic wraps or supportive stockings. Compression stockings worn long-term can facilitate flap contouring. Muscle flaps undergo a process of atrophy over 6 to 12 months; patient concerns regarding scaring or flap contour should not be addressed surgically until 12 to 24 months following the initial reconstructive surgery (Fig. 26-5).

COMPLICATIONS

Complications following the use of the gastrocnemius muscle flap include bleeding, infection, nerve injury, and flap loss. Bleeding (hematoma) and infection are most common, though rare if meticulous hemostasis is achieved at closure and aggressive debridement of the wound is performed prior to muscle flap transfer. Suction drains placed within the donor site at the time of closure will significantly minimize the risk of postoperative hematoma formation.

Partial flap necrosis or complete flap loss is usually associated with technical error, including injury to the vascular pedicle and/or excessive tension with secondary flap ischemia. If flap ischemia is suspected intraoperatively, the vascular pedicle should be examined for signs of kinking or injury to the sural artery. Small areas of skin graft loss may be seen postoperatively, but can be conservatively managed with topical ointments and wound care without the need for further surgical intervention.

Nerve injury is uncommon with meticulous dissection and nerve preservation. Injury to the sural nerve can occur during separation of the medial and lateral heads of the gastrocnemius muscle. Injury to the common perineal nerve may occur during elevation of the lateral gastrocnemius flap. Nerve injury is best avoided by clearly visualizing the nerve prior to flap transfer. The saphenous nerve may be ligated inadvertently with the saphenous vein during exposure of the posterior compartment; attempts should be made at nerve identification and preservation during flap dissection.

The gastrocnemius muscle provides plantar flexion of the foot and flexion of the knee joint. Removal of the muscle does not result in significant morbidity, although some loss of plantar flexion may lessen jumping and leaping ability. Either or both heads may be used with little functional deficit as long as the soleus muscle is preserved and uninjured.

RECOMMENDED READING

Arnold PG, Mixter RC. Making the most of the gastrocnemius muscles. *Plast Reconstr Surg.* 1983;72:38.

Bengston S, Carlsson A, Relanber M, et al. Treatement of the exposed knee prosthesis. *Acta Orthop Scand.* 1987;58:662.

Bos GD, Buehler MJ. Lower-extremity local flaps. *J Am Acad Orthop Surg.* 1994:2:342–351.

Dibbell DG, Edstrom LE. The gastrocnemius myocutaneous flap. *Clin Plast Surg.* 1983;7:43.

Ger R. The management of pretibial skin loss. *Surgery.* 1968:63:757–763.

Hersh CK, Schenck RC, Williams RP. The versatility of the gastrocnemius muscle flap. *Am J Orthop.* 1995;24(3):218–222.

McCraw JB, Arnold PG. *McCraw and Arnold's atlas of muscle and musculocutaneous flaps.* Norfolk: Hampton Press Publishing; 1986:491–543.

Pico R, Luscher NJ, Rometsch M, et al. Why the denervated gastrocnemius muscle flap should be encouraged. *Ann Plast Surg.* 1991;26:312–324.

Mathes SJ, Nahai F. *Reconstructive surgery principles, anatomy, and technique.* New York: Churchill Livingstone; 1997.

27 Revision and Infected Total Knee Arthroplasty

Henry D. Clarke, William J. Casey III, and Mark J. Spangehl

INDICATIONS/CONTRAINDICATIONS

Soft tissue management in revision and infected total knee arthroplasty (TKA) is an extremely important factor in determining the success or failure of the procedure. Without optimal wound healing, complication rates increase and the ultimate benefit of the operation may be diminished. Despite the critical role played by the soft tissues surrounding the knee, very little scientific data exist to help guide the practicing orthopaedic surgeon in this area. Rather, most of the recommendations and guidelines are based on extrapolations from other surgical fields and anecdotal experience from experts in knee arthroplasty. In this chapter, important factors that should be considered in the preoperative, intraoperative, and postoperative settings are reviewed. In addition, surgical techniques that may minimize potential soft tissue problems and help manage complications when they do occur are also presented. The soft tissues about the knee include skin and subcutaneous coverage, as well as the extensor mechanism; therefore, in this chapter management of both of these important components is addressed.

The very circumstances that necessitate revision TKA in the settings of either infection or aseptic failure require that every patient be considered at risk for soft tissue complications. Therefore, every patient in whom revision TKA is being considered should be thoroughly evaluated preoperatively. This allows all necessary plans to be addressed in order to meet individual needs. Indeed, absolute indications and contradictions are difficult to define: rather, all factors should be considered. While any patient who undergoes revision TKA should be considered at risk for soft tissue complications, some patients will have greater risks. A healthy patient with just one prior knee surgery, with aseptic loosening, is at less risk than a patient with diabetes and peripheral vascular disease who has a chronically infected total knee replacement. However, each patient should be carefully assessed. Certainly, once the risks have been evaluated, a decision to proceed with revision TKA surgery should be based on the individual circumstances. In each case, the current symptoms, including pain and disability, presence or absence of prosthetic infection, and age and activity demands of the patient, must be evaluated in the context of the potential risks. The potential increase in symptoms, time frame for deterioration, and additional surgical problems that may be encountered by delaying surgery should also be considered. Absolute contraindications for revision TKA include irreversible medical comorbidities that raise the risk of perioperative mortality to unacceptable levels, an avascular extremity where revascularization options have been exhausted, uncontrolled sepsis, and neurologic injuries with no motor function of the extremity. Relative contraindications include failed prior soft tissue flaps, massive bone loss, recurrent prosthetic infection, extensor mechanism disruption, and unstable medical comorbidities that require optimization. When the potential risks are too great, or when other rare circumstances are encountered, such as life-threatening sepsis or an avascular limb, alternative procedures including permanent resection arthroplasty, knee arthrodesis, or amputation may be required.

PREOPERATIVE PLANNING

Preoperative planning is critical for minimizing soft tissue problems about the knee. Both systemic factors and the characteristics of the knee and leg should be considered before revision knee surgery.

Systemic Factors

Patient-specific medical comorbidities should be assessed and treated before surgery (Table 27-1). While optimization of these conditions appears to reduce the risk of developing wound complications after revision TKA, the increased risk of wound problems in many cases is multi-factorial and does not return to baseline levels even when medical management is optimal. For example, the increased risks of delayed wound healing and infection noted in patients with diabetes appears to be caused by both the hyperglycemia, which has been shown to inhibit collagen synthesis, disrupt fibroblast proliferation, slow capillary in-growth, and deficiencies in polymorphonuclear neutrophil cell function. Furthermore, the increased risk of soft tissue complications in patients with rheumatoid arthritis is likely due to numerous factors including the long-term sequelae of corticosteroid use, which regulates macrophage function, reduces collagen synthesis, and delays vascular in-growth, as well as direct causes of the disease itself such as skin atrophy, decreased albumin, and vasculitis.

Another important risk factor in the pre- and postoperative periods is the use of tobacco products. Nicotine and its metabolites cause vasoconstriction, which interferes with micro-circulation; however, the effects on wound healing are more profound than from vasoconstriction alone. Other constituents of tobacco smoke, such as carbon monoxide, reduce the oxygen carrying capabilities of hemoglobin, which reduces tissue oxygenation. Nicotine also appears to have a direct effect on fibroblast and immune function. The optimal time for smoking cessation appears to be 4 to 8 weeks preoperatively, but even a week of abstinence appears to reduce the risk of complications. Abstinence in the entire postoperative period is also critical. For elective procedures, all patients who smoke and have other risk factors for wound healing must stop smoking before the procedure. In some cases, professional services must be used to achieve this end. The use of nicotine delivery substitutes are controversial, as these do not eliminate the patient's use of nicotine but do eliminate multiple other toxic substances that are inhaled in tobacco smoke, such as carbon monoxide and hydrogen cyanide. Therefore, while not an optimal solution, in certain circumstances these substitutes may be preferable to reduce the overall risk.

TABLE 27-1.   Complicating Comorbidities

Condition	Evaluation	Management
Diabetes	Blood glucose	Optimize diet and medication.
Malnutrition	Total lymphocyte count < 1,500 mm^3 Serum albumin < 3.4 g/dL	Nutritional supplements before surgery
Inflammatory arthritis	Review disease modifying medications	Hold medications, if possible, until wound healing has occurred.
Tobacco smoking	Serum kotinine level if poor abstinence/compliance	Avoid tobacco use 1 month before surgery.
Anemia	Hgb/Hct	Correct before surgery with erythropoietin injections.
Hypoxia	SaO^2	Optimize pulmonary function.
Peripheral vascular disease	Peripheral pulses, Doppler ultrasound, arteriogram	Revascularization prior to revision TKA
Obesity	BMI	Avoid significant weight loss in the immediate pre- or postoperative periods.
Cancer	History	Avoid elective surgery, if possible, while on chemotherapeutic agents.
Chronic corticosteroid use	History	> 2 years duration appears to increase risks of wound complications

BMI, body mass index; TKA, total knee arthroplasty.

The Knee

The local vascular anatomy of the knee can be unforgiving; in comparison to the hip, where wound necrosis is rarely a problem. Most of the perfusion to the skin is derived from perforator vessels that originate below the level of the deep fascia. Little subcutaneous communication occurs; rather, the perforating vessels connect at the level of the sub dermal plexus. Thus, when raising skin flaps about the knee, the dissection should be below the level of the deep fascia, rather than in the sub dermal plane to avoid damaging this superficial plexus. While the peri-patellar plexus formed by the medial and lateral, superior and inferior genicular arteries has been well described, the majority of the inflow to the skin appears to be derived from the medial side of the knee in the distribution of the saphenous and descending genicular arteries. Therefore, laterally based flaps should be avoided and any prior laterally biased vertical incision should be carefully considered when selecting the optimal incision. On the lateral side, the perforators from the superior and inferior genicular arteries are relatively more important, and it has been reported that use of a lateral patellar release with disruption of the superior genicular artery is associated with decreased tissue oxygenation and increased lateral wound problems. Some general guidelines for selection and placement of skin incisions follow.

A single, longitudinal anterior midline incision provides the most extensile exposure and is preferred for all revision and infected total knee replacement cases. Prior incisions about the knee should be carefully evaluated. Factors that are believed to be important, although little scientific data exist to support these suppositions, include age, orientation, length, and placement in relation to other or intended incisions. A single, transverse incision can be crossed by a new perpendicular anterior incision with relatively little concern. When a single, prior longitudinal anterior incision exists, this incision should be used. If placement of this prior incision is not directly midline, the proximal and distal ends of the incision may be extended back toward the midline to reduce tension on the wound. In these cases, subcutaneous dissection should be minimized; it is critical to maintain full-thickness flaps if the subcutaneous tissues must be mobilized to allow adequate exposure of the extensor mechanism. To preserve the sub dermal plexus, these flaps should be raised at the level of the deep fascia. If the prior incision is located far from the midline, and would necessitate creation of a large laterally based subcutaneous flap, one may consider using a new incision. In these circumstances, skin bridges greater than 3 to 5 cm should be maintained between the new and old incisions. When multiple incisions, or a single anterior incision located well away from the midline, are encountered, selection of the optimal incision should be carefully considered. In some circumstances where numerous prior incisions exist, or where the skin and subcutaneous tissues have been severely damaged by prior trauma, radiation exposure, infection, or are atrophic, due to systemic conditions, preoperative soft tissue management techniques that are described in following sections, such as soft tissue expansion or soft tissue flaps, may be required. Again, little definitive data exist to guide the surgeon when these interventions are absolutely required; rather, much of this assessment is subjective.

SURGERY

Soft Tissue Procedures

Sham Incision

TECHNIQUE   The sham incision or delay procedure is reviewed primarily for its historical significance as an early attempt to manage patients considered at risk for wound healing problems after TKA. Approximately 10 to 14 days before the planned knee procedure, the intended skin incision is made and extended to the level of the extensor mechanism. Next, the skin is undermined on both sides of the incision to expose the extensor mechanism, as required for the upcoming knee replacement, and then the incision is closed and observed. If the wound heals without complications, the intended knee procedure is subsequently performed. If skin necrosis occurs, a soft tissue flap is performed before knee replacement. The main advantage in these cases is that the knee joint has not been violated, and there is no prosthesis at risk for infection. Furthermore, increased collateral flow caused by the incision due to the delay phenomenon was felt to reduce the risk of subsequent wound healing problems. More contemporary soft tissue expansion techniques have, for the most part, eliminated the use of the sham incision.

RESULTS There is little except anecdotal evidence to support the use of this technique. Rothaus has detailed the outcomes in a small group of 12 patients, with multiple prior incisions, in whom this technique was used. In all 12 patients, the incisions healed and TKA was successfully performed without wound healing problems.

Soft Tissue Expanders

TECHNIQUE The concept of tissue expansion is not new and has been successfully used in a variety of soft tissue reconstructive procedures throughout the body. Despite the challenges posed by the unforgiving nature of the vascular supply around the knee, the use of tissue expanders is a relatively new concept with only a limited number of large patient series.

Tissue expansion has three important benefits that aid wound healing in the overlying soft tissues. First, and probably most important, it stimulates neo-vascularization of the overlying soft tissue; this improves the capillary in-flow that directly promotes healing. Second, it physically expands the overlying skin and subcutaneous tissue allowing larger areas, due to correction of malalignment or limb lengthening, to be covered. This also reduces the tension on the wound. This expansion is not simply a stretching and thinning of the overlying soft tissue, which would leave the flap less resilient, but actually a hypertrophy of the dermis and epidermis due to fibroblast stimulation, leading to an increase in the quantity of tissue available. Third, a fibrous capsule develops around the expander, and this thick, robust, vascular tissue is very useful as a "pseudo-fascial" layer to close over the joint and is particularly helpful in the area of the proximal medial tibia where the periosteum and soft tissue layer can be thin.

The technique for soft tissue expansion over the knee is begun approximately 6 to 8 weeks prior to the intended TKA (Fig. 27-1). Typically two to four 200 to 300 mL expanders are placed in pockets deep to the subcutaneous layer, just above the fascia (see Fig. 27-1C). These pockets are strategically placed based on the placement of prior incisions and characteristics of the overlying subcutaneous tissue and skin. The first step involves infiltrating the deep subcutaneous layer with a dilute solution composed of 1000 mL Ringer's lactate, 50 mL 1% lidocaine, and 1 mL 1:1000 epinephrine to create a pocket. Typically, injection of 250 to 300 mL of this solution is sufficient to produce the hydro-dissection that separates the skin and subcutaneous tissue from the underlying fascia to create a pocket. Also, use of the local anesthetic helps with postoperative pain relief. Next, through a short incision placed in one of the prior incisions, scissors are used to bluntly define and enlarge this plane within the deep subcutaneous tissue to create a pocket (see Fig. 27-1B). The un-inflated expander is then inserted through the same incision (see Fig. 27-1D). The access port to the expander is then tunneled through the subcutaneous tissue to an easily accessible site. The port should be accessed prior to skin closure and saline injected to ensure that the port is functional and that the expander was not damaged during the insertion. After this initial expansion, the incision is closed and a sterile dressing applied. Patients are typically placed in a knee immobilizer for a week and allowed to weight bear as tolerated. Most patients are admitted for an overnight stay and treated with 24 hours of intravenous antibiotics. Subsequently each week, about 10% to 15% of the volume of the expander is infused with the patient as an outpatient, via the access port. If at any time the overlying skin blanches and doesn't recover after a few minutes of observation, or if the patient experiences significant pain, saline must be removed until the problem is alleviated.

At the time of the intended TKA, the expanders are extracted through the incision used for the procedure (see Fig. 27-1F). The subcutaneous tissue and skin flaps should be protected during the TKA. At the end of the procedure, a superficial drain is placed in each individual expander pocket. These drains are removed individually once output is less than 10 mL per 8 hours or 30 mL per 24 hours. This protocol appears to reduce the risk of subcutaneous hematoma formation. Early in the experience of tissue expansion about the knee when subcutaneous drains were not routinely employed, hematomas occurred more frequently and occasionally had to be drained to reduce tension on the overlying tissue. During wound closure, the expansion process may have created excessive amounts of soft tissue that need to be excised. In these cases, the edge of the flap, especially focusing on old widened scars, can be trimmed or removed. However, the tension on the wound should not be increased by resecting too much surplus tissue.

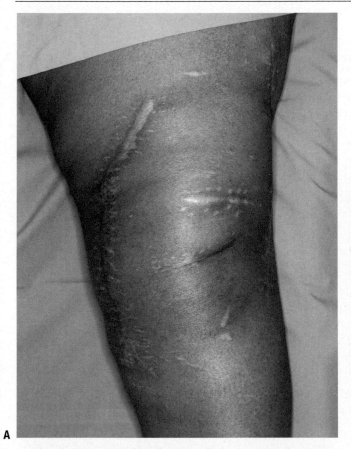

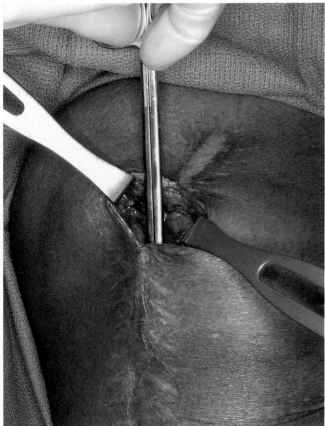

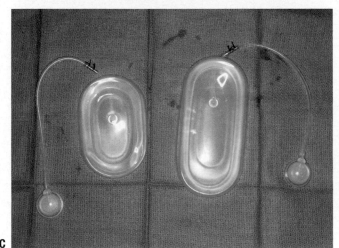

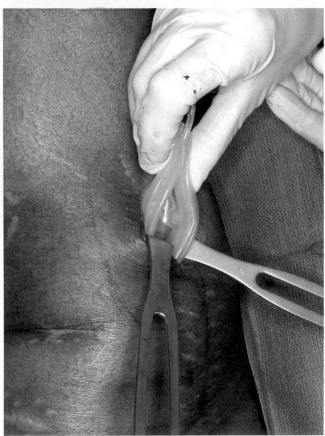

FIGURE 27-1

A: Knee with multiple prior vertical and horizontal incisions at risk for poor postoperative wound healing after TKA. **B:** Creation of subcutaneous pocket for soft tissue expander. **C:** Saline expanders demonstrating access portals for infusing saline. **D:** Insertion of the deflated saline soft tissue expander. *(Continued)*

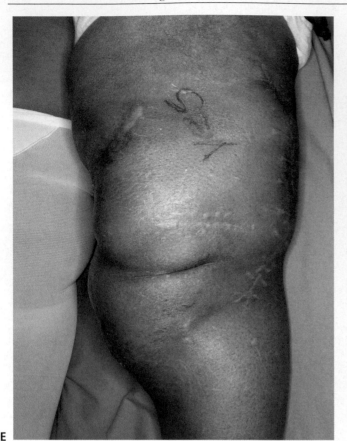

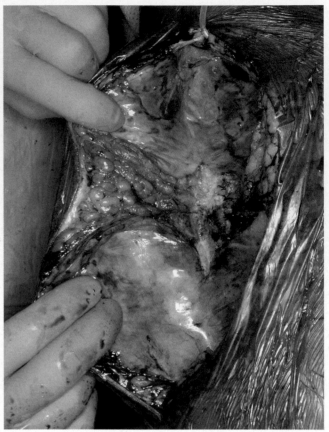

FIGURE 27-1

Continued **E:** Knee after tissue expansion process is complete. **F:** Fibrous, vascular membrane that surrounds the expander cavity after removal of the expander at the time of TKA.

RESULTS   Few large series of tissue expansion in association with TKA have been published, with most reports presenting only a handful of cases. The morbidity associated with the use of tissue expanders has been previously reported and includes infection, hematoma, expander rupture or deflation, and skin necrosis. Two significant papers have reported very favorable results. In an initial study, no significant complications occurred during the expansion process in a small group of 10 patients. In a second larger group of 29 knees, six (21%) minor wound complications occurred during expansion, including mild erythema or skin blistering. These complications were successfully managed by reducing the volume in the expander, and delaying further expansion until the problem resolved. In this same group, one major complication occurred after the insertion of the soft tissue expanders; this involved full-thickness skin necrosis in a patient with a history of radiation to the anterior knee. The knee replacement was subsequently not performed, as the patient declined to accept a prophylactic muscle flap, choosing to endure her arthritic symptoms.

Following the knee replacement, 5 (18%) of 29 patients experienced minor complications; three knees developed persistent drainage, and two knees developed subcutaneous hematomas. The persistent drainage resolved after wound compression and immobilization was initiated. The two subcutaneous hematomas required surgical evacuation, and it was these problems that prompted the use of subcutaneous drains in the expander pockets.

Soft Tissue Flap Coverage Procedures

Soft tissue flap procedures about the knee have been used both prophylactically and for salvage of wound complications about the knee. Although a large number of different techniques have been described, including simple skin grafts, random or axial pattern skin flaps, fasciocutaneous flaps, and rotational or free muscle flaps, the most reliable and most frequently used tissues about the knee include medial gastrocnemius muscle flaps, and free latissimus dorsi or rectus abdominus flaps. In addition to these techniques, the development of musculocutaneous perforator flaps during the past decade has provided another alternative for coverage about the knee. The principles involved in these three types of techniques are described following in ascending order of the extent of the area that can be adequately managed.

Musculocutaneous Perforator Flaps   The development of musculocutaneous perforator flaps in plastic surgery occurred during the 1990s as an extension of the generally very favorable experience with musculocutaneous flaps during the 1980s. Perforator flaps were based on the principle that neither the underlying fascial plexus, nor muscle, was required if the vessel that perforated through the muscle was carefully dissected. The major advantage of musculocutaneous perforator flaps versus musculocutaneous flaps is that the functional and cosmetic morbidity due to transfer of the underlying muscle could be avoided by transferring only the overlying skin.

Although perforator flaps can provide additional vascularized tissue in an area that may be deficient or fibrotic, their use in the setting of infection is controversial; and in these cases, traditional muscle flaps are preferred. Their use is best reserved for aseptic cases with a deficient or scarred soft tissue envelope.

TECHNIQUE   The wound is first debrided to remove all necrotic tissue (Fig. 27-2A,B). Next, elevation of the perforator flap requires careful microsurgical dissection of the musculocutaneous perforator vessels (Fig. 27-2C). Due to anatomical variability of these perforating vessels, Doppler ultrasound is used to locate the perforator before elevation of the flap. Once isolated, the perforator flap can be rotated about the vascular pedicle or transferred as a free flap (Fig. 27-2D). The donor site can be managed with either primary closure or split-thickness skin grafts depending on the specific perforator flap used (Fig. 27-2E). A number of perforator flaps have proven quite reliable for

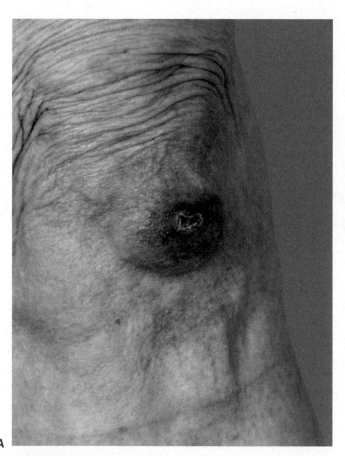
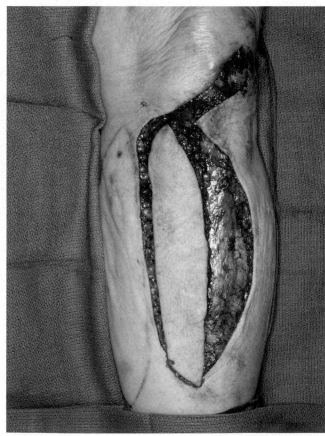

A   B

FIGURE 27-2

A: Pre-patellar bursa with central necrosis and recurrent infection that failed numerous attempts at local wound care. **B:** A perforator flap has been harvested after identifying the vessel, and the pre-patellar area has been debrided. *(Continued)*

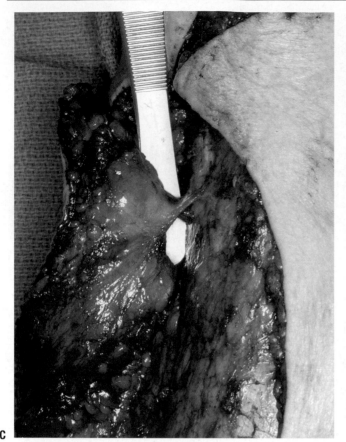

C

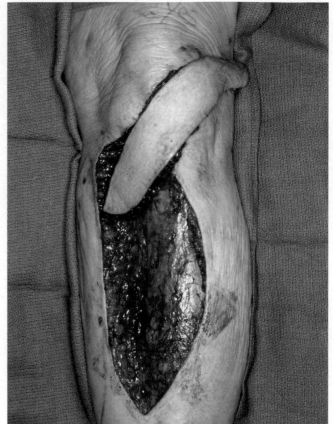

D

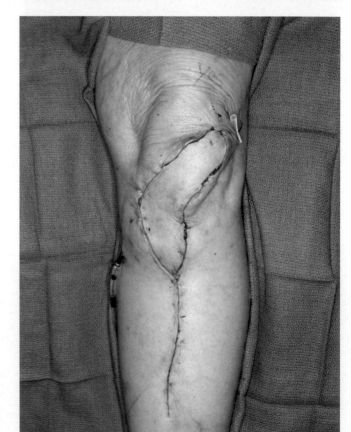

E

FIGURE 27-2

Continued **C:** Perforator vessel to flap. **D:** The flap is rotated 180 degrees on its pedicle and transferred to the area of the defect. **E:** Harvest site incisions have been closed primarily and the flap sutured in place.

managing soft tissue problems in the lower extremity; these include flaps based on the muscle perforators of the vastus lateralis, tensor fascia lata, sartorius, gracilis, and medial gastrocnemius. Unfortunately, due to the volume of tissue required in many cases associated with failed TKA, these muscle perforator flaps often would not provide enough soft tissue to cover the defect; in these circumstances, one of the alternative techniques must be considered.

Medial Gastrocnemius Flap

TECHNIQUE   Although both the lateral and medial heads of the gastrocnemius muscle can be used to provide soft tissue coverage about the knee, both the quantity of tissue provided by the lateral gastrocnemius, and its shorter vascular pedicle, restrict its use. The lateral head is generally 3 to 4 cm shorter than the medial head, and its transfer can place the common peroneal nerve at risk for injury as the muscle is passed across the proximal fibula. Therefore, the medial gastrocnemius rotational flap has been the preferred option for treating wound problems in association with total knee replacement (Figs. 27-3 and 27-4). First, the wound is debrided to healthy margins. Next, the medial

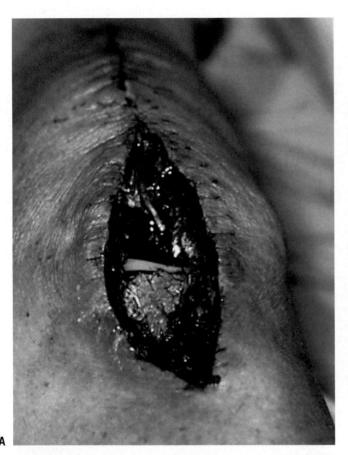

A

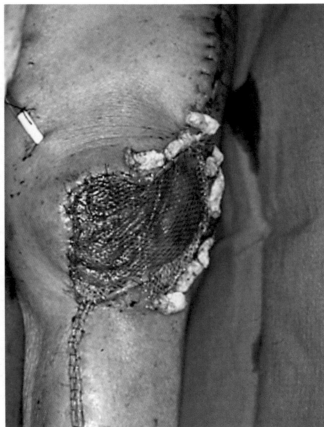

C

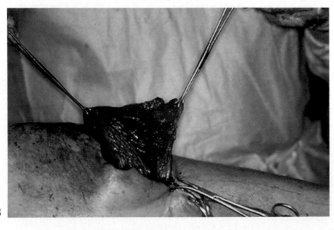

B

FIGURE 27-3

A: Debrided wound after full-thickness necrosis over proximal tibia after TKA. **B:** The medial gastrocnemius is harvested through a posteromedial incision of the calf and then tunneled under a skin bridge to the debrided area. **C:** The muscle flap is covered with a split-thickness skin graft.

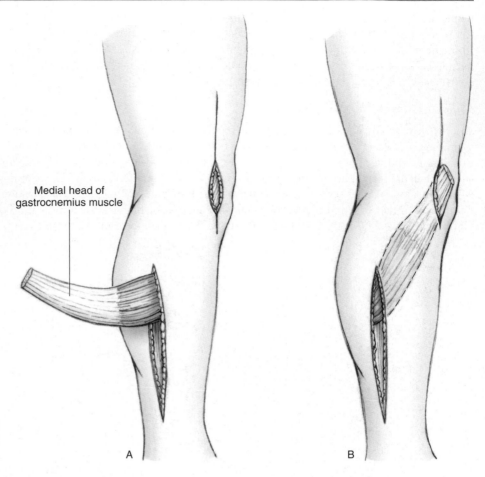

Medial head of gastrocnemius muscle

FIGURE 27-4

A: The medial head of the gastrocnemius muscle is harvested through a medial calf incision. **B:** The muscle is then rotated and delivered a skin bridge into the defect.

A

B

gastrocnemius muscle flap is developed through a posteromedial incision, separating the muscle belly away from the deep tissue superficially, and the underlying soleus muscle along its deep surface. The plantaris tendon provides an excellent landmark. The medial head is separated from the lateral head along its decussation, which does place the sural nerve at risk for injury. The vascular pedicle is based proximally on the sural artery, which is the first branch of the popliteal artery. The muscle is then divided distally at the musculotendinous junction and folded proximally. Next, the flap is tunneled under a medial skin bridge to cover the defect, where it is sutured in place (see Fig. 27-4). If added length is needed, radial scoring of the fascia along the undersurface of the muscle can be performed at 1-cm intervals to increase its arc of rotation. Once transferred, the muscle flap is covered with a split-thickness skin graft that can be performed either primarily, or at a later date; in most circumstances, the donor site can be closed primarily. Alternatively, the flap may be harvested as a musculocutaneous flap, where the entire soft tissue flap including the skin, subcutaneous tissue, fascia, and muscle is rotated about the vascular pedicle. In these cases the donor site must be skin-grafted (see Chapter 29).

RESULTS   In association with infected or exposed total knee prostheses where wound breakdown has occurred, use of medial gastrocnemius flaps has been quite successful, considering the complexity of the problems. In one series, Gerwin et al reported their experience from the Hospital for Special Surgery; successful salvage of an infected, or exposed total knee prosthesis with a medial gastrocnemius flap was achieved in 10 of 12 patients. Similar results have been reported by McPherson et al, with successful reimplantation in 20 of 21 patients who had chronically infected total knee replacements and compromised soft tissues about the knee.

Utilization of the gastrocnemius muscle for knee coverage results in little functional morbidity, with no significant deficits at walking speed, and only mild deficits as demand increases.

Free Latissimus Dorsi and Rectus Abdominus Muscle Flaps   In cases where the medial gastrocnemius flap has been previously used and failed, or when the extent of the soft tissue necrosis is large, alternative flaps must be considered. The free transfer of a latissimus dorsi or rectus abdominus muscle flap has been reliable in these difficult circumstances. The muscle is harvested with its vascular pedicle and the donor site primarily closed. The recipient site is debrided to healthy wound edges and then the free muscle is sutured into the defect after the vascular anastomosis is complete. The vascular anastomosis is typically performed to the popliteal vessels.

Postoperative Management of Soft Tissue Flap Coverage Procedures   Immobilization with elevation for 7 to 10 days to reduce venous congestion is common to all flap coverage procedures. Partial weight bearing and progressive range of motion are then begun on a case by case basis. Factors to be considered include any wound drainage, marginal necrosis, venous congestion, and success of the overlying skin graft. If the flap transfer is done prior to the TKA as a prophylactic measure, then the total joint replacement may be performed after the flap has matured, which is generally a minimum of 8 to 12 weeks.

Complications of Soft Tissue Flap Coverage Procedures   While successful retention or reimplantation of the knee prosthesis has been reported, the functional results associated with these so-called successful outcomes falls far short of knee replacement in association with uncomplicated wound healing. In addition to poor functional results, other complications associated with all types of flaps can include recurrent infection or recurrent wound problems, due to marginal necrosis or complete loss of the flap, as well as skin graft problems at the donor or graft sites. Weakness caused by transfer of the donor muscle can also occur. Due to loss of the medial gastrocnemius, patients have reduced plantar flexion strength of the involved ankle; however, given the extent of the associated knee problems, the functional limitations due to loss of the medial gastrocnemius may be relatively minor. Cosmesis can also be an issue as the flaps may be quite bulky; however, this concern must be considered relative to the presenting problem. Occasionally, debulking or thinning of a mature flap will be undertaken where atrophy of the muscle was less than anticipated.

Surgical Exposure

In addition to the specialized plastic surgery techniques that may be required in revision TKA, the orthopaedic surgeon must also be aware of the techniques that allow adequate surgical exposure to be obtained during the knee procedure in a manner that minimizes risks to the skin and extensor mechanism. If an intraoperative extensor mechanism disruption occurs during revision TKA, or if a preoperative extensor mechanism failure is known to exist, the surgeon must also be aware of the techniques used to address these problems. Simple repair, especially when associated with chronic extensor mechanism disruption, has a very poor track record, and the alternative reconstructive options are described following.

General principles to optimize wound healing and avoid complications include meticulous soft tissue handling in every case. Prolonged local tension from self-retaining retractors or from vigorous stretching due to attempts to perform mini-incision surgery should be avoided; in addition, undermining along the margins of the incision should be minimized. Intraoperatively, the importance of optimizing component positioning to avoid the need for a lateral patellar release that is associated with increased wound problems is also important. The use of a tourniquet is controversial, but evidence suggests that postoperative tissue oxygenation is reduced in patients in whom a tourniquet is used. Certainly, in patients with significant peripheral vascular disease, especially those in whom either a bypass has already been performed, or the lateral radiograph shows extensive calcification of the popliteal vessels, consideration should be made to perform the knee replacement without a tourniquet. In addition to the previously noted principles, numerous techniques exist for facilitating surgical exposure and relieving tension on the extensor mechanism to reduce the risk of iatrogenic tendon rupture or patellar fracture. These techniques, along with the results and complications that are specific to each, are reviewed following. All of these procedures, except where noted, are performed during revision TKA with the patient positioned in the supine position. The specific techniques are described generally progressing from less extensile to more extensile.

Medial Parapatellar Arthrotomy and Proximal Tibial Peel   The medial parapatellar arthrotomy allows the optimal exposure in revision TKA and is versatile as it is compatible with each of the more extensile exposures detailed in subsequent sections. The arthrotomy is begun at the proximal end of the quadriceps tendon approximately 6 to 8 cm proximal to the superior pole of the patella (Fig. 27-5). The arthrotomy is extended distally approximately 3 to 5 mm lateral to the medial border of tendon. At the superior pole of the patella, the arthrotomy is curved around the medial

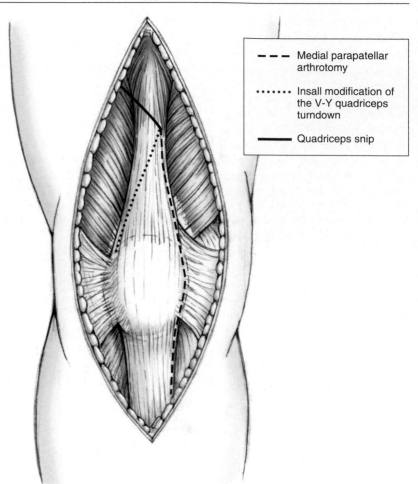

FIGURE 27-5

The medial arthrotomy (*dashed line*) is the standard exposure for revision TKA. This can be extended with a quadriceps snip (*solid line*) if the extensor mechanism is tight. The Insall modification of the V-Y quadriceps turndown (*dotted line*) allows extensile exposure in the stiff knee but is associated with postoperative extensor lag.

border of the patella and then continued distally along the medial edge of the patellar tendon. Next, the periosteum of the medial tibia is elevated sharply beginning at the medial border of the arthrotomy at the level of the joint. Working medially and distally, the entire medial periosteum is elevated approximately 5 to 7 cm distally. A periosteal elevator can be used once the flap of periosteum has been raised. At this stage the knee is flexed and the tibia is gradually externally rotated while the sub-periosteal elevation is continued all the way to the posteromedial corner. In many cases where this tissue plane was not violated in the primary replacement, the semi-membraneosus insertion on the posteromedial corner will be well defined, and this expansile insertion should be released in the sub-periosteal plane. As the dissection is continued to the posterolateral corner, and the tibia is externally rotated, the tibia will sublux from underneath the femur. In many cases, this will allow access to the modular tibial polyethylene. Once exposed, the tibial insert can be removed; this maneuver relaxes the flexion and extension gaps and usually improves the exposure. This exposure should be incorporated into every revision and provides the foundation for obtaining adequate visualization and access in order to safely remove the existing components and reconstruct the knee.

Quadriceps Snip

TECHNIQUE The quadriceps snip, originally promoted by Dr. John Insall, facilitates the exposure of stiff knees in the primary and revision setting. This technique is a proximal extension of a medial parapatellar arthrotomy (see Fig. 27-5). Beginning at the proximal apex of the standard arthrotomy, the incision is extended proximally and laterally at a 45-degree angle into the fibers of the vastus lateralis. This extension not only relieves the tension on the extensor mechanism in a stiff knee that can aid in exposure of the joint, but also allows the patella to be everted more easily during patellar preparation if this is required. The arthrotomy and this proximal extension are closed in routine fashion once the arthroplasty has been performed. In distinction to many of the alternative techniques for optimizing exposure in difficult cases, there is no need to modify or restrict postoperative rehabilitation. Indeed, patients in whom the quadriceps snip has been used may participate in standard TKA rehabilitation protocols. While this technique allows adequate exposure in most circumstances, in particularly stiff or difficult cases, additional measures may be required. In these extreme cases, a tibial tubercle osteotomy can be used even after a quadriceps snip has already been performed.

RESULTS   Insall's clinical experience in 16 patients who had bilateral TKA with a quadriceps snip on only on one side has been reported. In these patients, no differences in quadriceps strength were observed postoperatively between the two sides. In a similar study, no difference was identified between patients who had undergone a quadriceps snip, versus those in whom a standard medial parapatellar arthrotomy had been performed.

Tibial Tubercle Osteotomy   This technique, popularized by Whiteside, facilitates exposure in even very stiff knees. In addition, the tibial tubercle osteotomy can allow access to the tibial canal that may be helpful in revision or infected TKA when well-fixed stemmed, tibial components must be removed. This technique involves first incising the medial periosteum along the medial border of the patella tendon for approximately 6 to 7 cm distal to the joint line. The osteotomy is then performed with an oscillating saw from medial to lateral, creating a wedge of bone that is approximately 2 cm wide and 6 to 8 cm long. The osteotomized wedge should taper from a thickness of about 1 cm proximally, to the level of the anterior cortex distally. This minimizes the stress riser in the anterior tibia, especially at the distal end. In addition, at the proximal end, a step cut should be created about 1 cm distal to the joint line. This step acts as a buttress that helps to resist proximal migration of the osteotomized wedge after it has been reattached at the end of the case. Proximal migration is also resisted by the lateral periosteum and musculature that should remain attached to the osteotomized piece. During the revision knee arthroplasty, the lateral soft tissues act as a hinge that allows the osteotomized segment to be everted and displaced laterally. At the time of closure, three to four 18-gauge wires are used for fixation. The wires are passed through drill holes in the medial tibia and then brought up through the lateral aspect of the tubercle shingle. They are then brought distally and medially over the tibial crest and tightened on the medial side of the tibia. Tightening the wires pulls the osteotomy distally. The arthrotomy is then closed in a standard fashion. In most cases, we favor bypassing the tibial tubercle with a stemmed component. If a cemented stem is used, it is helpful to remember to pass the wires before insertion of cement.

RESULTS   Advantages of the tibial tubercle osteotomy versus the V-Y quadriceps turndown include a lower incidence of extensor lag and quadriceps weakness. Whiteside reported his experience with this technique in 136 patients; only two patients experienced a residual extensor lag. Another advantage of this technique is that if rigid fixation is obtained, full weight bearing and unrestricted range of motion are allowed postoperatively. Reported complications of tibial tubercle osteotomy that are not noted with the quadriceps turndown include proximal migration of the osteotomized tubercle, patellar tendon disruption, and tibial shaft fractures. Despite these unique problems, we favor the use of tubercle osteotomy when adequate exposure cannot be obtained with a standard arthrotomy and quadriceps snip.

V-Y Quadriceps Turndown

TECHNIQUE   The V-Y quadriceps turndown was originally described by Coonse and Adams and subsequently modified by Insall. In both techniques an inverted V-shaped flap incorporating the quadriceps tendon is created. Insall's modification described creating a second incision beginning at the apex of a standard medial parapatellar arthrotomy that is extended distally and laterally at a 45-degree angle along the tendinous portion of the vastus lateralis (see Fig. 27-5). In addition to allowing excellent exposure, the inverted V of tissue may be lengthened at the time of closure, forming an inverted Y shape.

RESULTS   Although this technique allows excellent exposure and releases excessive tension on the extensor mechanism during surgery, patients may develop an extension lag postoperatively. Trousdale et al reported the Mayo Clinic experience with this technique. Patients who had undergone bilateral TKA with a V-Y quadriceps turndown in one knee, and a standard medial parapatellar arthrotomy in the contralateral knee, underwent postoperative strength testing. In these patients, the results did not show any statistical differences between the strength of the two legs. However, 5 of 14 patients with the V-Y quadriceps turndown had a persistent extensor lag. Furthermore, use of the V-Y quadriceps turndown requires alterations in the postoperative rehabilitation protocol that includes restricted range of motion, use of a brace, and partial weight bearing for about 6 weeks. Due to the high rate of lag, and the increased recovery time associated with the use of the V-Y turndown, we favor the use of the tibial tubercle osteotomy when a quadriceps snip does not provide adequate exposure.

Femoral Peel

TECHNIQUE Windsor and Insall described the femoral peel as a useful technique for exposing an ankylosed knee. Initially, the proximal medial tibia is exposed subperiosteally, preserving the origin of the medial collateral ligament on the femur. Then, the distal femur is skeletonized by subperiosteal dissection, and the soft tissue sleeve is preserved medially and laterally.

RESULTS Although the soft tissue sleeve, including the medial and lateral stabilizing structures, is preserved, joint stability may be compromised by the extensive dissection; in these cases, a constrained knee prosthesis implant may be required.

Quadriceps Tendon Rupture

TECHNIQUE Fortunately, the incidence of quadriceps tendon rupture after TKA is very low with approximately 1 case per 1,000 reported, as this problem has proven to be difficult to manage. In distinction to the native knee, where primary repair of the tendon to its attachment on the superior pole of the patella with nonabsorbable sutures passed through vertical tunnels in the patella has proven quite successful, the same results have not been achieved in the setting of TKA. Therefore, the preferred technique includes a repair of the tendon with augmentation of the repair using autologous hamstring tissue or a synthetic mesh. First, the distal end of the tendon is resected back to healthy tissue. Then, two No. 5 nonabsorbable sutures are woven through the avulsed tendon in a Krackow-type technique and passed through vertical tunnels in the patella using a suture passer or straight needle. These sutures are then tied with the knee completely extended. An autologous semitendinosus or gracilis graft, or a synthetic surgical mesh, is then used to augment the repair. Postoperatively, the patient is immobilized in full extension for 6 to 8 weeks; motion is then increased by 30-degree increments at 2-week intervals, with the goal of 90 degrees by 3 months postoperatively. During this time, the leg is protected in a hinged brace. Patients with postoperative partial quadriceps tendon rupture after TKA can be adequately managed by the same nonoperative protocol as described for those patients with complete tears who have undergone surgical reconstruction.

RESULTS Patients with partial quadriceps tears after TKA treated nonoperatively, as described previously, have generally done well, with all seven patients in one recent large series achieving good results. In distinction, nonoperative treatment for patients with complete quadriceps tears has been poor, with patients generally requiring drop lock knee braces to ambulate. Furthermore, patients with complete tears treated with simple repair alone also had poor results. Six of 10 patients in this group had unsatisfactory outcomes, including four reruptures. Other complications included knee recurvatum and instability, and deep infection. These generally dismal results prompted the changes in surgical techniques noted previously.

Patellar Tendon Disruption

TECHNIQUE In association with TKA, postoperative patellar tendon rupture is an uncommon but potentially catastrophic complication that presents a difficult reconstructive problem. Nonoperative management is associated with loss of extensor power in the involved extremity, usually requiring the use of a drop lock brace or walker. Surgical intervention has also been associated with poor results when simple repair has been attempted. More recently, successful salvage of a functional extremity has been made possible with allograft reconstruction using an entire extensor mechanism. The technique is performed through a midline incision when possible. A midline arthrotomy passing over the medial patella allows the native patella to be shelled out from the retinaculum. If the prior patella has fragmented and there are numerous thin fragments of bone embedded in the soft tissue sleeve, these may be left in situ to prevent causing extensive damage to the retinaculum. Distally, over the proximal tibia the native tendon remnants and retinacular tissue should be elevated sub-periosteally, both medially and laterally, for a distance of 7 to 10 cm from the joint line to expose the entire tubercle area. This exposure creates two sleeves of tissue that will be closed over the allograft at the end of the procedure. If revision TKA needs to be simultaneously performed, the procedure is then performed at this stage. It is important to ensure that component positioning is optimal to minimize stress and shear forces on the graft.

Preparation of the host site begins with creating a trough about 6 cm long and just under 2 cm wide and deep with a burr, saw, or osteotome close to the location of the native tubercle. If possible, a bridge about 1.5 to 2 cm high should be left between the tibial surface proximally and the proximal end of the trough, although in some revision TKA cases this may not be possible when the bone is deficient. The proximal end of the trough should have an oblique cut that creates a small overhang that will lock in the bone block of the graft and resist proximal migration due to the pull from the quadriceps.

While the host site is being prepared, a second team prepares the allograft. The fresh frozen, extensor allograft must include a tibial bone block that is at least 6 to 8cm long and 2 cm wide and deep, the entire patellar tendon, the patella, and at least 5 to 6 cm of the quadriceps tendon. Distally, a block about 6 cm long and 2 cm wide and deep is prepared. The prepared block should be slightly larger than the trough in the host tibia to facilitate a solid press fit. The proximal end of the block should also have an oblique cut that is directed proximal and posteriorly that will help lock in the block, as previously noted (Fig. 27-6). In the proximal part of the allograft, two No. 5 nonabsorbable braided sutures are stitched through the medial and lateral portions of the quadriceps tendon using a Krackow technique. The free ends of the suture should exit from the proximal end of the quadriceps tendon.

Insertion of the graft begins by weaving two additional No. 5 nonabsorbable sutures into the distal end of the native medial and lateral quadriceps tendon remnants using a Krackow technique. Next, the bone block is gently press fit and tamped into the trough. The proximal portion of the bone block should first be wedged under the oblique step in the native bone, and then the distal end gently impacted to ensure the best fit. If the bone block needs to be trimmed at this stage, either a burr or bone rongeur can be used. Once the block is tapped in place, the block is fixed with two bicortical screws that should be countersunk. Certainly, use of screws creates stress risers in the graft and theoretically increases risk of graft resorption or weakening; however, loss of fixation anecdotally appears to be reduced. Alternatively, two or three 18-gauge wires can be used, as is customary with a standard tibial tubercle osteotomy. However, in these allograft cases, the surgeon must ensure that the proximal lock between the block and trough that is produced by the oblique cuts is solid, or proximal migration may occur. Lack of the native lateral soft tissue attachments that help resist proximal migration of the block with a standard tubercle osteotomy, as well as longer time to union, are perhaps reasons why the risk of migration may be higher in these allograft cases. After the block is secure, the sutures that were previously woven through the allograft quadriceps tendon are pulled

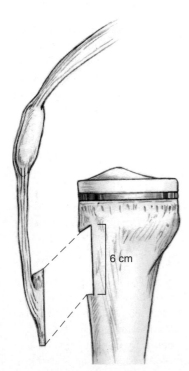

FIGURE 27-6

The trough in the host tibia should be made with a proximal overhang underneath which the oblique cut of the extensor allograft bone block can be wedged.

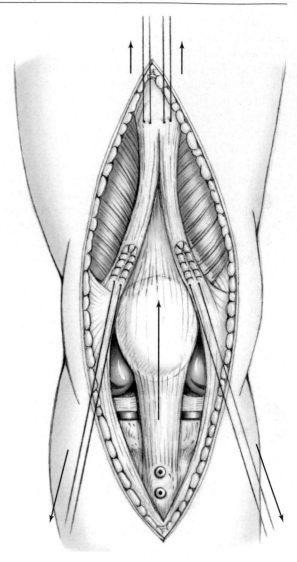

FIGURE 27-7

The extensor allograft should be tensioned and sutures tied with maximal proximal and distal directed forces applied to the allograft and native quadriceps, respectively.

proximally by an assistant. While under maximum tension, these sutures are passed under, and then up through the native quadriceps tendon remnants. The native tissues are simultaneously pulled distally using the other Krackow-type sutures that were previously woven through the medial and lateral sleeves (Fig. 27-7). While the knee is held in full extension and maximal proximal and distal forces are applied, the sutures that are attached to the allograft quadriceps tendon are tied. Additional No. 5 sutures are then placed into the native and allograft tendon to stitch the graft in place. The native medial and lateral tissue sleeves are then closed over the allograft in a "pants over vest" technique using a combination of 0 and No. 1 sutures.

Postoperatively, these patients are immobilized in full extension in a well-fitting brace or cylinder cast for 6 to 8 weeks. Factors including the patient compliance, shape of the leg, and wound care issues must be considered in selecting the optimal method of immobilization. Patients may ambulate with partial weight bearing during this period. After 6 to 8 weeks, flexion is advanced by 30 degrees every 2 weeks, with the goal of 0 to 90 by 3 months postoperatively. Typically, a hinged knee brace with flexion stops is used to protect the patient during this period and the brace is locked in full extension during ambulation.

RESULTS   The results of simple repair of patellar tendon ruptures after TKA have been poor with high failure rates. Furthermore, early attempts at patellar tendon reconstruction after TKA, using extensor allografts with techniques that tensioned the graft in varying degrees of flexion, have also been associated with high rates of extensor lag. Other complications of all techniques include infection and wound-healing problems. However, knee stiffness has not been a significant concern, and changes in the intraoperative technique, described previously, that emphasize tensioning the graft in maximal flexion, in conjunction with prolonged immobilization in extension postoperatively, have been associated with better results. Burnett et al reported clinical failures, with an average lag of 59 degrees, in all seven patients in whom the graft was minimally tensioned. In the subsequent 13 patients in whom the graft was maximally tensioned, all were successes with a mean of only 4 degrees lag.

POSTOPERATIVE MANAGEMENT

A number of factors have been reported to influence postoperative wound healing after TKA. Many of these factors include the same systemic conditions that need to be optimized preoperatively. Similarly, postoperatively, it is imperative that significant pulmonary disease and anemia, in addition to tobacco smoking, are aggressively managed to maintain optimal tissue oxygenation. Furthermore, nutritional requirements must be met, and management of diabetes should maintain blood glucose levels within tight control. When possible, immune-modifying medications should be held until primary wound healing has occurred. In addition to these factors, other factors specific to the postoperative period should be considered, especially in patients with other significant risks. Tight dressings should be avoided as these may compromise local capillary flow. Use of a continuous passive motion machine for extended periods should be avoided in any patient at risk for wound-healing problems, as flexion beyond 40 degrees is known to reduce the tissue oxygenation along the lateral wound, and greater than 60 degrees also compromises medial tissue oxygenation. Indeed, immobilization should be instituted in patients that develop problem wounds. Development of a significant postoperative hematoma may also reduce tissue oxygenation; in cases where wound-healing problems occur in conjunction with a hematoma, surgical drainage should be carefully considered.

When wound-healing problems occur, the problem should be carefully followed and aggressively managed to avoid secondary bacterial seeding of the joint. Small areas limited to 1 to 2 mm of marginal superficial skin necrosis that involves short segments of the wound (<1 to 2 cm) may be observed and treated with local wound care in the absence of infection. In these cases, immobilization should be used and activity minimized until the margins of the wound have declared themselves. Wound breakdown or full-thickness necrosis should be debrided early, and one of the previously described soft tissue coverage procedures should be used.

Prolonged wound drainage, without wound breakdown, should also be aggressively managed. Significant serous drainage beyond 3 or 4 days should be managed with a compressive (but not tight) dressing, immobilization, and bed rest. Failure to respond within 48 hours should prompt surgical drainage if a seroma is suspected. In cases where there is significant bloody drainage, initial treatment is the same as for serous drainage. However, in this second group of patients, persistent bloody drainage after TKA is suggestive of capsular dehiscence. Failure to respond to non-surgical treatment should prompt a return to the operating room for an evacuation of the hematoma and closure of the arthrotomy. Certainly, substantial drainage beyond a week from surgery should cause concern and requires careful observation and early intervention if quick resolution doesn't occur.

SUMMARY

In order for successful revision TKA to be accomplished, early wound healing is required. Numerous factors in the preoperative, intraoperative, and postoperative periods can influence this process. While many of these factors are beyond the control of the orthopaedic surgeon, many are not. Careful preoperative evaluation helps identify and manage potential problems to minimize the risks. Furthermore, the orthopaedic surgeon needs to be aware of the plastic and orthopaedic surgery techniques that not only help reduce complications, but also help salvage affected knees when these potentially devastating problems occur.

SUGGESTED READING

Adam RF, Watson SB, Jarratt JW, Noble J, Watson JS. Outcome after flap cover for exposed total knee arthroplasties. A report of 25 cases. *J Bone Joint Surg.* 1994;76B:750–753.

Barrack RL, Smith P, Munn B, Engh G, Rorabeck C. Comparison of surgical approaches in total knee arthroplasty. *Clin Orthop.* 1998;356:16–21.

Burnett SJ, Berger RA, Paprosky WG, Della Valle CJ, Jacobs JJ, Rosenberg AG. Extensor mechanism allograft reconstruction after total knee arthroplasty. A comparison of two techniques. *J Bone Joint Surg.* 2004;86-A:2694–2699.

Burnett SJ, Berger RA, Della Valle CJ, et al. Extensor mechanism allograft reconstruction after total knee arthroplasty: surgical technique. *J Bone Joint Surg.* 2005;87-A(suppl 1);Part 2:175–194.

Clarke HD, Craig-Scott S, Scott WN. Tissue expanders in total knee arthroplasty. *Tech Knee Surgery.* 2005;4:12–18.

Clarke MT, Longstaff L, Edwards D, Rushton N. Tourniquet-induced wound hypoxia after total knee replacement. *J Bone Joint Surg.* 2001;83B:40–44.

Colombel M, Mariz Y, Dahhan P, Kenesi C: Arterial and lymphatic supply of the knee integuments. *Surg Radiol Anat.* 1998;20:35–40.

Coonse K, Adams JD. A new operative approach to the knee joint. *Surg Gynecol Obstet.* 1943;77:344–347.

Dickhaut SC, DeLee JL, Pase CP. Nutritional statistics. Importance in predicting wound healing after amputation. *J Bone Joint Surg.* 1984;66A:71–75.

Dobbs RE, Hanssen AD, Lewallen DG, Pagnano MW. Quadriceps tendon rupture after total knee arthroplasty: prevalence, complications and outcomes. *J Bone Joint Surg.* 2005;87-A:37–45.

Garvin KL, Scuderi G, Insall JN. Evolution of the quadriceps snip. *Clin Orthop.* 1995;321:131–137.

Geddes CR, Morri SF, Neligan PC. Perforator flaps: evolution, classification, and applications. *Ann Plast Surg.* 2003;50:90–99.

Gerwin M, Rothaus KO, Windsor RE, Brause BD, Insall JN. Gastrocnemius muscle flap coverage of exposed or infected knee prosthesis. *Clin Orthop.* 1993;286:64–70.

Haertsch P. The surgical plane in the leg. *Br J Plast Surg.* 1981;34:464–469.

Haertsch P. The blood supply to the skin of the leg: a post-mortem investigation. *Br J Plast Surg.* 1981;34:470–477.

Hunt TK, Hopf HW. Wound healing and wound infection. What surgeons and anesthesiologists can do. *Surg Clin North Am.* 1997;77:587–606.

Johnson DP. Midline or parapatellar incision for knee arthroplasty. A comparative study of wound viability. *J Bone Joint Surg.* 1988;70B:656–658.

Johnson DP. The effect of continuous passive motion on wound healing and joint mobility after total knee arthroplasty. *J Bone Joint Surg.* 1990;78A:421–426.

Johnson DP, Eastwood DM. Lateral patellar release in knee arthroplasty: effect on wound healing. *J Arthroplasty.* 1992;7(suppl):407–431.

Manifold SG, Cushner FD, Craig-Scott S, Scott WN. Long-term results of total knee arthroplasty after the use of soft tissue expanders. *Clin Orthop.* 2000;380:133–139.

McMurray JF. Jr. Wound healing with diabetes mellitus. Better glucose control for better wound healing in diabetes. *Surg Clin North Am.* 1984;64:769–778.

McPherson EJ, Patzakis MJ, Gross JE, Holtom PD, Song M, Dorr LD. Infected total knee arthroplasty. Two-stage reimplantation with a gastrocnemius rotational flap. *Clin Orthop.* 1997;341:73–81.

Moller AM, Pedersen T, Villebro N, Munksgaard A. Effect of smoking on early complications after elective orthopaedics surgery. *J Bone Joint Surg.* 2003;85B:178–181.

Ranawat CS, Flynn WF Jr. Principles of planning and prosthetic selection for revision total knee replacement. In: Scott WN, ed. *The knee.* St. Louis: Mosby-Yearbook; 1994:1297–1303.

Rothaus KO. Plastic and reconstructive surgery. In: Insall JN, ed. *Surgery of the knee.* New York: Churchill-Livingstone; 1993:1200–1201.

Trousdale RT, Hanssen AD, Rand JA. V-Y quadricepsplasty in total knee arthroplasty. *Clin Orthop.* 1993;286:48–55.

Warner, DO. Preoperative smoking cessation: how long is long enough? *Anesthesiology.* 2005;102:883–884.

Weiss AP, Krackow KA. Persistent wound drainage after primary total knee arthroplasty. *J Arthroplasty.* 1993;8:285–289.

Whiteside LA. Exposure in difficult total knee arthroplasty using tibial tubercle osteotomy. *Clin Orthop.* 1995;321:32–35.

Windsor RE, Insall JN. Exposure in revision total knee arthroplasty: the femoral peel. *Techniques Orthop.* 1988;3:1–4.

28 The Pedicled Soleus Muscle Flap for Coverage of the Middle and Distal Third of the Tibia

Salvatore C. Lettieri and Steven L. Moran

Soft tissue defects involving the middle and lower third of the leg may occur following trauma, tumor extirpation, and osteomyelitis. Anteriorly the skin and subcutaneous tissue overriding the middle third and lower third of the tibia are thin and exposed bone and tendon may result from soft tissue injury or open fractures. Historically, middle third defects have been covered with the pedicled soleus muscle flap, while attempts have been made more recently to extend to soleus flap to cover defects of the lower third of the leg.

The soleus muscle, according to the Mathes and Nahai schema, is a type II muscle, containing dominant pedicles from the popliteal, peroneal, and posterior tibial arteries and minor segmental pedicles from the posterior tibial artery. The muscle lies in the superficial posterior compartment extending the entire length of the lower leg. The soleus originates from the posterior surface of the tibia, the interosseous membrane, and the proximal third of the fibula. The muscle runs deep to the gastrocnemius muscle in the upper third of the leg (Fig. 28-1). In the middle third of the leg, the muscle joins with the gastrocnemius muscle and is adherent to the calcaneal tendon. The soleus is a bipennate muscle with the medial and lateral muscle bellies each receiving an independent neurovascular supply; this allows the lateral and medial portions to be mobilized independently while preserving some function within the remaining soleus muscle. The medial head originates from the tibia and receives the majority of its blood supply from the posterior tibial artery. The lateral head originates from the fibula and receives the majority of its blood supply from the perineal artery, although 16% of muscles may be nourished entirely by the posterior tibial artery. The lateral and medial heads are fused proximally while a septum divides the muscle distally. This septum is an extension of the calcaneal tendon and soleus tendon. Dividing the muscle longitudinally at the level of the septum allows for the elevation of the medial and lateral hemi soleus flaps.

In the distal one third of the muscle, the soleus receives segmental arterial perforators from the posterior tibial artery (Fig. 28-2). These distal perforators may be absent in up to 26% of patients; in these cases distal perfusion to the muscle is provided by axial blood flow from more proximal perforators. The diameter and position of these distal perforators is variable but, if present and of large enough caliber, these perforators can allow for a portion of the muscle to be harvested in a reverse

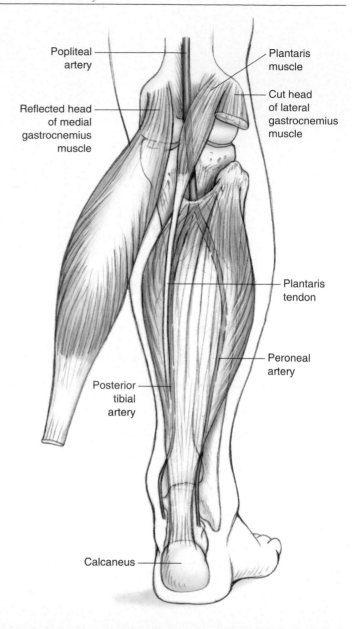

Popliteal artery

Plantaris muscle

Reflected head of medial gastrocnemius muscle

Cut head of lateral gastrocnemius muscle

Plantaris tendon

Peroneal artery

Posterior tibial artery

Calcaneus

FIGURE 28-1

Schematic anatomy of the posterior leg showing the soleus located deep to the gastrocnemius muscle bellies. The plantaris tendon helps define the plane between the soleus and the gastrocnemius muscle bellies. The blood supply to the soleus is from the popliteal, posterior tibial, and perineal arteries.

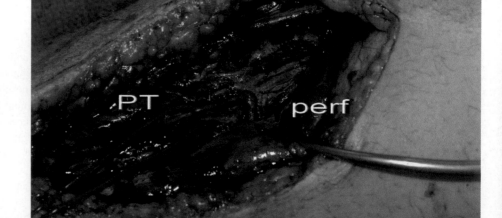

FIGURE 28-2

The posterior tibial artery (PT) as it approaches the ankle gives off several arterial perforators (perfs) to the distal soles muscle. If these perforators are of adequate caliber the muscle can be dissected free and rotated as a distally based flap.

fashion. The muscle may then be rotated 90 to 180 degrees, based on its distal perforators, allowing coverage of the lower third of the tibia and ankle region.

The soleus functions to stabilize the ankle and assist in plantar flexion. The muscle works synergistically with the gastrocnemius and tibialis posterior muscle to provide plantar flexion, while the flexor hallucis longus, flexor digitorum longus, and tibialis posterior all help to provide ankle stability and resist dorsiflexion.

INDICATIONS/ CONTRAINDICATIONS

The primary indication for the use of the soleus muscle flap is coverage of soft tissue defects in the middle third of the leg. Distal third defects have historically been covered with a free flap; however for small defects and in patients with significant comorbid disease, which would prohibit prolonged anesthesia times, a reverse soleus muscle flap may be considered as an alternative to free tissue transfer.

There are several factors which may prohibit the successful transfer of the soleus muscle and these are:

1. Size of the defect
2. Status of the muscle
3. Status of surrounding tissue and bone
4. Size and location of existing perforators

Size of the Defect

The soleus muscle has a limited surface area and a limited arc of rotation (Fig. 28-3). Large defects occupying the majority of the middle third and lower third of the leg are best covered with free tissue transfer. In addition, the distal aspect of the muscle can be unreliable if it must be stretched or inset under significant tension. In such cases, alternative methods of closure should be considered or the soleus may be used in conjunction with another flap.

The soleus can be used in conjunction with the medial or lateral gastrocnemius muscles for larger defects spanning the upper aspect of the lower leg, but this will compromise remaining plantar flexion (Fig. 28-4). When the defect is so large as to require more than just the soleus and medial gastrocnemius flaps, a free flap should strongly be considered as a means of soft tissue coverage and preservation of remaining posterior compartment function. Defects which are to be covered with a reversed soleus muscle flap should be less than 50 cm^2 while the standard soleus flap can cover most defects under 75 cm^2.

Status of the Muscle

Because the soleus muscle is closely adherent to the deep posterior surface of the interosseous membrane, tibia, and fibula, it can often be significantly traumatized following comminuted fractures of the tibia and fibula. During initial wound evaluation and debridement the muscle can often be inspected through the soft tissue defect. If the muscle is significantly lacerated by fracture fragments or contains a significant amount of intramuscular hematoma, it is most prudent to use another flap for soft tissue coverage. In addition, any associated injury to the popliteal, peroneal, or posterior tibial arteries can adversely affect the survival of the soleus muscle.

Status of Surrounding Tissue and Bone

Preexisting damage to the surrounding skin and deeper tissue of the middle third of the leg are also a relative contraindication to soleus muscle flap use. A history of previous radiation therapy, previous surgery, or penetrating trauma to the area surrounding the middle third of the leg should alert the surgeon to potential problems with the use of this flap. The soleus muscle has been shown to provide a source of collateral arterial flow between the posterior tibial and perineal arterial systems. In patients with vascular occlusions of the perineal or posterior tibial arteries, use of the soleus muscle may further compromise limb vascularity.

Size and Location of Existing Perforators

Indications for use of the soleus for distal third defects are based on the work of Pu and include (a) defect size less than 50 cm, (b) defects located over the anterior or medial portion of the distal tibia,

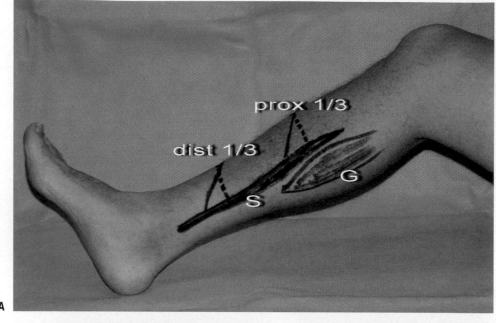

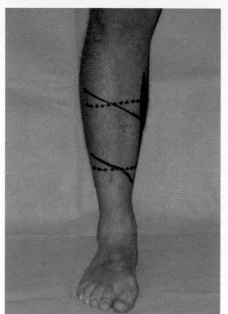

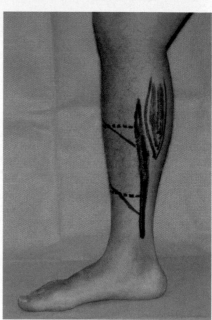

FIGURE 28-3

A-C: The soleus muscle (S) runs anterior to the gastrocnemius muscle (G) and to the area just proximal to the medial malleolus. The arc of rotation of the medially based soleus muscle is limited due to its deep origin and broad proximal attachments. This makes coverage of more laterally and inferiorly based middle third defects difficult. The solid red line shows the actual safe arc of rotation for the medially based soleus muscle flap, with the dashed line depicting the superior and inferior margins of the "middle third" of the leg.

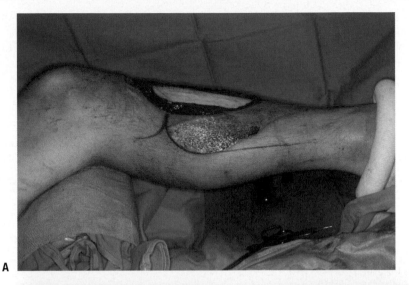

A

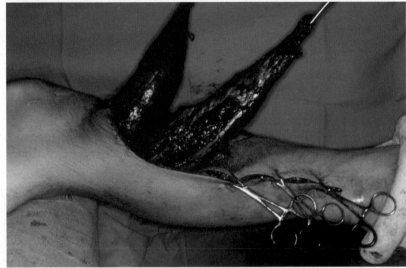

B

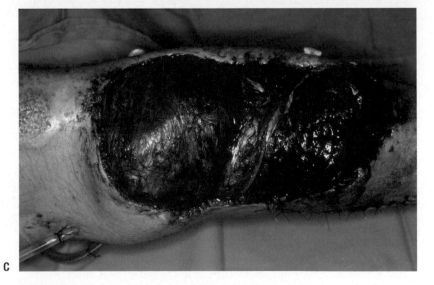

C

FIGURE 28-4

A-C: This large defect is easily covered by elevating both the medial gastrocnemius muscle and the soleus muscle.

(c) the presence of large perforators in distal 4 cm to 5 cm of muscle and (d) a soleus muscle which is nontraumatized on initial exploration (4–6). If these factors are met a reversed hemi soleus flap may be attempted for lower third defects, otherwise a free flap is chosen for distal third defects. In addition, patients who have a smoking history, peripheral vascular disease, and history of lower leg radiation therapy should be considered high risk for a reversed soleus muscle flap.

PREOPERATIVE PLANNING

Close inspection of the lower leg is necessary prior to surgery. Even though the soleus occupies the same compartment as the gastrocnemius, it can be more significantly damaged in open fractures due to its adherence to the tibia and interosseous membrane. If there is significant ecchymosis or swelling of the posterior compartment, in conjunction with significant displacement of the tibia and fibula on lateral radiographs, one must assume significant damage to the soleus muscle. In this case, free tissue transfer would provide a better alternative for coverage of the middle third of the tibia. If the patient has had previous surgeries, such as fasciotomies for trauma, this may also preclude reliable rotation of the flap, since the level of the fasciotomies and also the location of the injuries may have injured the underlying flap (Fig. 28-5).

A noninvasive vascular exam should be performed on the lower leg, verifying patency of the posterior, peroneal, and anterior tibial arteries. If the patient has a history of significant peripheral vascular disease or long standing diabetes, a CT angiogram may verify patency of the posterior and perineal arteries prior to flap transfer.

SURGERY

Patient Positioning and Surgical Preparation

The patient is placed in the supine position for anterior defects, the lateral decubitus position for lateral defects, and prone for posterior defect coverage. As part of the surgical preparation, the entire

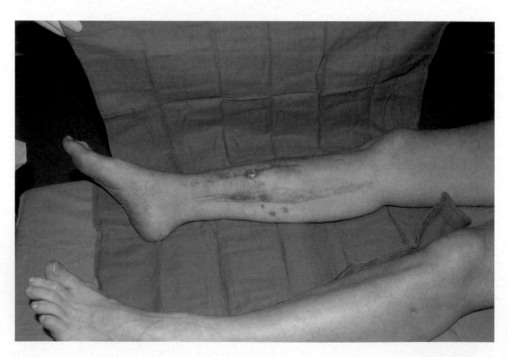

FIGURE 28-5

This patient had lower leg fasciotomies performed at the time of the original tibial injury. The patient now presents with osteomyelitis and exposed hardware over the middle third of the tibia. The defect is located within the arc of coverage of the medial soleus muscle flap; however, there is significant scarring and injury to the superficial posterior compartment secondary to the fasciotomies and previous split thickness skin grafting. Because of concerns of the reliability of the soleus muscle in this situation, this patient underwent coverage of exposed hardware with a free tissue transfer.

lower extremity is prepped and draped in the usual fashion. For anterior midtibial defects, a sterile "bump" is placed beneath the distal thigh region to allow for slight external rotation of the leg and bending of the knee; this can facilitate identification of the muscle. The muscle may be harvested with the use of spinal or general anesthetic. A tourniquet on the upper leg allows for a relatively bloodless field during muscle dissection.

Technique

Medial and proximally based soleus flap   The soleus is harvested through an incision which runs from the upper third of the leg to just above the medial malleolus. The incision is made 2 cm to 3 cm posterior to the medial palpable margin of the tibia. The defect site is incorporated into this incision (Fig. 28-6). Skin bridges are avoided. Dissection is carried down to the investing fascia of the superficial posterior compartment. The saphenous vein is identified and preserved during the dissection. The deep fascia is then opened longitudinally to expose the posterior compartment.

The muscle itself is most easily identified proximally deep to the gastrocnemius muscle. The plane between the two muscles is relatively avascular with the exception of some small perforators which may be ligated. The plantaris runs in the plane between the two muscles and can be used as a landmark in cases of severe trauma where hematoma may obscure the tissue planes.

The soleus fuses with the calcaneal tendon in the middle third of the leg. Here, sharp dissection is required to separate the soleus from the common calcaneal tendon as it extends towards the heel.

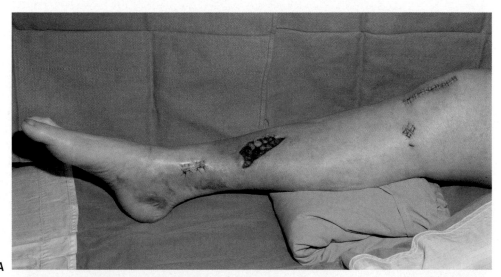

A

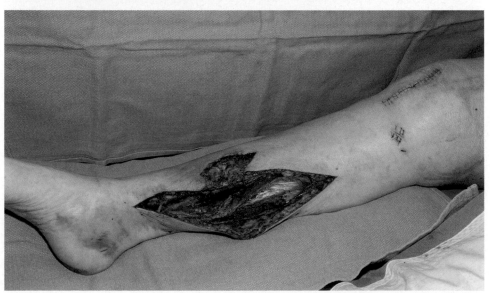

B

FIGURE 28-6

A: A middle third defect in the right leg of a 66 year old diabetic woman following a Gustilo type IIIB fracture of the tibia. The fracture has been stabilized with an intramedullary rod and the wound has been covered with an antibiotic beads pouch following initial debridement at the time of fracture fixation. **B:** An incision is made slightly posterior to the medial tibial margin and then carried inferiorly. The open wound is incorporated into the incision to avoid creating a skin bridge. *(Continued)*

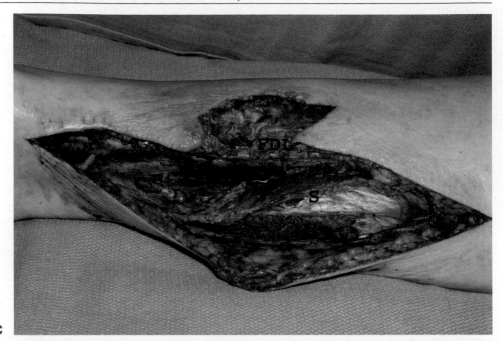

C

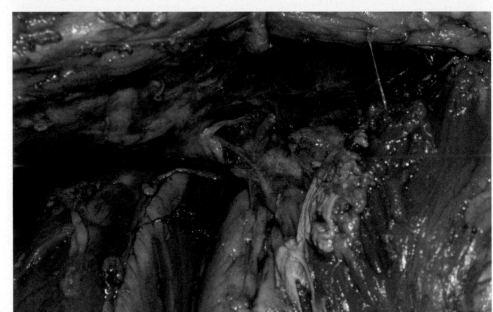

D

FIGURE 28-6

Continued **C:** The soleus muscle (S) has been dissected free of the calcaneal tendon (C) and separated from the gastrocnemius muscle (G) and flexor digitorum longus muscle (FDL). **D:** Large perforators from the posterior tibial artery can be seen entering the muscle. **E:** The muscle is now divided at its distal attachment and pedicled to cover the open defect. Because the soleus is elevated off the common calcaneal tendon the superficial surface of the muscle is devoid of fascia. The muscle is "fanned out" and inset with half buried absorbable sutures. *(Continued)*

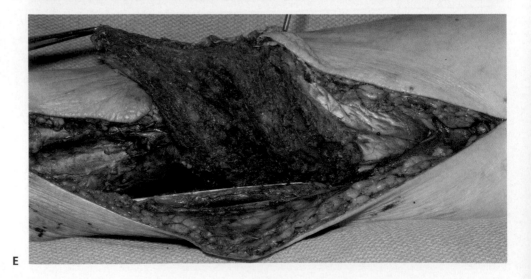

E

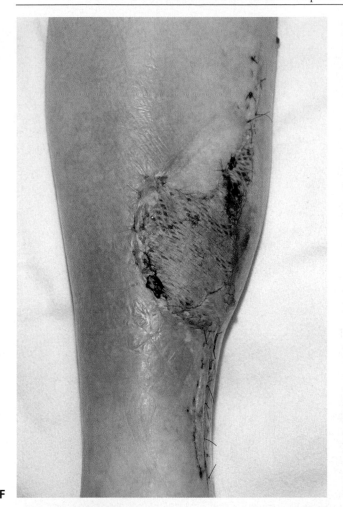

F

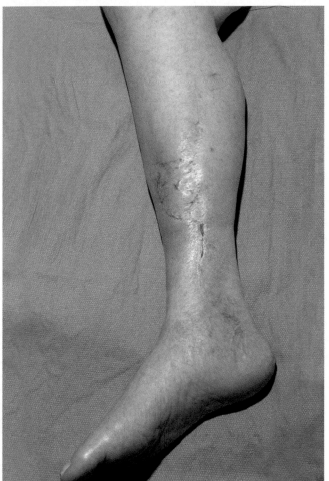

G

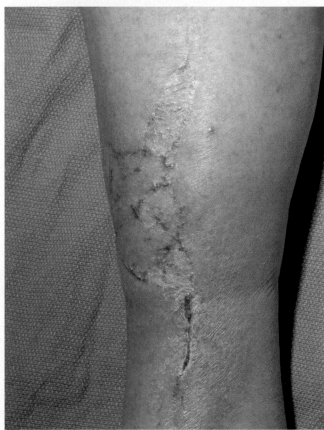

H

FIGURE 28-6

Continued **F:** The donor incision is closed up to the rotated muscle and the exposed muscle is covered with a split thickness skin graft. **G,H:** At 2 months the patient has a well healed wound with excellent contour.

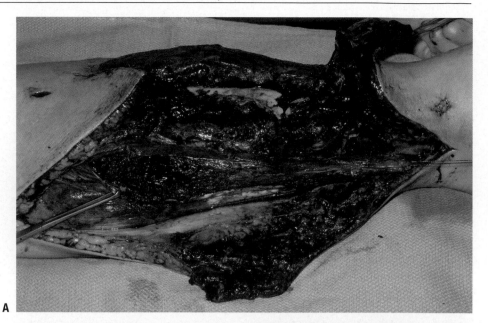

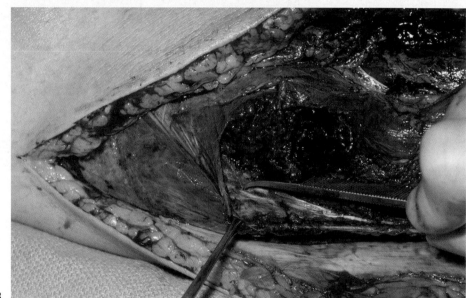

FIGURE 28-7

A: Picture of a middle to lower third Gustilo IIIB injury following a motor vehicle accident in a 58 year old man. The soleus has been separated from the flexor digitorum longus as well as the gastrocnemius muscle. The muscle has just been divided distally and a stay suture has been placed in the distal aspect of the muscle. **B:** A Carroll elevator is used to facilitate dissection of the soleus muscle off the common calcaneal tendon as medial traction is applied to the edge of the tendon with Alice clamps. **C:** The muscle is dissected proximally until enough length is available for defect coverage. Large arterial perforators from the posterior tibial artery are preserved to perfuse the flap (p). *(Continued)*

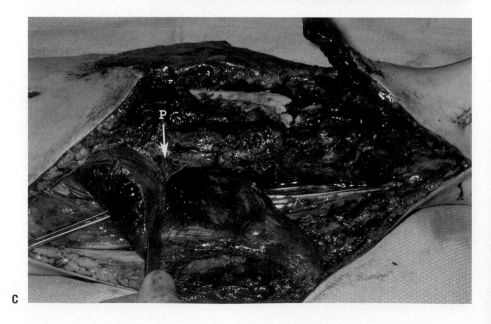

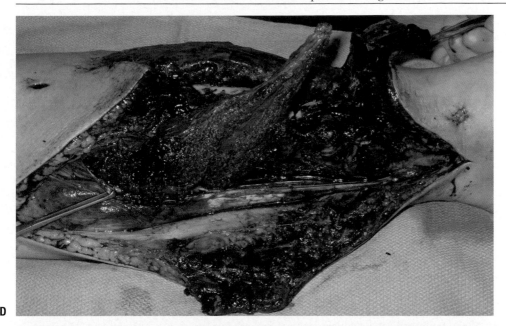

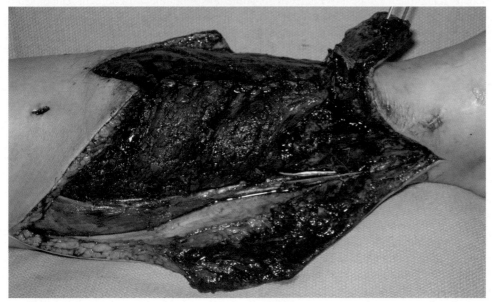

FIGURE 28-7

Continued **D,E:** The flap is then pedicled into position and covered with a split thickness skin graft.

This dissection is aided by placing medial traction on the edge of the Achilles tendon with the use of several clamps (Fig. 28-7). In the distal aspect, the muscle readily separates from the calcaneal tendon. Dissection from the calcaneal tendon is carried to the midline raphe for hemisoleus elevation. The midline septum does not extend the entire length of the muscle but should be used as guide for hemisoleus elevation. Once the soleus is elevated from the calcaneal tendon, the space between the gastrocnemius muscle and the soleus muscle is easily entered and there is a transverse junction point which is easily cut with scissors or a knife. This will free the entire posterior aspect of the soleus muscle.

The posterior tibial artery is identified in the plane between the soleus and flexor digitorum longus. Inferiorly a finger can be passed beneath the soleus muscle but superficial to the posterior tibial vessels. A cautery is then used to separate these medial attachments of the soleus to the tibia. Once the medial aspect of the muscle is mobilized, the space between the soleus and the deep posterior compartments is readily opened with blunt dissection and the lateral aspect of the muscle is identified.

Once the posterior tibial artery and nerve are identified and the superficial and deep attachments of the muscle have been mobilized, the muscle may be divided distally. Distal perforators from the posterior tibial artery and perineal vessels are then sequentially ligated to allow for mobilization of the muscle. There can be multiple small diameter perforators off the posterior tibial artery; these vessels should be clipped or ligated and not cauterized, as thermal injury may be propagated to the posterior tibial vessels.

Once the muscle has been completely elevated, it is rotated into position to cover the defect. Generally, the fascia on the deep surface is left attached to the muscle, but there will be no fascia on the superficial surface. Multiple half buried absorbable sutures can be used to "fan out" the muscle and inset it into the defect site. The distal incision is closed over a drain up to the point of muscle rotation. The muscle should not be tunneled as this can contribute to distal venous congestion within the flap (Figs. 28-6 and 28-7).

The muscle flap is then immediately covered with a meshed skin graft taken from the upper thigh. Vaseline impregnated gauze or a Xeroform dressing are used to cover the skin graft. The leg is then placed in a large Robert-Jones type dressing with the addition of a posterior splint. A window is left in the dressing overlying the muscle so flap checks may be performed while the patient is recovering on the ward.

Lateral and proximally based soleus flap   Though the arc of rotation for this muscle is limited, the lateral approach can be advantageous for some lateral middle third defects. The incision is made just inferior to the lateral border of the fibula. The deep fascia is incised just below the fibula and the plane between the gastrocnemius muscle and soleus are created with blunt dissection. Distally the soleus is again sharply dissected from the calcaneal tendon. Deep proximal dissection involves separating the soleus from its tough attachments to the fibula. During proximal dissection one must be cognizant of the common perineal nerve running close to the fibular head. Once elevated, the muscle is inset as previously described.

Reverse soleus muscle flap   The reverse soleus muscle flap modification (Fig. 28-8) is used to cover small distal defects over the medial anterior aspect of the tibia or medial superior aspect of the medial malleolus (Fig. 28-9). The success of this operation is predicated on the presence of adequate caliber distal perforators from the posterior tibial artery. If during the surgical procedure these perforators are injured or are of insufficient quality the procedure must be abandoned and the defect should be covered with a free tissue transfer. A preoperative angiogram has been recommended by some authors to verify the position of the distal perforator prior to surgery.

Dissection is performed under tourniquet control. The same incision is made as for the proximally based soleus flap (Fig. 28-9). The incision is 2 cm medial to the medial border of the tibia. The existing wound is incorporated into the incision. The medial portion of the soleus is identified as described above and is separated from the gastrocnemius muscle, calcaneal tendon, and the flexor digitorum longus muscle. The posterior tibial artery is identified and the distal perforators are examined. As many distal perforators should be preserved as possible but the authors have had success with the preservation of one or two perforators alone if they are of adequate caliber (vein greater than 1.5 mm and artery of 1 mm or greater). Once the perforatus are determined to be of adequate size, the soleus is then split at the level of the central raphe and divided at the junction of the proximal and middle third. The muscle is then divided longitudinally using the cautery or scissors until the inferior perforator is reached. The muscle is then rotated 90 degrees to 180 degrees. Additional arterial pedicle dissection may be required to prevent vessel kinking. The flap is then inset into the defect with half buried mattress sutures and covered with a split thickness skin graft (Fig. 28-9).

POSTOPERATIVE MANAGEMENT

The patient should be maintained on bed rest in a posterior splint or knee immobilizer for one week. The bolster dressing may be removed on postoperative day 5 to ensure adequate skin graft "take." Until this time the flap ay be monitored through a window in the postoperative dressing. If the skin graft is adherent to the underlying muscle, the patient may begin to mobilize and bear weight as tolerated, barring any underlying fractures. Gentle range of motion should then begin, increasing the motion by 5 or 10 degrees per day. Ambulation can begin on the 10th post-surgical day. If the

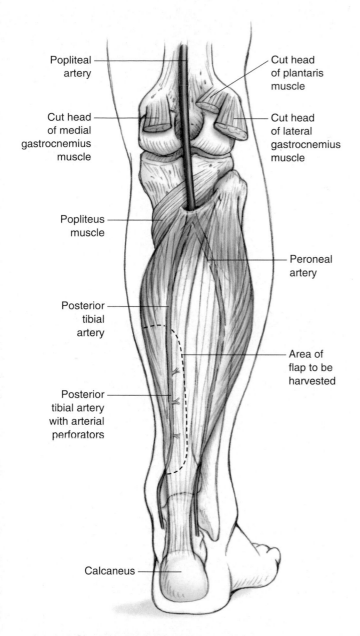

Popliteal artery

Cut head of plantaris muscle

Cut head of medial gastrocnemius muscle

Cut head of lateral gastrocnemius muscle

Popliteus muscle

Peroneal artery

Posterior tibial artery

Area of flap to be harvested

Posterior tibial artery with arterial perforators

Calcaneus

FIGURE 28-8

Schematic drawing of the distally based reverse soleus flap. The flap's arterial supply is from perforators found at the distal portion of the posterior tibial vessels. If present these vessels may be used to supply a strip of soleus muscle which is cut from the medial margin of the soleus muscle.

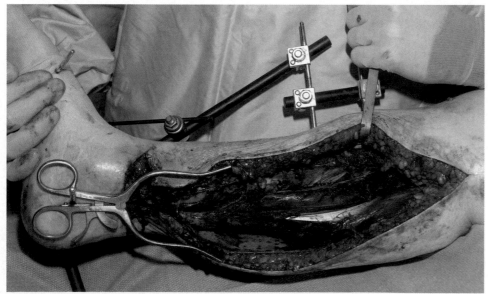

A

FIGURE 28-9

A: A 61 year old female with a distal defect overlying the superior medial margin of the malleolus. An incision was made at the medial posterior margin of the tibia. *(Continued)*

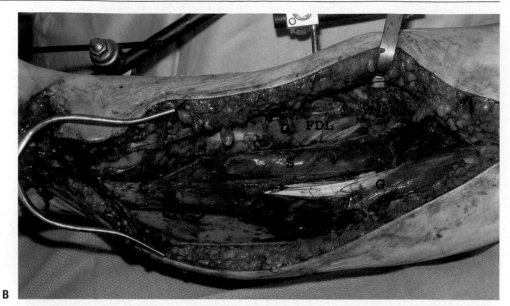

B

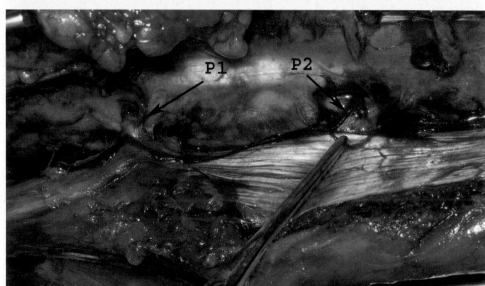

C

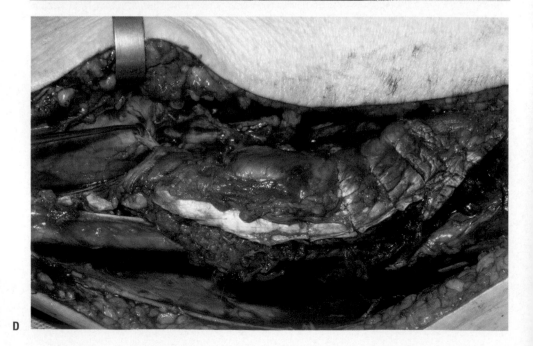

D

FIGURE 28-9

Continued **B:** The gastrocnemius (G), soleus (S) flexor digitorum longus (FDL) and calcaneal tendon (C) are identified. **C:** Exploration of the posterior tibial vessels, in preparation for free tissue transfer, revealed that the patient had two (p1 and p2) large distal perforators to the soleus muscle. Because of this the patient was felt to be an excellent candidate for a distally based soleus muscle flap. **D:** A medial strip of soleus is then elevated from the common calcaneal tendon, gastrocnemius muscle and flexor digitorum longus muscle. The nerve hook points to the preserved distal perforator. *(Continued)*

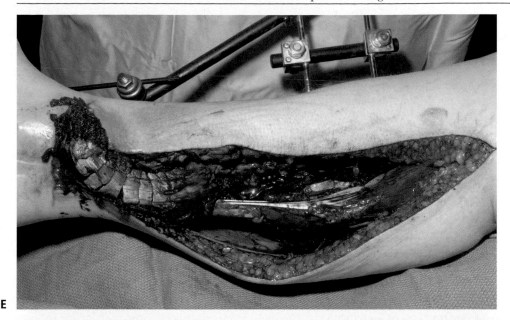

E

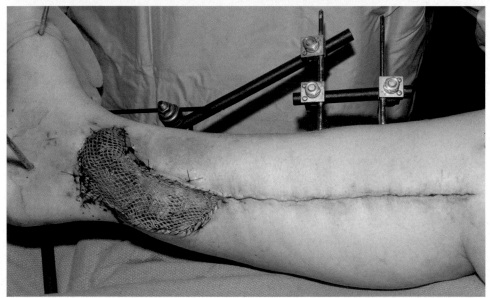

F

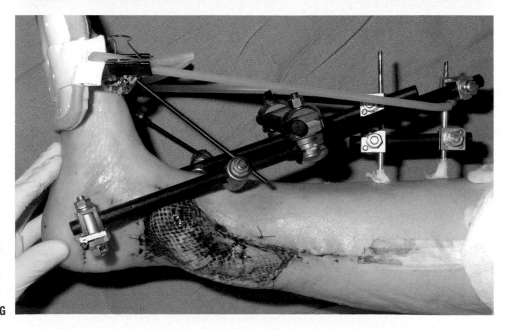

G

FIGURE 28-9

Continued **E:** The muscle is then rotated 180 degrees to cover the distal defect. Care is taken to dissect the proximal perforator back to its origin on the tibial artery to prevent kinking of the artery or vein. **F,G:** The muscle is covered with a split thickness skin graft and the remaining portion of the external fixator is attached to provide needed stabilization.

flap is inset under tension or if the healing environment is less than ideal, the knee immobilizer can be maintained for an additional week to prevent undue tension on the margins of the muscle flap. The drains are removed once drainage is less than 30 cc a day.

Once the original dressing is removed from the skin graft, dressings may be changed daily. This should include the application of topical antibiotic ointment and nonadherent gauze followed by a lightly compressive wrap to minimize edema. Dependent leg position is limited to 30 minutes an hour for the first 2 weeks to minimize edema. On the third postoperative week the patient is fitted for compressive stockings which help the patient continue to manage lower extremity edema and help in the flap contouring.

Rehabilitation

Knee and ankle motion may begin once the skin graft is adherent to the underlying muscle bed. Weight bearing status is determined by the stability of the underlying fractures.

Results

In a study by Hallock of 29 soleus flaps, 24 of 29 flaps were used for coverage of high energy impact defects. All soleus muscle flaps in this study were based on a proximal pedicle. Complication rates were low (13.8%) and there were no cases of total flap loss (1,2). Similar results were reported by Pu, who found no cases of total flap loss when the flap was based on a proximal pedicle for coverage of middle third tibial defects (3,4,7,8).

COMPLICATIONS

Major complications include total and partial flap necrosis. Total flap loss can occur from injury to the vessels at the time of dissection, use of a flap which has been significantly injured with the surrounding bony trauma, or use of the flap in a situation where the posterior tibial vessels and peroneal vessels were compromised or injured. In such cases a free tissue transfer is often needed for leg salvage.

Partial necrosis most often occurs at the distal most margin of the flap. If the partial flap necrosis results in exposure of vital structures, another flap will be required for coverage; most commonly a free flap is used but local fasciocutaneous advancement flaps may be used to cover smaller defects. If the bone is completely covered and the defect is just along the periphery, the wound may be debrided and treated with dressing changes. The remaining wound can then heal through secondary intention.

Skin graft loss may occur due to infection or sheering. Such cases are treated with dressing changes until the underlying muscle bed appears capable of accepting another skin graft. Other minor complications include hematoma in the donor bed and injury to the tibial nerve or the posterior tibial vessels during flap dissection. Both complications may be avoided with meticulous hemostasis and clear identification of the anatomical landmarks prior to muscle division. Limitations in plantar flexion are minimized if the muscle is taken in isolation.

RECOMMENDED READING

Beck JB, Stile F, Lineaweaver W. Reconsidering the soleus muscle flap for coverage of wounds of the distal third of the leg. *Ann Plast Surg*. 2003;50;631–635.

Kauffman CA, Lahoda LU, Cederna PS, et al. Use of the soleus muscle flaps for coverage of distal third tibial defects. *J Reconstr Micro*. 2004;20:593–597.

REFERENCES

1. Bos GD, Buehler MJ. Lower Extremity local flaps. *J Am Acad Orthop Surg*. 1994;2:342–351
2. Hallock GG. Getting the most from the soleus muscle. *Ann Plast Surg*. 1996;36;139–146.
3. Mathes S, Nahai F. Reconstructive Surgery: Principles, anatomy and technique, 1st ed. New York: Churchill Livingstone; 1997:1473–1487.
4. Pu LLQ. Soft tissue reconstruction of an open tibial wound in the distal third of the leg. *Ann Plast Surg*. 2007;58:78–83.
5. Pu LLQ. The reversed medial hemi soleus muscle flap and its role in reconstruction of an open tibial wound in the lower third of the leg. *Ann Plast Surg*. 2006;56:59–64.
6. Pu LLQ. Medial hemi soleus muscle flap: a reliable flap for soft tissue reconstruction of the middle third tibial wound. *Int. Surg*. 2006;91:194–200.
7. Taylor GI, Gianoutsos MP, Morris SF. The neurovascular territories of the skin and muscles: anatomic study and clinical implications. *Plast Reconstr Surg*. 1994;94:1–36.
8. Tobin GR. Hemi soleus and reversed hemi soleus flaps. *Plast Reconstr Surg*. 1985;76:87–96.

29 The Sural Artery Flap

Michael Sauerbier and Thomas Kremer

INDICATIONS/CONTRAINDICATIONS

Soft tissue defects of the lower one-third of the leg and the calcaneal region remain crucial issues. This area is easily susceptible to trauma, and defects of this area are commonly experienced in orthopaedic and trauma surgery.

This region is characterized by tightness and limited mobility of the skin and, frequently, by poor circulation. Thus, chronic and diabetic ulcers, pressure sores, unstable scars, or chronic infection following Achilles tendon rupture or trauma surgery often occur in the distal parts of the leg. Furthermore, exposure of viable structures such as neurovascular bundles, tendons, bone, or osteosynthesis material is a common clinical occurrence due to the superficial course of these structures in the lower one-third of the leg.

In these patients, vascularized soft tissue reconstruction is necessary if further soft tissue damage, with subsequent infection and a potential risk of osteitis, is to be prevented. Relatively few procedures for cutaneous coverage have demonstrated real effectiveness and an acceptable morbidity. In recent years, free microvascular tissue transplantation has become a reliable option among patients suffering from acute or chronic defects in the lower one-third of the leg. Free flaps such as the gracilis flap or the latissimus dorsi flap, as well as fasciocutaneous flaps (e.g., anterolateral thigh flap, parascapular flap, lateral arm flap, and free groin flap) are frequently performed for limb salvage. Despite the fact that free microvascular transplantation possesses the disadvantages of extensive surgery, sophisticated equipment, general anesthesia, and high costs, this procedure often remains the only option for reconstruction of large defects in this region for limb salvage (Fig. 29-1).

For the coverage of smaller defects, alternative options such as pedicled flaps (e.g., flexor digitorum communis flap, medial plantar flap, [hemi-] soleus muscle flap, abductor hallucis flap, peroneal brevis flap, and lateral supramalleolar flap) have been developed (Table 29-1). In 1992, Masquelet et al. published their experimental work involving skin island flaps supplied by the vascular axis of sensitive superficial nerves. The distally based sural artery flap, which is perfused by reverse flow through the anastomosis between the superficial sural artery and the lowermost perforator of the peroneal artery, forms part of this group. One of the advantages of this thin fasciocutaneous flap is that it permits skin coverage with ideal contouring. Other advantages are that it can be performed quickly, the soft tissue coverage is durable, postoperative discomfort and donor site morbidity are minimal, and it is unnecessary to sacrifice major vessels. This flap has been used for the successful coverage of defects of the posterior and inferior surface of the heel, the Achilles tendon, the middle and distal one-third of the leg, and the dorsum of the foot and the lateral—as well as medial—malleolus (Tables 29-2 and 29-3; Figs. 29-2 through 29-4).

The sural artery flap is insensate and is not an option in cases in which sensitivity is an issue. Furthermore, the sacrifice of the sural nerve results in hyposensitivity of the lateral border of the foot.

Because perfusion of large sural artery flaps (>9 × 12 cm) is unreliable, it is not deemed suitable for coverage of extensive defects of the lower one-third of the leg. Moreover, higher complication rates have to be anticipated in patients with comorbidities such as peripheral artery disease, diabetes mellitus, and venous insufficiency. The sural artery flap is contraindicated in patients with destruction of the vascular pedicle or the lowermost perforator of the peroneal artery (see Table 29-2).

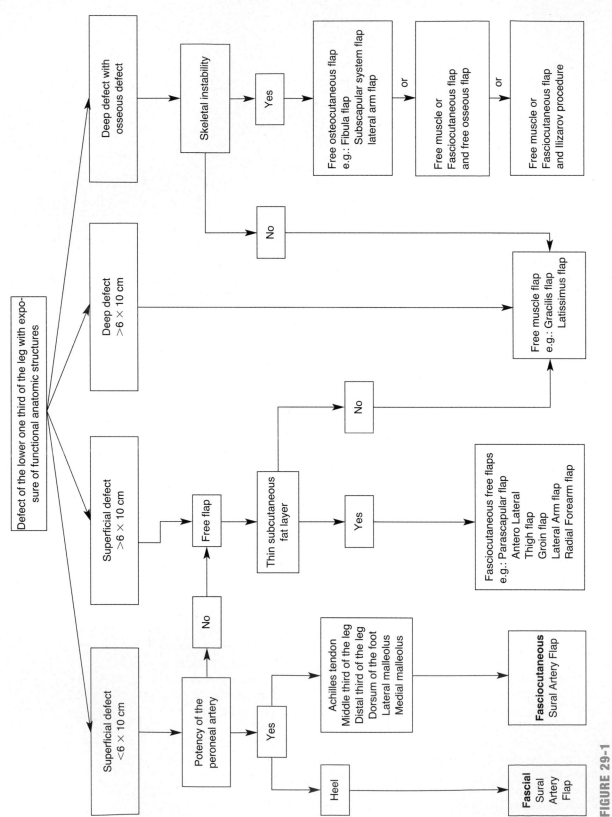

FIGURE 29-1

Treatment algorithm. Small superficial defects of the lower one-third of the leg can be treated by a sural artery flap if the defect size is smaller than 6 × 10 cm. Larger superficial defects can be reconstructed by fasciocutaneous free flaps, whereas deep defects, especially in combination with osseous, defects should be reconstructed by muscle flaps. Defects in the weight bearing area of the heel should be reconstructed by fascial sural artery flaps to prevent pathologic movement of the subcutaneous layer. For alternative pedicled flaps to the lower limb, see Table 29–1.

TABLE 29-1.   Flaps and Their Indications According to Location

Flap	Indications
Soleus flap	Middle third of the leg
Flexor digitorum communis flap	Distal third of the leg
Flexor hallucis longus flap	Distal third of the leg
Peroneus flap	Achilles tendon
Lateral supramalleolar flap	Dorsum of the foot/heel (non-weight bearing)
Dorsalis pedis flap	Foot/distal third of the leg
Extensor digitorum brevis flap	Premalleolar area/dorsum of the foot and toes
Medial plantar flap	Heel (weight bearing)

TABLE 29-2.   Advantages and Disadvantages of the Sural Artery Flap

Advantages	Disadvantages
Constant anatomy	Increased morbidity in patients with comorbidities
Thin flap with ideal contouring	Sacrifice of the sural nerve
Quick procedure	Susceptible to venous congestion
Durable soft tissue coverage	Insensate flap
Low donor site morbidity	Split thickness skin grafts for donor site closure in large
Acceptable donor site scar in small flaps (<4 cm)	flaps (>4 cm)
No sacrifice of major vessels	

TABLE 29-3.   Indications for Sural Artery Flap Reconstruction

Healthy patients with no comorbidities (diabetes mellitus, peripheral artery disease, venous insufficiency)
Skin and soft tissue defects up to 9 × 12 cm:
    Chronic and diabetic ulcers
    Pressure sores
    Chronic infection
    Traumatic defects
    Unstable scars
    Exposure of viable structures (neurovascular bundles, tendons, bone, osteosynthesis material)
One of the following locations:
    Middle and lower third of the leg
    Posterior surface of the heel
    Inferior surface of the heel
    Achilles tendon
    Dorsum of the foot
    Lateral malleolus
    Medial malleolus

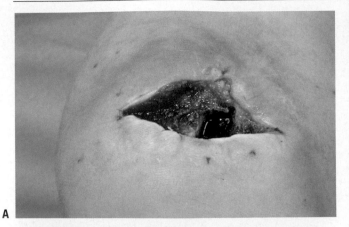

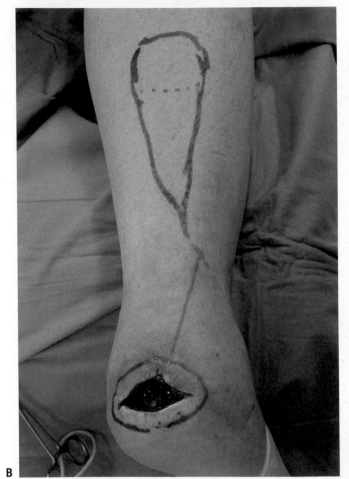

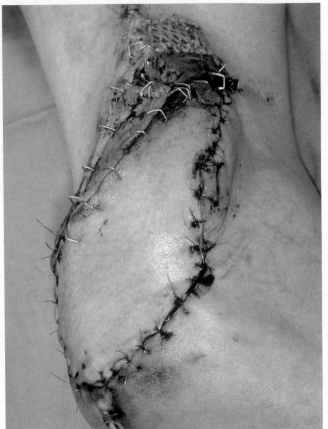

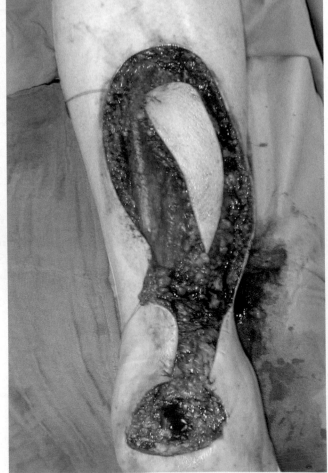

FIGURE 29-2

Male patient suffering from a combined soft tissue and osseous defect in the heel **(A)**. After debridement, soft tissue reconstruction was planned by a sural artery flap **(B)**. Flap transposition was performed to the defect **(C)** after flap harvest **(D)**. *(Continued)*

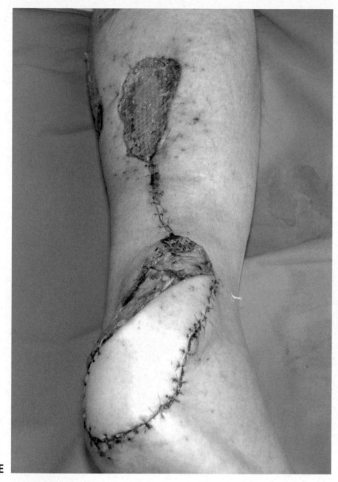
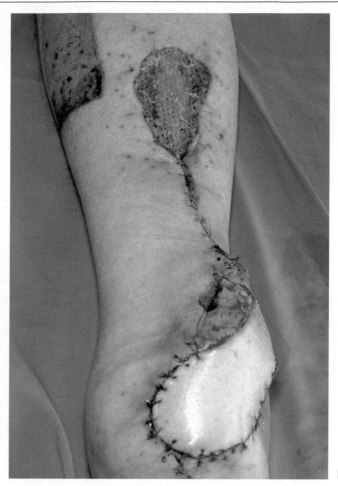

E

F

FIGURE 29-2

Continued Split thickness skin grafting of the donor site was necessary. Postoperative course and wound healing were uneventful **(E,F)**.

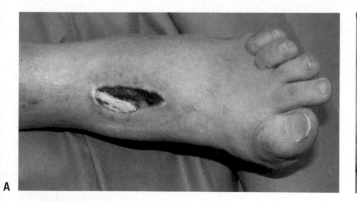
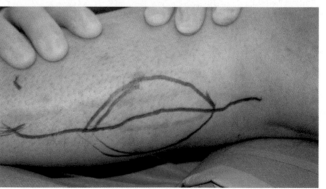

A

B

FIGURE 29-3

A 34-year-old man with a chronic ulcer of the dorsum of the foot. A sural artery flap was planned to reconstruct the defect with exposed tendons **(A,B)**. *(Continued)*

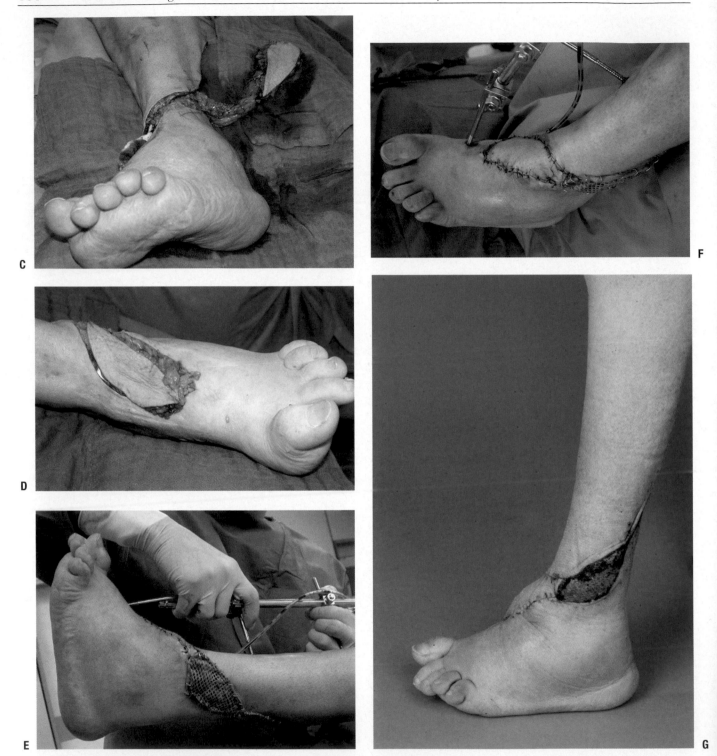

FIGURE 29-3

Continued After complete flap harvest, the skin island is transposed to the defect **(C,D)**. The skin over the pedicle is incised and split thickness skin grafted to reduce pressure on the nutrient vessels **(E,F)**. The functional and aesthetic results are excellent 2 weeks post surgery **(G)**. *(Continued)*

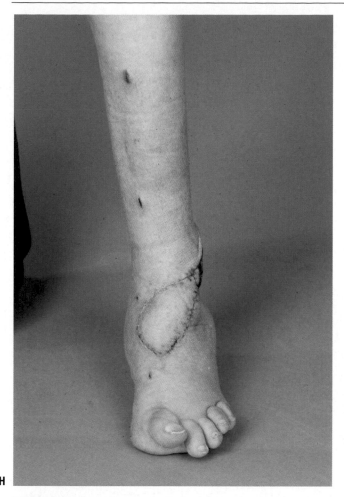
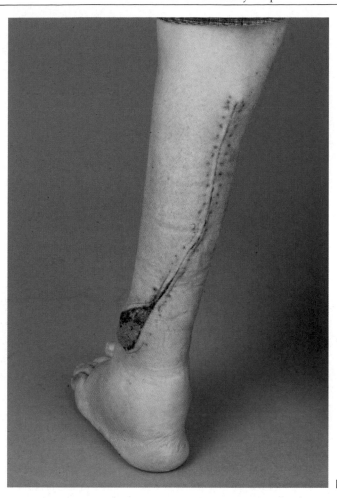

H

I

FIGURE 29-3

Continued The functional and aesthetic results are excellent 2 weeks post surgery **(H,I)**.

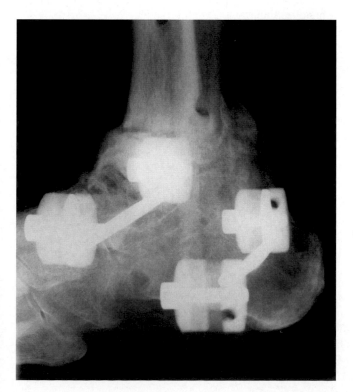

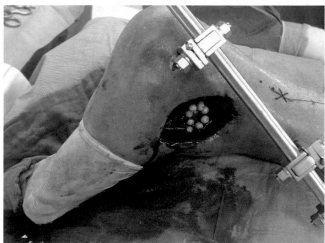

FIGURE 29-4

A 36-year-old woman with osteitis (above left). After debridement and application of an antibiotic chain (above right). *(Continued)*

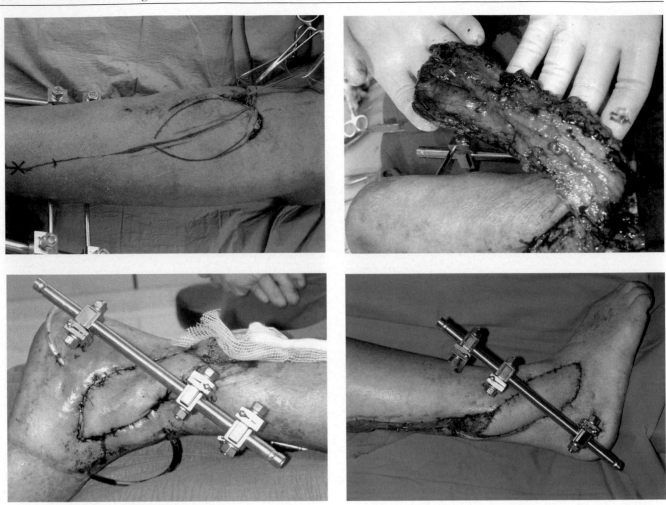

FIGURE 29-4

Continued Defect reconstruction was planned by a sural artery flap (upper left). After complete flap harvest, the pedicle is visible through the cural fascia, which has to be included in the flap (upper right). After transposition to the defect, wound healing was uneventful (below).

PREOPERATIVE PLANNING

A thorough clinical and radiologic examination of the donor and the recipient sites is mandatory, and it is first necessary to estimate the size of the recipient site defect. There are no studies regarding maximum flap dimensions with regard to safety, but small and moderate-sized defects can usually be covered satisfactorily. Defects up to 9 × 12 cm have been successfully reconstructed using sural artery flaps. Radical debridement may result in an enlargement of the defect, and this should be taken into account in the preoperative planning.

An examination of the patient's peripheral function should be performed to determine the total extent of the injury. Depending on the size and location of the defect, various functional structures may be exposed or destroyed. Changes in the normal resting position of the foot and toes will help identify the loss of continuity of lower extremity tendons, and traditional functional tests will confirm the loss of active range of motion. A careful examination of sensitivity and muscle function helps to evaluate the extent of the defect in terms of destruction of sensor or motor nerve components. Additionally, peripheral perfusion should be ascertained by simple palpation of pulses or by Doppler probe. If in doubt, an angiogram should be performed. If any of these structures have been destroyed, additional reconstruction procedures must be planned. In patients suffering from chronic or infected wounds or diabetic gangrene, additional osteitis or osteomyelitis must be considered and conventional radiographs and/or magnetic resonance imaging (MRI) scans can help to prove the existence or extent of altered osseous structures.

TABLE 29-4.   Preoperative Planning for Sural Artery Flap Reconstruction

Clinical examination
   Defect size (after debridement)
   Peripheral function (to determine destruction of functional structures [nerves, tendons, blood vessels])
MRI or conventional radiographs of the recipient site (fractures, extension of osseous or soft tissue defects, osteitis)
Examination of patency of the lesser sapheneous vein and peroneal artery
   Doppler ultrasound probe in healthy patients
   Conventional angiogram or MRI-angiogramm in comorbid patients
Detailed information of the patient
   Sacrifice of the sural nerve (hyposensitivity of the lateral border of the foot)
   Neuroma formation
   Split thickness skin grafting of the donor site

The sural artery flap pedicle should be examined preoperatively. In all patients the patency of the peroneal artery and the lesser saphenous vein is examined by palpation of pulses and Doppler probe. Additionally, the lowermost perforators between the peroneal artery and the flap pedicle can be examined 4 to 7 cm proximal to the tip of the lateral malleolus. In patients with comorbid conditions such as diabetes mellitus and peripheral vessel disease, flap perfusion may be particularly unreliable. In these patients, a conventional angiogram or an MRI-angiogram can be helpful in preoperative planning procedures.

Finally, the surgeon should provide the patient with a detailed account of the surgical procedure. Information regarding the postoperative function, the possibility of persisting complaints, and donor site morbidity should be given. In particular, the loss of sensitivity of the lateral border of the foot and the possibility of neuroma formation as well as the potential necessity of donor site closure by split thickness skin grafting should be discussed (Table 29-4).

SURGERY

Anatomy

The reverse flow sural artery flap is based on the vascular network along the sural nerve. The nutritient artery is the superficial sural artery (SSA), which arises from the popliteal artery proximal to the medial and lateral sural arteries in about 65% of cases, directly from the medial (20%) or lateral (8%) sural artery, or sometimes from the common stem of origin of the two. The artery courses posteriorly for 2 to 3 cm before joining the medial sural nerve descending between the two heads of the gastrocnemius muscle. The medial sural nerve anastomoses with the communicating branch of the lateral sural nerve to become the sural nerve. Both the medial sural nerve and the SSA pierce the crural fascia at the junction of the proximal and middle thirds of the leg to become subcutaneous. The SSA courses alongside the sural nerve to the lateral malleolus in 65% of all patients; in 35% of cases the artery fades into a vascular net at the distal one-third of the leg. Regardless of the termination, the SSA has a constant distal anastomosis from the lateral malleolar arteries, which in turn arises from the peroneal artery. The distally based sural artery flap is dependent on this anastomosis, and its perfusion is reverse flow through the SSA and its cutaneous branches at the distal two-thirds of the leg.

The venous drainage of the sural artery flap is dependent on small commitant veins and mainly on the short saphenous vein which accompanies the sural nerve at the distal two-thirds of the leg. Theoretically, a reverse flow in this vein is impossible due to of the presence of valves; however, clinical findings disprove this theory. Duplex scans of the small saphenous vein generally show a continuous or phasic reverse flow postoperatively. Several theories exist regarding these findings. Some authors stress the existence of bridges between the short saphenous vein and the commitant veins, thus bypassing the valves. Moreover, denervation of the short saphenous vein due to the surgical procedure and increased venous pressure due to the altered flow are thought to be responsible for venous dilatation, which renders the valves insufficient.

Overall, the sural artery flap exhibits a constant anatomy with reliable arterial perfusion and venous drainage.

Surgical Procedure

Surgery is performed in general anesthesia; however, in elderly patients or because of comorbidities, epidural or spinal anesthesia is also possible. Depending on the defect location, the patient is placed in prone position or in a ventral or lateral decubitus position.

The recipient site is first prepared. In patients with chronic wounds, infection, diabetic gangrene, or wound colonization, a radical debridement is mandatory. Analogous to the principles of oncologic resections, a complete resection of the entire infected or altered tissue must be performed. An insufficiently radical debridement renders the reconstructive attempts unsuccessful; therefore, compromises are unacceptable. If, after debridement, the recipient defect is too large for a sural artery flap reconstruction, a temporary wound closure (e.g., vacuum-assisted closure [VAC] therapy) should be performed and other therapeutic options such as free flaps should be planned. For this reason, it can be useful to include the possibility of free flap reconstruction in the initial preoperative patient briefing so that a one-step reconstruction can be carried out.

The authors prefer to perform flap harvest under pneumatic tourniquet (500 mm Hg) to make visualization of the anatomy easier. In addition, the surgeon should use 2.5 to 4 times magnification loupes.

As mentioned previously, the short saphenous vein and the arterial perforators of the peroneal artery on the lateral aspect of the distal leg have to be located using a Doppler ultrasound probe. Following debridement, the defect size is measured and a skin island with adequate dimensions is planned with its center along the line of the short saphenous vein. The proximal limit of the flap should not exceed a boundary of 20 cm proximal to the lateral malleolus, due to the fact that the portion of the flap that exceeds the suprafascial (subcutaneous) portion of the nerve behaves like a random extension, and thus its reliability is unsure. The skin island is planned in the middle or distal third of the leg, according to the pedicle length required (Fig. 29-5). Because of its thicker subcutaneous tissue, the skin island should be designed to be slightly larger than the recipient defect to facilitate skin-to-skin closure of the defect. The maximum size of the skin island should not exceed 9 × 12 cm. The pivot point is marked 5 cm above the tip of the lateral malleolus to include the branches that anastomose with the peroneal artery. The skin incision starts distally along the line of the pedicle to localize the vein. If the skin island is not centered over the short saphenous vein, correction of the flap position is still possible. When the pedicle has been located, the dissection proceeds in the proximal extreme of the flap; again, the short saphenous vein and the sural nerve are identified suprafascially. At this point, the short saphenous vein, the suralis nerve, and the SSA are ligated, divided, and included into the flap. The proximal stump of the nerve is coagulated and buried in the surrounding gastrocnemius musculature to avoid a troublesome neuroma over the donor area. Some authors report raising the flap and sparing the sural nerve to prevent neuroma formation and foot hyposensitivity. In our opinion this strategy is too risky for the vascular supply of the flap and is unnecessary because the morbidity of harvesting the flap with the sural nerve is minimal. In the literature, several series show no significant alteration in foot sensitivity, and in most cases, patients exhibit improved sensitivity over time.

Dissection proceeds distally at the plane below the deep fascia, so that inclusion of the pedicle in the flap is easily accomplished and the nutrient anastomosis of the flap can be preserved. Two to three constant and direct perforators from the gastrocnemius muscle to the vascular axis of the sural nerve are identified and ligated with ligature clips, because electrocoagulation of these perforators increases the risk of pedicle destruction. The fascial and subcutaneous pedicle, which includes the SSA, the sural nerve, and the short saphenous vein, should be at least 3 cm in width. The paratenon of the sural triceps muscle should be carefully preserved, especially when split thickness skin grafting of the donor site defect is necessary. The flap procedure remains simple if care is taken to avoid dissection too close to the pedicle and if dissection is only extended to the demarcated limit of 5 cm above the tip of the lateral malleolus. During elevation of the flap, near this inferior limit of dissection, efforts should be made to preserve the large perforating septocutaneous vessels.

When flap harvest is completed, transposition of the skin island to the recipient defect can be performed. Under normal conditions (e.g., a sufficient amount of elastic skin), the flap can be transposed through a subcutaneous tunnel. However, when there is any sign of tight skin or venous congestion, a decompression of the pedicle must be performed. The risk of pedicle compression increases with edema formation, surrounding scars, or skin induration and/or thick and inelastic skin. In patients with this risk profile, two approaches should be considered. First, skin extensions (the "cutaneous tail") overlying the pedicle can facilitate defect closure and reduction of pressure on

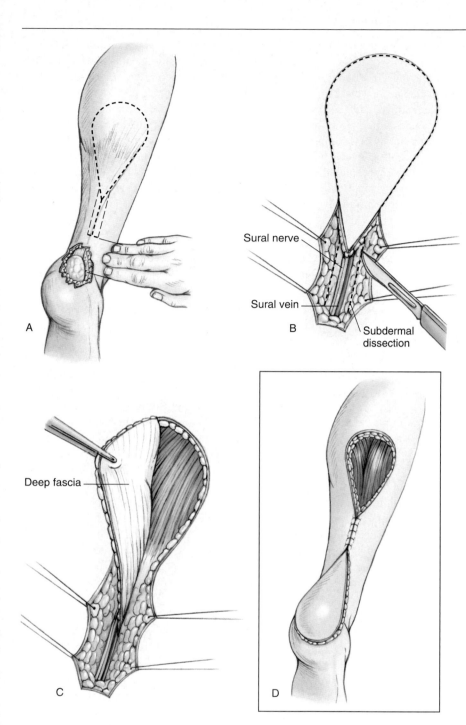

Sural nerve

Sural vein

Subdermal
dissection

Deep fascia

A

B

C

D

FIGURE 29-5

The skin island has to be planned according to the size of the defect with its center along the line of the short saphenous vein. The pivotal point is three fingers breadth to the tip of the lateral malleolus **(A)**. The skin incision starts distally along the line of the pedicle to localize the vein. The subcutaneous pedicle should be at least 3 cm wide (**B**; 1—sural vein and nerve; 2—subdermal dissection). Dissection proceeds along the plane below the deep fascia; thus, inclusion of the pedicle in the flap is easily possible and the nutrient anastomosis can be preserved (**C**: 3—deep fascia included). After complete flap elevation, the flap is transposed to the recipient site **(D)**.

the pedicle after transposition. Second, the bridge over the subcutaneous tunnel can be incised and a split thickness skin graft can be used to cover the pedicle. In the literature, the possibility of using the "distally based sural artery interpolation flap" is described. This involves transposition of the flap to the defect without tunneling, and the pedicle is exteriorized and skin grafted. In a second procedure, after randomization, the pedicle is removed. The authors have no experience using this approach, but there appears to be no distinct advantage of this approach over other options. Indeed, it has the disadvantage of a two-step procedure.

If signs of insufficient perfusion or venous drainage occur after flap transposition and if decompression of the pedicle is unsuccessful in resolving this problem, a suralis flap delay procedure is possible. In this procedure, the flap is replaced into its donor site bed, a powder-free glove is placed between the elevated fascia and the gastrocnemius muscle, and transposition is performed 2 to 4 days later.

In some cases, the reverse flow sural artery flap can be modified. Hence, muscle tissue can be included in the flap when the perforating vessels from the gastrocnemius muscle to the vascular axis of the sural nerve (see previous discussion) are preserved. Flap harvest is similar to the procedure described previously. The only difference is that a fragment of the gastrocnemius muscle is taken from the lower part of the muscle without separating the fascia from the muscle fragment. Another option is to elevate the flap as a fascial flap without a skin island; this is the preferred approach of some authors in patients with heel defects. In these cases, the flap is covered by split thickness skin grafting. Furthermore, some authors describe the possibility of reconstructing defects distant from the sural artery flap donor site by performing a free microvascular sural artery flap.

Donor site closure is possible primarily when a skin island of less than 4 cm in width is harvested. In these cases, the donor site is acceptable in terms of function as well as aesthetics. Larger donor site defects have to be closed by split thickness skin grafting. In these cases, the acceptability of the donor site scar is questionable, particularly among obese patients and females.

POSTOPERATIVE MANAGEMENT

The most important postoperative issue is prevention of compression of the vascular pedicle. This can be achieved either by an adequately elevated position of the leg and/or by the use of conventional splints with a gap over the flap; however, the authors prefer using an external fixation device. External fixation incorporates the treatment of concomitant fractures and prevention of an equinus, as well as elevated positioning of the leg.

The administration of anticoagulants in the postoperative period after pedicled flap reconstruction remains controversial. To the authors' knowledge, there is no scientific evidence of beneficial effects of an anticoagulation therapy in terms of flap survival or thrombosis rates. Moreover, one could postulate that anticoagulants increase perioperative morbidity due to bleeding and hematoma. Nevertheless, in our center, as in many other centers, we usually use an postoperative regimen of hydroxyethyl starch (HAES 10%; 500 mL in 24 hours for 5 days) and heparin or low-molecular-weight heparin (Clexane). Moreover, all patients are treated with antibiotics (cephalosporin) perioperatively. Antibiotic treatment is prolonged if the patient shows an increased risk of postoperative wound infection or persistent infection.

Surveillance of flap perfusion in terms of arterial as well as venous flow must be performed regularly during the first postoperative days. In the authors' department, the capillary refill is tested every hour for the first 48 hours. Thereafter, the intervals between testing are increased.

A revision procedure should be performed if any signs of poor arterial perfusion or venous congestion are identified. New positioning of the vascular pedicle or decompression of the nutrient vessels may facilitate flap salvage. Moreover, the flap may be laid back in the donor site bed if these options fail.

The patient has complete bed rest for a minimum of 5 days. After this period compression bandages are applied to the treated leg and mobilization begins. The regimen begins with hanging down the leg for 5 minutes. The tolerance of the flap to this treatment (as well as accompanying injuries) determines the next stages of mobilization. If signs of venous congestion or poor perfusion are recognized, the mobilization regimen is prolonged. In most cases, the patient is completely mobilized after 10 days. The further use of a compression garment is obligatory for a period of at least 1 year after discharge to improve contouring of the flap and avoid hypertrophic scarring. Secondary corrections at the recipient as well as the donor site should not be performed until at least 6 months post surgery.

COMPLICATIONS

Partial or complete necrosis of the sural artery flap remains the most important issue concerning the success or failure of this reconstructive method. Necrosis rates between 5% and 36% have been described in the literature. A detailed analysis of the study cohorts helps to explain these different findings. When patients with comorbidities are excluded, the patient's age alone has been found to be a significant risk factor for flap necrosis. Furthermore, systemic diseases such as diabetes mellitus, peripheral arterial disease, and venous insufficiency are considered to be negative predictors for flap survival. Therefore, necrosis rates should always be interpreted in relation to the risk profile of the individual patient.

However, comorbidity with any of the above-mentioned diseases does not present an absolute contraindication to this approach, especially in view of the limited alternatives. First, it should be kept in mind that the flap does still have a chance of success; second, the sural artery flap often represents the last chance of limb salvage in multi-morbid patients who are not suitable candidates for a free flap transfer. Some authors suggest that in cases of partial and even complete necrosis, the sural artery flap can serve as a valuable biologic dressing, so that the reconstructive surgeon sometimes experiences a well-vascularized granulating wound after debridement of the necrotic flap that allows successful split thickness skin transplantation. It seems that vascularization improves under the flap, which facilitates a skin graft on a wound bed that initially would not have been possible.

Several technical guidelines should be followed to prevent perioperative morbidity, particularly among patients with an increased risk of flap necrosis. The first of these guidelines is the use of the Doppler ultrasound in preoperative planning. Then, as described previously, the sural nerve should be included in the flap and the surgeon should pay attention to the subcutaneous layer. It can cause the flap to be bulky at the recipient site and, therefore, increases the risk of pedicle compression. The solution is to plan the flap slightly larger than the defect to facilitate skin-to-skin closure or to perform extensive mobilization of the surrounding skin, although this in turn can cause wound healing disturbances. We recommend the use of an external fixation device to prevent pedicle compression and to facilitate postoperative care, especially in less compliant patients. Tunneling of the vascular pedicle should only be performed if elastic skin surrounds the defect; otherwise, the pedicle should be grafted or the skin paddle should be planned in a teardrop shape to facilitate pedicle coverage (see previously). Furthermore, it should be taken into consideration that the more proximal the donor site is planned, the greater the risk of necrosis.

Further complications described in the literature are not specific to sural artery flaps but relate to the underlying defect or the surgical procedure, respectively. Wound infection or persistent infection are common findings as well as hematoma, delayed healing, or persistent osteitis (which itself is usually due to incomplete debridement). As described previously, inelastic skin and induration are familiar findings especially in patients with comorbidities. Therefore, the skin surrounding the flap margins or the pedicle may require skin grafting for wound closure. Edema formation is common, especially in patients with venous insufficiency. In these cases, application of compression bandages may help improve local trophicity.

Donor site morbidity is generally low. The most common findings are neuroma of the sural nerve and scarring. In these patients, secondary corrections should be performed. Neuromas have to be resected, and the nerve stump has to be buried in the surrounding musculature.

RECOMMENDED READING

Almeida MF, da Costa PR, Okawa RY. Reverse-flow island sural flap. *Plast Reconstr Surg.* 2002;109:583-591.

Arnez ZM, Kersnic M, Smith RW, et al. Free lateral arm osteocutaneous neurosensory flap for thumb reconstruction. *J Hand Surg [Br].* 1991;16:395–399.

Baumeister SP, Spierer R, Erdmann D, et al. A realistic complication analysis of 70 sural artery flaps in a multimorbid patient group. *Plast Reconstr Surg.* 2003;112:129–140.

Bocchi A, Merelli S, Morellini A, et al. Reverse fasciosubcutaneous flap versus distally pedicled sural island flap: two elective methods for distal third leg reconstruction. *Ann Plast Surg.* 2000;45:284–291.

Cavadas PC, Bonanad E. Reverse-flow sural island flap in the varicose leg. *Plast Reconstr Surg.* 1996;98:901-902.

Cormack GC, Lamberty BG. A classification of fascio-cutaneous flaps according to their patterns of vascularisation. *Br J Plast Surg.* 1984;37:80–87.

Costa-Ferreira A, Reis J, Pinho C, et al. The distally based island superficial sural artery flap: clinical experience with 36 flaps. *Ann Plast Surg.* 2001;46:308–313.

Dolph JL. The superficial sural artery flap in distal lower third extremity reconstruction. *Ann Plast Surg.* 1998;40:520–522.

Donski PK, Fogdestam I. Distally based fasciocutaneous flap from the sural region. A preliminary report. *Scand J Plast Reconstr Surg.* 1983;17:191–196.

Erdmann D, Gottlieb N, Humphrey JS, et al. Sural flap delay procedure: a preliminary report. *Ann Plast Surg.* 2005;54:562–565.

Fraccalvieri M, Verner G, Dolcet M, et al. The distally based superficial sural flap: our experience in reconstructing the lower leg and foot. *Ann Plast Surg.* 2000;45:132–141.

Germann G, Bickert B, Steinau HU, et al. Versatility and reliability of combined flaps of the subscapular system. *Plast Reconstr Surg.* 1999;103:1386–1399.

Germann GK. Invited discussion. The simple and effective choice for treatment of chronic calcaneal osteomyelitis: neurocutaneous flaps. *Plast Reconstr Surg.* 2003;111:761–762.

Goldberg JA, Adkins P, Tsai TM. Microvascular reconstruction of the foot: weightbearing pattern, gait analysis and long term follow-up. *Plast Reconstr Surg.* 1993;93:904–911.

Hasegawa M, Torii S, Katoh H, et al. The distally based superficial sural artery flap. *Plast Reconstr Surg.* 1994;93:1012–1020.

Huisinga RL, Houpt P, Dijkstra R, et al. The distally based sural artery flap. *Ann Plast Surg.* 1998;41:58–65.

Hyakusoku H, Tonegawa H, Fumiiri M. Heel coverage with a t-shaped distally based sural island fasciocutaneous flap. *Plast Reconstr Surg.* 1994;93:872–876.

Imanishi N, Nakajima H, Fukuzumi S, et al. Venous drainage of the distally based lesser saphenous-sural-venoneuroadipofascial pedicled fasciocutaneous flap: a radiographic perfusion study. *Plast Reconstr Surg.* 1999;103:494–498.

Jeng SF, Wei FC. Distally based sural island flap for foot and ankle reconstruction. *Plast Reconstr Surg.* 1997;99:744–750.

Jeng SF, Hsieh CH, Kuo YR, et al. Distally based sural island flap. *Plast Reconstr Surg.* 2003;111:840–841.

Katsaros J, Tan E, Zoltie N, et al. Further experience with the lateral arm free flap. *Plast Reconstr Surg.* 1991;85:902–910.

Koshima I, Fukuda H, Utunomiya R, et al. The anterolateral thigh flap; variations in vascular pedicle. *Br J Plast Surg.* 1989;42:260.

Le Fourn B, Caye N, Pannier M. Distally based sural fasciomuscular flap: anatomic study and application for filling leg or foot defects. *Plast Reconstr Surg.* 2001;107:67–72.

Lin SD, Lai CS, Chiu CC. Venous drainage in the reverse forearm flap. *Plast Reconstr Surg.* 1984;74:508–512.

Lin TS, Jeng SF, Wei FC. Temporary placement of defatted plantar heel skin in the calf and subsequent transfer to the heel using distally based sural artery flap as a carrier. *Plast Reconstr Surg.* 2002;109:1358–1360.

Maffi TR, Knoetgen Jr, Turner NS, et al. Enhanced survival using the distally based sural artery interpolation flap. *Ann Plast Surg.* 2005;54:302–305.

Masquelet AC, Romana MC, Wolf G. Skin island flaps supplied by the vascular axis of sensitive superficial nerves: anatomic study and clinical experience in the leg. *Plast Reconstr Surg.* 1992;89:1115–1121.

McGregor IA, Jackson IT. The groin flap. *Br J Plast Surg.* 1972;24:3.

Mueller JE, Ilchmann T, Lowatscheff T. The musculocutaneous sural artery flap for soft tissue coverage after calcaneal fracture. *Arch Orthop Trauma Surg.* 2001;121:350–352.

Nakajima H, Imanishi N, Fukuzumi S, et al. Accompanying arteries of the lesser saphenous vein and sural nerve: anatomic study and its clinical applications. *Plast Reconstr Surg.* 1999;103:104–120.

Nassif TM, LV, Bovet JL, et al. The parascapular flap: a new cutaneous microsurgical free flap. *Plast Reconstr Surg.* 1982;69:591–597.

Ögun TC, Arazi M, Kutlu A. An easy and versatile method of coverage for distal tibial soft tissue defects. *J Trauma.* 2001;50:63–69.

Ponten B. The fasciocutaneous flap: Its use in soft tissue defects of the lower leg. *Br J Plast Surg.* 1981;34:215–220.

Price MF, Capizzi PJ, Watterson PA, et al. Reverse sural artery flap: caveats for success. *Ann Plast Surg.* 2002;48:496–504.

Rajacic N, Darweesh M, Jayakrishnan K, et al. The distally based superficial sural flap for reconstruction of the lower leg and foot. *Br J Plast Surg.* 1996;49:383–389.

Satoh K, Fukuya F, Matsui A, et al. Lower leg reconstruction using a sural fasciocutaneous flap. *Ann Plast Surg.* 1989;23:97–103.

Sauerbier M, Erdmann D, Bruner S, et al. Covering soft tissue defects and unstable scars over the achilles tendon by free microsurgical flap-plasty. *Chirurg.* 2000;71:1161–1166.

Shepler H, Sauerbier M, Germann GK. The distally pedicled suralis flap for the defect coverage of posttraumatic and cronic soft tissue lesions in the "critical" lower leg (in german). *Chirurg.* 1997;68:1170–1177.

Singh S, Naasan A. Use of distally based superficial sural island artery flaps in acute open fractures of the lower leg. *Ann Plast Surg.* 2001;47:505–510.

Song R, Song Y, Yu Y, et al. The upper arm free flap. *Clin Plast Surg.* 1982;9:27–35.

Song R, Gao Y, Song Y, et al. The forearm flap. *Clin Plast Surg.* 1982;9:21–26.

Torii S, Namiki Y, Mori R. Reverse-flow island flap: clinical report and venous drainage. *Plast Reconstr Surg.* 1987;79:600–609.

Touam C, Rostoucher P, Bhatia A, et al. Comparative study of two series of distally based fasciocutaneous flaps of the lower one-fourth of the leg, the ankle and the foot. *Plast Reconstr Surg.* 2001;107:383–392.

Yilmaz M, Karatas O, Barutcu A. The distally based superficial sural artery island flap: clinical experiences and modifications. *Plast Reconstr Surg.* 1998;102:2358–2367.

30 Fasciotomies of the Lower Extremity

Christopher J. Salgado, Amir A. Jamali, and Jason Nascone

INDICATIONS/CONTRAINDICATIONS

Compartment syndrome is the most common indication for fasciotomy. Compartment syndrome is a clinical condition with elevated tissue pressure within a closed anatomic compartment. Muscles are contained within an osseofascial compartment that has a limited capacity to expand. The causes of compartment syndrome can be divided into two major categories: decreased compartment size and increased compartment volume. Decreases in compartment size can be due to extrinsic factors such as tight dressings or casts or due to intrinsic causes such as bleeding into a compartment after injury or a postoperative coagulopathy. Increased compartment volume can occur at the macroscopic or microscopic level. Bleeding or iatrogenic infiltration of intravenous fluid into a closed compartment are both common causes of compartment syndrome. At the microscopic level, compartment volume can be increased in proportion to either increased capillary permeability and/or capillary pressure. Conditions associated with tissue damage such as burns, ischemia/reperfusion, and trauma can all lead to increased capillary permeability. Increased capillary pressure is the underlying cause of compartment syndrome due to venous obstruction or exercise.

The underlying pathologic condition leading to compartment syndrome is an elevated tissue pressure which leads to decreased arteriolar perfusion. At this point shunting occurs, bypassing the capillary circulation which then worsens the tissue ischemia, and in turn, increases the capillary permeability and interstitial tissue pressure. This vicious cycle can quickly lead to permanent tissue damage if not treated expediently. The tissues most at risk in compartment syndrome are the nerves and muscles. If untreated, compartment syndrome can lead to Volkmann's contracture, a permanent paralysis of muscles in the compartment with scarring in a shortened position leading to the term "contracture." Assessment of an injured lower extremity must include a thorough evaluation of factors, which can contribute either directly or indirectly to compartment syndrome. A list of such factors is given in Table 30-1. The treatment of compartment syndrome is the correction of the underlying pathologic state and the performance of a fasciotomy. Fasciotomy is the incision of fascial compartments in order to expand the size of the compartment and to restore tissue perfusion to the contents of the compartment.

PREOPERATIVE PLANNING

Preoperative planning of a fasciotomy is based on an accurate and timely diagnosis of compartment syndrome. The most important data guiding this decision is the clinical examination. In the setting of an awake, unsedated patient, the diagnosis can commonly be made based on clinical grounds. The classical clinical signs of compartment syndrome are the six P's: pain, pressure, paresthesia, paralysis, pallor, and pulselessness. Note that significant muscle damage occurs prior to the onset of pallor, pulselessness, and paralysis, and that these are late findings of a missed compartment syndrome. The most sensitive clinical sign of compartment syndrome is pain. This is often described as being out of proportion to the injury. In the author's experience, the variability of pain threshold among

TABLE 30-1. Compartment Syndrome Risk Factors

History	Injury	Treatment
Crush injury	Open and closed fractures	Fluid administration
Entrapment	Arterial injury	Tourniquets
Ischemia	Venous injury	Positioning
Shock/hypotension	Gunshot wounds to extremity	MAST
Overdose/unconsciousness	Coagulopathy	Arthroscopy pumps
Tight ski boots	Shock	Jet lavage
Coumadin	Deep vein thrombosis	Revascularization
Weightlifting/overuse	Burns	Vein ligation
Knee arthroscopy	Muscle tear	Fracture tables
	Snake envenomation	Tight wound closures
	Ruptured Baker's cyst	Constrictive dressings
		Regional anesthesia

MAST, Military anti-shock trousers

patients can make the assessment of "expected level of pain" somewhat arbitrary. The presence of a greater than expected level of pain does not indicate definitive compartment syndrome and the absence of pain does not rule out the diagnosis, particularly in the setting of a possible neurologic injury. The use of sedatives and analgesics, a history of central nervous system trauma, and the possibility of peripheral nerve injury highlight the need for a high index of suspicion and the need for early intracompartmental pressure measurements. Passive stretching of muscles within the compartment leads to elevated pressures and increased pain, another valuable tool in establishing a clinical diagnosis. Other signs of compartment syndrome include paresthesias and paralysis. Paresthesias are due to ischemic damage to the peripheral nerves running in the compartment. Decreased 2-point discrimination is the most consistent early finding. Correlation has also been reported between diminished vibration sense (256 cycles per sec) and increasing compartment pressure. On deep palpation, a firm wooden feeling is a specific sign when present. Bullae may also be observed. In later stages, the paresthesias can progress to complete anesthesia in the distribution of the peripheral nerve.

Paralysis can be due to muscle ischemia, nerve ischemia, direct injury to these structures, or secondary to pain inhibition. Pulselessness is uncommon in an isolated compartment syndrome and heralds a probable vascular injury. Laboratory testing revealing a creatine kinase (CK) of 1,000 to 5,000 U/mL or higher or the presence of myoglobinuria may alert the physician to the occurrence of compartment syndrome. When the clinical picture is borderline, compartment pressure measurements must be performed as soon as possible.

A number of techniques have been employed to determine compartment pressures, including variations in size and needle design. At our institution all compartment measurements are performed with a side-port needle attached to a commercially available pressure monitor (Stryker, Kalamazoo, MI) or a standard arterial line pressure transduction line (Fig.30-1). The Stryker pressure tonometer is widely used, and pressure measurements from the Stryker device are within 5 mm Hg of the slit catheter for 95% of all readings. Measurements with a standard 18-gauge needle are not accurate and are not recommended. Pressure measurements should be performed within all compartments and at multiple sites.

The compartment pressure data can be viewed in isolation or in relation to the patient's diastolic blood pressure. Although there is no absolute minimum compartment pressure value, most current literature indicates that the ΔP value from measured compartment pressure to diastolic blood pressure is a more valuable guide in performance of a fasciotomy. Studies suggest that the ischemic threshold of muscle is a perfusion pressure of at least 20 mmHg between the compartment pressure and the diastolic pressure. The ΔP is a direct measure of the pressure gradient between diastolic blood pressure and the tissue pressure within the compartment, indicating the presence of shunting. At our institution, a ΔP of 30 mmHg combined with increased palpable pressure is a strong indication and a ΔP of 20 mmHg an absolute indication for fasciotomy.

Therapy is begun for the treatment of compartment syndrome while preparations are made for actual surgical decompression. The affected limb(s) are placed at the level of the heart. Elevation is

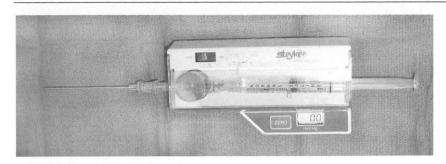

FIGURE 30-1
Stryker pressure monitor (Stryker, Kalamazoo, MI) with side-port needle.

contraindicated because it decreases arterial inflow and narrows the arterial-venous pressure gradient and thus worsens the ischemia. If a cast is on the affected extremity, releasing one side of the plaster cast can reduce compartment pressure by 30%; bi-valving can produce an additional 35% reduction; and cutting the cast padding may further decrease compartmental pressure by 10% to 20%. In cases of snake envenomation, administration of antivenom may reverse a developing compartment syndrome. Hypoperfusion may be corrected with crystalloid and blood products, and mannitol may reduce compartment pressures and lessen reperfusion injury.

Hyperbaric oxygen (HBO) is a valuable adjunct in the treatment of compartment syndrome. It promotes hyperoxic vasoconstriction, which reduces swelling and edema and improves local blood flow and oxygenation. It also increases tissue oxygen tensions and improves the survival of marginally viable tissue. The best results are obtained when therapy is started early after fasciotomy. Twice-daily treatments at 2.0 atmospheres absolute (ata) to 2.5 ata for 90 to 120 minutes for 5 to 7 days, with frequent examinations of the affected area, may be beneficial. This may be more practical in centers familiar with the use of hyperbaric oxygen therapy.

Vacuum-assisted closure devices (VAC) have a number of advantages in the treatment of post-fasciotomy wounds. They reduce interstitial edema and provide a one-way flow of exudate from the wound. Additionally, this therapy increases granulation tissue formation and may lead to an earlier ability to close or skin graft the wound.

FASCIOTOMY OF THE THIGH

Thigh and gluteal compartment syndromes are uncommon and may often go unrecognized. The pathophysiology and the principles of diagnosis and treatment, however, are the same as those for other compartment syndromes. Gluteal compartment syndromes are often associated with substance abuse and a prolonged period of unconsciousness or recumbency and can occur in the absence of any obvious trauma. As a result of the large muscle mass involved, systemic manifestations of a crush syndrome are usually present. Altered mental status and metabolic abnormalities may distract from the primary problem, resulting in delayed diagnosis and treatment. The proximity of the sciatic nerve can result in compression-induced neuropathy.

Clinical Findings

Thigh compartment syndrome is rare because of the large volume required to cause a pathologic increase in the interstitial pressure. It may occur in the setting of high-energy thigh trauma such as femur fractures with an associated crush component. These patients often have pain and swelling after fixation, which may confound the diagnosis. In addition, these trauma patients are often obtunded and require substantial fluid resuscitation, increasing the risk of compartment issues. The fascial compartments in the thigh blend anatomically with muscles of the hip, potentially allowing extravasation of blood outside these compartments. Anticoagulation can be a major risk factor leading to bleeding into the thigh compartments and the development of a compartment syndrome.

Patient Positioning

The approach to thigh compartments may be medial or lateral depending on the area of injury or suspected hematoma. The thigh should be prepared from the iliac crest to the knee joint with the patient in either the lateral decubitis position or supine.

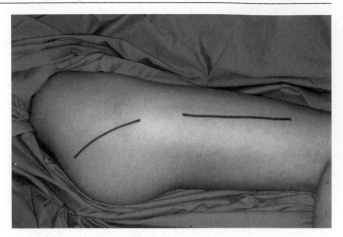

FIGURE 30-2

Skin markings for gluteal and thigh (anterior and posterior) compartment release.

Technique

For lateral and posterior compartment syndromes, the skin and subcutaneous tissues are incised beginning just distal to the intertrochanteric line and extending to the lateral epicondyle of the femur to expose the iliotibial band or fascia lata (Fig. 30-2). The iliotibial band is incised for the length of the incision. The vastus lateralis muscle is reflected superiorly and medially to expose the lateral intermuscular septum, which is incised for the length of the incision, thus freeing the posterior compartment. Caution is required to control the perforating branches of the descending branch of the lateral femoral circumflex artery traversing the lateral intermuscular septum (vessels which supply the anterolateral thigh skin), since these may retract and bleed during this portion of the decompression (Fig. 30-3). After the anterior and posterior compartments have been released, measure the pressure of the medial compartment. If elevated, then the compartment can be approached through a separate medial incision. The incision is carried along the course of the saphenous vein. Reflect the sartorius muscle superiorly, and incise the medial intermuscular septum. Intramuscular hematomas may require release through gentle muscle splitting. The wounds are packed open and a large bulky dressing applied or, alternatively, a vacuum-assisted closure device is applied.

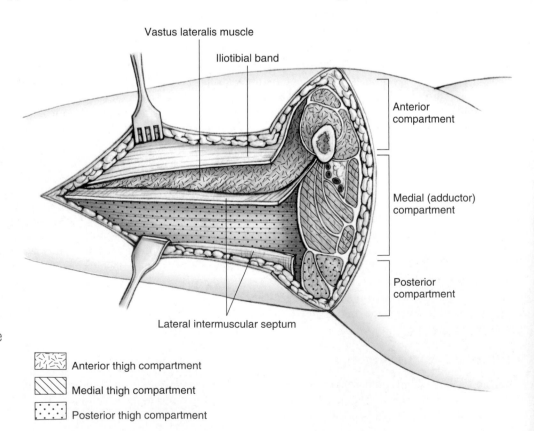

FIGURE 30-3

Schematic lateral view showing decompression of anterior compartment performed by incising the fascia latae longitudinally. The vastus lateralis is retracted medially to expose the lateral intermuscular septum, which is incised to decompress the posterior compartment.

Vastus lateralis muscle

Iliotibial band

Anterior compartment

Medial (adductor) compartment

Posterior compartment

Lateral intermuscular septum

Anterior thigh compartment

Medial thigh compartment

Posterior thigh compartment

Two to three days later, the patient is returned to the operating room for debridement of any non-viable tissue. If there is no evidence of necrotic tissue, the skin is either loosely closed, packed once again for closure at a later date, or again covered with a vacuum-assisted closure device. Often a medial thigh fasciotomy is not needed once a lateral release is performed.

Results

Because this diagnosis is not always obvious, the surgeon must maintain a high index of suspicion. Early treatment by operative compartment release follows anatomic tracts and produces good results.

FASCIOTOMY OF THE LEG

The framework of the lower leg is composed of two long bones, the fibula and tibia, which are arranged in parallel and connected along their length by a fibrous membrane termed the interosseous membrane. These three structures together divide the leg into two anatomic sections, the anterior and posterior compartments. The anterior compartment is further divided into anterior and lateral by a thick anterior intermuscular septum. The lateral leg compartment is separated from the posterior compartment by the posterior intermuscular septum.

The anterior compartment has four muscles, the (a) extensor digitorum longus, (b) extensor hallucis longus, (c) peroneus tertius, and (d) the tibialis anterior. These muscles are supplied by the anterior tibial vessels and are innervated by the deep peroneal nerve, all traveling deep to the muscles along the interosseous membrane. The posterior compartment is divided into superficial and deep compartments by a thin fascia termed the transverse intermuscular septum. Three muscles are located in the superficial compartment: the gastrocnemius, soleus, and plantaris. The gastrocnemius and soleus join together at midcalf to form the Achilles tendon, which inserts into the calcaneal bone. The plantaris is a thin, small muscle, the tendon of which medially follows the bigger Achilles tendon to insert into the calcaneal bone. All of these muscles flex the foot in a plantar direction (the gastrocnemius also flexes the knee) with slight inversion. The muscles are vascularized by branches from the popliteal and posterior tibial artery and innervated by branches of the tibialis nerve from the popliteal fossa. The deep posterior leg compartment contains four muscles: the popliteus, flexor digitorum longus, flexor hallucis longus, and tibialis posterior. The lateral compartment contains two muscles, the peroneus longus and brevis. Their action consists of extension and eversion of the foot. They are vascularized by vessels from the peroneal artery and innervated by the superficial peroneal nerve (Fig. 30-4).

The posterior tibial artery, after branching from the popliteal artery, descends posterior to the tibia, within the deep posterior compartment. Distally in the lower third of the leg it is more superficial, covered only by the skin and superficial fascia and parallel to the medial border of the Achilles tendon. The peroneal artery originates from the posterior tibial artery and runs laterally and downward along the posterior fibula providing four to six segmental, circular arterial branches around the fibula, nourishing the bone, periosteum, and surrounding muscles. The anterior tibial artery commences at the bifurcation of the popliteal artery passing forward between the tibialis posterior muscle and through the interosseous membrane to the deep aspect of the anterior leg compartment. After perforation of the interosseous membrane, the artery descends adjacent and along the membrane, gradually approaching the extensor retinaculum of the ankle. At the bend of the ankle joint, it becomes superficial and known as the dorsalis pedis artery.

Patient Positioning

In cases of isolated compartment syndrome of the leg, the patient is positioned in the supine position on a standard operating table. A general anesthetic is employed in most cases. A tourniquet is applied to the thigh and isolated with broad tape or a plastic isolation dressing. The leg is prepared and draped in the standard fashion. A stockinette or isolation sheet is applied to the foot to maintain the sterile field. The tourniquet is not inflated unless active arterial bleeding is encountered.

Technique

The technique for fasciotomy of the leg can be performed using either a one incision or two incision technique (Table 30-2). The two incision technique is the gold standard. Regardless of the technique,

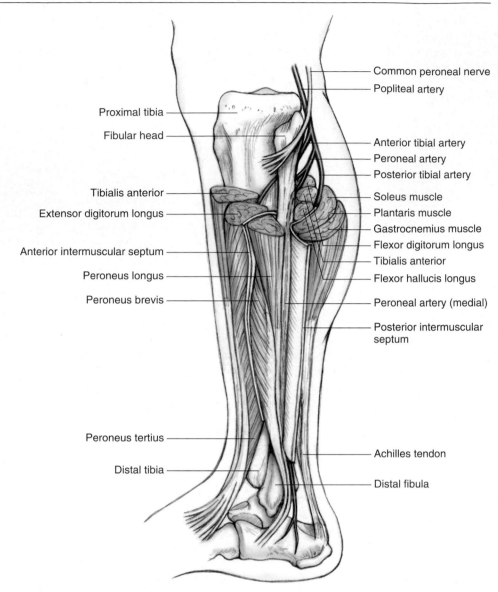

Common peroneal nerve

Popliteal artery

Proximal tibia

Fibular head

Anterior tibial artery

Peroneal artery

Posterior tibial artery

Tibialis anterior

Soleus muscle

Extensor digitorum longus

Plantaris muscle

Gastrocnemius muscle

Anterior intermuscular septum

Flexor digitorum longus

Tibialis anterior

Peroneus longus

Flexor hallucis longus

Peroneus brevis

Peroneal artery (medial)

Posterior intermuscular septum

Peroneus tertius

Distal tibia

Achilles tendon

Distal fibula

FIGURE 30-4
Lateral leg.

the skin incisions must be of adequate length to decompress all affected compartments. The performance of percutaneous fasciotomies is not recommended, particularly with compartments deformed by soft tissue edema, since this technique can be fraught with complications such as iatrogenic nerve injury. In addition, the skin itself has been shown to exert a constrictive effect on the muscle compartments in the leg.

One Incision Fasciotomy   The planned incision is marked in line with the fibula extending to 5 cm short of either end of the fibula along the anterolateral leg. The initial step is the identification of the lateral intermuscular septum separating the lateral and anterior compartments. Make a transverse incision to expose this septum and to identify the superficial peroneal nerve just deep to the septum. Separate fasciotomies of the compartments are performed with Metzenbaum scissors. The anterior compartment is released proximally by aiming for the patella and distally by aiming for the center of the ankle in line with the tibialis anterior. Then, perform a longitudinal fasciotomy of the lateral compartment in line with the fibular shaft (Fig. 30-5). Extreme care is taken in the distal aspect of the lateral compartment at the junction of the middle and distal thirds, where the superficial peroneal nerve emerges from the lateral compartment. Direct the scissors toward the posterior lateral malleolus to stay posterior to the superficial peroneal nerve. In the case of acute compartment syndrome, we avoid subcutaneous fasciotomies. The use of the "sliding scissor" technique decreases the ability to perform a controlled fasciotomy and should be avoided. Once the anterior and lateral compartments have been decompressed, the fibula is identified after posterior undermining of the

---

TABLE 30-2.   Pearls for Fasciotomy of the Leg

- Check intracompartmental pressures at multiple levels within each compartment.
- Threshold for fasciotomy is intracompartmental pressure within 20 mm Hg of the diastolic blood pressure.
- Beware of compartment syndrome secondary to intraoperative positioning of uninjured extremities.
- Pulselessness is NOT a common finding in compartment syndrome unless a concurrent vascular injury exists.
- Fasciotomy should not be performed more than 12 hours after a compartment syndrome is established.
- Compartment syndrome can occur with a late onset 2 to 4 days after the underlying event.
- Compartment pressure measurements with a standard 18-gauge needle are consistently higher than those obtained with specialized needles with a side-port needle or slit catheter.
- Compartment pressures can vary among several different points in each compartment at risk.
- In any patient at risk, baseline compartment pressures are necessary in the case of a suspicion of compartment syndrome in the future.

Two Incision Feg Fasciotomy (Gold Standard)

- Mark both incisions before making the first surgical incision.
- Beware of the superficial peroneal nerve as it emerges anteriorly within the lateral compartment at the junction of the middle and distal one-third of the fibula.
- Beware of the use of vessel loops or other elastic forms of skin tension applied at the time of fasciotomy, as these may lead to recurrence of the compartment syndrome if excessively tight.
- Close medial wound before the lateral wound to avoid need for soft tissue coverage.

One Incision Leg Fasciotomy

- Obtain complete visualization of the release of the deep posterior compartment, as extensive bleeding can occur secondary to perforating vessels on the posterior aspect of the fibula.
- Extend incision to within 5 cm of either end of the fibula on the anterolateral leg.
- Beware of the superficial peroneal nerve at the junction of the middle and distal one-third of the leg.

---

skin for release of the deep posterior compartments. The lateral compartment musculature is elevated off the fibula, demonstrating the posterior intermuscular septum. A longitudinal incision of this septum exposes the superficial posterior compartment. Posterior retraction of the soleus and gastrocnemius muscles then exposes the deep posterior compartment for its decompression. We have found that surgical exposure of the posterior aspect of the fibula is critical in the avoidance of bleeding from the perforating branches of the peroneal artery. Release of all four compartments through one incision, however, is not commonly performed at our institutions, and we recommend a two incision fasciotomy.

Two Incision fasciotomy   The two incision fasciotomy is the gold standard treatment for compartment syndrome of the leg, particularly in the hands of surgeons with limited previous experience and limited assistance in the operating room. The positioning and preparation are identical to that of the one incision fasciotomy. It is crucial to mark the medial and lateral skin incisions before making the incision to ensure an adequate skin bridge is maintained. After one single incision is made, the

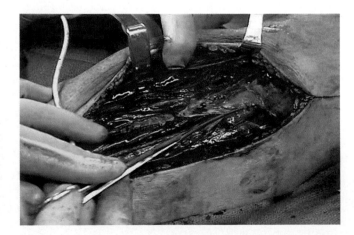

FIGURE 30-5

Intraoperative view after anterior and lateral compartment decompression. Note the intermuscular septum separating the anterior and lateral compartments.

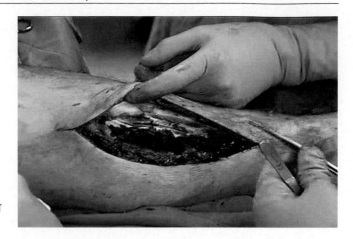

FIGURE 30-6

Intraoperative view after release of superficial posterior compartment and before release of deep posterior compartment.

skin envelope will retract in the opposite direction resulting in a narrow skin bridge anteriorly, and marking these incisions will avoid this complication. After performance of the anterior and lateral fasciotomies, a separate incision is made along the posteromedial leg, 1 to 2 cm posterior to the tibia, measuring at least 15 cm in length. The greater saphenous vein and saphenous nerve are identified and retracted anteriorly. The fasciotomy is extended as far as possible proximally and distally to the level of the medial malleolus. The soleus is then released from the posteromedial tibia with a concurrent release of the deep posterior compartment (Fig. 30-6). A common pitfall is to not adequately release the soleus muscle insertion thereby adequately releasing the deep posterior compartment. Care should be exercised when releasing the deep compartment ligating or cauterizing branches traversing the soleus muscle. The posterior tibial neurovascular bundle is just deep to this transverse intermuscular septum, which separates the deep from posterior compartments and is therefore in close proximity to the release. The skin incisions can also be slightly staggered, with the lateral more proximal (the anterior and lateral compartments are largely tendonous at their distal extent) and the medial incision made more distally. Finally, the fascia and skin are then re-evaluated for adequacy of release.

After either type of fasciotomy, compartment pressures are again checked using a sterile side-port needle attached to the non-sterile pressure monitor held by an unscrubbed assistant or, alternatively, using an arterial pressure monitor setup. The wounds are then copiously irrigated with crystalloid. Devitalized tissue if present is debrided. Vessel loops can be applied to the skin edges to prevent marked skin retraction but must be used judiciously to avoid a recurrence of the compartment syndrome. At our institution, we routinely employ a vacuum-assisted closure device over all open fasciotomy wounds to maintain a one-way flow of extravasated fluid, to encourage the formation of granulation tissue, and potentially to minimize the area needed for later skin grafting. The patient is returned to the operating room at 2 to 3 days for a repeat irrigation and debridement and partial closure. At or around postoperative day 7, the wound is again treated with irrigation and debridement. At that time, definitive closure is performed with additional skin coverage obtained with a split-thickness skin graft. We usually strive to close the medial wound first to provide bony coverage and avoid the need for soft tissue coverage, whereas the lateral wound may be easily skin grafted if appropriate. It is imperative to maintain the foot in a neutral position to avoid equinus contracture either with external fixation or external splinting.

Results

The primary goal of fasciotomy is to prevent permanent nerve and muscle damage leading to Volkmann's contracture. The results of fasciotomy can be analyzed based on two endpoints: muscle and nerve function, and wound- or incision-related complications. A number of studies have demonstrated that the majority of patients have normal leg function if the fasciotomy is performed within 12 hours of the onset of compartment syndrome. In our experience, prompt recognition and early treatment of the compartment syndrome leads to minimal long-term complications. Despite early and aggressive fasciotomy, however, nearly 20% of patients may have persistent motor deficits at 1 year follow-up. Wound complications associated with fasciotomy include numbness and persistent ulceration at the fasciotomy site. The risk of sensory changes has been reported to be as high as 70% in some reports. The use of a VAC dressing may contribute to a lower risk of hematoma and edema and an expeditious granulation of fasciotomy wounds that are not able to be closed. Little or no return of function can be expected when diagnosis and treatment are delayed. Tendon transfers and foot stabilization may be indicated as late treatment; but in most patients, enough scarring and contracture eventually develop in the anterior musculature to prevent foot drop. A foot drop brace (ankle foot orthosis) is indicated for the first few months until fibrosis occurs. Some patients experience persistent gastrocnemius and soleus muscle weakness thought to be due to the loss of the supporting compartment fascia.

FASCIOTOMY OF THE FOOT

Anatomically, the foot consists of well-demarcated osseofascial spaces that subdivide the foot into discrete compartments. These compartments are filled with muscles, nerves, and tendons and are lined by a tight membrane (the fascia). There are four clinically relevant compartments known as the medial, central, lateral, and interosseous (Fig. 30-7). Other anatomic compartments of the foot may be identified with dyes or injection studies but are not clinically relevant. Muscles within the medial compartment are the abductor hallucis and flexor hallucis brevis, and within the central (calcaneal) compartment lay the flexor digitorum brevis, quadratus plantae, and adductor hallucis muscle. There are four dorsal and plantar interosseous muscles between the first and fifth metatarsals, and these comprise the interosseus (intrinsic) compartment. The lateral compartment houses the abductor digiti minimi and flexor digiti minimi brevis muscle.

Compartment syndrome in the foot is commonly due to severe local trauma after fairly significant industrial, agricultural, and motor vehicle accidents in which crushing of the foot occurs. The trauma leads to bleeding from injured bones or muscles and avulsed vasculature. When the bleeding and inflammation of the muscle becomes significant, it will exceed the capacity of blood flow in and out of the small compartments.

Clinical Findings

Tense tissue bulging may be the most reliable symptom in compartment syndrome of the foot, and in the presence of this massive swelling pulses are usually not palpable. Increased pain on passive dorsiflexion of metatarsophalangeal joints is another key finding that indicates myoneural ischemia in the foot intrinsic muscles. It is imperative to maintain a high clinical suspicion based on the severity of the traumatic incident. Compartment syndromes of the foot are often associated with compartment syndromes of the deep posterior compartment.

Patient Positioning

The patient position is supine to allow easy access to the dorsum and medial aspect of the foot. A tourniquet may be used, but is not insufflated unless there is active arterial bleeding. The knee should be included in the preparation to enable better mobility of the limb during the procedure.

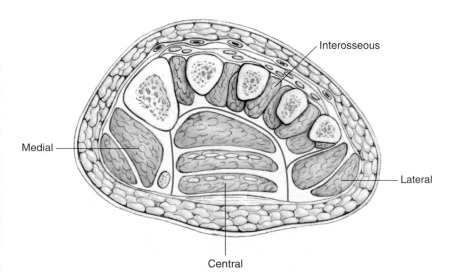

Interosseous

Medial

Lateral

Central

FIGURE 30-7

Schematic coronal section of right foot through base of metatarsals. Medial, central, lateral, and interosseus compartments are shown.

Technique

The same principles that apply to fasciotomy of the thigh and leg apply to the foot. Appropriate treatment for a suspected compartment of the foot is immediate fasciotomy. Debridement of marginal tissue at the time of initial fasciotomy is not advised because it is very difficult to determine muscle viability and contractility in the foot. Once the muscle is decompressed, much of it may recover after compartmental release.

Medial Approach Effective decompression of all four compartments can be accomplished through a medial longitudinal (Henry) approach or through an additional two parallel dorsal incisions along the length of the second and fourth metatarsal bones (more common). The medial approach can be used to decompress the medial and central compartments as well as the remaining foot compartments (lateral and interosseous). The incision is made 3 cm from the sole of the foot and extends from a point below the medial malleolus to the proximal aspect of the first metatarsal (Fig. 30-8). The posterior tibial neurovascular bundle is identified and preserved. This may be very difficult in a massively swollen foot. The fascia overlying the abductor hallucis and flexor hallucis brevis is released. Dissection is continued adjacent and deep to the first metatarsal toward the medial intermuscular septum, separating the medial compartment from the central compartment, which is opened longitudinally. The lateral plantar neurovascular bundle is found between the flexor digitorum brevis and quadratus plantae muscles and preserved. Downward retraction of the flexor digitorum brevis along with lateral dissection will allow access to the lateral intermuscular septum separating the central compartment from the lateral compartment. This septum is divided to release the lateral compartment. Blunt dissection dorsally via the central compartment will release the interosseous compartment. Scissors or sharp instruments are not used during this portion of the dissection, since it is essentially blind to avoid injury to the neurovascular bundle.

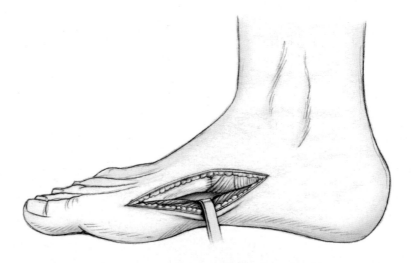

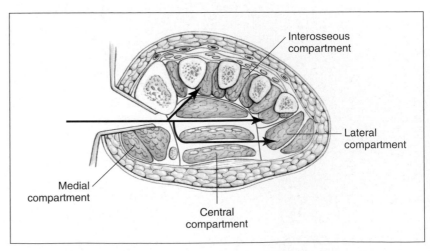

FIGURE 30-8

Medial approach for four-compartment release of foot compartment syndrome.

Dorsal Approach   This approach is more commonly used when there are concomitant metatarsal or Lisfranc fractures. Two parallel dorsal incisions are centered just medial to the second metatarsal and lateral to the fourth metatarsal shafts, maximizing the intervening skin bridge. The dorsal veins and the subcutaneous tissues are elevated laterally and medially to expose the respective interosseous musculature. Injury to the sensory nerves and extensor tendons is avoided. Caution should be used when making the incision between first and second metatarsal to avoid iatrogenic injury to the dorsalis pedis artery. The superficial fascia is incised longitudinally, and the interosseous muscles are elevated off the metatarsals. The first dorsal and plantar interossei are stripped from the medial aspect of the second metatarsal shaft, which is then retracted medially, and the fascia of the central and medial compartment is released longitudinally deep within the inner space. The interosseous musculature is decompressed by releasing the fascia between the second and third metatarsals also through this medial incision. The lateral incision is used to decompress the interosseous muscles between the third and fourth, and fourth and fifth metatarsals, in addition to allowing access to release the central and lateral compartments (Fig. 30-9). More commonly, a separate medial incision as described previously is used to release the medial (adductor) compartment, since the medial approach only to all four compartments carries an increased risk of damage to the neurovascular bundles in the plantar aspect of the foot. These fasciotomy incisions are sometimes used for fracture fixation.

Results

Controversy exists in what results with a missed compartment syndrome of the foot. Predominately patients end up with clawing of the toes that needs to be corrected at a later date. The argument against the release is that it complicates the soft tissue envelope, limits possible incisions for reconstruction, and carries the risk of iatrogenic neurovascular injury.

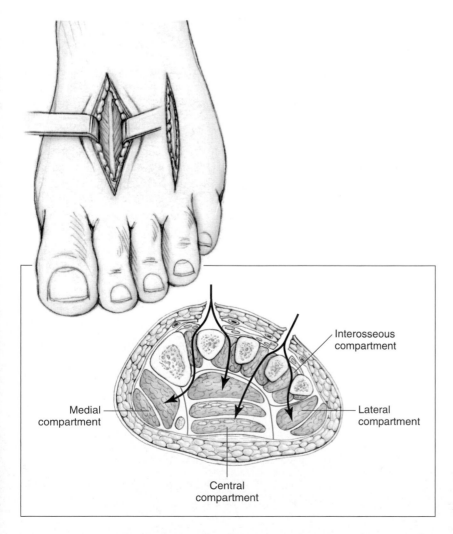

FIGURE 30-9

Dorsal approach for compartment release of foot compartment syndrome.

Treatment of a foot compartment syndrome with "benign neglect" is not advised, and early decompression as in the thigh and leg is recommended. A delay in diagnosis is a potentially devastating occurrence. Early reduction of dislocations and some fractures facilitates reduction in edema in the foot and decreases tissue breakdown due to pressure necrosis. Desire to obtain an early reduction must be weighed heavily against whether the soft tissue envelope of the injured foot will tolerate additional incisions. The fasciotomy incisions may be used to facilitate reduction and fracture fixation, but caution is warranted to avoid excessive undermining of the soft tissues. Delayed fixation is feasible, but usually not before 7 to14 days post injury, due to soft tissue edema. In addition, liberal use of external fixation, particularly in the setting of a mangled foot, is advised for stabilization and edema control.

POSTOPERATIVE MANAGEMENT

Fasciotomy sites are dressed with a wound vacuum-assisted closure sponge, and wet to dry dressing changes with normal saline solution or silver sulfadiazine depending on the degree of contamination. The patient is returned to the operating room several days later to attempt closure. When muscle necrosis ensues, the patient is brought to surgery earlier for debridement. Wound closure should not be performed until all necrotic tissue is debrided. Direct closure can be attempted when the wound approximates without tension. When the wound edges will not oppose easily, either the wound is treated conservatively with dressing changes or a vacuum-assisted closure device. The patient is brought back to the operating room at a later date for definitive closure or skin grafting. Increased intramuscular pressure can occur with closure of fasciotomy wounds secondarily and, therefore, skin grafting of the wounds is often a safer option. Hypesthesia and painful dysesthesia resulting from compartment syndrome typically resolve slowly with time. This type of neuropathic pain can by treated with diphenylhydantoin (Dilantin), gabapentin (Neurontin), or carbamazepine (Tegretol).

COMPLICATIONS

Although a fasciotomy incision does result in patient morbidity, the incompletely released compartment, delayed diagnosis, or unrecognized compartment syndrome has substantially higher risks. Systemic complications including acute renal failure, sepsis, and acute respiratory distress syndrome (ARDS) have been reported in some cases. Most fatalities are due to prolonged intensive care admissions with sepsis and multisystem organ failure. If fasciotomy is done within 12 hours after the onset of compartment syndrome, the prognosis is typically good. Despite early intervention, approximately 1% to 10% of all cases of compartment syndrome develop Volkmann's contracture. Little or no return of function can be expected when the diagnosis and treatment are delayed. In no instance was benefit from fasciotomy reported after 2 or 3 days. When the procedure is done late, severe infections have been shown to develop in the necrotic tissues of many patients, frequently leading to amputations. In these situations, clinically evident by complete absence of demonstrable muscle function in any segment of the involved limb, the extremity should be splinted to maintain a functional position as muscle fibrosis and contracture develop.

ACKNOWLEDGMENTS

The authors express their gratitude to the Department of Orthopaedics at the University of Maryland Shock Trauma and the Surgery Audio Visual Department at Cooper University Hospital (Paul Rogers) for their assistance and efforts in the preparation of this chapter.

RECOMMENDED READING

Azar FM, Pickering RM. Traumatic disorders. In: Canale ST, ed. *Campbell's operative orthopaedics*. 10th ed. St. Louis: Mosby; 2003:1405–1411.

Boody AR, Wongworawat MD. Accuracy in the measurement of compartment pressures: a comparison of three commonly used devices. *J Bone Joint Surg Am.* 2005;87:2415–2422.

Cohen MS, Garfin SR, Hargens AR, Mubarak SJ. Acute compartment syndrome. Effect of dermotomy on fascial decompression in the leg. *J Bone Joint Surg Br.* 1991;73:287–290.

Finkelstein JA, Hunter GA, Hu RW. Lower limb compartment syndrome: course after delayed fasciotomy. *J Trauma*. 1996;40:342–344.

Fitzgerald AM, Gaston P, Wilson Y, Quaba A, McQueen MM. Long-term sequelae of fasciotomy wounds. *Br J Plast Surg*. 2000;53:690–693.

Garcia-Covarrubias L, McSwain NE Jr, Van Meter K, Bell RM. Adjuvant hyperbaric oxygen therapy in the management of crush injury and traumatic ischemia: an evidence-based approach. *Am Surg*. 2005;71:144–151.

Goldsmith AL, McCallum MI. Compartment syndrome as a complication of the prolonged use of the Lloyd-Davies position. *Anaesthesia*. 1996;51:1048–1052.

Gulli B, Templeman D. Compartment syndrome of the lower extremity. *Orthop Clin North Am*. 1994;25:677–684.

Heckman MM, Whitesides TE Jr, Grewe SR, Rooks MD. Compartment pressure in association with closed tibial fractures. The relationship between tissue pressure, compartment, and the distance from the site of the fracture. *J Bone Joint Surg Am*. 1994;76:1285–1292.

McQueen MM, Court-Brown CM. Compartment monitoring in tibial fractures. The pressure threshold for decompression. *J Bone Joint Surg Br*. 1996;78:99–104.

McQueen MM, Gaston P, Court-Brown CM. Acute compartment syndrome. Who is at risk? *J Bone Joint Surg Br*. 2000;82:200–203.

Meyer RS, White KK, Smith JM, et al. Intramuscular and blood pressures in legs positioned in the hemilithotomy position: clarification of risk factors for well-leg acute compartment syndrome. *J Bone Joint Surg Am*. 2002;84-A:1829–1835.

Myerson MM. Soft tissue trauma. Acute and chronic management. In: Coughlin MJ, Mann RA, eds. *Surgery of the foot and ankle*. St. Louis: Mosby; 1999:1340–1344.

Olson SA, Glasgow RR. Acute compartment syndrome in lower extremity musculoskeletal trauma. *J Am Acad Orthop Surg*. 2005;13:436–444.

Schwartz JT Jr, Brumback RJ, Lakatos R, et al. Acute compartment syndrome of the thigh. A spectrum of injury. *J Bone Joint Surg Am*. 1989;71:392–400.

Sheridan GW, Matsen FA III. Fasciotomy in the treatment of the acute compartment syndrome. *J Bone Joint Surg Am*. 1976;58:112–115.

Slater RR Jr, Weiner TM, Koruda MJ. Bilateral leg compartment syndrome complicating prolonged lithotomy position. *Orthopedics*. 1994;17:954–959.

Strecker WB, Wood MB, Bieber EJ. Compartment syndrome masked by epidural anesthesia for postoperative pain. Report of a case. *J Bone Joint Surg Am*. 1986;68:1447–1448.

Templeman D, Lange R, Harms B. Lower-extremity compartment syndromes associated with use of pneumatic antishock garments. *J Trauma*. 1987;27:79–81.

Wiger P, Tkaczuk P, Styf J. Secondary wound closure following fasciotomy for acute compartment syndrome increases intramuscular pressure. *J Orthop Trauma*. 1998;12:117–121.

31 Amputation and Stump Management

Norman S. Turner and Thomas C. Shives

INDICATIONS/CONTRADICTIONS

Amputation is one of the oldest surgical procedures. Early amputations consisted of severing the extremity, and hemostasis was obtained by dipping the stump in hot oil. Techniques have dramatically improved and most of the advances have occurred during war time. Prosthetic technology now allows for amputees to run, jump, ski, swim, and be involved in competitive sports.

The indications for above and below knee amputation include life-threatening infections, malignant tumors, burns, extensive frost bite, congenital anomalies, ischemic pain, osteomyelitis, extensive trauma (including a tibial nerve ilaceration or unreconstructable vascular injury) and chronic pain. The most common indications for a below knee or above knee amputation are complications of diabetes. Functionally, the patients with below knee amputation are able to walk with prosthesis, with most patients walking within 3 months after surgery. Amputation should not be viewed as a limb salvage failure, but as a reconstructive procedure to improve function.

There are few contraindications to amputations; however, a contraindication to a below knee amputation is a non-ambulatory patient. A non-ambulating patient with a below knee amputation is at high risk for developing a flexion contracture, which can result in increased pressure on the stump and cause ulceration. Therefore, when a patient is wheelchair bound and is not a candidate for prosthetic fitting, an above knee amputation should be considered.

PREOPERATIVE PLANNING

It is imperative that these patients be evaluated preoperatively to determine the vascular status of the limb. The majority of patients undergoing a below knee amputation or above the knee amputation have diabetes and have some component of peripheral vascular disease. Preoperative noninvasive vascular studies, including ankle brachial indexes, are important to determine the level of amputation. An ankle brachial index is determined by measuring the ankle systolic pressure and dividing it by the brachial systolic pressure using Doppler detection of the pulses. The severity of the arterial disease is related to decreased value of the ankle/brachial index (ABI), and a value of less than .5 is considered abnormal in people with diabetes. Also, noninvasive vascular studies using transcutaneous oxygen tension measurement (TcPo2) are useful in assisting with amputation levels. Amputations are likely to heal if the TcPo2 measurements are greater then 40 mm Hg. Patients with TcPo2 values less than 20 mm Hg are at higher risk for not healing and should be evaluated with further vascular testing and possibly an angiogram before surgical intervention. A vascular surgery consult is almost always indicated before performing an amputation. With the advances in distal bypass surgery and invasive radiologic procedures, certain patients can be successfully treated with limb salvage after vascular reconstruction.

Imaging studies are important in determining the underlying pathology. Imaging of the tibia or femur is important if there is a question regarding extension of tumor or infection into the tissues or bone adjacent to the intended level of amputation or if there is a prosthetic device such as a total knee arthroplasty or internal fixation device in place, which may alter the surgical procedure.

If amputation is contemplated, optimizing the patient's medical condition before surgery is recommended. Literature has shown that patients with a serum albumin less than 3.5 g/dL or true lymphocyte count less than 1,500 cells per mL are at high risk for wound-healing difficulties.

Determination of the amputation level is important for both healing and function. The more distal the amputation level, the less energy required to ambulate. In elderly patients, a more proximal amputation may not allow for ambulation secondary to energy requirements. If a patient has good cognitive function, balance, and strength, then the most distal level with a realistic chance of healing should be attempted.

SURGERY

In order for the below knee amputation to be performed correctly, proper attention to detail is important to improve the quality of the result. Gentle handling of the soft tissues, especially in diabetic patients, is important to minimize wound complications. The level of the amputation is determined by the extent of the infection, tumor, or the level that would provide optimal function with prosthesis. In general, the patient is positioned in the supine position for above or below knee amputations.

Full-thickness flaps should be used to minimize skin edge necrosis. Meticulous hemostasis and use of a drain is imperative to decrease the risk of a hematoma. The nerves should be divided sharply under tension to minimize the risk of a symptomatic neuroma. Also the bone ends are rasped until smooth to prevent bony prominences.

An open amputation is performed in patients with grossly contaminated wounds or in patients with extensive infection. These patients will require further surgeries to optimize the soft tissues around the stump, and then a definitive closure can be performed once this is accomplished.

Technique

Below Knee Amputation   Below knee amputation is the most commonly performed lower extremity amputation. A long posterior flap is used and brought anteriorly to cover the distal stump of the tibia, which should be 8.5 to 12.5 cm in length (Fig. 31-1). The flaps, if planned properly, will have minimal redundant skin in the corners, or "dog ears." This will provide a good prosthetic fit.

The patient is placed supine on the operating room table. A nonsterile tourniquet is used and the leg is prepared and draped in the usual fashion. A skin marker is used to plan the flaps (see Fig. 30-1), and the flaps are drawn so that the posterior flap begins two-thirds of the way posterior to the anterior aspect of the tibia and then extends distally and posteriorly so that the distance will be long enough to cover the tibia (Fig. 31-2). A tourniquet can be used at the discretion of the surgeon. The incision is then made through the skin and subcutaneous tissues down to the fascia. The subcutaneous nerves including the saphenous and sural nerve can be identified and divided under tension. The fascia is then incised. The anterior compartment musculature is cut with a cautery (Fig. 31-3) down to the deep peroneal nerve, which is identified and cut under tension (Fig. 31-4), and the anterior tibial artery is identified and tied with silk suture (Fig. 31-5). The superficial peroneal nerve is identified and cut under tension. The periosteum is reflected off the tibia (Fig. 31-6), and the tibia is cut 1 cm proximal from the skin incision (Fig. 31-7). A segment of the fibula is then resected 1 cm proximal to the tibial bone cut (Figs. 31-8 through 31-10). Traction is applied, and an amputation knife is used to perform the remaining portion of the amputation (Fig. 31-11). Dissection is carried deep until blood from the posterior tibial artery and vein is identified, and then the cut is beveled distally until the fascia is cut (Fig. 31-12). The anterior aspect of the tibia is beveled (Fig. 31-13). The remaining edges are rasped until smooth. The tibial nerve is identified and transected under traction (Fig. 31-14). The tibial artery and vein are identified and tied with silk sutures (Fig. 31-15). The wound is then copiously irrigated. If a tourniquet is used, it is deflated at this time. Hemostasis is obtained. The wound is then closed in layers over a drain with sutures in the fascia (Fig. 31-16). The subcutaneous layer is closed with monofilament suture, and the skin is then closed with nylon sutures in a vertical mattress fashion (Fig. 31-17). A sterile dressing is applied, and then a compressive Robert Jones dressing is applied with plaster in full extension (Fig. 31-18).

Above Knee Amputation   Above knee amputation is the second most frequently performed lower extremity amputation. Stump length is important for the lever arm control of the prosthesis.

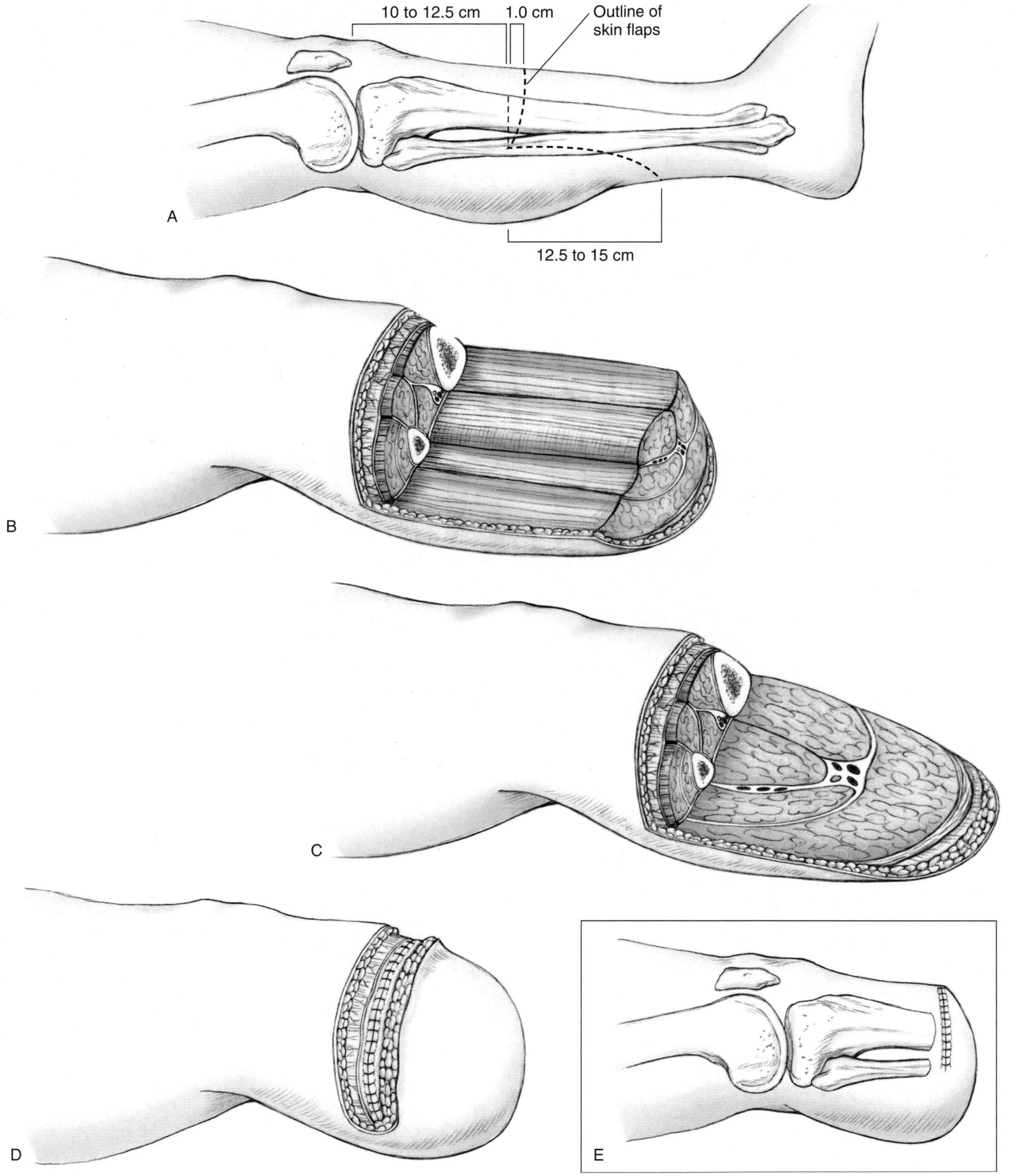

FIGURE 31-1

Below knee amputation. **A:** Planning of short anterior and long posterior skin flaps. **B:** Amputation of distal leg. **C:** Tailoring of posterior muscle to form flaps. **D:** Closure of flap to deep fascia. **E:** Closure of skin flaps. (Redrawn after Burgess EM, Zettl JH. Amputations below the knee. *Artif Limbs.* 1969;13:1. With permission.)

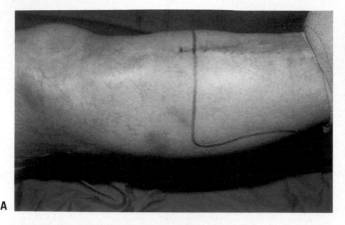

FIGURE 31-2

A,B: The long posterior flap is planned.

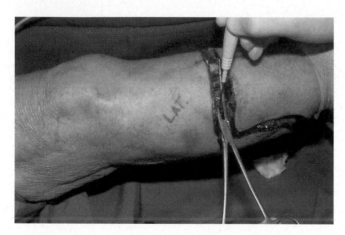

FIGURE 31-3

The anterior compartment muscle is dissected with cautery.

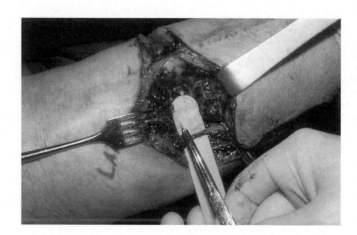

FIGURE 31-4

The deep peroneal nerve is identified and sharply transected.

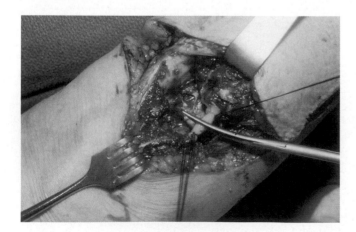

FIGURE 31-5

The anterior tibial artery and vein are ligated.

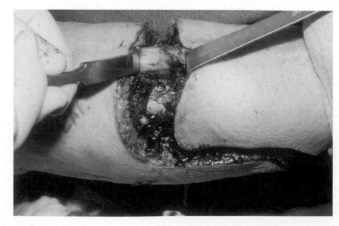

FIGURE 31-6

The periosteum is reflected off the tibia.

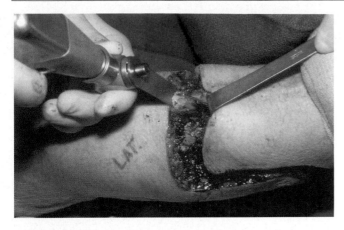

FIGURE 31-7

The tibia is osteotomized 1 cm proximal to skin incision.

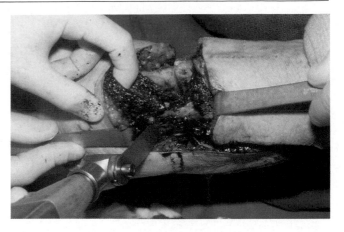

FIGURE 31-8

The fibula is identified and osteotomized 1 cm proximal to tibia osteotomy.

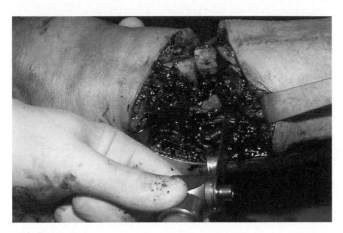

FIGURE 31-9

A second fibula osteotomy is performed 2 to 3 cm distal.

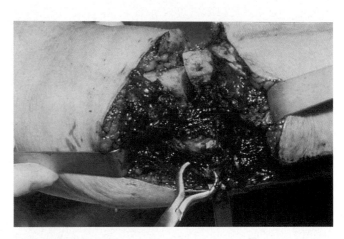

FIGURE 31-10

The segment of the fibula is removed.

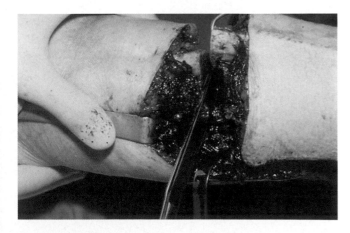

FIGURE 31-11

The amputation knife is used to sharply dissect the posterior compartment muscle.

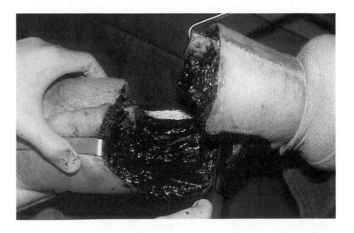

FIGURE 31-12

The posterior compartment muscle is beveled to minimize bulk.

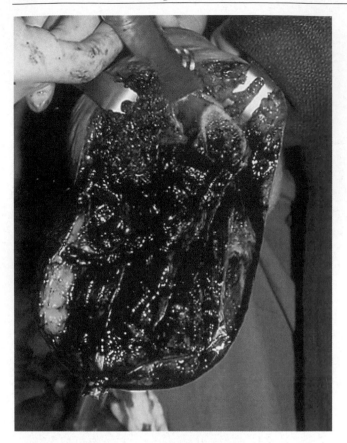

FIGURE 31-13
The saw is used to bevel the anterior tibia.

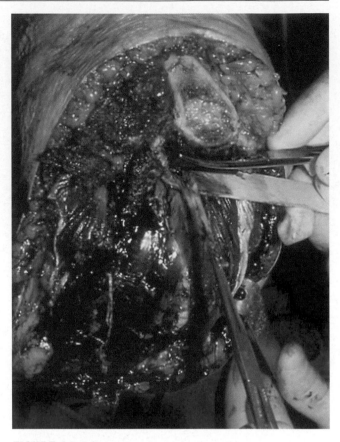

FIGURE 31-14
The tibial nerve is identified and sharply removed.

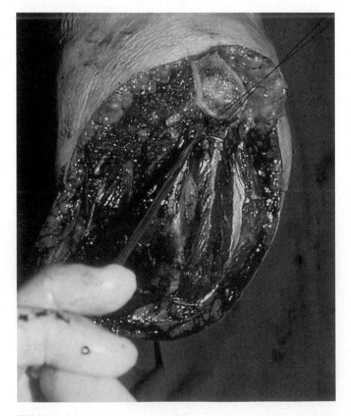

FIGURE 31-15
The tibial artery and vein are ligated.

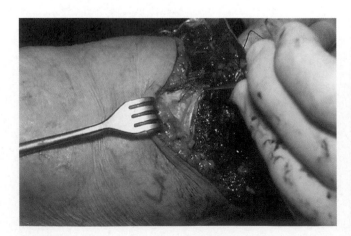

FIGURE 31-16
The fascia is closed with interrupted suture.

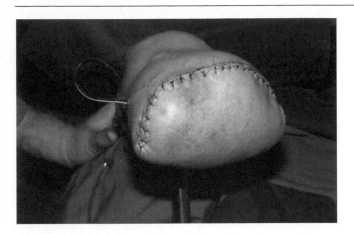

FIGURE 31-17

The skin is closed with interrupted vertical mattress suture.

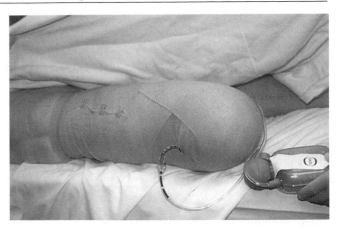

FIGURE 31-18

A compressive bulky dressing with plaster is applied with the knee in full extension.

Too long of a femoral stump, however, can lead to difficulty with fitting the prosthetic knee joint. Therefore, the bone cut should be 10 to 12 cm proximal to distal femoral articular surface.

For non-ambulatory patients with ischemic disease, above knee amputations are performed with equal anterior and posterior flaps, and myodesis is not performed to prevent further vascular compromise. For patients with adequate vascular supply and the potential to ambulate, a myodesis is performed. Above knee amputation is performed with the patient in a supine position. Skin flaps are marked with a long medial flap and a shorter lateral flap (Fig. 31-19). A sterile tourniquet can be used at the discretion of the surgeon. Dissection is carried through the skin and subcutaneous tissues and down to the muscle. The muscles are then identified. The quadriceps is detached proximal to the patella, retaining some of its tendinous portion (Fig. 31-20). The vastus medialis is reflected off of the intermuscular septum, and the adductor magnus (Fig. 31-21) is detached from the adductor tubercle by sharp dissection and reflected medially, exposing the femoral shaft. The vessels are identified (Fig. 31-22) at the level of Hunter's canal, and the artery and vein are ligated. The femur is then exposed proximally 12 to 14 cm above the condylar level and is cut with an oscillating saw approximately 10 to 12 cm above the joint line. The remaining edges are smoothed with a saw or rasp (Fig. 31-23). Small drill holes through the remaining distal femoral cortex are made with a 2.5-mm drill (Fig. 31-24). The adductor magnus tendon is then sutured with nonabsorbable suture to the lateral femur through the drill holes (Fig. 31-25). The femur is held in maximum adduction while this is being sutured to the bone as a myodesis (Fig. 31-26). The quadriceps is then brought over the bone and anchored to the posterior aspect of the femur through the drill holes (Fig. 31-27). The hip is in extension when this is done to try to minimize hip flexion. The fascia lata is then sutured to the medial fascia. Subcutaneous tissue is closed with monofilament suture, and the skin is closed with nylon suture (Fig. 31-28). Sterile dressing is applied, as well as a compressive wrap to minimize swelling.

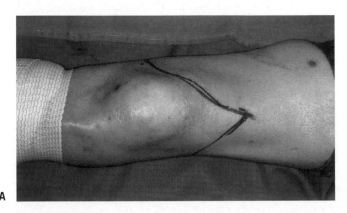

A   B

FIGURE 31-19

A,B: Skin flaps are marked with a long medial and shorter lateral flap.

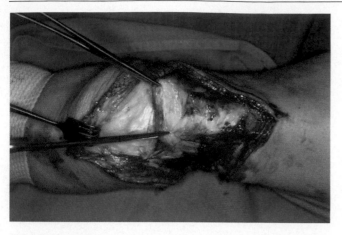

FIGURE 31-20

The quadriceps muscle is detached proximally to the patella, preserving some of the tendinous insertion.

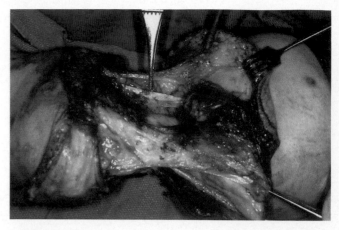

FIGURE 31-21

The adductor magnus is identified and reflected off the femur.

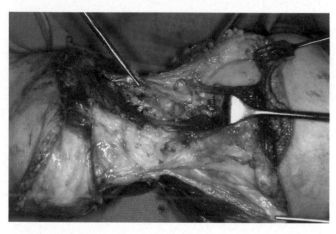

FIGURE 31-22

The femoral vessels at the level of Hunter's canal are identified and ligated.

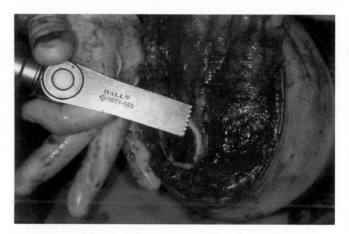

FIGURE 31-23

The femur is osteotomized and the end is rasped until smooth.

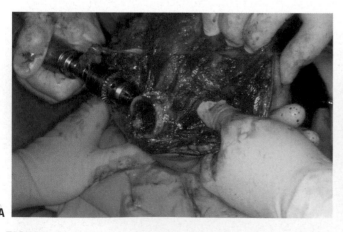

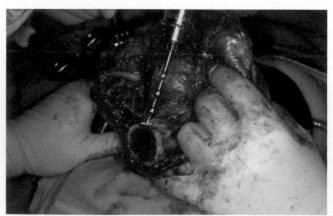

FIGURE 31-24

A,B: Four drill holes are made in the femoral stump for the myodesis.

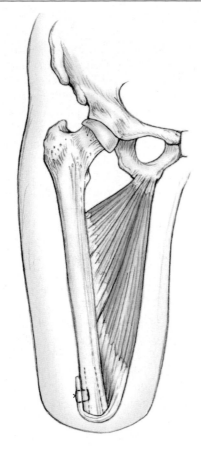

FIGURE 31-25

Attachment of adductor magnus to lateral femur. (Redrawn from Gottschalk F. Transfemoral amputations. In: Bowker JH, Michael JW, eds. *Atlas of limb prosthetics: surgical, prosthetic, and rehabilitation principles.* 2nd ed. St Louis: Mosby; 1992.)

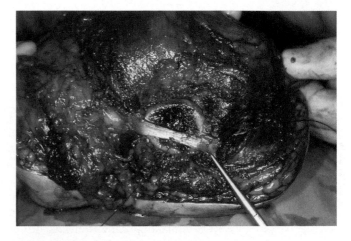

FIGURE 31-26

The adductor magnus tendon is sutured to the femur through the drill holes.

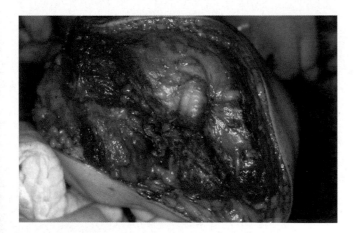

FIGURE 31-27

The quadriceps tendon is brought over the femoral stump and sutured through the drill holes.

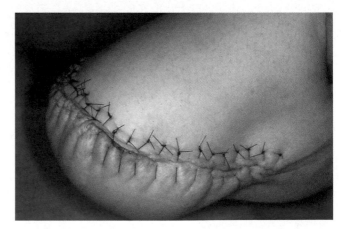

FIGURE 31-28

The skin is closed with interrupted vertical mattress suture.

POSTOPERATIVE MANAGEMENT

For both a below knee and an above knee amputation, a compressive dressing is used to minimize swelling. The patient is kept in bed for 24 hours. The suction drain is kept in for at least 24 hours or until the drainage has decreased to minimal output. For a below knee amputation, a compressive Robert Jones dressing is removed approximately 48 hours after the surgery. If the swelling is well controlled and the wounds are in good condition, a pilon cast can be applied with a temporary prosthetic foot. The patient is restricted to minimal weight bearing but is allowed to be up and ambulating with gait aids. The pilon cast is removed at 2 weeks after surgery and another one can be placed. At 4 weeks after surgery, the pilon cast is removed completely. Sutures are removed at 2 to 4 weeks depending on the healing of the wound. A stump protector is used between 4 to 6 weeks. Shrinker socks are used to shrink the stump, and once the stump volumes have stabilized, a permanent prosthesis can be fitted.

Above knee amputations are initially treated with a compressive dressing and a stump protector. At approximately 2 to 3 weeks after surgery, if the wounds are healed, the sutures are removed. These patients also use shrinker socks as well as a protector. Once their stump volume has stabilized, they can be fitted for their prosthesis.

COMPLICATIONS/RESULTS

The most common complications of amputation surgery are soft tissue or wound healing problems. These can lead to superficial infections that can ultimately cause deep infection, and possibly progress to osteomyelitis. Such complications may result in more proximal amputations.

The treatment of wound complication initially begins with dressing changes, and frequently these patients will heal with local wound care. Occasionally, a vacuum-assisted closure device can be helpful in increasing the granulation tissue to improve the healing in a more timely fashion. Long-term complications include difficulty with prosthetic fitting, which usually can be managed by an experienced prosthetist.

RECOMMENDED READING

Dickhaut SC, DeLee JC, Page CP. Nutritional status: importance in predicting wound-healing after amputation. *J Bone Joint Surg.* 1984;66A:71.

Gottschalk F. Transfemoral amputation: surgical procedures. In: Bowker JH, Michael JW, eds: *Atlas of limb prosthetics: surgical, prosthetic, and rehabilitation principles.* 2nd ed. St. Louis: Mosby; 1992.

Gottschalk F. Transfemoral amputation: biomechanics and surgery. *Clin Orthop.* 1999;361:15.

Harris IE, Leff AR, Gitelis S, Simon MA. Function after amputation, arthrodesis, or arthroplasty for tumors about the knee. *J Bone Joint Surg.* 1990;72A:1477.

Heck. RK Jr, Carnesale PG. General principles of amputations. In: Canale ST, ed. *Campbell's operative orthopaedics.* 10th ed. St. Louis: Mosby; 2003.

Pinzur MS. Amputations and prosthetics. In: Beaty JH, ed: *Orthopaedic knowledge update 6.* Rosemont, IL: American Academy of Orthopaedic Surgeons, 1999.

Pinzur MS, Bowker JH, Smith DG, Gottschalk FA. Amputation surgery in peripheral vascular disease. *AAOS Instr Course Lect.* 1999;48:687.

Pinzur MS, Gottschalk F, Smith D, et al. Functional outcome of below-knee amputation in peripheral vascular insufficiency: a multicenter review. *Clin Orthop.* 1993;286:247.

Smith DG, Ehde DM, Legro MW, et al. Phantom limb, residual limb, and back pain after lower extremity amputations. *Clin Orthop.* 1999;361:29.

Smith DG, Fergason JR. Transtibial amputations. *Clin Orthop.* 1999;361:108.

Waters RL, Perry J, Antonelli D, Hislop H. Energy cost of walking amputees: the influence of level of amputation. *J Bone Joint Surg.* 1976;58A:42.

Wyss CR, Harrington RM, Burgess EM, Matsen FA. Transcutaneous oxygen tension as a predictor of success after an amputation. *J Bone Joint Surg.* 1988;70A:203.

PART VI

SOFT TISSUE MANAGEMENT AROUND THE FOOT AND ANKLE

32 Soft Tissue Management of Ankle Fractures and Use of the Gracilis Muscle Flap

S. Andrew Sems, Matthew DeOrio, and Steven L. Moran

S oft tissue management of injuries around the distal tibia and ankle region will often dictate and drive the timing and methods of definitive fixation. Injuries in this region vary from low energy ankle fractures to high energy tibial pilon fractures. The soft tissue injuries often reflect the amount of energy that was involved in creating the bony injury. Regardless of the radiographic appearance of the fractures, certain initial treatment principles hold true for both low and high energy injuries. Early fracture reduction to restore limb alignment, rotation, and appropriate limb length combined with fracture immobilization will allow sooner resolution of soft tissue swelling and impairment that might otherwise prevent or delay early internal fixation.

ANKLE FRACTURES

Indications/Contraindications

Operative treatment is generally recommended for all unstable ankle fractures in which the talus is unable to be maintained in a position beneath the tibial plafond by closed reduction. Nonoperative management is appropriate for stable ankle fractures in which there is no lateral subluxation of the talus within the ankle mortise.

Comorbidities   Open reduction and internal fixation can generally be safely performed on most patients regardless of associated comorbidities. In patients with severe peripheral vascular disease, preoperative transcutaneous pressure oximetry measurements should be obtained to assess the likelihood of the patient healing the surgical wounds. TcPO2s less than 30 mm Hg have a higher risk of wound failure and fracture nonunion. Involving Vascular Medicine to assist with maximizing lower extremity perfusion is reasonable if vascular disease is a concern. The implications of insulin dependent diabetes mellitus and peripheral neuropathy should also be considered when determining operative versus nonoperative treatment but are not contraindications to surgery. Postoperative soft tissue management should be modified in patients with high risks of developing wound complications. Longer periods of cast immobilization and protected weight bearing may be indicated for patients with these comorbidities.

Nonoperative management of fractures in the nonambulatory patient is reasonable provided the fracture does not cause deformity which would result in subsequent skin breakdown. Modified techniques of internal fixation in patients who are nonambulatory may be utilized in order to maintain the anatomy around the ankle joint to prevent soft tissue compromise.

Preoperative Planning

Plain radiographs should be obtained in all patients with unstable ankle fractures prior to surgical intervention. Anteroposterior (AP), mortise, and lateral views are necessary to assess the fracture orientation. Ankle fractures tend to include the medial malleolus, lateral malleolus, and occasionally, the posterior malleolus. Recognition of the three-dimensional plane in which each fracture occurs is important so that surgical incisions are placed appropriately and the correct internal fixation is selected. While computed tomography is utilized more often for pilon type tibial fractures, it may be used if there is not a clear understanding of the fracture pattern.

Surgical approach selection for treatment of ankle fractures depends on the location of the fractures and the quality of the surrounding tissues. Fractures of the medial malleolus are typically approached with an anteromedial incision overlying the medial malleolus. This incision can be adjusted anteriorly or posteriorly depending on the size and orientation of the medial malleolar fragment. Fractures which include both the anterior and posterior caliculus may require slight posterior adjustment of the incision while fractures that only involve the anterior caliculus may be approached through a more anteromedial incision. Fibular fractures are typically treated with a direct lateral approach, although a posterolateral approach is useful for fibula fractures which occur in the coronal plane or in cases of associated posterior malleolus fragments that may be addressed through this same incision.

The timing of surgery is dictated by the state of the soft tissue envelope. For ankle fractures, immediate fixation within the first 24 to 48 hours is feasible so long as the swelling will not compromise wound healing. Patients who present to the clinic or emergency department with ankle fractures within 48 hours from injury can often be treated with immediate open reduction and internal fixation prior to the onset of the maximal amount of soft tissue swelling. Surgery should be delayed when soft issue is so edematous that the surgeon is unable to create skin wrinkles by gently pinching the skin over both the medial and lateral malleolus. Open fractures require immediate surgical intervention for debridement of all contaminated soft tissues. Antibiotic cement bead pouches or Vacuum Assisted Closure (VAC) devices may be used until definitive fixation or final wound closure. External fixation may be necessary to restore length, alignment, and rotation of both the soft tissues and the bone prior to definitive internal fixation.

Ankle fractures should ideally be treated within 3 weeks of injury prior to early callus formation, which can create significant difficulty in fracture reduction. Patients who present in the first week following an ankle fracture and whose soft tissues are not amenable to immediate surgical fixation should be treated with a Robert Jones type compressive dressing with plaster immobilization. These patients should be encouraged to maintain strict elevation of their limb at all times. They are then seen back in the clinic or preoperative area approximately 7 to 10 days after their injury for soft tissue evaluation prior to surgical intervention. This dressing should be taken down and the skin should be evaluated prior to any type of anesthetic administration. In patients who are admitted to the hospital, sequential compression boots can be applied to the foot prior to the application of the Robert Jones dressing. These pneumatic boots are usually well tolerated so long as they do not extend up past the ankle.

SURGERY

Medial/Lateral Approaches

Patient Positioning   The patient is positioned supine on a radiolucent table with a thigh high pneumatic tourniquet and a small bump (towel) placed under the ipsilateral hip to prevent excessive external rotation of the limb. The bump placed underneath the hip area should be adjusted so that the foot points vertically when in its resting position. A foam block or bump of towels can be utilized underneath the leg and ankle area so as to elevate the operative limb from the nonoperative limb. This facilitates obtaining lateral radiographs without manipulation of the operative leg. The intraoperative fluoroscopy unit is brought in from the contralateral side, and it is positioned perpendicular to the long axis of the patient.

Prophylactic antibiotics are utilized for internal fixation of ankle fractures. They should be administered prior to inflation of the tourniquet. Once the tourniquet is inflated, it should be maintained as long as necessary, but not for more than 2 hours. If it is impossible to complete the procedure in the allotted 2 hours, the tourniquet should be deflated and hemostasis should be obtained, and the procedure should be completed without the aid of a tourniquet. If small vessel bleeding continues to be an issue, consider moving the operative bed into a Trendelenburg position and asking the anesthesiologist to decrease the systolic blood pressure within safe limits.

Technique

ANATOMIC LANDMARKS—MEDIAL APPROACH   Palpate the medial malleolus to define the location of the anterior aspect of the anterior caliculus, the posterior aspect of the posterior caliculus, as well as the fracture location. The leg should be palpated to determine the longitudinal axis of the tibia.

INCISION AND SURGICAL APPROACH   The incision is made along the midlateral axis of the distal tibia. Beyond the tip of the medial malleolus the incision may be slightly curved anteriorly (Fig. 32-1). Be aware that excessive curvature of the incision may create difficulties in placing internal fixation in the medial malleolar fragment. Dissection should be carried through the skin and subcutaneous and hemostasis obtained as this is performed (Fig. 32-2). Care should be taken to preserve and protect the saphenous vein and nerve throughout the case. In this location, the saphenous vein is often very subcutaneous and an aggressive skin incision may lacerate the vein. With the saphe-

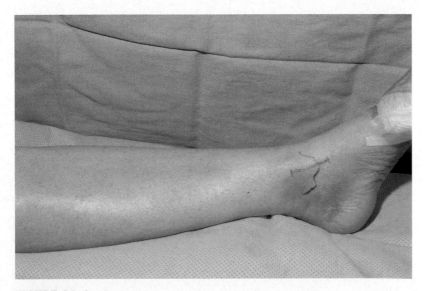

FIGURE 32-1

The incision is made along the mid-lateral axis of the distal tibia, curving anteriorly beyond the tip of the medial malleolus.

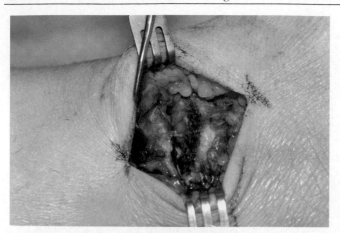

FIGURE 32-2

Exposure of the medial malleolar fracture line prior to elevation of the periosteum along the fracture edges.

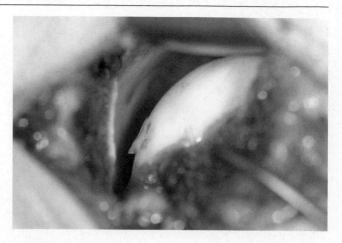

FIGURE 32-3

Retraction of the medial malleolus allows exposure of the talus and ankle joint.

nous vein and nerve protected, the medial malleolar fragment can be retracted distally with sharp bone hooks to allow inspection of the ankle joint (Fig. 32-3). A 15 blade, used to elevate the periosteum along the fracture edges, can be utilized to ensure that the fracture is reduced in an anatomic position. Preservation of the soft tissue and minimal periosteal stripping is recommended. Following internal fixation, the subcutaneous tissue can be closed using a 2-0 absorbable suture, and the skin closed with a nonabsorbable monofilament suture (Fig. 32-4).

Lateral Approach—Lateral Malleolar Fixation The direct lateral approach to the fibula allows placement of fixation along the lateral aspect of the fibula. This incision is positioned in line with the longitudinal axis of the fibula and may be curved anterior distally to allow access for reduction of a Chaput-Tillaux fragment (Fig. 32-5). If plate fixation along the posterior aspect of the fibula is desired, such as in a situation when an anti-glide plate is used, rather than committing excessive soft tissue stripping via a direct lateral approach, the incision can be adjusted posteriorly. The superficial peroneal nerve may cross the surgical approach in a subcutaneous location; therefore the skin incision should go no deeper than the skin (Fig. 32-6). Dissection through the subcutaneous tissues should be performed using combinations of sharp and blunt dissection with care to identify and protect the superficial peroneal nerve if encountered. Periosteal elevation at the fracture edges with a 15 blade is recommended to ensure an anatomic reduction of the fibular fracture.

For long spiral oblique fractures in which lag screw only fixation of the fibula is to be used, this incision can be altered with an apex anterior curve along the midportion of the incision. This "wave" in the incision will allow anterior retraction of the soft tissues and appropriate directional placement of lag screws across the fracture site. The same concerns remain with regards to protection of the superficial peroneal nerve when this modification is performed.

Following internal fixation, closure is performed with interrupted 2-0 absorbable sutures in the subcutaneous tissue followed by nonabsorbable monofilament sutures in the skin (Fig. 32-7).

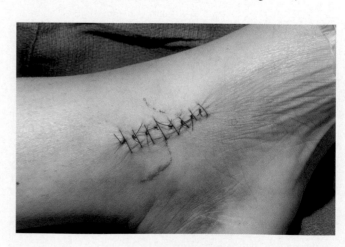

FIGURE 32-4

Skin closure is performed using a nonabsorbable monofilament suture.

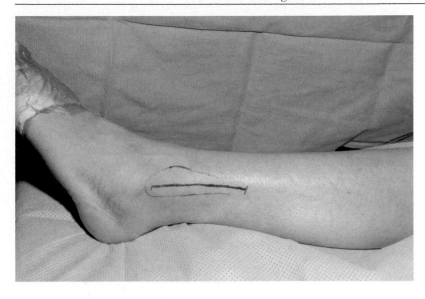

FIGURE 32-5

The incision is positioned in line with the longitudinal axis of the fibula, curving anteriorly at the distal end to allow access for reduction of a Chaput-Tillaux fragment.

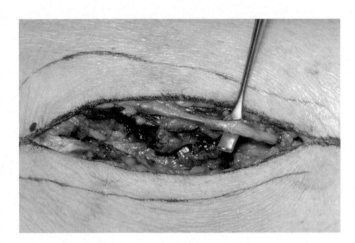

FIGURE 32-6

The superficial peroneal nerve may cross the incision, and care should be taken to identify and protect this structure.

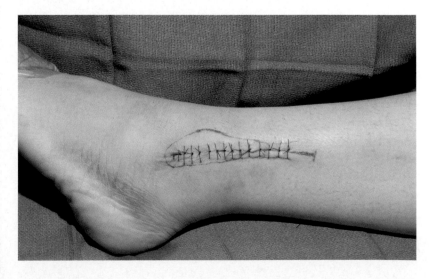

FIGURE 32-7

Skin closure is performed using a nonabsorbable monofilament suture.

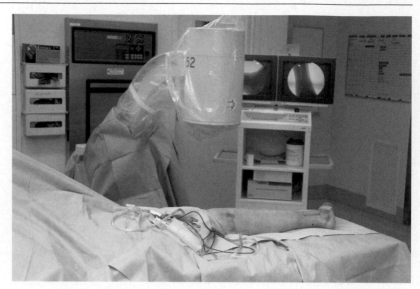

FIGURE 32-8

Intraoperative fluoroscopy can be utilized in either the lateral or prone position, and image quality should be confirmed prior to incision.

Posterolateral Approach—Posterior Malleolus Fractures

PATIENT POSITIONING   Fractures which require fixation of the posterior malleolus can be approached through a posterolateral incision. Controversy exists regarding the size of the fragment, but internal fixation is typically recommended for fractures which include 20% to 30% of the articular surface. This approach requires the patient to be in either a lateral or prone position (Fig. 32-8). The prone position allows direct visualization and better stabilization of the limb during the approach and is therefore preferred. The patient should be placed on a well-padded radiolucent table with care to be taken to prevent hyperextension of the shoulders and neck. If the arms are placed in an abducted position, care should be taken to avoid direct compression of the ulnar nerve at the cubital tunnel. A thigh high tourniquet is utilized and can be placed prior to prone positioning. Once the patient is in the prone position, they are translated towards the foot of the bed so that the hindfoot is slightly hanging off the end of the bed to aid with reduction and fixation. The C-arm fluoroscopy unit is placed perpendicular to the longitudinal axis of the patient and intraoperative films can be used on the patient's uninjured side to guarantee symmetry following reduction.

TECHNIQUE   Palpation of the fibula and Achilles tendon is possible due to the subcutaneous location of these structures. The incision is made midway between the posterior border of the lateral malleolus and the lateral border of the Achilles tendon and will need to extend to the tip of the fibula distally and as far proximally as necessary to obtain visualization of the fibular fracture and the posterior malleolar fracture (Fig. 32-9). The short saphenous vein and sural nerve are located immediately behind the lateral malleolus and the incision is placed posterior and medial to these structures. The deep fascia of the leg is split in line with the incision and the peroneal retinaculum is incised to release the peroneus longus and brevis (Fig. 32-10). The peroneal tendons and muscles are retracted laterally and the flexor hallucis longus is elevated from its origin on the fibula and retracted medially (Fig. 32-11). This allows access to the posterior aspect of the tibia for reduction and fixation (Fig. 32-12). The peroneal tendons are retracted medial or lateral depending on the location of the fracture. For fibular fractures which require a more proximal exposure, dissection to the lateral aspect of the peroneal tendons and muscles is necessary.

Following internal fixation of the posterior malleolus fragment and/or lateral malleolar fracture through the posterolateral approach, the peroneal retinaculum is repaired utilizing a 2-0 absorbable suture (Fig. 32-13). If possible, the deep fascia of the leg is also reapproximated using the same absorbable suture. Subcutaneous tissues are closed with a 2-0 absorbable suture and the skin is closed in interrupted fashion using a 3-0 or 4-0 nylon suture (Fig. 32-14).

Postoperative Management

Following internal fixation, the patient is placed in a well-padded Robert Jones splint to provide further postoperative immobilization (Fig. 32-15). The splint is applied with the knee flexed to allow dor-

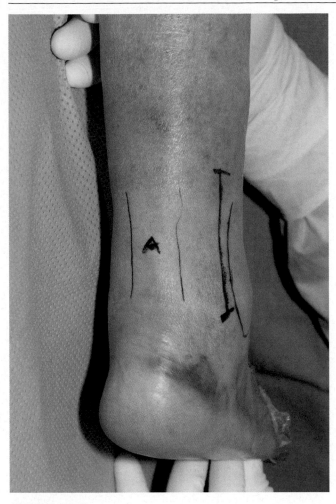

FIGURE 32-9

The incision is made midway between the posterior border of the lateral malleolus and the lateral border of the Achilles tendon.

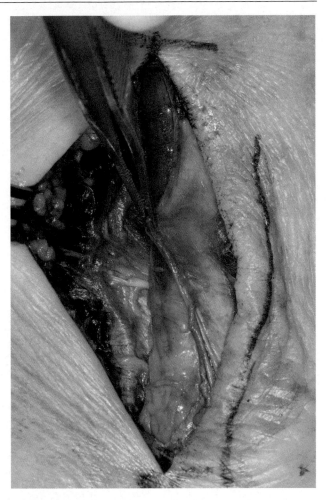

FIGURE 32-10

The deep fascia of the leg is split in line with the incision and the peroneal retinaculum is incised to release the peroneus longus and brevis.

siflexion of the ankle to a neutral position and avoidance of equinus positioning. This splint is maintained for the first 10 days to allow for postoperative swelling. The patient is then converted to either a short-leg cast or a fracture boot following this initial Robert Jones dressing. The sutures are removed 2 to 3 weeks from the date of surgery, however they should remain in place if there is any concern of delayed wound healing. Weight bearing restrictions are tailored to the individual fracture pattern and in patients with excellent bony quality and excellent healing potential weight bearing may be started at 6 weeks. In patients with multiple comorbidities, poor bone quality, or concerns for delayed fracture healing, weight bearing may be limited for up to 3 months post-operatively.

Complications

Postoperative wound dehiscence   With appropriate soft tissue management and timing of internal fixation of ankle fractures, postoperative wound dehiscence should be a relatively infrequent complication. Due to the relatively subcutaneous location of the internal fixation, any wound complication involving full thickness skin dehiscence or necrosis should be considered to communicate with the hardware and appropriate aggressive surgical intervention involving debridement and dressing changes should be performed.

Patients with partial skin necrosis or minor wound dehiscence that is located away from the hardware, particularly on the medial side, can be treated with local wound care including wet-to-dry dressing changes. If this is noted prior to suture removal, the sutures should be kept in place during these dressing changes, particularly near the portion of the wound adjacent to the dehiscence. Surrounding cellulitis should be treated with appropriate antibiotics.

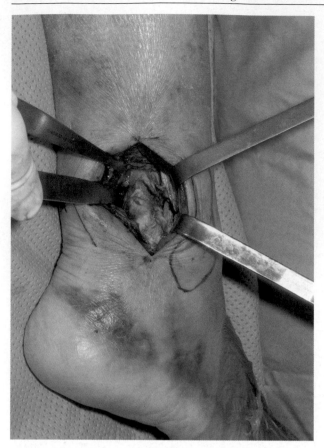

FIGURE 32-11

The peroneal tendons and muscles are retracted laterally and the flexor hallucis longus is elevated from its origin on the fibula and retracted medially.

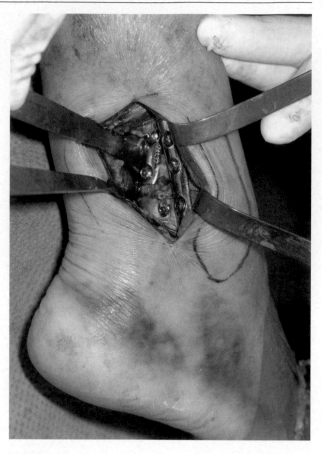

FIGURE 32-12

Following exposure, the reduction and fixation of the posterior malleolar fragment may be completed.

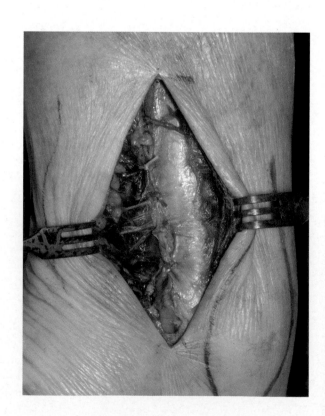

FIGURE 32-13

The peroneal retinaculum is repaired using an absorbable suture.

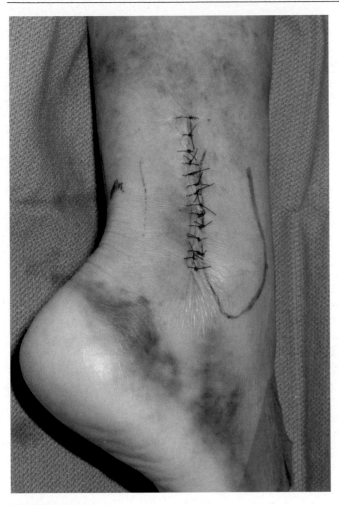

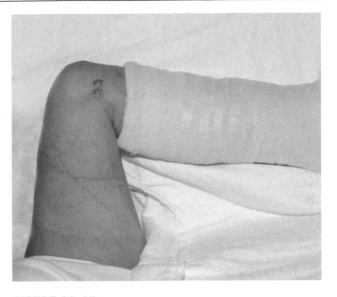

FIGURE 32-15

A well-padded Robert Jones splint is placed to provide further postoperative immobilization.

FIGURE 32-14

The skin is closed using a nonabsorbable monofilament suture.

TIBIAL PILON FRACTURES

The "personality" of tibial pilon fractures is much different from that of ankle fractures. Tibial pilon fractures usually represent a much higher energy injury with more involvement of the surrounding soft tissues. While immediate open reduction and internal fixation of some ankle fractures is feasible, the same is not true for pilon fractures. The skin around the distal tibia is not very tolerant of excessive swelling with early operative fixation and therefore allowing sufficient time for solution of swelling is necessary. Initial series of tibial pilon fractures treated with immediate open reduction and internal fixation had significantly higher rates of postoperative wound complications compared with later series in which a staged protocol was utilized. Initial management of pilon fractures is with limited internal fixation of the fibula and spanning external fixation to gain appropriate limb alignment and length. This will provide appropriate soft tissue stabilization to allow for resolution of the swelling that will inevitably occur following tibial pilon fractures.

Preoperative Planning

Initial evaluation of tibial pilon fractures consists of AP and lateral x-rays of the tibia as well as AP, lateral, and mortise radiographs of the ankle. When a pilon fracture has an associated fibula fracture, there is often shortening of the limb. After appropriate soft tissue evaluation, management consists of initial open reduction and internal fixation of the fibular fracture through a lateral or posterolateral approach in addition to application of an external fixator from the tibia to the calcaneus. This external fixator should be positioned so that the limb length is restored and the tibiotalar joint is reduced. Distraction of the joint may be necessary to prevent "cartilage necrosis" if the articular surface is comminuted and irregular. Preoperative planning is important because the incision for fibular fixation should be tailored to the anticipated approach for the tibial internal fixation. A posterolateral approach to the fibula may be utilized when a future anterolateral approach to the tibia is planned. When an anteromedial approach to the tibial pilon fracture is anticipated, a direct lateral approach to the fibula is appropriate. By utilizing a posterolateral approach to the fibula, an appropriate 5 or 6 mm skin bridge can be preserved between this approach and an anterolateral approach to the tibia. A direct lateral approach to the fibula should not be combined with an anterolateral approach to the tibia because the proximity of the incisions and resultant narrow skin bridge may result in skin necrosis between the incisions.

Once careful preoperative planning has determined the initial approaches for fibular stabilization, the patient should be positioned on a radiolucent table. A thigh high pneumatic tourniquet may be utilized during the initial fibular reduction and stabilization. Fixation of the fibula is generally performed prior to application of the external fixator. In the acute setting, fibular reduction is usually easily obtainable as the soft tissues have not yet contracted. In situations when difficulty is encountered gaining fibular length, the external fixator may be applied before fibular reduction. Careful construction of the external fixator will allow access to the fibula during internal fixation.

If the initial stabilization is performed within 24 hours, there is frequently minimal to moderate soft tissue swelling and fibular fixation can be performed. In the polytrauma setting, when fibular fixation may not be performed within 48 hours, careful soft tissue evaluation should be made before planning internal fixation. If the skin does not wrinkle when performing the pinch test, then fibular fixation should be delayed; however, spanning external fixation from the tibial to the calcaneus should not be delayed and this should be performed at the first possible time following injury. The external fixator improves length, angulation, and rotation of the fracture, but more importantly, it restores the appropriate soft tissue tension and can prevent further soft tissue compromise and development of fracture blisters. Tibial pin placement should be proximal enough that anticipated tibial plate fixation will not be contaminated by the pin tracts. A calcaneal transfixion pin is frequently utilized, however pins may also be placed in the talar neck or metatarsals to provide further support to the foot to prevent equinus positioning of the foot.

Following initial spanning external fixation, the patient's lower extremity should be elevated at all times to decrease soft tissue swelling. Deep venous thrombosis prophylaxis should be utilized for these now relatively immobile patients who have joint spanning external fixators in place. Repeat clinical evaluation should be performed on a weekly basis to monitor progression of a soft tissue injury. Once the swelling has subsided to the point that soft tissue wrinkles are attainable over the planned surgical incisions, internal fixation may be performed. There is frequently a 2 to 3 week interval between initial injury and resolution of soft tissue swelling. Once the soft tissues are amenable to surgical intervention, a duplex ultrasound screening examination should be performed on the injured extremity prior to removal of the external fixator and planned internal fixation. Avoidance of tourniquet should be considered in patients who have developed deep venous thrombosis in the injured extremity.

Once the soft tissue swelling has subsided, careful preoperative planning is required to determine appropriate patient positioning, operative approach, and implant choice for internal fixation. Planning consists of reviewing imaging studies, which should include a post reduction CT scan once limb length has been restored with the use of the external fixator and/or fibular fixation. Operative approaches should be selected which allow access to the fracture segment that requires anatomic reduction. Pilon fractures with an associated medial malleolar fracture or coronal split which extends to the fibula are often best approached through a medial or anteromedial approach. Pilon fractures with significant articular comminution, particularly in the anterolateral area, can be approached through an anterolateral approach. Fractures with significant posterior comminution are best approached through a posterolateral approach as previously described for ankle fracture fixation. Two incisions are often necessary and preoperative planning is required to ensure that there is a minimum 6 cm skin bridge between the incisions to prevent skin necrosis.

Posterolateral Approach to the Distal Tibia and Fibula

The patient is positioned in a prone position on a radiolucent operative table. The patient should be translated towards the foot of the bed so that the midfoot and toes are hanging off the bed so the foot is free. A well-padded pneumatic tourniquet may be placed around the thigh and should be placed prior to placing the patient in a prone position. The landmarks of the lateral malleolus and Achilles tendon are identified by palpation. A longitudinal skin incision is made half-way between the lateral border over the Achilles tendon and the posterior border of the lateral malleolus. The incision should extend distally until it reaches the level of the tip of the lateral malleolus. The deep fascia of the leg is incised in line with the incision, and the peroneal musculature and tendons are identified and retracted laterally. The peroneal retinaculum is incised distally to allow lateral retraction of these tendons. The flexor hallucis longus is elevated from its origin on the fibula and retracted medially to gain access to the posterior aspect of the tibia. Once reduction and fixation have been completed, the peroneal retinaculum and deep fascia of the leg are closed utilizing an absorbable suture. The subcutaneous tissue is closed with a 2-0 resorbable suture and the skin is then closed utilizing either 3-0 or 4-0 nonabsorbable monofilament sutures such as nylon.

Anterolateral Approach to the Distal Tibia

Patient Positioning   The patient is positioned supine on a radiolucent operating table and a well-padded pneumatic tourniquet is placed around the thigh. A bump is placed under the operative hip so that the foot rests vertically in the neutral position. The intraoperative C-arm is positioned on the uninjured side perpendicular to the long axis of the patient. A foam block or several folded towels can be utilized to elevate the operative limb higher than the nonoperative limb to provide a clear image with fluoroscopy. This also minimizes frequent manipulation of the leg that could potentially compromise the reduction.

Surgical Technique   For the anterolateral approach, a longitudinal skin incision is made in line with the fourth metatarsal. The incision is extended proximally as far as necessary to expose the tibia for application of a plate of the appropriate length and distally will end over the talus. The superficial peroneal nerve should be protected and retracted laterally in the wound. The subcutaneous nature of the superficial peroneal nerve requires careful skin dissection and blunt dissection once the skin has been incised. The fascia and extensor retinaculum are incised in line with the skin incisions with care taken to avoid undermining the skin flaps. The extensor digitorum longus is retracted medially and the peroneal muscles are retracted laterally. During medial dissection, avoid injury to the deep peroneal nerve and anterior tibial artery as they cross the ankle joint.

Following reduction and fixation through the anterolateral approach, the superior and inferior extensor retinaculum is repaired utilizing absorbable suture. Once the retinaculum and fascia have been reapproximated, the wound is closed with 2-0 absorbable subcutaneous sutures followed by interrupted vertical mattress nylon sutures in the skin.

Anteromedial Approach to the Distal Tibia

Preoperative Planning   The patient is positioned supine on a radiolucent operating room table and a thigh high pneumatic tourniquet is used. A foam block or set of folded towels is put under the operative leg to elevate it higher than the nonoperative leg for lateral intraoperative fluoroscopic imaging. The foot should rest in a slightly externally rotated position; therefore; placement of bumps underneath the ipsilateral hip is unnecessary. Preoperative templating to select the appropriate implant and length prevents miscalculation and unnecessary delays in the operating room.

Technique   The skin incision parallels the tibialis anterior tendons and extends proximal enough to allow application of an appropriate length of plate. Distally, the incision curves slightly medially over the ankle joint towards the talonavicular joint. The extensor retinaculum over the tibialis anterior is incised in line with the incision, and the tibialis anterior is retracted laterally. Dissection should continue beneath the tibialis anterior on the anterior aspect of the tibia, elevating the hallucis longus and extensor digitorum tendons which are retracted laterally with the tibialis anterior. The dissection may also be carried medially towards the medial malleolus to expose fractures that extend into this region. Following open reduction and internal fixation, repair the extensor retinaculum over the tibialis anterior utilizing an absorbable size 0 suture. The subcutaneous tissue is closed using an 2-0 resorbable suture, and the skin is then closed using an interrupted vertical mattress nylon suture.

Postoperative Management

Following sterile dressing application, a bulky Robert Jones type dressing utilizing both a posterior splint, as well as a stirrup-type splint, provide added stability. The patient is hospitalized until adequate pain control has been achieved. Careful postoperative evaluation should be performed to monitor for development of possible compartment syndromes in the leg following internal fixation of pilon fractures. The patient is maintained in the initial postoperative dressing for the first 7 to 10 days, which can then be exchanged for a short leg cast for further protection of both the bony and soft tissue elements. Sutures may be removed approximately 2 to 3 weeks postoperatively once the wound has healed. Depending on the bone quality and the quality of fixation, the patient is transitioned into a fracture boot or cast when rigid fixation is a concern. Once the soft tissues have healed, the patient should be encouraged to remove the walking boot multiple times per day to begin range of motion of the ankle. Weight bearing is not permitted until radiographic evidence of healing is seen, usually at 12 weeks from surgery. Initial weight bearing begins in a walking boot and once the patient is comfortable in the boot, they wean into a regular shoe over a several week period. After progression of weight bearing, radiographs should be obtained in 3 to 4 weeks to assure there is no displacement of the fractures.

Complications

Delayed Wound Healing/Wound Dehiscence Soft tissue complications can be minimized when an appropriate protocol of external fixation followed by delayed internal fixation is respected. In the event that delayed wound healing with dehiscence occurs, sutures should be left in place if it is a superficial skin dehiscence. Often, these can be treated often with dressing changes and occasionally oral antibiotics if there is surrounding cellulitis. In the event that there is deep or full thickness necrosis of either the posterolateral or anterolateral approaches, careful clinical inspection should be performed to determine whether the infection communicates with the deep hardware. Due to the relatively subcutaneous nature of the anteromedial approach, full thickness break-down should be treated as a deep infection with formal irrigation, debridement, and antibiotic treatment. Full thickness dehiscence of the anterolateral or posterolateral exposures should be inspected to determine if there is communication with the deep hardware. In the event that the subcutaneous and retinacular layers appear intact, appropriate treatment methods include local debridement and dressing changes. Any infection that communicates deep with the hardware needs to be treated aggressively with formal surgical debridement and postoperative dressing changes to obtain closure. Alternatively, VAC devices may be used in open wounds to help gain granulation tissue prior to an impending soft tissue coverage operation. With any type of wound dehiscence, range of motion exercises should be halted until resolution of the wound complication. While a cast boot is convenient for inspection of the wounds, a formal cast application with window cut-outs is more effective at immobilizing the limb and allows resolution of the soft tissue complications. In the event of early deep infections, repeat serial irrigation and debridements are necessary with intravenous antibiotic treatment to obtain suppression of the infection until union has occurred. If the infection persists following fracture union, then the hardware may be removed and further soft tissue coverage provided as necessary.

GRACILIS FREE MUSCLE FLAP FOR EXTENSIVE TISSUE LOSS FOLLOWING ANKLE INJURIES

Despite the best attempts at atraumatic tissue handling during the surgical exposure soft tissue defects surrounding the ankle may still occur. Whether due to initial soft tissue loss, or due to tissue devitalization following fixation, soft tissue deficits surrounding the ankle often require urgent coverage to avoid the complications of hardware infection, nonunion, and osteomyelitis.

For soft tissue closure of ankle defects there are many options, including the reversed soleus flap, the sural artery flap, and free latissimus dorsi muscle flap. Our preference however, in these situations, is the use of the gracilis free muscle flap. This flap provides a great deal of versatility, contours well to the ankle, and produces minimal donor site morbidity.

Indications/Contraindications

Any defect surrounding the ankle can be considered for flap coverage. The flap is limited in terms of surface area, and is not well suited for circumferential coverage of the ankle and Achilles tendon region. Also the pedicle length can be limited if a wide zone of injury requires the use of recipient vessels higher than the midcalf.

Patient factors which may increase the risk of flap failure include atherosclerosis, smoking status, and renal failure but these are not considered absolute contraindications to surgery. Absence of adequate recipient vessels is the only absolute contraindication for flap transfer.

Preoperative Planning

Often following significant lower extremity trauma a CT angio-gram is obtained to evaluate the arterial inflow to the ankle. In severe ankle trauma the posterior or anterior tibial arteries may be occluded or transected, limiting recipient vessel options: either vessel may be used as a recipient vessel for successful flap transfer. If an angiogram is not to be performed prior to surgery a careful assessment of the posterior and anterior tibial vessels must be performed with the use of a hand held Doppler probe.

SURGERY

Patient Positioning

The patient is placed supine on the operating room table with the leg in mild abduction and the knee slightly bent. Depending on the extent of the concomitant trauma either the ipsilateral or contralateral gracilis may be used. If possible we prefer to harvest the gracilis from the same leg as the original ankle trauma.

Technique

The gracilis receives its blood supply from the medial femoral circumflex artery which originates from the profunda femoral artery. The major pedicle can be identified approximately 8 to 10 cm inferior to the pubic tubercle. The flap also has a minor arterial pedicle which enters the muscle at the level of the mid thigh. This artery originates from the superficial femoral artery. The muscle receives its nervous innervation from the anterior branch of the obturator nerve. This branch of the obturator nerve can be harvested with the muscle if there are requirements for functional muscle transfer (Fig. 32-16).

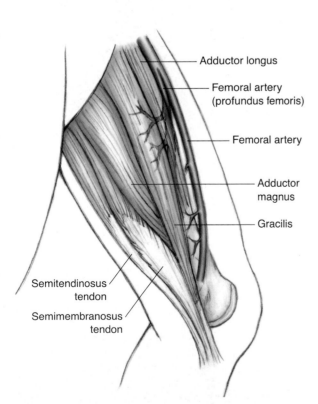

Adductor longus

Femoral artery
(profundus femoris)

Femoral artery

Adductor magnus

Gracilis

Semitendinosus tendon

Semimembranosus tendon

FIGURE 32-16

The gracilis muscle lies in the medial thigh. Its major pedicle is a branch of the medial femoral cutaneous artery which is a branch of the profunda femoris artery. The major pedicle can be identified entering the muscle 8 to 10 cm inferior to the pubic tubercle.

The muscle is exposed through a medial thigh incision. The incision is made 3 cm posterior to a line connecting the pubic tubercle and the medial condyle of the femur. A single long incision provides the most expedient means of identification of the gracilis muscles; however the resultant scar can be unsightly. Alternatively the muscle may be harvested through two separate smaller incisions; a 10 to 12 cm incision may be created over the area of the vascular pedicle and a second 5 cm incision can be created at the level of the medial femoral condyle which allows for division of the muscle insertion (Fig. 32-17).

Proximally the gracilis muscle lies between the adductor longus medially and the semitendinous muscle inferiorly. It lies superficial to the adductor magnus. The pedicle lies deep to the adductor longus but runs along the superficial surface of the adductor magnus.

Once the skin incision has been made the muscle is carefully identified inferiorly at the level of the knee. Inferiorly the muscle lies posterior to the sartorius muscle and anterior to the insertion of the semimembranous and semitendinous muscles (Fig. 32-18). The gracilis can be confused with the sartorius muscle. It may be differentiated from the sartorius and semimembranous tendon by looking for the musculotendinous portion of the gracilis. At the level of the medial femoral condyle the gracilis consists of both muscle and terminal tendon, the semimembranosus is entirely composed of tendon and the sartorius is entirely muscle. Once the gracilis is identified it may be rapidly separated from the surrounding tissue with blunt dissection to the level of the minor pedicle. The minor pedicle is not divided until the major pedicle is clearly visualized (Fig. 32-19).

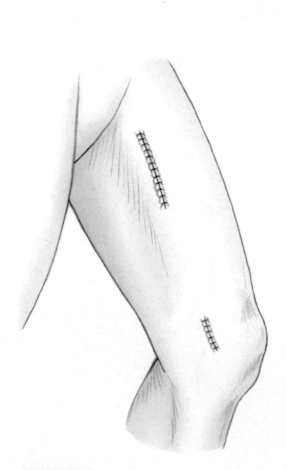

FIGURE 32-17

The muscle may be harvested through a long medial incision, or alternatively through two smaller incisions; a 10 to 12 cm incision may be created over the area of the vascular pedicle and a second 5 cm incision can be created at the level of the medial femoral condyle which allows for division of the muscle insertion.

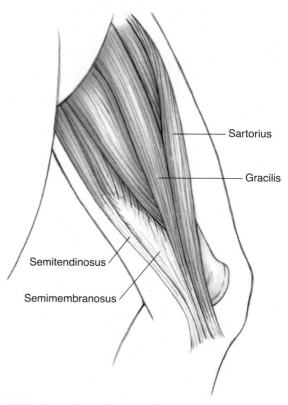

FIGURE 32-18

Inferiorly the muscle lies posterior to the sartorius muscle and anterior to the insertion of the semimembranous and semitendinous muscles. The gracilis can be confused with the sartorius muscle. It may be differentiated from the sartorius and semimembranous tendon by looking for the musculotendinous portion of the gracilis. At the level of the medial femoral condyle the gracilis consists of both muscle and terminal tendon, the semimembranosus is entirely composed of tendon, and the sartorius is entirely muscle.

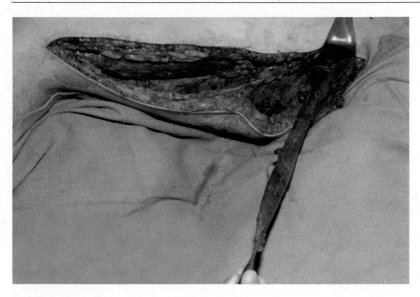

FIGURE 32-19

The muscle may be rapidly elevated back to the major pedicle. The pedicle can be seen inferior to the soft tissue retractor. The saphenous vein has been preserved as it crosses the incision midway down the thigh.

The major pedicle is identified running at the proximal lateral margin of the muscle approximately 8 to 10 cm from the pubic tubercle. The adductor longus is retracted laterally to expose the major pedicle. The fascia of the adductor magnus must be divided to allow for mobilization of the pedicle significantly. The pedicle is traced back to its origin at the profunda femoris vessels. Multiple perforating branches to the adductor muscles must be divided to gain exposure to the profundus artery, thus maximizing pedicle length of up to 6 cm. Dissection and visualization is aided with the use of lighted retractors; alternatively the adductor longus may be mobilized and retracted medially allowing visualization of the pedicle origin deep to the muscle (Fig. 32-20).

Once the major pedicle is identified and determined to be adequate for microvascular anastomosis the secondary pedicle is divided. The origin of the muscle and branch of the obturator nerve is now divided. The muscle is left to perfuse on its major pedicle until the recipient vessels have been prepared for microvascular anastomosis.

Prior to muscle transfer a final definitive debridement of the defect site is performed. The recipient vessels are then exposed away from the original zone of injury (Fig. 32-21). Donor vessel prepa-

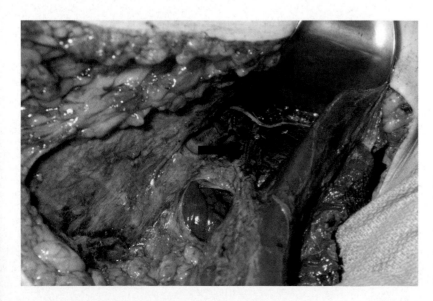

FIGURE 32-20

The pedicle (*black arrow*) is dissected back to its origin at the profunda femoris. This allows for a significant improvement in pedicle length. A branch of the obturator nerve can be seen running on top of pedicle and the adductor magnus muscle.

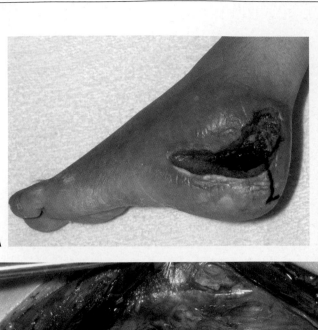

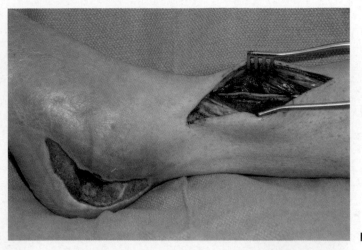

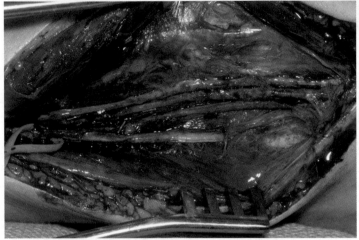

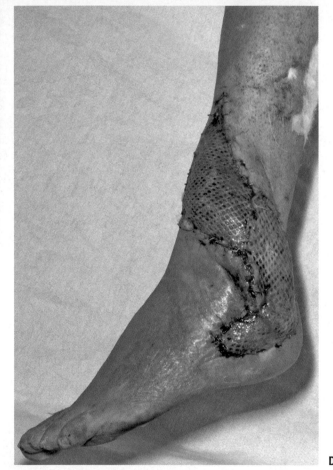

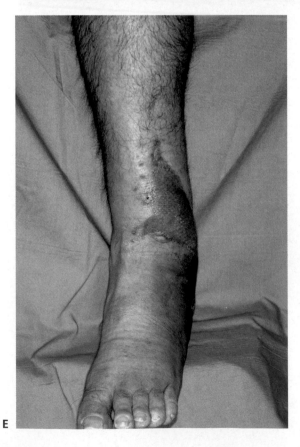

FIGURE 32-21

A: A lateral malleolar defect has developed in a 48-year-old gentleman following stabilization of a complex malleolar and calcaneal fracture. **B:** The anterior tibial vessels are exposed away from the zone of injury in preparation for free tissue transfer. **C:** The anterior vessels are identified just lateral and deep to the anterior tibialis muscle. The perineal nerve is surrounded with a vessel loop and gently freed from the underlying vessels. **D:** The flap at one week shows good take of the skin graft. **E:** Four month view shows excellent contouring of the flap with stable wound coverage allowing for normal shoe wear.

ration is performed with the use of high powered operative loop magnification or the microscope to verify that the vessels are adequate for microvascular anastomosis. The anterior tibial artery is used as a recipient vessel for lateral malleolar defects while the posterior tibial artery is preferentially used for medial defects (Fig. 32-22). End to side anastomosis to the artery is preferred while an end to end anastomosis to the venous comitantes is performed in most settings. If two veins are present within the arterial pedicle both of the venous comitantes to the gracilis muscle are anastomosed to minimize the chances of postoperative venous insufficiency.

Once the anastomosis is complete the muscle is allowed to reperfuse for 20 minutes as the donor site is closed. An implantable Doppler probe is placed circumferentially around one of the two veins to allow for evaluation of anastomotic patency postoperatively. Donor site closure is performed with deep dermal sutures and an absorbable subcutaneous monofilament suture. A closed suction drain is also used to prevent postoperative seroma or hematoma formation. Flap insetting is then performed. Muscle insetting is facilitated with the use of half buried absorbable sutures placed within the muscle and pulled beneath the native skin. The epimysium of the muscle is often excised to allow for expansion of the muscle's surface area. This allows for improved contouring over the malleolus. At the

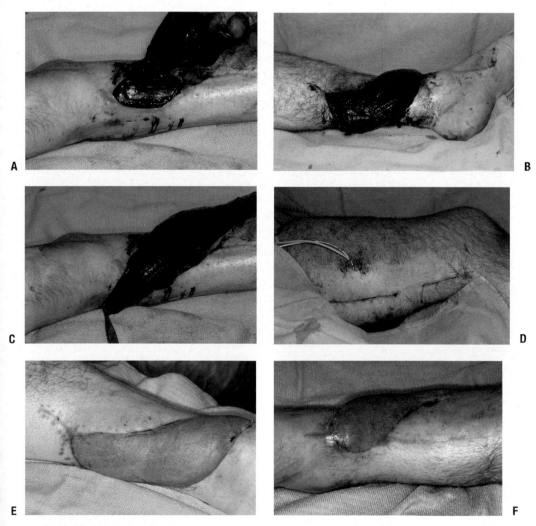

FIGURE 32-22

A: A 32-year-old gentleman presents with a defect of the lower margin of the tibia which developed following treatment of a malleolar fracture. **B,C:** In this case the gracilis muscle is anastomosed to the posterior tibial vessels and brought anteriorly to cover the bone and soft tissue defect. **D:** The muscle was harvested through two limited incisions over the medial thigh. The inferior incision is used for division of the muscle insertion while the superior incision is used for dissection of the vascular pedicle and division of the muscle origin. **E,F:** The wound is stable at 6 months with no further drainage or signs of ongoing infection.

completion of insetting the muscle is covered with a meshed split thickness skin graft. The flap is covered with a Xeroform and the patient's leg is then loosely wrapped in sterile cotton and placed into a posterior splint for postoperative comfort. A large window is created in the dressing for postoperative flap monitoring. A single suture is placed superficially within the muscle over the pedicle so that anastomotic patency can be evaluated postoperatively with the use of a hand held Doppler device.

Postoperative Management

Flap monitoring may be performed with either the use of an implantable Doppler probe, or with the use of a hand held Doppler probe at the bedside. Evaluation of perfusion is performed every hour for the first 24 hours by a skilled microsurgical nursing staff who are familiar knows the signs of arterial insufficiency and venous thrombosis.

On postoperative day 4 or 5 the entire dressing is removed and skin graft survival is assessed. At this point the patient may be placed into a loose Robert-Jones dressing or a removal posterior splint. The donor site drain is removed once output is less than 30 cc a day.

Complications/Results

The most devastating complication following any free tissue transfer include partial flap loss and total flap loss. If arterial insufficiency or venous insufficiency occurs postoperatively, immediate re-exploration is recommended. At the time of surgical exploration thrombosis may be identified at the anastomotic site. In such cases early revision of the anastomosis will often allow for flap salvage. If the flap is unsalvageable and flap loss occurs, an additional flap will be required. In such cases a secondary free flap, pedicled flap, or cross-leg flap can be considered. In cases of partial flap loss, occasionally the flap may be advanced distally to cover critical structures. Alternatively small areas of distal necrosis may be managed with dressing changes, skin grafting, or pedicle flap coverage.

In an examination of 50 acute traumatic and post-traumatic wounds, Redett and colleagues found the gracilis muscle effective for covering defects up to 165 cm^2. Successful free tissue transfer was performed in 93% of patients, and limb salvage was possible in 96%. Studies by Hallock have shown that the vascular pedicle is of adequate length for reconstruction of defects extending over the calcaneus and lateral malleolus (Fig. 32-21). For defects which exceed the limits of a gracilis transfer a latissimus free muscle flap can be considered. We have found the gracilis to contour nicely over time allowing for normal shoe wear following reconstruction.

RECOMMENDED READING

Blauth M, Bastian L, Krettek C, et al. Surgical options for the treatment of severe tibial pilon fractures: a study of three techniques. *J Orthop Trauma*. 2001;15(3):153–60.

Gopal S, Majumder S, Batchelor AG, et al. Fix and flap: the radical orthopaedic and plastic treatment of severe open fractures of the tibia. *J Bone Joint Surg Br*. 2000;82(7):959–66.

Hallock GG, Arangio GA. Free-flap salvage of soft tissue complications following the lateral approach to the calcaneus. *Ann Plast Surg*. 2007;58(2):179–81.

Redett RJ, Robertson BC, Chang B, et al. Limb salvage of lower-extremity wounds using free gracilis muscle reconstruction. *Plast Reconstr Surg*. 2000;106(7):1507–13.

Sirkin M, Sanders R, DiPasquale T, et al. A staged protocol for soft tissue management in the treatment of complex pilon fractures. *J Orthop Trauma*. 1999;13(2):78–84.

33 Calcaneal Fractures/Talar Neck Fractures

Michael P. Clare and Roy W. Sanders

Fractures of the calcaneus and talus are among the most complex and challenging of fractures for the orthopaedic surgeon to effectively manage, in that both are three-dimensionally unique structures with highly specialized biomechanical function and a distinctly limited surrounding soft tissue envelope. Fractures of the calcaneus and talus are generally the result of high-energy trauma, such as a motor vehicle accident or a fall from a height, and as such, the severity of fracture displacement and the extent of soft tissue disruption are directly proportional to the amount of force and energy absorbed by the limb.

FRACTURES OF THE CALCANEUS

Indications/Contraindications

General Considerations   Operative treatment is generally indicated for displaced intra-articular fractures involving the posterior facet as demonstrated on computed tomography (CT) scanning. Nonoperative treatment is best reserved for non- or minimally-displaced extra-articular calcaneal fractures, and truly non-displaced intra-articular fractures as determined on CT scan.

Comorbidities   While nicotine use/dependence is not a contraindication to operative treatment, all patients who are smokers are counseled at length as to the associated risks and encouraged to discontinue tobacco use. We consider heavy smoking (≥2 packs per day) as a relative contraindication to surgery. Specific contraindications for operative treatment include fractures in patients with insulin-dependent diabetes mellitus, severe peripheral vascular disease, or other major medical comorbidities precluding surgery, as well as fractures in elderly patients who are minimal (household) ambulators. Because many older patients are healthy and active well into their 70s, chronologic age itself is not necessarily a contraindication to surgical treatment.

Delayed Treatment by Necessity   Operative treatment may also be contraindicated if initial evaluation has been delayed beyond 3 or 4 weeks from the date of injury, or in certain situations in which injury severity prohibits early surgical intervention, including fractures associated with severe fracture blisters or prolonged edema; fractures with large open wounds; and fractures in patients with life-threatening injuries. Operative treatment following a prolonged delay (>4 weeks) from initial injury to definitive treatment is complicated by the fact that early consolidation of the fracture has occurred, making the fracture fragments increasingly difficult to separate to obtain an adequate reduction, and the articular cartilage may delaminate away from the underlying subchondral bone. In these instances, delayed treatment by necessity is used whereby the fracture is allowed to heal and is later managed as a calcaneal malunion following resolution of the prohibitive factors.

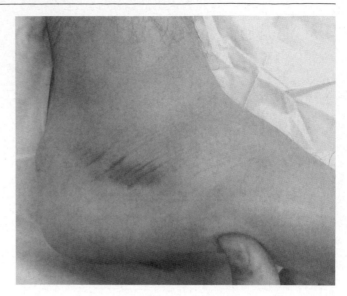

FIGURE 33-1

Preoperative "wrinkle" test. Note presence of skin creases indicating that surgery may now be safely undertaken.

Preoperative Planning

In completing preparations for surgery, the surgeon should thoroughly review the plain radiographs and CT scans to gain a preliminary understanding as to the "personality" of the fracture pattern, which then allows for planning of patient position and surgical approach, as well as anticipation of specific technical steps in obtaining fracture reduction, and the necessary implants for definitive stabilization. While multiple surgical approaches have historically been described, the general consensus currently favors the extensile lateral approach for most displaced intra-articular calcaneal fractures. Percutaneous reduction techniques, such as the Essex-Lopresti maneuver, are particularly ideal for certain tongue-type fracture (Sanders type II-C) patterns.

Surgery is ideally completed within the first 3 weeks of injury before early fracture consolidation; however, surgery should not be attempted until the associated soft tissue swelling has sufficiently dissipated as demonstrated by a positive wrinkle test. The test involves assessment of the lateral calcaneal skin with passive dorsiflexion and eversion of the injured foot. A positive test is confirmed by the presence of skin wrinkling without residual pitting edema, such that surgical intervention may be safely undertaken (Fig. 33-1). A variety of modalities may used to decrease swelling in the affected extremity. We prefer initial elevation and immobilization in a bulky Jones dressing and supportive splint, with later conversion to an elastic compression stocking and fracture boot locked in neutral flexion as the acute swelling begins to dissipate in the ensuing few days.

EXTENSILE LATERAL APPROACH

Surgery

Patient Positioning/General Considerations   The procedure requires use of a radiolucent table and a standard C-arm. For isolated injuries, we prefer placing the patient in the lateral decubitus position on a beanbag. The lower extremities are positioned in a scissor configuration, whereby the operative ("up") limb is flexed at the knee and angles toward the posterior, distal corner of the operating table, and the nonoperative ("down") limb is extended at the knee and positioned away from the surgical field to facilitate intraoperative fluoroscopy. Protective padding is placed beneath the contralateral limb for protection of the peroneal nerve, and an operating "platform" is created with blankets and foam padding to elevate the operative limb (Fig. 33-2). The prone position may alternatively be used in the event of bilateral injuries.

The patient is given prophylactic preoperative antibiotics, and a pneumatic thigh tourniquet is used. The procedure should be completed within 120 to 130 minutes of tourniquet time, so as to minimize wound complications. If the procedure extends beyond that time, the tourniquet should be released and the remainder of the procedure performed without it. In allocating tourniquet time, the surgical approach should be completed within 20 minutes, allowing up to 60 minutes for fracture reduction, 20 minutes for implant placement, and 20 minutes for wound closure.

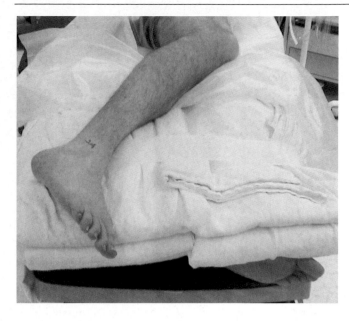

FIGURE 33-2
Lateral decubitus position. Note scissor-like limb configuration to facilitate intraoperative fluoroscopy.

Technique

ANATOMIC LANDMARKS   Wound complications following surgical management of calcaneal fractures remain a major source of morbidity with these injuries. The soft tissues overlying the lateral hindfoot receive blood supply from a confluence of three arterial branches: the lateral calcaneal artery, the lateral malleolar artery, and the lateral tarsal artery. Borrelli and Lashgari determined that the majority of the full-thickness flap with an extensile lateral approach is supplied by the lateral calcaneal artery, typically a branch of the peroneal artery. At the level of lateral malleolus, the artery courses parallel to the Achilles tendon and lies approximately 11 to 15 mm anterior to the terminal Achilles tendon and its insertion. Thus, strict attention to detail with respect to placement of the incision and gentle handling of the soft tissues is of paramount importance.

INCISION AND SURGICAL APPROACH   The extensile lateral incision is then outlined on the skin with a marking pencil (Fig. 33-3). The incision begins approximately 2 cm proximal to the tip of the lateral malleolus, just lateral to the Achilles tendon extending toward the plantar foot. In this manner, the vertical limb of the incision will course posterior to the sural nerve and the lateral calcaneal

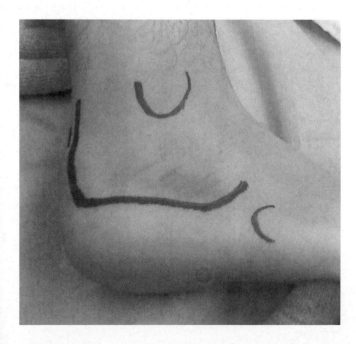

FIGURE 33-3
Planned extensile lateral incision.

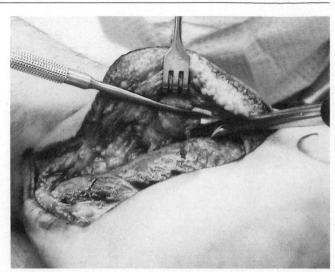

FIGURE 33-4

Full-thickness subperiosteal flap. Note peroneal tendons contained within the flap.

artery, thereby avoiding devascularization of the lateral calcaneal flap. The horizontal limb of the incision is drawn along the junction of the skin of the lateral foot and heel pad, the demarcation of which can be identified by compressing the heel. We prefer to substitute a gentle curve where these two lines intersect to form a right angle, primarily to avoid necrosis of the apical skin. The terminal portion of the horizontal limb includes a gentle curve anteriorly along the skin creases, extending over the calcaneocuboid articulation.

With a sterile bolster placed beneath the medial ankle, the incision begins at the proximal portion of the vertical limb, becoming full-thickness at the level of the calcaneal tuberosity; dissection is specifically taken from "skin to bone" at this level while avoiding any beveling of the skin. Scalpel pressure is again lessened beyond the apical curve, roughly at the midpoint of the horizontal limb, at which point a layered incision is again developed.

A full-thickness subperiosteal flap is then developed starting at the apex. Any use of retractors should be avoided until a sizeable flap has been raised, so as to avoid separation of the skin from the subcutaneous tissues and periosteum. The calcaneofibular ligament and inferior peroneal retinaculum are released sharply, thus exposing the peroneal tendons. Both tendons are identified and released from the peroneal tubercle through the cartilaginous pulley, and further gently mobilized distally with a periosteal elevator, thereby exposing the anterolateral calcaneus and calcaneocuboid joint. In this manner, the peroneal tendons and sural nerve are contained entirely within the subperiosteal flap (Fig. 33-4).

Deep dissection continues anteriorly to the sinus tarsi and anterior process, and posteriorly to the superior-most portion of the calcaneal tuberosity for "window visualization" of the posterior facet, so as to prevent rotational malalignment of the posterior facet articular surface in the sagittal plane. Three 1.6-mm Kirschner wires are then placed for retraction of the subperiosteal flap using the "no touch" technique. In this technique, one wire is placed into the distal fibula as the peroneal tendons are slightly subluxed anteriorly; a second wire is placed in the talar neck; a third wire is placed in the cuboid as the peroneal tendons are levered away from the anterolateral surface of the calcaneus with a periosteal elevator. Thus, each Kirschner wire retracts its respective portion of the peroneal tendons and subperiosteal flap (Fig. 33-5). A small Bennett-type retractor may additionally be used at the distal margin of the sinus tarsi for further exposure of the anterolateral calcaneus.

ASSESSMENT OF THE PERONEAL TENDONS   Following fracture reduction, definitive stabilization, and final fluoroscopic images, the wound is copiously irrigated. As the previously placed Kirschner wires are manually removed, the peroneal tendons should easily reduce into the peroneal groove at the posterior border of the lateral malleolus. A Freer elevator is introduced into the tendon sheath, advanced proximally to the level of the lateral malleolus, and levered anteriorly to assess the stability of the peroneal tendon sheath and superior peroneal retinaculum. If the tendon sheath is detached from the lateral malleolus and therefore incompetent, the elevator will easily advance anterior to the lateral malleolus, indicating that a retinacular repair is required. A 3-cm incision is then made along the posterior margin of the lateral malleolus, exposing the tendon sheath and retinaculum. With the peroneal tendons held reduced in the peroneal groove, one to two suture anchors are

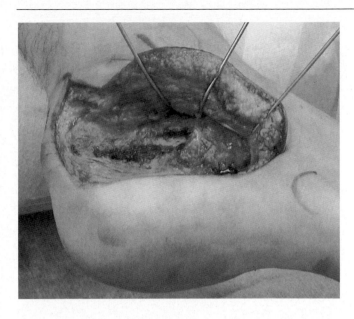

FIGURE 33-5

"No touch" technique: K-wire placement for retraction of the full-thickness flap.

placed in the lateral malleolus to secure the detached tendon sheath and retinaculum. Tendon stability is then reassessed with a Freer elevator in the same manner.

CLOSURE TECHNIQUE A deep drain is placed exiting proximally in line with the vertical limb of the incision. Deep No. 0 absorbable sutures are then passed in interrupted, inverted fashion starting with the apex of the incision. Sutures are placed thereafter at the proximal and distal ends of the incision, and progressing toward the apex of the incision, while attempting to advance the flap toward the apex. The suture ends are temporarily clamped until all sutures have been passed (Fig. 33-6). The sutures are then hand tied in sequential fashion, starting at the ends proximally and distally, progressing toward the apex of the incision to minimize tension at the apex.

ALLGÖWER-DONATI SUTURE The skin layer is closed with 3-0 monofilament suture using the modified Allgöwer-Donati technique, again starting at the ends and working toward the apex (Fig. 33-7). The suture technique is a modified vertical mattress stitch, whereby the far end passes subcutaneous to the skin edge to minimize tension on the skin margin. Alternatively, the sutures may be passed in modified horizontal mattress fashion. In the context of an extensile lateral approach, the

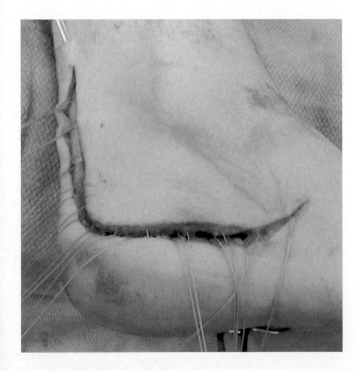

FIGURE 33-6

Deep closure. Note placement of all sutures prior to sequential tying (different patient).

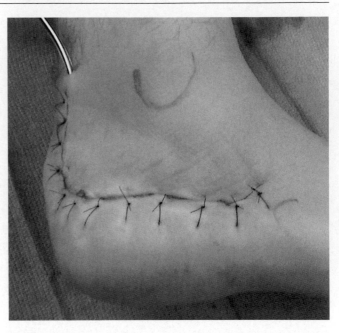

FIGURE 33-7

Skin closure using modified Allgöwer-Donati technique.

knots are placed along the periphery of the incision, avoiding violation of the skin margin of the subperiosteal flap.

The suture is placed initially into the wound edge of the near end, and the needle is then reversed in the needle driver. The suture is introduced into the subcuticular edge of the far end and extended through the subcutaneous tissue of the near end, exiting approximately 1 cm from, and in line with, the initial entry point. A single reverse throw is passed to maintain the skin bridge between the entry and exit point, and the knot is slightly tensioned to approximate the skin edges. A second reverse knot is passed to allow the knot to slide and gently evert the wound edges, followed by a forward knot to lock the stitch in place (Fig. 33-8). Following completion of wound closure, the tourniquet is deflated and sterile dressings are applied, followed by a Jones-type bulky cotton dressing and Weber splint.

Postoperative Management

The patient remains in the hospital overnight for pain control, and is converted to a short-leg nonweight bearing cast prior to discharge. The patient is converted back into an elastic compression stocking and fracture boot at 2 to 3 weeks postoperatively, and subtalar range of motion exercises are initiated. The sutures are removed once the incision is fully sealed and completely dry, typically at 3 to 4 weeks; however, they should not be removed until the wound is fully healed. We prefer that the patient sleep in the fracture boot at night until weight bearing is begun to prevent an equines contracture. Weight bearing is not permitted until 10 to 12 weeks postoperatively, at which point the fracture should be radiographically healed. The patient is then gradually transitioned to a regular shoe, and activities are advanced. In our experience, the patient should be able to return to a moderately active job at approximately 4 to 6 months postoperatively.

Complications

Delayed Wound Healing/Wound Dehiscence   Delayed wound healing or wound dehiscence is the most common complication following surgical management of a calcaneal fracture, and may occur in up to 25% of cases. Risk factors for wound complications include smoking, diabetes mellitus, open fractures, high body mass index, and a single layered wound closure. While the extensile lateral incision approximates relatively easily at the time of initial closure, wound separation may later occur—typically at the apex of the incision, and even up to 4 weeks postoperatively (Fig. 33-9). The vast majority of wounds, however, will ultimately heal; deep infection and osteomyelitis develop in only 1% to 4% of closed fractures.

In the event of a wound dehiscence, all range of motion activities are discontinued to prevent further dehiscence of the wound. We prefer a fairly aggressive approach to the wound, with a manage-

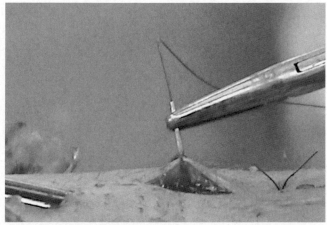

A

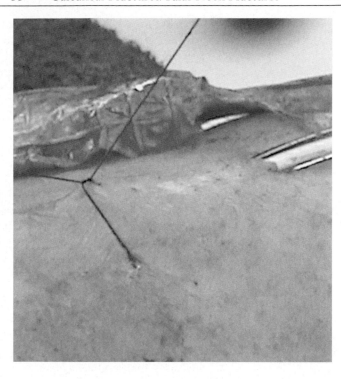

B

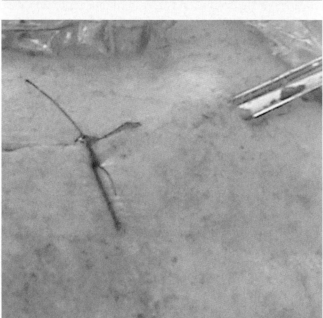

C

FIGURE 33-8

Allgöwer-Donati technique. Note reverse throw **(B)** to maintain skin bridge between suture ends.

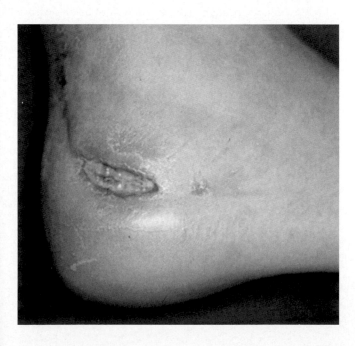

FIGURE 33-9

Apical wound dehiscence at 4 weeks postoperatively.

ment regimen of daily whirlpool treatments, damp-to-dry dressing changes, and oral antibiotics. Other granulation-promoting wound agents may also be beneficial in this instance. Alternatively, the limb may be immobilized in a short leg cast, with a window overlying the wound for access for dressing changes. These treatment regimens will typically prove successful, so long as the wound necrosis is limited to partial thickness of the skin layer. Range of motion exercises are re-initiated once the wound seals and remains dry with the patient off antibiotics.

We prefer use of a negative-pressure device (Vacuum-Assisted Closure®, KCI, Inc., San Antonio, TX) to promote healing in the event of a recalcitrant wound; if all other treatment methods fail, a low-profile fasciocutaneous flap such as a lateral arm flap may be required for wound coverage.

Peroneal Tendon Adhesions   Peroneal tendon adhesions and scarring may develop in up to 18% of cases, either from the extensile lateral exposure itself or from prominent screwheads adjacent to the tendons, particularly surrounding the anterior process of the calcaneus. Nonoperative treatment includes tendon massage, stretching, strengthening, and other local modalities. Peroneal tenolysis or removal of the symptomatic hardware may be required in refractory cases.

Cutaneous Nerve Injury   The most common neurologic complication with surgical treatment of calcaneal fractures is iatrogenic injury to a sensory cutaneous nerve, particularly the sural nerve. Sural nerve injury occurs in up to 15% of cases and ranges from a stretch neuropraxia, which can be transient or permanent, to complete laceration of the nerve. Clinically, the patient may experience decreased or complete loss of sensation in the lateral hindfoot, or perhaps even a painful neuroma. Initial treatment includes gabapentin or amitriptyline, shoe modifications or soft accommodative inserts, and physical therapy modalities. In the event of a painful neuroma refractory to these measures, surgical neurolysis and resection may be considered, including burial of the proximal stump into deep tissues.

FRACTURES OF THE TALAR NECK

Indications/Contraindications

Operative treatment is generally indicated for all displaced fractures of the talar neck, and these fractures have traditionally been considered a surgical emergency, due to the high incidence of osteonecrosis associated with displaced fractures. More recent studies have indicated that a delay in surgical management beyond 6 to 8 hours from the time of injury does not necessarily increase the risk of osteonecrosis, such that definitive stabilization within the first 24 hours following injury is now gaining acceptance as standard of care.

Severely displaced fractures or fracture-dislocations, however, may produce sufficient tension and pressure on the surrounding skin acutely to impair local circulation and result in skin necrosis and slough, potentially leading to a catastrophic deep infection and/or osteomyelitis. Thus, a timely attempt at closed reduction of the involved fracture fragment or dislocation is of paramount importance in minimizing soft tissue complications associated with these injuries, particularly if a delay in definitive stabilization is anticipated.

Nonoperative management is reserved for truly non-displaced fractures as confirmed on CT scan. Because of the high-energy nature of these injuries, displaced talar neck fractures occur most commonly in young adults. Thus in the majority of cases, the primary contraindication to surgery is the presence of severe life-threatening injuries where the patient is too medically unstable to tolerate surgery. In this instance, however, an attempt at closed reduction or manipulation of any dislocated fragments should be made in the emergency room to minimize the risk of skin necrosis.

Preoperative Planning

The surgeon should thoroughly review the plain radiographs and CT scans to gain an initial understanding of the fracture pattern, which then allows for appropriate preoperative planning, including: the surgical approach, anticipation of specific technical steps in obtaining fracture reduction, and the necessary implants for definitive stabilization. While we commonly use up to eight different surgical approaches in the management of talar fractures in general, we prefer dual anteromedial and anterolateral approaches for talar neck fractures.

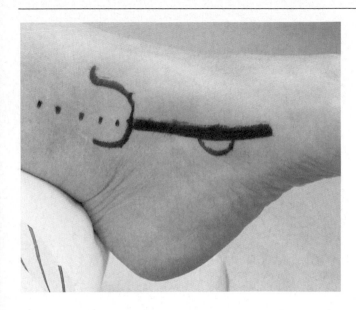

FIGURE 33-10
Planned anteromedial incision.

Surgery

Patient Positioning/General Considerations

DUAL ANTEROMEDIAL AND ANTEROLATERAL APPROACHES   The procedure requires use of a radiolucent table and a standard C-arm. For isolated injuries, we prefer placing a non-sterile bolster beneath the ipsilateral hip and pelvis to allow sufficient limb exposure both medially and laterally. Protective padding is placed beneath the contralateral limb for protection of the peroneal nerve, and the contralateral limb is secured to the operating table to allow for axial plane rotation as needed for surgical exposure. The patient is given prophylactic preoperative antibiotics, and a pneumatic thigh tourniquet is employed. The procedure should be completed within 120 to 130 minutes of tourniquet time to minimize wound complications.

Technique

INCISION AND SURGICAL APPROACH   The dual anteromedial and anterolateral incisions are outlined on the skin with a marking pencil. Medially, the talar neck is isolated approximately a thumb-breadth distal to the anterior tip of the medial malleolus, or midway between the medial malleolus and navicular tubercle. Thus, the anteromedial incision extends from the tip of the medial malleolus in line with the medial column of the foot to a point approximately 1 cm beyond the navicular tubercle (Fig. 33-10). In this manner, the deep dissection will course through the "soft spot" between the anterior and posterior tibial tendons, and posterior to the saphenous nerve and vein. The approach is potentially extensile, as it can be extended proximally to allow for a medial malleolar osteotomy for talar neck fractures extending into the talar body or posteromedial process, as well as distally for access to the entire medial column of the foot as necessary (Fig. 33-11).

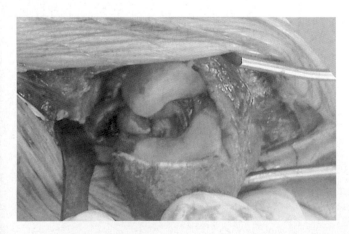

FIGURE 33-11
Medial malleolar osteotomy: anteromedial approach extended proximally for exposure of talar body (different patient).

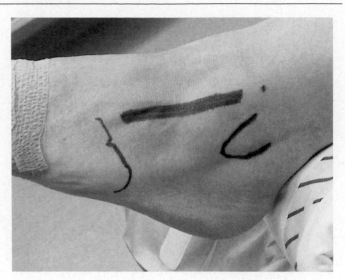

FIGURE 33-12

Planned anterolateral incision.

Laterally, the talar neck is found immediately dorsal to the sinus tarsi in line with the extensor digitorum longus and peroneus tertius tendons. The anterolateral incision actually consists of the Böhler approach, coursing from the anterolateral corner of the ankle joint in line with the extensor digitorum longus and peroneus tertius tendons toward the base of the fourth metatarsal (Fig. 33-12). This approach is also considered extensile, as it can be extended proximally to allow for exposure of the lateral talar dome, with or without a lateral malleolar osteotomy, and distally for exposure of the entire lateral column of the foot as necessary.

We prefer completing the anterolateral approach first because the majority of the comminution is typically found medially; thus, the most accurate initial indication of the extent of fracture displacement or rotational malalignment is found laterally. With sterile bolsters placed beneath the knee and ankle, the anterolateral approach is initiated, and superficial dissection continues to the extensor retinaculum and tendon sheath of the extensor digitorum longus and peroneus tertius tendons. Care is taken to avoid violation of the superficial peroneal nerve proximally, although the proximal portion of the incision rarely extends proximal enough to visualize the nerve before it begins coursing medially toward the first dorsal web space.

The tendon sheath is incised at the lateral margin of the tendons, and deep dissection is continued to the deep capsule of the ankle and subtalar joints proximally, and the extensor digitorum brevis muscle distally. The extensor brevis muscle is then traced to its origin beneath the tendons working dorsally, and subsequently reflected plantarly, thereby exposing the lateral capsule of the talonavicular joint and distal portion of the talar neck. The deep capsules of the ankle and subtalar joints are then released in line with and including the talonavicular joint capsule extending dorsally and plantarly, thereby completing a full-thickness flap (Fig. 33-13). In this manner, the foot may be adducted to expose the lateral portion of the talar head, thereby facilitating eventual placement of screws,

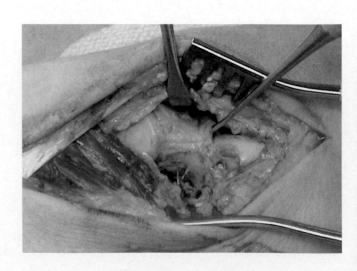

FIGURE 33-13

Anterolateral approach. Note full-thickness flap with simultaneous exposure of ankle, subtalar, and talonavicular joints.

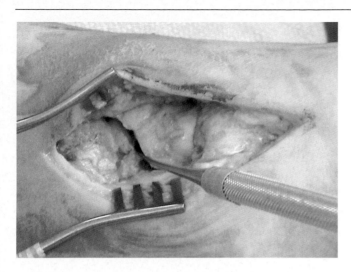

FIGURE 33-14

Anteromedial approach. Note full-thickness flap with simultaneous exposure of ankle, subtalar, and talonavicular joints.

which may be countersunk within the talar head. We make a conscious effort to limit the extent of subperiosteal dissection into the sinus tarsi, exposing only what is necessary to obtain an anatomic reduction, to minimize further compromise of the already precarious blood supply to the talar body.

The anteromedial approach is then initiated, and superficial dissection continues to the extensor retinaculum and deep capsules of the ankle and subtalar joints proximally, and dorsal margin of the posterior tibial tendon sheath distally. The extensor retinaculum and deep capsules are longitudinally incised, continuing along the dorsal edge of the posterior tibial tendon through the underlying talonavicular joint capsule and spring ligament. Care is taken to avoid violation of the deltoid ligament fibers at the proximal margin of the incision.

The talonavicular joint capsule is then elevated in subperiosteal fashion off of the navicular tubercle, extending roughly to the midpoint of the navicular dorsally. The dorsal-most portion of the posterior tibial tendon insertion may also be reflected plantarly to ease soft tissue tension as necessary (Fig. 33-14). In this manner, the foot may be abducted to expose the medial portion of the talar head, again facilitating eventual screw placement. We again limit the extent of subperiosteal dissection along the undersurface of the talar neck medially in an attempt to preserve the vascular anastamoses extending into the tarsal canal. At the completion of the anterolateral and anteromedial approaches, the fracture patterns traversing the dorsal portion of talar neck should be easily visualized.

CLOSURE TECHNIQUE   Following fracture reduction, definitive stabilization, and final fluoroscopic imaging, the wound is copiously irrigated. The deep capsular layers are closed medially and laterally with interrupted No. 0 absorbable sutures placed in figure-of-eight fashion. Laterally, the extensor digitorum brevis muscle is gently approximated distally with interrupted 2-0 absorbable sutures in similar fashion, as is the extensor retinaculum and extensor digitorum longus and peroneus tertius tendon sheath more proximally. Medially, the extensor retinaculum and posterior tibial tendon sheath are closed in identical fashion with interrupted 2-0 absorbable sutures. The subcutaneous and subcuticular layers are closed with inverted, interrupted 2-0 absorbable sutures. The tourniquet is then deflated, and the skin layers are approximated with interrupted 3-0 monofilament suture, again using the modified Allgöwer-Donati technique. Sterile dressings are applied, followed by a Jones-type bulky cotton dressing and Weber splint with the ankle in neutral dorsiflexion-plantar flexion.

Postoperative Management

The patient remains in the hospital overnight for pain control, and is converted to a short-leg non-weight bearing cast before discharge. The patient is converted back into an elastic compression stocking and fracture boot at 2 to 3 weeks postoperatively, and ankle and subtalar range of motion exercises are initiated. The sutures are removed once the incision is fully sealed and completely dry, typically at 3 to 4 weeks; however, they should not be removed until the wound is fully healed. We prefer that the patient sleep in the fracture boot at night until weight bearing is begun to prevent an equines contracture.

Weight bearing is not permitted until 10 to 12 weeks postoperatively, and the patient is gradually transitioned to a regular shoe, and activities are advanced. Postoperative radiographs are carefully

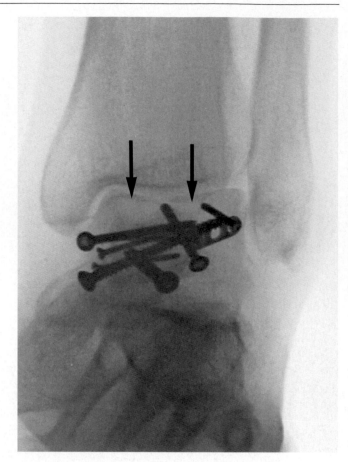

FIGURE 33-15

Hawkins sign: anteroposterior radiograph of the ankle demonstrating subchondral atrophy (*arrows*) at 8 weeks postoperatively following open reduction and internal fixation of a displaced talar neck fracture.

scrutinized beginning at 6 weeks following surgery for the presence of a Hawkins sign (Fig. 33-15), suggesting revascularization of the talar body. The absence of a Hawkins sign at that time, however, does not necessarily indicate osteonecrosis, as revascularization of the talar body may not occur for up to 2 years following surgery.

Complications

Delayed Wound Healing/Wound Dehiscence/Infection Delayed wound healing or wound dehiscence following open reduction and internal fixation occurs in a relatively small percentage of patients, ranging from 0% to 4%. In the event of a wound dehiscence, all range of motion activities are discontinued to prevent further dehiscence of the wound. We prefer a fairly aggressive approach to the wound, with management regimen of daily whirlpool treatments, damp-to-dry dressing changes, and oral antibiotics. Other granulation-promoting wound agents, or use of a negative-pressure device may also be beneficial in this instance. Alternatively, the limb may be immobilized in a short leg cast, with a window overlying the wound for access for dressing changes. These treatment regimens typically are successful, as long as the wound necrosis is limited to partial thickness of the skin layer. Range of motion exercises are re-initiated once the wound seals and remains dry with the patient off antibiotics.

Deep infection and osteomyelitis rates are similarly low, occurring in up to 5% of closed fractures. Open injuries, however, are associated with markedly higher rates of deep infection and osteomyelitis, up to 38% in some series. Deep infection and osteomyelitis may also result from skin necrosis and slough from an unreduced closed fracture or fracture-dislocation due to excessive tension on the surrounding soft tissue envelope. Management of a deep infection includes serial surgical debridements, with local or flap coverage as needed, and long-term intravenous antibiotics. In the event of osteomyelitis, partial or complete talectomy with staged salvage arthrodesis is usually required.

OSTEONECROSIS Osteonecrosis of the talar body is frequent complication following a displaced talar neck fracture, owing to the inherently tenuous blood supply. Historically, osteonecrosis rates for displaced fractures (Hawkins type II, III, and IV fractures) treated with closed reduction and casting or pinning have ranged from 70% to 100%. Because of these factors, treatment of a displaced talar neck fracture has traditionally been considered a surgical emergency. Despite modern advances in internal fixation techniques and implants, osteonecrosis still develops in up to 30% to 50% of displaced fractures. It is well established in the literature that osteonecrosis is most related to the extent of initial fracture displacement; recent reports have suggested that the timing of definitive fixation has little influence on the risk of osteonecrosis.

RECOMMENDED READING

Abidi NA, Dhawan S, Gruen GS, Vogt MT, Conti SF. Wound-healing risk factors after open reduction and internal fixation of calcaneal fractures. *Foot Ankle Int.* 1998;12:856–861.

Benirschke SK, Kramer PA. Wound healing complications in closed and open calcaneal fractures. *J Orthop Trauma.* 2004; 18:1–6.

Benirschke SK, Sangeorzan BJ. Extensive intraarticular fractures of the foot. Surgical management of calcaneal fractures. *Clin Orthop.* 1993;291:128–134.

Böhler L. Diagnosis, pathology and treatment of fractures of the os calcis. *J Bone and Joint Surg.* 1931;13:75–89.

Borrelli J Jr, Lashgari C. Vascularity of the lateral calcaneal flap: a cadaveric injection study. *J Orthop Trauma.* 1999;13: 73–77.

Canale ST, Kelly FB Jr. Fractures of the neck of the talus: long-term evaluation of seventy-one cases. *J Bone Joint Surg Am.* 1978; 60:143–156.

Carr JB, Hamilton JJ, Bear LS. Experimental intra-articular calcaneal fractures: anatomic basis for a new classification. *Foot Ankle.* 1989;10:81–87.

Clare MP, Lee WE III, Sanders RW. Intermediate to long-term results of a treatment protocol for calcaneal fracture malunions. *J Bone Joint Surg Am.* 2005;87:963–973.

Crosby LA, Fitzgibbons T. Computerized tomography scanning of acute intra-articular fractures of the calcaneus. *J Bone and Joint Surg Am.* 1990;72:852–859.

Essex-Lopresti P. The mechanism, reduction technique, and results in fractures of the os calcis. *Br J Surg.* 1952;39:395–419.

Folk JW, Starr AJ, Early JS. Early wound complications of operative treatment of calcaneus fractures: analysis of 190 fractures. *J Orthop Trauma.* 1999;13:369–372.

Gould N. Lateral approach to the os calcis. *Foot Ankle.* 1984;4:218–220.

Haliburton RA, Sullivan CR, Kelly PJ, Peterson LFA. The extra-osseous and intra-osseous blood supply of the talus. *J Bone Joint Surg Am.* 1958;40:1115–1120.

Harvey EJ, Grujic L, Early JS, Benirschke SK, Sangeorzan BJ. Morbidity associated with ORIF of intra-articular calcaneus fractures using a lateral approach. *Foot Ankle Int.* 2001;22:868–873.

Hawkins LG. Fractures of the neck of the talus. *J Bone Joint Surg Am.* 1970;52:991–1002.

Herscovici D Jr, Sanders RW, Infante A, Dispasquale T. Bohler incision: an extensile anterolateral approach to the foot and ankle. *J Orthop Trauma.* 2000;14:429–432.

Herscovici D Jr, Sanders RW, Scatudo JM, Infante A, DiPasquale T. Vacuum-assisted wound closure (VAC therapy) for the management of patients with high-energy soft tissue injuries. *J Orthop Trauma.* 2003;17:683–688.

Herscovici D Jr, Widmaier J, Scaduto JM, Sanders RW, Walling A. Operative treatment of calcaneal fractures in elderly patients. *J Bone Joint Surg Am.* 2005;87:1260–1264.

Howard JL, Buckley R, McCormack R, Pate G, Leighton R, Petrie D. Complications following management of displaced intra-articular calcaneal fractures: a prospective randomized trial comparing open reduction internal fixation with nonoperative management. *J Orthop Trauma.* 2003;17:241–249.

Levin LS, Nunley JA. The management of soft-tissue problems associated with calcaneal fractures. *Clin Orthop.* 1993;290: 151–160.

Lim EV, Leung JP. Complications of intraarticular calcaneal fractures. *Clin Orthop.* 2001;391:7–16.

Lindvall E, Haidukewych G, Dipasquale T, Herscovici D Jr, Sanders R. Open reduction and stable fixation of isolated, displaced talar neck and body fractures. *J Bone Joint Surg Am.* 2004;86:2229–2234.

Marsh JL, Saltzman CL, Iverson M, Shapiro DS. Major open injuries of the talus. *J Orthop Trauma.* 1995;9:371–376.

Mulfinger GL, Trueta J. The blood supply of the talus. *J Bone Joint Surg Br.* 1970;52:160–167.

Palmer I. The mechanism and treatment of fractures of the calcaneus. *J Bone and Joint Surg Am.* 1948;30:2–8.

Sanders R. Intra-articular fractures of the calcaneus: present state of the art. *J Orthop Trauma.* 1992;6:252–265.

Sanders R. Fractures and fracture-dislocations of the calcaneus. In: Coughlin MJ, Mann RA, eds. *Surgery of the foot and ankle.* 7th ed. St. Louis: Mosby: 1999:1422–1464.

Sanders R. Fractures and fracture-dislocations of the talus. In: Coughlin MJ, Mann RA, eds. *Surgery of the foot and ankle.* 7th ed. St. Louis: Mosby: 1999:1465–1518.

Sanders R. Displaced intra-articular fractures of the calcaneus. *J Bone Joint Surg Am.* 2000;82:225–250.

Sanders R, Fortin P, DiPasquale T, Walling A. Operative treatment in 120 displaced intraarticular calcaneal fractures. Results using a prognostic computed tomography scan classification. *Clin Orthop.* 1993;290:87–95.

Stephens HM, Sanders R. Calcaneal malunions: results of a prognostic computed tomography classification system. *Foot Ankle Int.* 1996;17:395–401.

Thordarson DB, Krieger LE. Operative vs. nonoperative treatment of intra-articular fractures of the calcaneus: a prospective randomized trial. *Foot Ankle Int.* 1996;17:2–9.

Tornetta P III. The Essex-Lopresti reduction for calcaneal fractures revisited. *J Orthop Trauma.* 1998;12:469–473.

Vallier HA, Nork SE, Barei DP, Benirschke SK, Sanjeorzan BJ. Talar neck fractures: results and outcomes. *J Bone Joint Surg Am.* 2004;86:1616–1624.

White RR, Babikian GM. Tibia: shaft. In: Reudi TP, Murphy WM, eds. *AO principles of fracture management.* New York: Thieme; 2000:525–526.

34 Flap Coverage for the Foot

L. Scott Levin and Alessio Baccarani

The goals of soft tissue reconstruction for the foot and ankle region are satisfactory wound coverage and restoration of function. Ancillary considerations include acceptable appearance and minimal donor site morbidity. For soft tissue coverage alone, muscle and axial fasciocutaneous flaps remain primary choices in the lower extremity. Random pattern cutaneous flaps and musculocutaneous flaps usually have more limited applications, but should be considered. Free flaps are generally the soft tissue coverage of choice for most extensive defects of the foot and of the lower third of the leg. Amputations and fillet flaps always represent a fourth possibile option when the limb cannot be preserved in its entirety. Finally, procedures such as osteotomies and/or ostectomies for the production of soft tissue "gain" and resultant coverage of the defect are becoming more common.

INDICATIONS

Each anatomic region of the foot has certain characteristics that will influence selection of the flap to be transferred for reconstruction. The foot has special requirements for shoeing and ambulation. The reconstructive ladder for injury to the foot is based on whether there is a fracture, what part of the foot is exposed, and whether the area is weight bearing or non–weight bearing. The ankle and the dorsum of the foot require thin, pliable soft tissue coverage for exposed tendons, bones, or joints. The plantar skin is thick and heavily keratinized, designed to resist high stress, and anchored to underlying bones and ligaments by thick fibrous connective tissue.

Topographically, the forefoot includes the dorsal areas of the metatarsals and toes. The plantar aspect includes the metatarsal heads and the instep. The hindfoot can be divided into the plantar aspect, instep, and lateral aspect of the calcaneus. The ankle can be divided into the area of the Achilles tendon and the anterior aspect of the tibiotalar joint. In the forefoot, the dorsum and the area over the toes are primarily skin and subcutaneous tissue, making the exposure of tendons and joints more probable with high-energy injury. The plantar forefoot is prone to avulsion because of the vertically oriented septa that bridge from the plantar fascia to the dermal elements of the skin. The heel pad is a very unique structure that contains cushion-like shock-absorbing chambers of fat that are not easily replaced if loss is due to such an avulsion injury.

Achilles Tendon Area

The Achilles tendon area is characterized by thin skin with little or no subcutaneous layer. Among local flaps, we consider the sural fasciocutaneous flap one of the best options for covering this area. Other flaps options include lateral supramalleolar and lateral calcaneal artery.

Ankle and Foot Dorsum

Most shallow wounds on the foot dorsum may be safely closed with a split-thickness skin graft. If necessary, exposed extensor tendons may be resected and the skin graft may be applied to the underlying periosteum, providing a simple and quick solution to the clinical problem. For management of larger wounds with bone or tendon exposure, flaps may be required. The most common local flaps used for coverage of this area are abductor hallucis–abductor digiti minimi muscle flaps, extensor digitorum brevis muscle flap, lateral supramalleolar flap, and sural fasciocutaneous flap.

Plantar Forefoot

Local flaps play a major role in the management of deep wounds of the distal third of the foot. Severe injury or infection to a single toe may be best managed by toe or ray amputation, and subsequent closure by means of a plantar or of a dorsal skin flap. If additional skin is required, an adjacent toe may be filleted and trasposed for closure. Ray amputation may be necessary if the metatarsal bone is infected, injured, or devascularized. Metatarsal head ulceration is the most frequent lesion occurring in this area, especially in patients presenting with peripheral neuropathy and associated arthropathy. Many local flaps have been described to treat plantar forefoot defects. The most commonly used are neurovascular island flap (Moberg's flap), toe fillet flap, V-Y plantar flap, and suprafascial flaps medially or laterally based.

Transmetatarsal amputation provides a functional option when three or more rays have been seriously damaged, expecially in post-traumatic, ischemic, or neuropathic patients. No prosthetic or orthotic device would be necessary, and the patient may be able to wear normal shoes. Achilles tendon lenghtening should be performed in conjunction with transmetatarsal amputation to avoid equinus deformity and stump ulceration.

Plantar Midfoot

The midfoot is defined as the region between the midshaft of the metatarsals and the proximal tarsal row. It comprises the medial non-weight bearing arch as well as the more lateral weight bearing area. Small wounds in this region may be reconstructed with a variety of reconstructive options. Split-thickness skin grafts may provide adequate coverage if the transverse arch of the foot has been maintained, thus allowing the midfoot to remain a largely non–weight-bearing region. Local flap options for reconstruction of defects in this area include neurovascular island flap, V-Y advancement flap, and medially or laterally based suprafascial flaps.

Wounds larger than 4 to 6 cm generally require either free flap reconstruction or midfoot amputation to achieve a stable coverage. Clearly amputation would represent the second option if foot salvage is not indicated or possible with free tissue transfer. The two most common forms of midfoot amputation are the Lisfranc amputation and the Chopart amputation. The Lisfranc amputation is the amputation at the tarso-metatarsal joint and is associated with a high rate of equinovarus deformity. The Chopart procedure requires an intertarsal resection, just distal to the cuboid and navicular bone. Both types of midfoot amputations will affect the patient's ability to dorsiflect and evert the residual limb because of disruption of the insertions of the peroneal and tibialis anterior tendons.

Plantar Hindfoot

Hindfoot soft tissue repair is the most challenging to the reconstructive surgeon. Reconstruction should provide durable soft tissue for safe weight-bearing, while permitting a normal ankle motion. The dualism of form and function represents a mandatory principle to be considered in the management of wounds in this area. Damage to the neurovascular and tendinous structures beneath the flexor retinaculum is an event that may impair permanently the patient's gait, mandating a below-knee amputation.

Many local flaps have been described to restore healing in the hindfoot area. The most common are intrinsic muscle flaps (abductor hallucis AH, flexor digitorum brevis FDB, abductor digiti minimi ADM); medial plantar artery flap; heel pad flaps; and sural fasciocutaneous flap. With the only exception being the sural artery fasciocutaneous flap, all the regional flaps listed require antegrade blood flow through the posterior tibial artery and its branches. Those procedures are therefore often not possible in patients affected by peripheral vascular disease.

Large hindfoot defects greater than 5 to 6 cm in patients devoid of the posterior tibial vessels should be considered for microsurgical reconstruction. Many neurosensory flaps have been described for microvascular transplantation in an effort to provide sensation to the plantar reconstruction. Lateral arm and deltoid represent two useful donor sites because of their reliable neurovascular anatomy, the ability to recover protective sensation, and because of their thickness; however, a correlation between the presence of flap sensation and the success of hindfoot reconstruction has never been established. Microvascular transplantation of muscle with skin graft coverage can provide succesful outcomes if the surgeon remembers to remove the underlying bone prominences, educates the patient on proper shoe wear, and performs frequent follow-up. We believe the use of muscle to obliterate dead space and aid in delivering antibiotics to the region is important for successful

TABLE 34-1. Surgical Reconstructive Options

Foot Region	Locoregional Flaps	Free Flaps	Amputation and Ancillary Procedures
Achilles tendon region	Sural fasciocutaneous Lateral calcaneal artery	Fasciocutaneous	Syme Below knee
Ankle and dorsum	Intrinsic muscle flaps (AH, ADM, EDB) Sural fasciocutaneous Lateral supramalleolar	Fasciocutaneous Myocutaneous	Syme Below knee
Plantar forefoot	Toe fillet flap Neurovascular island flap V-Y advancement Suprafascial flaps	Fasciocutaneous Myocutaneous Muscle	Ray Transmetatarsal
Plantar midfoot	Neurovascular island flap V-Y advancement Suprafascial flaps	Fasciocutaneous Myocutaneous Muscle	Lisfranc Chopart
Plantar hindfoot	Intrinsic muscle flaps (AH, FDB, ADM) Medial plantar artery flap Sural fasciocutaneous Suprafascial flaps (heel pad flaps)	Fasciocutaneous Myocutaneous Muscle	Syme Calcanectomy

outcomes in cases of osteomyelitis. Because of its proximity to the wound margin, the posterior tibial artery is usually the preferred recipient vessel in hindfoot reconstruction. For hindfoot coverage, it is important to avoid scarring around the posterior tibial nerve and around the posterior tibial tendon, which may become exposed or trapped during the healing process.

Syme's amputation has a well-established role in the management of complex hindfoot deformities, especially in diabetic patients. The procedure involves the use of the heel pad as a soft tissue cover over the distal end of the residual tibia and fibula. Table 34-1 summarizes the main surgical reconstructive options for each region of the foot.

PREOPERATIVE PLANNING

Evaluation of the patient with soft tissue injury should include determination of the time of injury, mechanism, energy absorption, fracture configuration, systemic injuries, damage to the soft tissue envelope, vascularity of the extremity, sensibility, ultimate ability to salvage the foot (which is both functional and sensate), and underlying medical conditions of the patient. The principles of evaluation of orthopaedic trauma are the same for any basic medical evaluation. These principles apply whether in the outpatient clinic, emergency room, or trauma unit. An evaluation of the perfusion of the traumatized limb is of paramount importance, and if vascular (arterial) injury is suspected, a vascular surgery or microsurgery consultation should be obtained. Compartment syndrome should be considered and ruled out in any injured extremity, particularly after crush injuries. A general motor examination including the active and passive range of motion as well as a detailed sensory examination should be performed. A nerve deficit may be secondary to a spinal cord injury, nerve laceration, compartment syndrome, traction injury, or entrapment between bony fragments. The radiologic evaluation starts with standard plain radiographic examination. Computed tomography (CT) is indicated in complex foot injuries and may give valuable information regarding soft tissue damage as well.

The wound should be inspected once, and the wound pattern and contamination noted. The next inspection of the wound should then be in the operating room under sterile conditions. Repetitive examination of open wounds in the emergency room has led to higher rates of wound infections and osteomyelitis and should be avoided. In cases of open fractures in polytrauma patients, workup of other injuries may take several hours, not to mention the need for emergent lifesaving visceral surgery that may precede definitive care for open fractures. Prophylactic antibiotics are administered and given on a regular basis until definitive wound debridement and fracture stabilization can be performed.

In summary, with any lower extremity reconstruction, three basic principles are of great importance and should therefore be carefully optimized before undertaking any reconstructive effort:

- Evaluation of underlying skeletal architecture, stabilization, and management of associated orthopaedic injuries
- Adequate wound preparation, which includes full debridement and control of any local infection prior to coverage
- Overall assessment of the patient's suitability for reconstruction and rehabilitation, including the opportunity of restoring some degree of protective sensation to the limb

Recipient Vessels   If free tissue transfer is required for wound coverage, then the last point of consideration prior to surgery should be the selection of recipient vessels for microvascular transfer as this will influence patient positioning within the operating room. A general agreement on which vessels to use has not yet been reached. Conflicting data have been reported on the survival and outcome of the transferred flaps, depending on the vessel used or the location of anastomosis proximal or distal to the zone of injury. For example, the anterior tibial vessels may be preferred for their easy accessibility, whereas the posterior tibial vessels are strongly advocated by others due to their larger diameter.

The most important factors influencing the site of recipient vessel are the site of the injury and the vascular status of the lower extremity; it is best to ensure adequate arterial inflow and adequate venous outflow before surgery. Intraoperatively, it is imparative that the anastomosis be performed outside the zone of injury. The type of flap used, method, and type of microvascular anastomosis represent less important factors in determining the recipient vessels.

SURGERY

Locoregional Flaps

As discussed in the Indications section, locoregional flaps play a very important role into the management of foot wound coverage.

Toe Fillet Flap

ANATOMY   The flap is based on the medial and lateral neurovascular bundles of the toe to be amputated.

FLAP DESIGN   The toe adjacent to the wound is outlined. This island flap is better disssected with the patient in supine position under tourniquet control.

TECHNIQUE   The flap is elevated beginning distally, off the distal phalanges and flexor tendons. The medial and lateral bundles are identified in the associated web spaces. A connecting incision to the wound is made. The toe is thus disarticulated at the metatarsophalangeal joint, and the dorsal skin is used for donor site closure. The flap is then rotated to the defect, ensuring a safe placement of the neurovascular structures (Fig. 34-1).

Neurovascular Island Flap

ANATOMY   The flap is based on the great toe neurovascular bundle on the fibular side.

FLAP DESIGN   The flap is designed on the fibular side, centerd over the area of the neurovascular bundle. These flaps may cover wounds up to 2 to 3 cm in diameter. The use of a tourniquet facilitates a safe dissection. The donor site often requires a skin graft closure.

TECHNIQUE   The flap is elevated on the lateral plantar aspect of the great toe at the level of the phalangeal periosteum. The vascular bundle can be proximally dissected in the web space to allow a longer arc of rotation. An incision is made to connect the web space to the wound, and the flap is thus transposed to the defect.

V-Y Advancement Plantar Flaps

ANATOMY   These flaps are based on vertical perforating vessels throughout the plantar aspect of the foot.

FLAP DESIGN   Many V-Y advancement flaps may be designed with different orientation on the plantar foot. The use of a tourniqut facilitates a safer dissection.

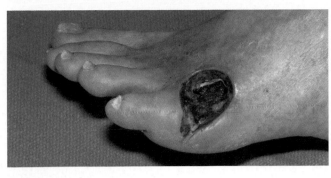
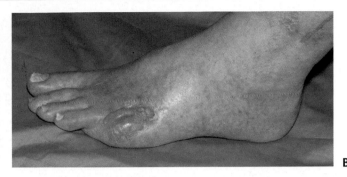

A   B

FIGURE 34-1

Dorsal forefoot diabetic ulcer covered with fifth toe fillet flap shown before **(A)** and after **(B)** surgery.

TECHNIQUE   The skin ajacent to the defect is incised in a V fashion (Fig. 34-2). The plantar fascia about the circumference of the flap must be incised as well. Septal attachments to the underlying metatarsal may be divided to provide further advacement. Two V-Y opposing flaps may be combined in the management of a larger wound.

Suprafascial Flaps

ANATOMY   Medially or laterally based flaps of plantar skin and fat may be advanced, rotated, or transposed to cover plantar defects. Although popular in the 1970's as random flaps, they have been largely supplanted by the other techniques described. Their vascularization is based on cutaneous branches from the medial or lateral plantar arteries (Fig. 34-3).

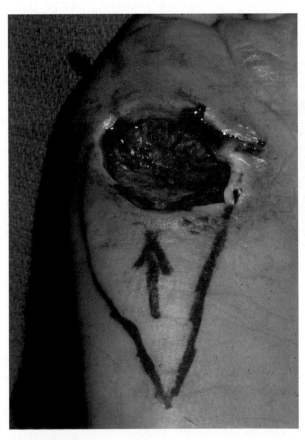
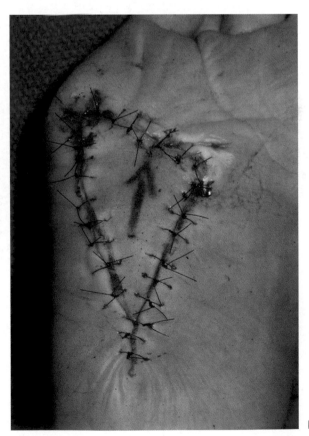

A   B

FIGURE 34-2

Plantar forefoot pressure sore in a myelodysplastic patient treated with a V-Y advancement flap shown before **(A)** and after **(B)** surgery.

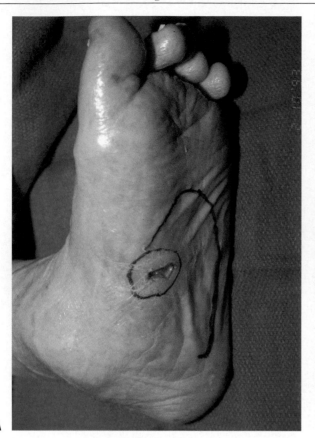
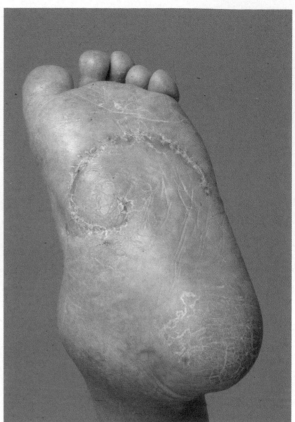

A

B

FIGURE 34-3

Plantar midfoot diabetic ulcer covered with a suprafascial rotation flap medially based shown before **(A)** and after **(B)** surgery.

FLAP DESIGN   The design of a suprafascial flap varies largely according to location of the defect. The donor site often requires a skin graft for coverage.

TECHNIQUE   Medially based flaps are raised by incising laterally and elevating the subcutaneous tissues off the abductor digiti minimi muscle and plantar fascia from lateral to medial. Branches from the medial plantar nerve and artery should be preserved as they emerge from the cleft between the plantar fascia and the abductor hallucis muscle.

For the laterally based flap, the dissection is similar but requires the sacrifice of the branches from the medial plantar artery, to allow rotation or transposition.

If the flap is designed on the heel pad to cover a small wound over the weight-bearing and posterior heel, a calcanectomy may be associated to remove bone prominences and to simplify the closure.

Intrinsic Muscle Flaps: Abductor Hallucis, Flexor Digitorum Brevis, Abductor Digiti Minimi, and Extensor Digitorum Brevis

ANATOMY   The abductor hallucis muscle (AH) is vascularized proximally by branches off the medial plantar artery. The flexor hallucis brevis (FHB) is also vascularized by analogue branches. The flexor digitorum brevis (FDB) is the largest of the foot muscles, and is very useful for heel pad reconstructions. It is vascularized by branches off both the medial and lateral plantar arteries, the lateral usually being dominant.

The abductor digiti minimi (ADM) is the smallest of the muscle flaps that can be harvested. It is innervated and vascularized by the lateral plantar neurovascular bundle through branches entering its proximal portion.

The extensor digitorum brevis (EDB) is a dorsal muscle. It is vascularized by the lateral tarsal artery, which is a branch off the dorsalis pedis artery, at the level of the distal edge of the extensor retinaculum.

FLAPS DESIGN   The AH muscle with or without the medial head of the FHB and the ADM can be used to close small proximal dorsal foot wounds, but it is better qualified in the management of plantar hindfoot defects. The use of an ADM flap alone is not recommended because of its small dimensions and its short arc of rotation.

The FDB is especially qualified in heel pad reconstruction.

The EDB muscle is usually transposed proximally to cover the ankle, the dorsal foot, and the malleoli provided that the anterior tibial artery has antegrade blood flow.

TECHNIQUE   When harvesting the AH, a medial foot incision is placed on the non–weight-bearing surface. The tendon is devided distally, and the muscle is separated from the medial head of the FHB, if the latter component is not required to enhance the flap dimensions. If an increase in the arc of rotation is needed, the medial plantar artery is ligated and divided distal to the branches to the abductor, and a more proximal dissection of the medial plantar artery to its origin can be accomplished.

When harvesting the FDB, a midline plantar foot incision is used to expose the muscle. The skin is elevated laterally and medially, and detached from the plantar fascia. The fascia is usually elevated with the muscle to add bulk. The four tendons are divided distally and the muscle is turned on itself, after detaching it from the quadratus plantae. The lateral plantar artery may be ligated after it passes beneath the muscle, if further mobilization is required to reach the defect. The division of the origin of the AH also increases the arc of rotation of this flap.

When harvesting the ADM, a lateral foot incision is made onto the non–weight-bearing skin. The muscle is detached from the fifth metatarsal and the tendinous insertion is divided, allowing posterior rotation of the flap. Further rotation is obtained ligating the lateral plantar artery distal to the branches to the muscle and dissecting the pedicle proximally after dividing the FDB and the AH.

When harvesting the EDB, a curvilinear incision is made on the dorsum of the foot, in continuity to the defect to be repaired. The entire dorsalis pedis pedicle is divided distally to the origin of the lateral tarsal vessels to provide the needed arc of rotation for muscle transposition. The long extensors are then dissected off the underlying short extensors muscle slips. The dissection proceeds proximally ligating the medial tarsal branches. The lateral tarsal vessels are elevated with the muscle while the origin and the tendinous extensions of the muscle are divided. The muscle may thus be rotated to the defect.

Lateral Supramalleolar Flap

ANATOMY   This flap is vascularized by a perforating branch off the peroneal artery as it pierces the interosseus membrane 5 cm proximal to the tip of the lateral malleolus. Cutanous vessels then course upward, anterior to the fibula, and anastomose with the vascular network that accompanies the superficial peroneal nerve.

FLAP DESIGN   The flap is qualified in the coverage of defects over the lateral malleolus and anterior ankle. The flap should be distally based, with the pedicle centered onto the perforator artery. Flap width includes the tissue between the fibula and tibia. The length should be 6 to 8 cm or more according to the defect. Often the flap is harvested only in its fascial component; then turned over to the defect in a book page fashion; then skin grafted. If designed in this way, the donor site can be closed directly.

TECHNIQUE   The skin incision is made so that skin flaps may be elvated off the underlying fascia. The fascia is then incised anteriorly and reflected until the perforating branch is visualized. Branches of the superficial peroneal nerve are divided to allow elevation. The posterior margin is eventually incised and released from the septum between the anterior and lateral compartment of the leg.

Medial Plantar Artery Flap

ANATOMY   This is a true neurosensory type A fasciocutaneous flap supplied by cutaneous fascicles from the medial and lateral plantar nerves. It is vascularized by the medial plantar artery and its vena comitans. The flap provides an invaluable amount of specialized skin that configures its chief value in heel reconstruction, because of its nonshearing, well-padded, adherent qualities.

FLAP DESIGN   Patency of anterior and posterior tibial arteries should be assessed prior to surgery. The presence of a Charcot deformity with midfoot collapse contraindicates the flap harvest. In this deformity, the instep area should remain covered by specialized plantar skin. For heel reconstruction, the flap is designed as an island centered on the medial plantar artery. It has to be outlined 2 to

3 cm proximal to the metatarsal heads, distal to the heel and medial to the lateral midsole weight bearing area. The donor site is usually closed with a split-thickness skin graft.

TECHNIQUE   The flap is incised distally, exposing the medial plantar artery and nerves. After ligation of the artery, the dissection continues proximally beneath the plantar aponeurosis, including the medial plantar artery and the neurovascular bundles to the overlying fascia and skin. This requires an intraneural dissection of the midsole cutaneous branches from those fascicles supplying three and one-half digits. Often, the second common digital nerve is included with the branches to the flap because of difficulties encountered in separation. The flap is thus elevated in a distal to proximal direction in the plane between the plantar fascia and the first layer of muscles. Fascial comunications to the clefts between the underlying muscles (AH, FDB, and ADM) are cut.

Fascicles from the lateral plantar nerve may also be included in the flap following an intraneural dissection. The medial plantar artery and the fascicles from the medial plantar nerve are traced proximally to the AH muscle, which may be cut if a longer pedicle is required.

Sural Artery Fasciocutaneous Flap

ANATOMY   This type A fasciocutaneous flap is innervated by the medial sural cutaneous nerve (S1-2). Its dominant vascular supply is a direct cutaneous sural artery branch that arises in the distal popliteal fossa between the two heads of the gastrocnemius muscle, and minor muscolocutaneous perforators from the gastrocnemius muscle. In most patients, the arterial supply will not be an identifiable vessel, but a "vascular network" that also anastomoses with the peroneal artery. The most relevant of these connections is located approximately 5 cm cephalad to the lateral malleolus. The lesser saphenous vein and its branches provide venous drainage.

FLAP DESIGN   The flap is centered between the popliteal fossa and the midposterior leg with a width up to 12 cm, but the length can be extended 20 cm to the Achilles tendon. The donor site is usually closed with a split-thickness skin graft.

TECHNIQUE   The flap is raised from distal to proximal in the plane beneath the deep fascia and the above gastrocnemius muscle. The sural nerve and the lesser saphenous vein are divided distally and elevated with the flap. The pedicle is carefully dissected proximally, leaving abundant fascio-subcutaneous tissues around the neurovascular structures. It can be dissected up to 7 to 9 cm from the lateral malleolus, according to the location of the defect to be reached. After flap rotation to the defect, the skin over the pedicle is usually not sutured to avoid compression, and a skin graft is usually applied to provide coverage. Flap delay procedures and/or venous supercharging should be evaluated to avoid congestion, which commonly complicates the postoperatory course (Fig. 34-4).

Free Flaps

Latissimus Dorsi   This flap is based on the thoracodorsal artery as the major pedicle and on branches of the intercostals and lumbar arteries as secondary segmental branches. The pedicle length is 8 to 10 cm. The latissimus is innervated by the thoracodorsal nerve, which is a direct branch of the brachial plexus and enters the muscle 10 cm from the apex of the axilla. This flap's consistent anatomy and long vascular pedicle make it a common flap choice for larger defects of the foot and Achilles tendon region. For more details on flap dissection, see Chapter 11, Pedicled and Free Latissimus Flap for Elbow and Forearm Coverage. Some of the technical problems associated with this flap for lower extremity reconstruction include difficulty in positioning the patient to allow for flap elevation and simultaneous recipient site preparation. If the anterior tibial system is to be used as a recipient vessel, the ipsilateral latissimus is usually harvested; if the posterior tibial system is to be used, the contralateral latissimus should be harvested to allow for simultaneous flap elevation and recipient site exposure. In addition, in obese patients the musculocutaneous flap may be excessively thick for smooth contour over the foot (Fig. 34-5).

Rectus Abdominis   The rectus abdominis can be harvested with the patient in a supine position. This vertically oriented muscle extends between the costal margin and the pubic region and is enclosed by the anterior and posterior rectus sheats. It is a type 3 muscle (two dominant pedicles) based on the superior epigastric artery and vein and inferior epigastric artery and vein. The pedicle length is 5 to 7 cm superiorly and 8 to 10 cm inferiorly.

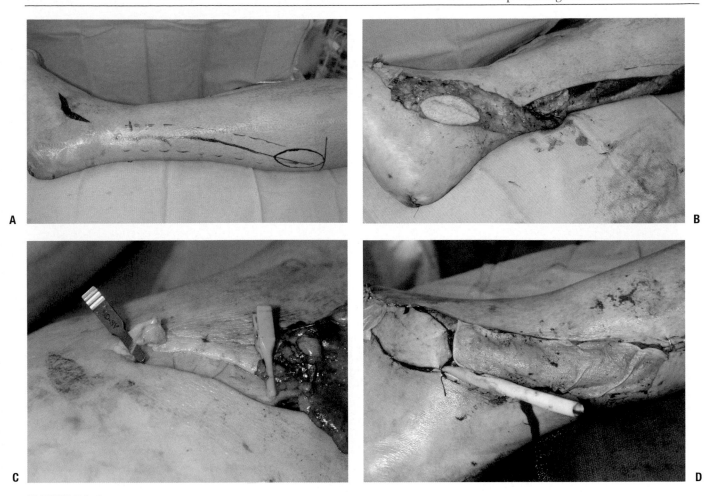

FIGURE 34-4

Wound dehiscence post triple ankle arthrodesis covered with a distally based sural flap. **A:** Preoperative view and flap design**.** **B:** The flap is transposed to the defect. **C:** The flap will be turbo-charged to improve the venous outflow (lesser saphenous vein to superficial dorsal vein). **D:** The pedicles are protected with split-thickness skin grafts.

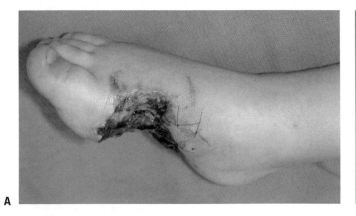
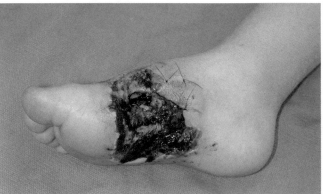

FIGURE 34-5

Medial plantar midfoot traumatic defect in a pediatric patient (lawnmower injury). The defect is reconstructed with a free latissimus dorsi flap shown before **(A)** and after **(B)** surgery. *(Continued)*

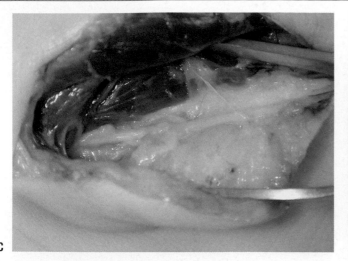

C

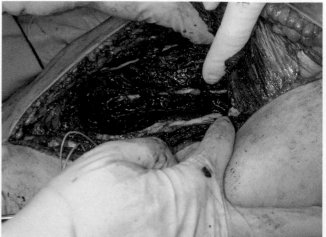

D

FIGURE 34-5

Continued Medial plantar midfoot traumatic defect in a pediatric patient (lawnmower injury). The defect is reconstructed with a free latissimus dorsi flapshown before **(A)** and after **(B)** surgery. **C,D:** Latissimus dorsi flap harvesting. **E:** The flap is revascularized and sutured to the defect.

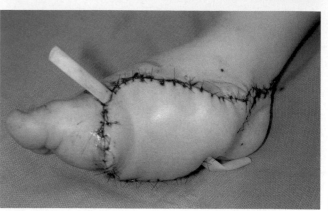

E

Each of the dominant pedicles supplies just over one-half of the muscle. There is an anastomosis between these vessels that is usually sufficient to support the nondominant half if one of the two pedicles is ligated. Because of the larger size and easier dissection of the inferior epigastric vessel, it is usually used for free tissue transfer.

The motor innervation is supplied by segmental motor nerves from the seventh through twelfth intercostal nerves that enter the deep surface of the muscle at its middle to lateral aspects. The lateral cutaneous nerves from the seventh through twelfth intercostal nerves provide sensation to the skin territory of the rectus abdominis muscle. The size of the muscle is up to 25×6 cm^2. The skin territory that can be harvested is 21×14 cm^2 and is based on musculocutaneous perforatore (Fig. 34-6).

Gracilis The gracilis is a smaller transplant and is useful for defects requiring less bulk than the latissimus or rectus. The gracilis muscle is a type 2 muscle (with a dominant pedicle and several minor pedicles). It is a thin, flat muscle that lies between the adductor longus and sartorius muscle anteriorly and the semimembranosus posteriorly. The dominant pedicle is the ascending branch of medial circumflex femoral artery and venae comitantes. The length of the pedicle is 6 cm and the diameter of the artery is 1.6 mm. The minor pedicles are one or two branches of the superficial femoral artery and venae comitantes. Their length is 2 cm and their diameter is 0.5 mm.

Motor innervation is via the anterior branch of the obturator nerve, which is located between the abductor longus and magnus muscles, and it usually enters the muscle above the level of the dominant vascular pedicle. The anterior femoral cutaneous nerve (L2–3) provides sensory innervation to the majority of the anterior medial thigh.

This muscle functions as a thigh adductor. The presence of the adductor longus and magnus makes it an expendable muscle.

The size of the muscle is 6×24 cm^2. The skin territory is 16×18 cm^2, but the skin over the distal half of the muscle is not reliable when the flap is based on its dominant vascular pedicle with division of the minor vascular pedicles. In obese patients, the musculocutaneous flap may be too bulky, necessitating use of a skin graft placed on the muscle (Fig. 34-7) (see Chapter 32).

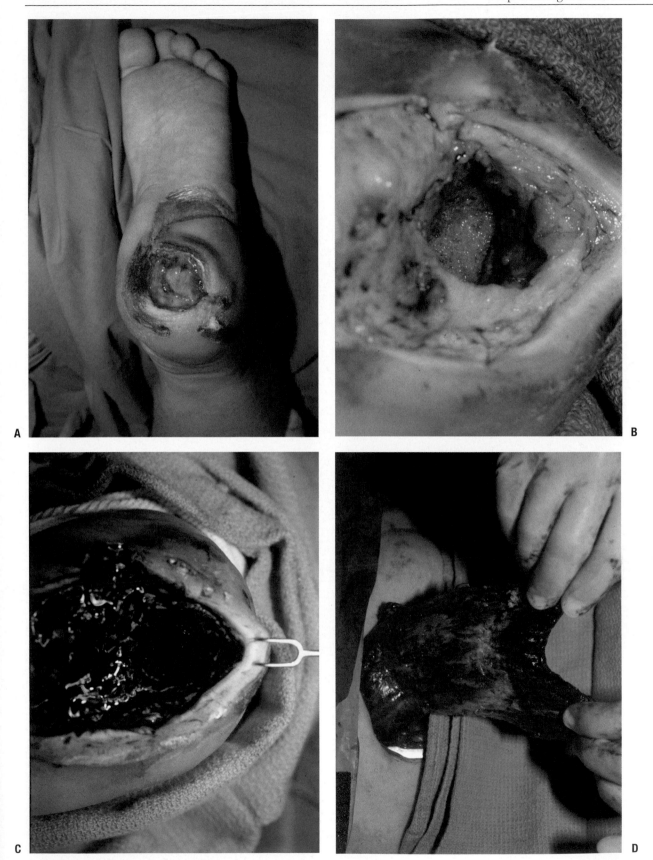

FIGURE 34-6

Calcaneal osteomyelitis on a diabetic foot. The defect was reconstructed with a free rectus abdominis flap. **A,B:** Preoperative view. **C:** After debridement. **D:** The rectus muscle is harvested from the abdomen. *(Continued)*

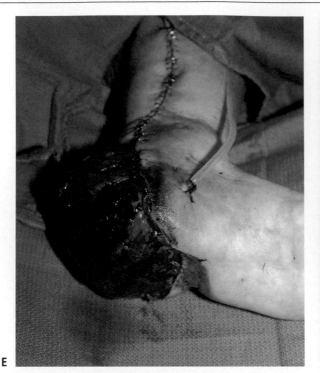
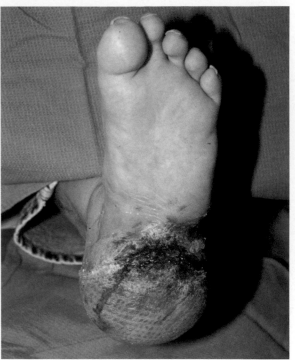

FIGURE 34-6

Continued **E:** The flap is tailored to the defect and revascularized. **F:** Late postoperative view showing calcaneal salvage.

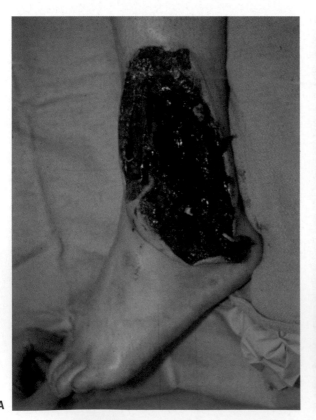
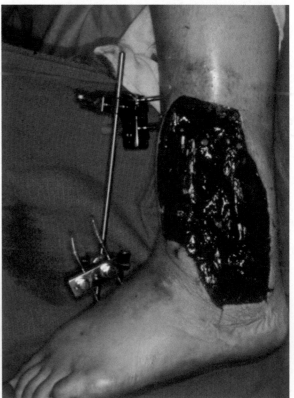

FIGURE 34-7

Gunshot wound to the distal leg-hindfoot. The defect is reconstructed with a free gracilis flap. **A:** Significant soft-tissue and bony defects are present. **B:** Debridement and external fixation. *(Continued)*

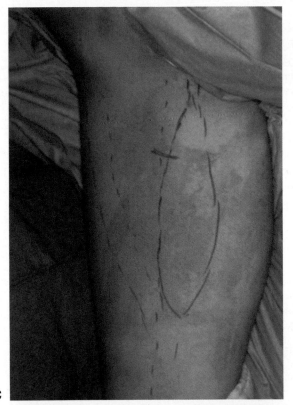

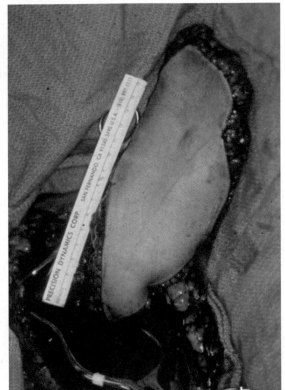

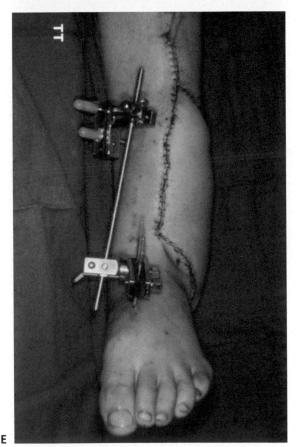

FIGURE 34-7

Continued **C:** A myocutaneous free gracilis flap is planned. **D:** The free flap is harvested. **E:** The flap is inset to the defect and revascularized.

Radial Forearm Flap   This is a thin, well-vascularized fasciocutaneous flap on the ventral aspect of the forearm that was widely used in China before it was popularized in the Western literature. The flap is based on the radial artery, which can achieve a 20-cm pedicle and has a diameter of 2.5 mm. This length of the pedicle facilitates the microsurgical anastomosis out of the zone of injury. The venous drainage is through the venae comitantes of the radial artery, but the flap can include the cephalic vein, the basilic vein, or both. The flap can contain the lateral antebrachial cutaneous nerve or the medial antebrachial cutaneous nerve and then serve as a neurosensory flap. The size of the flap can be 10×40 cm².

A portion of the radius can be included as a vascularized bone with this flap. The advantages of this flap are a long pedicle and potential sensory innervation. The quality of the bone from the radius is mainly cortical and not of any substantial volume. Including the bone in the radial forearm flap may lead to stress fracture of the donor radius. Preliminary tissue expansion will increase the flap dimensions, and more importantly, it will allow direct closure of the donor defect (Fig. 34-8).

Scapular and Parascapular Flap   The scapular flap remains the workhorse of skin flaps. It is a thin, usually hairless, skin flap from the posterior chest and can be de-epithelialized and used as subcutaneous fascial flap, pedicled or free.

The flap is perfused by the cutaneous branches of the circumflex scapular artery (CSA) and drained by its venae comitantes. The CSA is the main branch of the subscapular artery and the main blood supply to the scapula, the muscles that attach to the scapula, and the overlying skin. The length of the pedicle is 5 cm and the diameter of the artery is 2.5 mm. The vascular pattern of this territory makes it possible to raise multiple skin flaps on a single vascular pedicle or to harvest the lateral border of the scapula as an osteocutaneous flap for a complex reconstruction.

The cutaneous territory can be 20×7 cm² and can be divided in two components—a horizontal territory (horizontal scapular flap) and a vertical territory (parascapular flap)—based on the branches of the CSA after the vessel courses through the triangular space. Preliminary expansion of the territory of the scapular flap will increase the flap dimensions and permit direct donor-site clo-

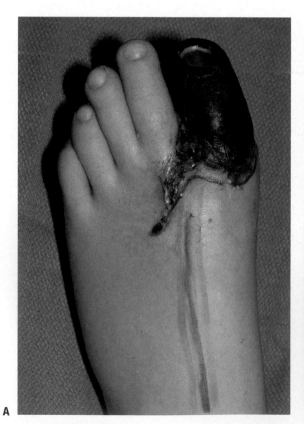
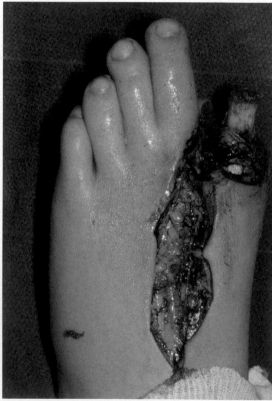

A
B

FIGURE 34-8

Post-traumatic left great toe necrosis. After debridement the soft tissue defect is restored with a free radial forearm flap. **A:** Preoperative view. **B:** After debridement. *(Continued)*

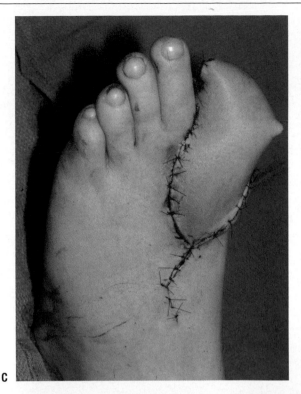

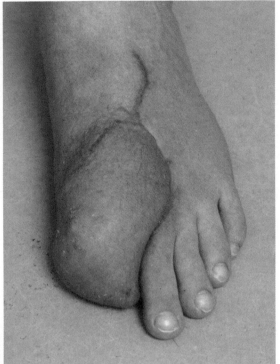

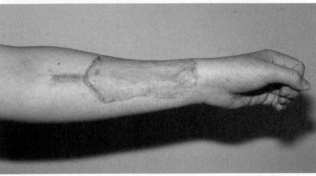

FIGURE 34-8

Continued **C:** Radial forearm flap is tailored to cover the exposed phalanx. **D,E:** Four weeks postoperative showing toe salvage and flap donor site.

sure. This flap can be combined with other flaps based on subscapular blood supply and may greatly facilitate certain complex reconstructions. These include the latissimus dorsi and serratus anterior flaps, which can supply additional skin, muscle, and bone (rib) if necessary. The primary indication for the scapular flap is a defect requiring a relatively thin, large cutaneous flap. These kinds of defects are often found in the foot. The osteoseptocutaneous free scapular flap reconstruction has been described in the lower extremity (Fig. 34-9).

POSTOPERATIVE MANAGEMENT

The success of a reconstructive foot surgery importantly relies on well-planned multidisciplinary postoperative management and rehabilitation. A non–weight-bearing regimen for at least 3 weeks is mandatory for every patient carrying plantar sutures. Elevation is required for 3 to 8 days after a local flap or a skin graft, and for 2 to 3 weeks after a free flap. Heparin regimen is advisable while the patient is in the aforementioned bed rest phase. Elastic wraps may be useful in controling edema once the patient's limb is permitted in a dependent position. Clinical findings should dictate the use of antibiotics.

The L'Enard splint (Fig. 34-10) is a useful tool to provide immobilization of the foot and ankle, and in keeping the posterior heel off the bed. It is also useful when the patient begins non–weight-bearing ambulation with crutches. Local care of all weight bearing surfaces is also recommended after suture removal, together with a frequent multidisciplinary follow-up that involves the plastic surgeon, the orthopaedic surgeon, the podiatrist and, if required, the prosthetist.

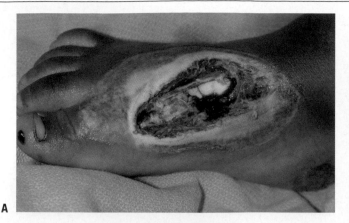

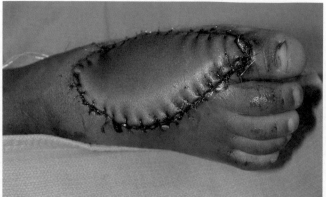

FIGURE 34-9

Dorsal foot avulsion injury in a pediatric patient (go-cart trauma). The dorsal aspect of the foot is reconstructed with a free scapular-parascapular flap. **A:** After debridement. **B:** Free scapular-parascapular flap is inset to the defect and revascularized. **C:** Two months postoperative view.

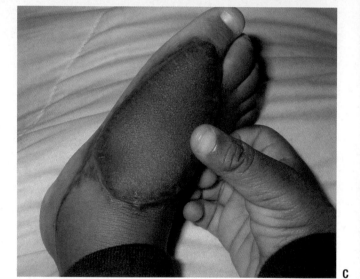

Postoperative care of free tissue transfer patients requires the patients to be adequately hydrated. Maintenance of proper body temperature and hematocrit is also important. Routine heparinization and anticoagulation are not used.

Flaps are usually monitored for a minimum of 5 days with a laser Doppler in addition to clinical observation. While the immediate postoperative period of 24 to 48 hours is critical, there have been occasional late failures; thus, laser Doppler monitoring should be continued for 4 or 5 days.

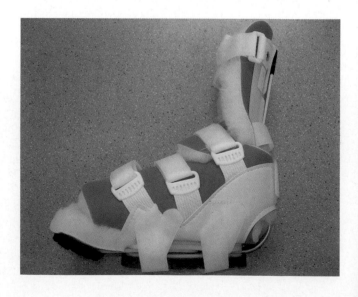

FIGURE 34-10
L'Enard splint.

COMPLICATIONS

Any flap failure requires a new detailed evaluation of the patient's local and general conditions before undertaking a new reconstruction. If a locoregional flap fails, and no other local option is available, the next step on the reconstructive ladder would be a free flap.

The success of free tissue transfer should be on the order of 95% to 99%. Acute complications usually occur in the first 48 hours and include venous thrombosis, arterial thrombosis, hematoma, hemorrhage, and excessive flap edema. Arterial insufficiency can be recognized by decreased capillary refill, pallor, reduced temperature, and the absence of bleeding after pinprick. This complication can be caused by arterial spasm, vessel plaque, torsion of the pedicle, pressure on the flap, technical error with injury to the pedicle, a flap harvested that is too large for its blood supply, or small vessel disease (due to smoking or diabetes). Management of arterial compromise requires prompt surgical intervention to restore the blood flow. Pharmacologic intervention at the time of exploration includes use of vasodilators, calcium channel blockers, and systemic anticoagulants for flap salvage presenting with arterial insufficiency. Ultimately, if these pharmacologic agents do not relieve spasm at the level of the arterial inflow, the anastomosis should be redone to rule out intra-arterial thrombus.

Venous outflow obstruction can be suspected when the flap has a violaceous color, brisk capillary refill, normal or elevated temperature, and production of dark blood after pinprick. Venous insufficiency can occur due to torsion of the pedicle, flap edema, hematoma, or tight closure of the tissue over the pedicle. The venous outflow obstruction can result in extravasation of red blood cells, endothelial breakdown, microvascular collapse, thrombosis in the microcirculation, and finally flap death. Given the irreversible nature of the microcirculatory changes in venous congestion that occur even after short periods of time, the surgeon must recognize venous compromise as early as possible.

These complications can occur alone or in any combination. The clinical observation and the monitoring of the patient (such as with laser Doppler) should alert the surgeon who has to decide between conservative and operative intervention. Conservative treatment may include drainage of the hematoma at the bedside with release of a few sutures to decrease pressure. In cases of venous congestion, leeches may be helpful if insufficient venous outflow cannot be established despite a patent venous anastomosis. The leeches inject a salivary component (hirudin) that inhibits both platelet aggregation and the coagulation cascade. The flap is decongested initially as the leech extracts blood and is further decongested as the bite wound oozes after the leech detaches.

The donor site should be given the same attention as the recipient site during the postoperative period. Complications of the donor site include hematoma, seroma, sensory nerve dysfunction, and scar formation.

Occasionally free flaps, despite early return to the operating room for vascular compromise, do fail. Options for management include the performance of a second free tissue transfer, noting the technical or physiologic details that led to initial failure. Most of the time, free tissue transfers that fail are due to technical errors in judgment, whether they be flap harvest, compromise of the pedicle during the harvest, improper microvascular technique during anastomosis, improper insetting resulting in increased tissue tension and edema, or postoperative motion of the extremity resulting in pedicle avulsion. The next decision made by the operating surgeon as to the management of this patient is based on several factors. If a patient required a free flap in the first place, a second free flap should be considered. If a decision is made not to redo the flap, it could be left in place using the Crane principle to see if underlying granulation will be sufficient such that skin grafting can be performed once the necrotic flap is removed.

The Crane principle can be applied to cases where a local flap or free tissue transfer that necrotizes in part or totally acts as a biologic dressing or eschar over a wound bed. If there is no infection, the eschar can be left on the wound bed to see if some healing in the form of granulation occurs underneath it. Ultimately, the eschar is removed and the granulation bed skin grafted, obviating another free tissue transfer. If wound observation shows that such a bed is not produced, then a second flap must be considered.

It is usually our preference not to follow this course, as the flap can become a source of sepsis and further compromise local tissues. Necrotic nonviable flaps should be removed and a temporary wound dressing such as an antibiotic bead pouch or wound vacuum-assisted closure (VAC) should be used. Occasionally when flaps fail in a severely compromised extremity, consideration should be given to amputation. If a second free flap is considered, errors that lead to flap compromise need to be recognized and avoided. It may be prudent to obtain an arteriogram, evaluate the coagulation profile, and research other issues that might have led to failure.

RECOMMENDED READING

Arnold PG, Yugueros P, Hanssen AD. Muscle flaps in osteomyelitis of the lower extremity: a 20-year account. *Plast Reconstr Surg.* 1999;104:107.

Attinger CE, Ducic I, Zelen C. The use of local muscle flaps in foot and ankle reconstruction. *Clin Podiatr Med Surg.* 2000;17(4):681.

Colen L, Uroskie T. Foot reconstruction. In: Mathes SJ, ed. *Plastic surgery.* 2nd ed. Vol.6. Philadelphia: Elsevier; 2006.

Follmar KE, Baccarani A, Levin LS, Erdmann D. The distally based sural flap. *Plast Reconstr Surg.* 2007;119(6):138e–148e.

Fraccalvieri M, Verna G, Dolcet M. The distally based superficial sural flap: our experience in reconstructing the lower leg and the foot. *Ann Plast Surg.* 2000;45:132.

Heller L, Levin LS. Lower extremity microsurgical reconstruction. *Plast Reconstr Surg.* 2001;108:1029.

Levin LS. Foot and ankle soft-tissue deficiencies: who needs a flap? *Am J Orthop.* 2006;1:11–19.

35 Soft Tissue Coverage of the Pelvis and Sacrum: Hemipelvectomy and Pedicled Flap Coverage

Alex Senchenkov, Robert Esther, Franklin H. Sim, and Steven L. Moran

Extensive defects of the pelvis and sacrum can result from tumors, ablation, and severe trauma. Due to limited amounts and relative immobility of the pelvic soft tissue, these defects may pose a serious reconstructive challenge. Until the late 1970s, the majority of large pelvic tumors were treated with external hemipelvectomy. Advances in imaging, chemotherapy, and radiation therapy, as well as improvements in resection and reconstructive techniques, have greatly reduced the need for radical lower extremity amputations, allowing limb preservation in a majority of cases.

Historically, buttock tumors were not amenable to a classic hemipelvectomy and just a few decades ago were considered unresectable. Likewise, extensive buttock defects inflicted by trauma, infection, or end-stage pressure ulcers in paraplegics could not be effectively reconstructed. Secondary intention healing frequently resulted in protracted hospital course, extensive scarring, contractures, and unstable soft tissue coverage. Many of these patients were bound to years of ongoing wound care and immobility.

External hemipelvectomy denotes removal of the hemipelvis with affected lower extremity by disarticulation of the pubic symphysis and the sacroiliac joint. Because external hemipelvectomy resulted in major functional impairment, limb-sparing procedures removing part or all innominate bone with preservation of the extremity have been advocated. These pelvic resections are referred to as internal hemipelvectomies.

Large, composite pelvic defects associated with internal hemipelvectomies are more challenging to reconstruct than the soft tissue defect typically created in external hemipelvectomy patients for two main reasons. First, following removal of bony hemipelvis in external hemipelvectomy, a large amount of soft tissue of the buttock or proximal thigh becomes available for reconstruction. Second, a decrease of the pelvic volume obliterates the dead space.

Sacral resections are performed as a part of extended external hemipelvectomy for musculoskeletal sarcomas and, as such, reconstructed as a part of hemipelvectomy closure. Isolated sacral defects result from composite pelvic resections for locally advanced anal and rectal malignancies or tumors intrinsic to the sacrum such as sacral chordomas and sarcomas.

INDICATIONS/CONTRAINDICATIONS

When embarking on treatment of pelvic sarcomas, three important questions should be borne in mind.

1. Is this patient operable, i.e., can the individual medically withstand a major oncologic resection?
2. Is this tumor resectable, i.e., can this patient be rendered disease-free surgically?
3. Can the residual defect or deformity from the proposed resection be reconstructed in a functionally satisfactorily manner with stable soft tissue coverage?

The answers to these questions have to be determined during preoperative evaluation by the surgical oncologist, reconstructive surgeon, and anesthesiologist. Resection of the tumor with negative margins is the only reliable means of obtaining a cure in cases if tumor.

Internal hemipelvectomy is indicated in cases of localized tumor where margin negative resection of the tumor is possible with preservation of the lower extremity. If clean margins cannot be achieved, external hemipelvectomy should be performed. Main indications for external hemipelvectomy are: large tumors involving multiple compartments unresponsive to neoadjuvant therapies, contamination of compartments from pathologic fracture, or failed previous resection, a nonviable extremity. Nononcologic external hemipelvectomy may be performed in the cases of uncontrolled pelvic osteomyelitis, traumatic hemorrhage, and failed aorto-femoral revascularizations (Table 35-1).

Wound complication rates following hemipelvectomy are notoriously high and have been reported to range from 20% to 80%. Proper technical execution of the procedure and the use of well-designed skin and muscle flaps can minimize postoperative wound morbidity.

Although infrequently, pelvic and sacral resections are performed en bloc with pelvic visceral structures for locally advanced rectal and gynecologic malignancies eroding or invading the skeletal pelvis. When such pelvic resection involves removal of a part of the pelvis or sacrum, it is referred to as *composite resection*. Any type of external hemipelvectomy performed in continuity with

---

TABLE 35-1. Basic Tumor Flap Principles

- Safe oncologic margins are the primary requirement
- Reconstruction does not take precedence over adequate, safe resection
- Adequate soft tissue coverage of bony reconstruction/prosthesis and neurovascular structures
- Healed surgical wound
- Durable
- Minimal donor morbidity
- Appropriate function, contour

visceral structures is known as *compound hemipelvectomy*. Due to the aggressive nature of these tumors, the disease has to be limited to the pelvis and extensive imaging is required to select the patients that can benefit from these extensive operations.

Primary sacral tumors such as chordomas and sarcomas are relatively uncommon. The majority of these tumors are low-grade malignancies. They infrequently metastasize and therefore local control becomes important. Reconstruction of these defects with flaps facilitates optimal postoperative wound healing.

PREOPERATIVE PLANNING

Prior to surgical resection, patients should undergo local and systemic staging studies. Musculoskeletal malignancies have a propensity to pulmonary spread. Therefore, a chest CT is mandatory to screen for systemic disease. An MRI (and plain radiographs for primary bone tumors) is sufficient for gauging the local extent of disease and response to treatment. A CT of the pelvis is often useful to complement the MRI as this area is difficult to image. Surgical planning relies on MRI images taken before and after neoadjuvant therapies. Pretreatment MRI images may be helpful in distinguishing radiation-induced reactive changes from actual tumor tissue.

Most patients with high grade bone malignancies will undergo some form of neoadjuvant treatment, including chemotherapy and/or radiation therapy prior to tumor resection. Typically, primary bone sarcomas such as osteosarcoma are treated with several cycles of preoperative chemotherapy, surgery, and then several additional cycles of chemotherapy. Radiation therapy also has an established role in treatment of soft tissue sarcomas.

The treatment team must choose between pre- and postoperative radiation therapy. Both approaches have advantages and shortcomings. Preoperative treatment requires a smaller area of treatment, creation of a fibrous rind around the tumor, and often causes tumor shrinkage, leading to an improved ability to obtain wide margins without sacrificing vital structures. Preoperative radiation's disadvantages include a higher rate of wound problems and less viable tumors available for pathologic examination. Postoperative radiation has the advantage of earlier surgery, viable tumors for pathologic study, and fewer wound complications. Treatment volumes however are increased and there is a delay in administering treatment to allow time for adequate healing of operative wounds. We prefer preoperative radiation for pelvic and retroperitoneal sarcomas.

Brachytherapy requires proper reconstruction planning so that flaps do not interfere with catheter placement (Fig. 35-1). Afterloading catheters should be evenly spaced and sutured in place to the tumor bed with fast absorbable sutures to prevent their displacement during postoperative therapy. Alternatively, VAC dressing can be used as a temporary coverage of brachytherapy catheters, followed by delayed primary reconstruction of the defect after completion of brachytherapy. Intraoperative radiation therapy (IORT) is another means of augmenting a preoperative radiation therapy regimen, allowing for directed treatment at close intraoperative margins.

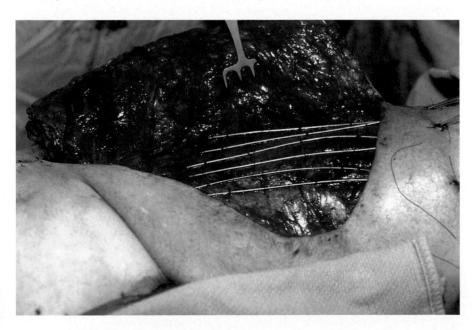

FIGURE 35-1

Placement of afterloading brachytherapy catheters under inferiorly based TRAM flap in treatment of recurrent sarcoma of the thigh.

TABLE 35-2. Principles of Pelvic Reconstruction

- Routine use of preoperatively placed ureteral stents aids in the identification of ureters intraoperatively.
- Patients should receive both antibiotic and mechanical bowel prep.
- Standard hemipelvectomy flaps provide adequate soft tissue coverage, and there is no difference in postoperative wound complications related to flap design.
- Abdominal and pelvic wall reconstruction is not necessary if the muscle with its investing fascia is a component of an external hemipelvectomy flap, but the abdominal wall should be reconstructed in cases of internal hemipelvectomy.
- Omentum should be interposed between the intestine and hemipelvectomy flap whenever possible to wall off intra-abdominal contents in the event of hemipelvectomy flap necrosis.
- Precise surgical technique, thorough hemostasis throughout the entire hemipelvectomy wound, wide drainage with multiple closed suction drains, débridement of all nonviable tissue off hemipelvectomy flap, and meticulous layered closure of the operative wound are the key to successful postoperative healing.
- Hemipelvectomy wound complications are common and related to the extensive nature of the procedure and the level of vascular ligation. Infected wounds have to be aggressively débrided until control of the wound is achieved.
- Secondary intention healing with wet-to-moist dressing changes and VAC® therapy is the most common approach to complicated hemipelvectomy wounds.
- Tertiary closure is reserved for the patients with healthy granulating wounds and extensive defects who are otherwise good operative candidates.
- Local tissue rearrangement by advancement of the skin flaps is the most common form of tertiary intention closure.
- Contralateral inferiorly based rectus abdominis muscle or musculocutaneous flap is the flap of choice for tertiary closure of large hemipelvectomy wounds. To preserve contralateral rectus abdominis muscle, contralateral ostomies should be avoided by careful preoperative planning and communication between different surgical specialties involved in this procedures.
- Hemipelvectomy reconstruction with a microvascular fillet flap obtained by ex-vivo anatomic exploration of an amputated extremity is an underutilized reconstructive option and should be considered in the cases of paucity or poor quality of local tissues and vascular ligation above the bifurcation of common iliac vessels that is plagued with the high rate of flap necrosis rate.

Preoperatively, the patients with large pelvic tumor undergo mechanical bowel preparation and intravenous antibiotic coverage. Ostomy sites must be preoperatively marked in accordance with anticipated flap use because inappropriate colostomy or ileostomy placement may burn an important reconstructive bridge and prevent rectus abdominis flap elevation. Involvement of several surgical services such as urological, colorectal, vascular, spine, and plastic surgery is common. The patient is positioned on a bean bag prior to induction of general anesthesia. Large bore intravenous access is established in an event of rapid blood loss. We liberally use ureteral stents that facilitate intraoperative identification of the ureters. After placement of the stents and Foley catheter, the patient is placed in the "sloppy" lateral decubitus position and is secured with the bean bag. This position is preferred for internal or external hemipelvectomy because it permits a wide skin preparation and an easy access to the abdomen, buttock, and perineal regions. If additional procedures on spine, sacrum, or rectum need to be performed, intraoperative repositioning of the patient will be required (Table 35-2).

Low sacral resection can also be performed in the "sloppy" lateral decubitus position (**abdominolateral sacral portion**) or a full lateral position with the hip and knee joints in 90-degree flexion. When combined abdominal exploration may be required to deal with the intrapelvic anterior component of the tumor, we start the abdominal portion of the operation supine and later reposition the patient for the posterior, sacral stage of the procedure. Plastic surgeon performs an initial marking and flap dissection as dictated by an anticipated defect.

SURGERY

External Hemipelvectomy Reconstruction

Pelvic reconstruction following external hemipelvectomy is principally accomplished with three pedicled flap designs: posterior, long anterior, and total thigh fillet flaps. The vast majority of hemipelvectomy defects can be closed with these flaps which constitute the *first choice for hemipelvectomy flap reconstructions*. If these standard hemipelvectomy flaps are unusable due to very proximal vascular ligation, causing flap ischemia, division of the flap origin during tumor resection or previous procedure, or extensive radiation damage, then alternative flaps must be used for coverage. These *second-line reconstructive options* include contralateral inferiorly based vertical rectus musculocutaneous (VRAM) flaps, microvascular lower extremity fillet flaps, or standard free flaps depending on the de-

TABLE 35-3.   Purpose of Soft Tissue Flaps in Tumor Surgery
• Covers exposed neurovascular structures
• Coverage for endoprostheses or allografts
• Addresses functional deficits (neurotized flaps)
• Obliterates dead space
• Enhances healing of irradiated wounds

fect configuration. Likewise, the second-line reconstructive options are useful for closure of hemipelvectomy wounds in the setting of postoperative wound complications (Table 35-3).

Posterior Hemipelvectomy Flap

The classic hemipelvectomy technique relies on pelvic exploration, ligation of the common iliac vessels, division of the pelvic rim by disarticulation of the pubic symphysis and the sacroiliac joint, and creation of the posterior fasciocutaneous flap to achieve soft tissue closure. It was initially recommended that gluteal muscles be left with the specimen. This fasciocutaneous hemipelvectomy flap was based on relatively poor random blood supply due to ipsilateral ligation of the common iliac vessels and was further compromised by removal of the gluteal muscles that greatly increased wound complication rates.

Three modifications of this classic technique aimed to decrease high wound complication rates:

1. Incorporation of gluteal muscles in the hemipelvectomy flap
2. Whenever oncologically appropriate, ligation at the level of external iliac vessels with reservation of the internal iliac vessels to improve the flap blood supply
3. Limited resection of the bony pelvis that allows preservation of the sacral perforators

With these modifications, the posterior hemipelvectomy flap is designed as a musculocutaneous flap based on the superior and inferior gluteal vessels (Fig. 35-2). Preservation of the gluteal muscle decreases posterior flap necrosis rates and makes the construction of a long, viable posterior flap that would reach up to or above the level of umbilicus possible. Impact of the level of vascular ligation on hemipelvectomy wound outcomes has been a point of controversy. Several reports from Karakousis et al suggested that the level of vascular ligation does not affect the posterior hemipelvectomy flap viability and the rate of postoperative wound complications. These authors believed that there was an adequate blood supply of the gluteal muscle through small arterial branches along its sacral origin, which was sufficient to sustain the viability of the flap unless resection of the edge of the sacrum was oncologically necessary. In our experience, we found 2.7-fold higher rates of posterior hemipelvectomy flap necrosis in the patients that had ligation at the level of common iliac vessels. This finding was independent from sacral resection performed during extended hemipelvectomy in some of these patients (1).

Long Anterior and Total Thigh Fillet Hemipelvectomy Flaps

One of the major limitations of the posterior flap external hemipelvectomy is its inability to deal with the advanced tumors of the buttock and posterior pelvis in an oncologically sound manner. In 1953, Bowden et al described utilization of the skin of the femoral triangle based on the preserved segment of the superficial femoral artery for closure of the hemipelvectomy performed for the sarcoma of the buttock. However, it was the critical need for soft tissue reconstruction of the advanced decubiti and the infection of bony pelvis in paraplegic patients that led to increased utilization of the soft tissue obtained from high amputations. The total thigh flap was proposed by Georgiade et al as a last-resort reconstructive option for such patients in the 1950s and subsequently gained wide-spread use. This principle was subsequently applied for coverage of the hemipelvectomy defects whereby a musculocutaneous flap of the anterior thigh compartment was elevated based on the superficial femoral artery. The technique was further refined by Sugarbaker et al, who also demonstrated that the anterior flap can be used as a sensate island flap based on the superficial femoral vessels and saphenous nerve.

Standard long anterior flap hemipelvectomy includes the bulk of quadriceps femoris muscle (Fig. 35-3). A total thigh fillet flap utilizing the majority of the thigh musculature can also be designed as a variation of the anterior hemipelvectomy flap technique (Fig. 35-4). Anterior hemipelvectomy flap is an axial pattern musculocutaneous flap based on the branches of femoral vessels, including lateral

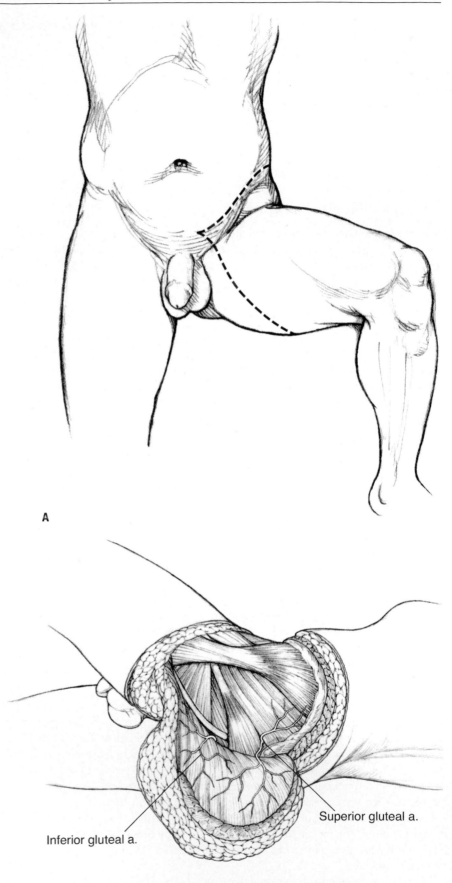

A

B

FIGURE 35-2

A: Skin markings of external hemipelvectomy with utilization of the posterior flap. **B:** Musculocutaneous design of the posterior hemipelvectomy flap based on the superior and inferior gluteal vessels.

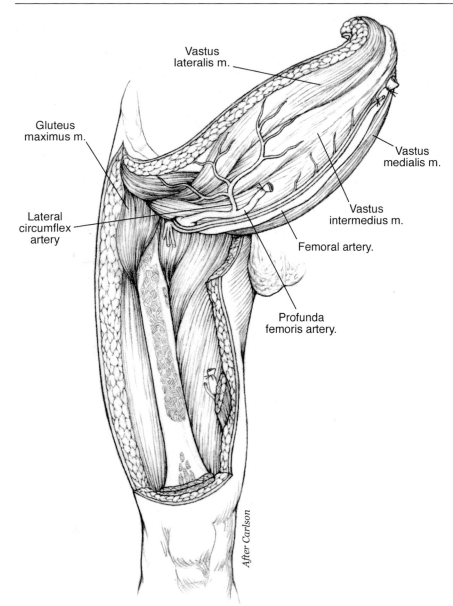

Vastus
lateralis m.

Gluteus
maximus m.

Lateral
circumflex
artery

Vastus
medialis m.

Vastus
intermedius m.

Femoral artery.

Profunda
femoris artery.

After Carlson

FIGURE 35-3

Long anterior hemipelvectomy flap based
on the branches of profunda femoris and
superficial femoris vessels.

and medial circumflex arteries which arise from branches from the profundus femoris artery. The
latter perforate the adductor magnus muscle to the posterior and lateral compartments of the thigh
and play a role in supporting a total thigh fillet flap.

The skin of the anterior thigh down to the knee is innervated by the lateral and anterior femoral cutaneous nerves. These nerves can be preserved to provide sensory flap coverage of the hemipelvectomy
defect. Both anterior flap and total thigh fillet flap hemipelvectomy provide well-vascularized and sensate immediate coverage of the hemipelvectomy defect. An effort should be made to preserve innervation of this flap by protecting sensory nerves during the dissection (Fig. 35-5). Both long anterior and
total thigh fillet hemipelvectomy flaps are sufficient to cover even very extensive hemipelvectomy defects (as well as spinopelvic resections) with tissues that have rich axial-pattern blood supply.

Second-Line Hemipelvectomy Reconstructions

Standard hemipelvectomy flaps either posteriorly or anteriorly based provide reliable reconstruction
in a vast majority of the cases because removal of the hemipelvis creates relative soft tissue excess
for three reasons:

1. Reduction of pelvic volume decreases requirement for the size of soft tissue envelop.
2. Skeletal resection eliminates the issue of the dead space.
3. Tissues or the proximal part of the amputated lower extremity can be used for hemipelvectomy
   defect reconstruction.

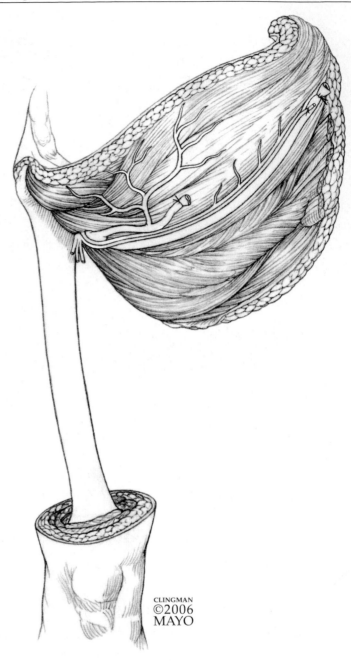

FIGURE 35-4

Total thigh fillet flap utilizes the majority of the thigh musculature.

For these reasons, external hemipelvectomy itself is the ultimate solution to soft tissue coverage problems. The difficulty arises when common iliac vessels have to be ligated for oncologic reasons, which precludes creation of the anterior hemipelvectomy flap, and, at the same time, tissues of the buttock are not suitable for posterior flap design due to tumor involvement or sequela of previous operations or radiation therapy. In the past, such patients were considered unresectable. With the advent of microvascular tissue transfer however, a suitable and tumor-free block of tissue can be recovered by ex-vivo anatomic exploration of an amputated extremity and transferred as a free flap to achieve coverage of the hemipelvectomy defect.

Internal Hemipelvectomy Reconstruction

Internal hemipelvectomy involves total or partial removal of the innominate bone with preservation of the lower extremity. This operation provides good local tumor control and acceptable functional outcome. Several types of internal hemipelvectomy as proposed by Enneking and Dunham exist based on the part of innominate bone resected: Type 1—ileum; Type 2—periacetabular region; Type 3—pubic bone; and, described by some, Type 4—ileum and sacral ala (Fig. 35-6). This clas-

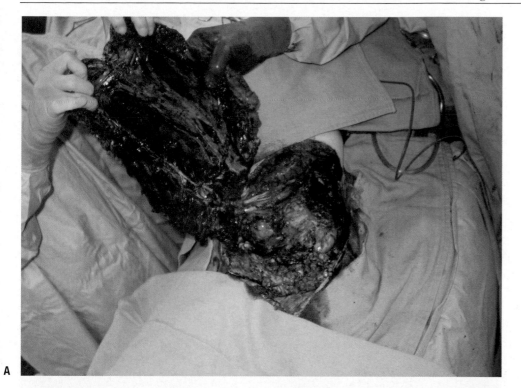

A

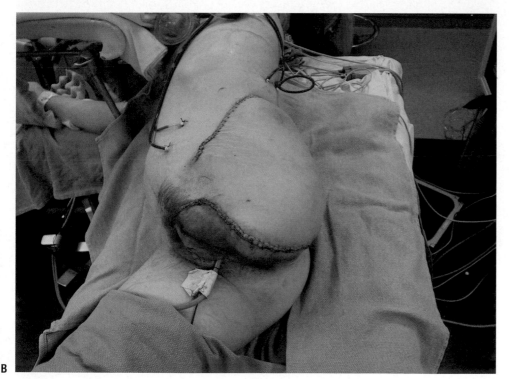

B

FIGURE 35-5

A: Total thigh fillet flap provides abundance of well vascularized soft tissue. **B:** The flap provides excellent contour and adequate posterior reach. *(Continued)*

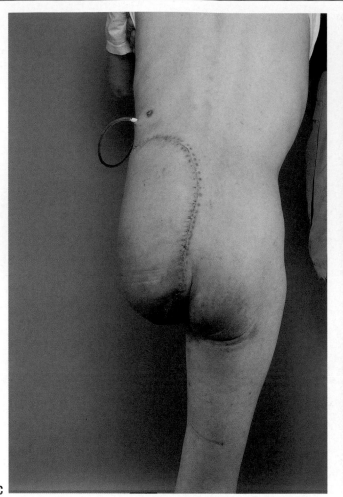

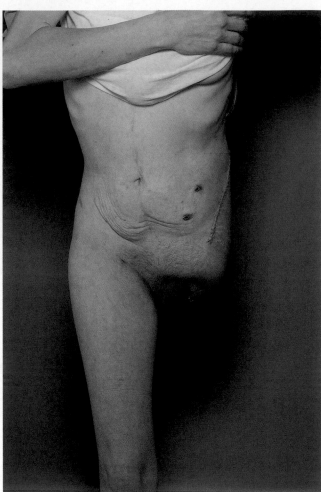

FIGURE 35-5

Continued **C,D:** Postoperative result following extended hemipelvectomy for the tumor of the buttock.

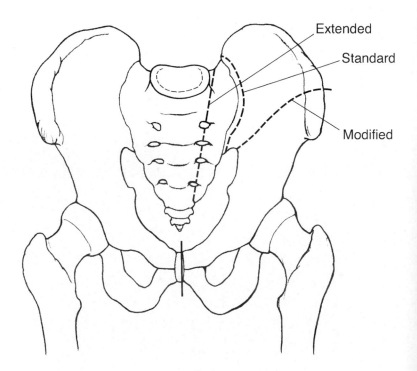

FIGURE 35-6

Schematic drawing of the pelvis showing osteotomy lines for standard modified and extended hemipelvectomies.

sification provides the basis for the surgical oncologic approaches to malignant tumors of the non-visceral pelvis.

Introduction of internal hemipelvectomies increases requirements for soft tissue reconstruction since the pelvic volume is not reduced and lower extremity cannot be filleted. Additionally, a large amount of the dead space is created and often requires obliteration with a flap, especially in the settings of preoperative radiation. Several regional pedicled flap options for filling these defects exist (Table 35-4). Muscle flaps and de-epithelialized musculocutaneous flaps can be used effectively for dead space obliteration. De-epithelialized flaps create more bulk and are used for filling larger defects. Because fat is a part of the skin paddle, the flap retains volume long term. In addition to dead space obliteration, these flaps bring blood supply into relatively ischemic radiated tissues of the operative site and thus enhance stable coverage and promote wound healing. Although flap demands for bony sarcomas without soft tissue extension are not high, however, in the cases of soft tissue sarcomas or soft tissue involvement from the bony sarcomas, flap reconstruction becomes critical for the coverage of exposed skeletal structures. Musculocutaneous, muscle pedicled, or free flaps can be used. When the skin is not part of such a flap, a split-thickness skin graft can be used for coverage of exposed muscle of the flap.

Sacral Reconstruction

Primary sacral tumors are often low-grade lesions such as chordoma. They do not metastasize, but have a tenacious local course. Chordomas and locally-advanced rectal cancers are the two most commonly encountered sacral tumors. Sacral surgery presents a major challenge due to regional anatomic complexity, technical difficulty in obtaining clear margins, functional impairment, and an often prolonged postoperative course due to poor wound healing. Sacrectomy is a procedure that is uncommon outside of specialized cancer centers. Although distal sacral resections are safely performed through the posterior approach, larger tumors, tumors of rectal origin, and resections proximal to S3 require an initial abdominal exploration to dissect visceral and neurovascular structures, perform formal visceral resection when required, assure hemostasis, and complete anterior sacrectomy dissection. Sacrectomy is completed through the posterior approach.

Soft tissue reconstruction becomes important in preventing postoperative wound complication following sacrectomy. Two flaps are commonly utilized: pedicled omentum and rectus abdominis muscle/musculocutaneous flaps. **Omentum** is preferred for smaller defects (the defects *smaller than the surgeon's fist*), and the rectus flap is used for larger ones. Inferiorly based vertical rectus abdominis musculocutaneous (VRAM) flap is the most commonly used reconstructive technique.

The flap accomplishes two main objectives: it obliterates large dead space and provides tension-free closure of the sacrectomy wound. In the cases of preoperative radiation, well-vascularized tissue of the flap enhances local circulation and further promotes wound healing. Implementation of this practice in our institution led to a marked decrease in sacrectomy wound complication rates. Careful preoperative planning and communication between different services is critical in executing these operations. VRAM flap as a reconstructive option must always be borne in mind in the light of previous abdominal incisions as well as ostomies, drains, and feeding tube placements. The VRAM flap represents a very important surgical technique in oncologic pelvic reconstruction.

If soft tissue defect is too large for sole VRAM coverage, fasciocutaneous V-to-Y advancement flap provides additional recruitment of the local tissues. If aforementioned techniques are not sufficient to achieve an immediate coverage of sacrectomy-buttockectomy defect, microvascular tissue

---

TABLE 35-4.   Flap Options for Internal Hemipelvectomy Defect Reconstruction

- Rectus abdominis muscle based are inferiorly based ipsilateral or contralateral:
  - Vertical rectus abdominis musculocutaneous (VRAM) flap
  - Transverse rectus abdominis musculocutaneous (TRAM) flap
  - Rectus abdominis muscle flap with or without skin graft
- Rectus femoris muscle flap
- Latissimus dorsi muscle or musculocutaneous flap
- Vastus lateralis muscle flap
- Tensor fascia lata muscle or musculocutaneous flap
- Anterolateral thigh flap

transfer should be performed with a free flap of appropriate dimensions. Finally, anterior flap external hemipelvectomy is reserved as a last resort reconstructive operation.

Technical Elements of Pelvic Flap Surgery

Omentum Pedicled Flap   Omentum is readily available during laparotomy although it can also be harvested laparoscopically. Its blood supply is based on the right or left gastroepiploic artery. Significant mobilization and extent of reach can be gained by basing the flap on left gastroepiploic vessels, dividing the short gastric vessels along the greater curvature of the stomach, and further dividing middle omental artery to release a long vascular pedicle (Fig. 35-7). The latter maneuver releases omentum to its fullest length, which may be important for the reconstruction of the larger pelvic defects in the event that the VRAM flap is unavailable.

Rectus Abdominus Muscle and Musculocutaneous Flaps   The rectus abdominus muscle can be elevated alone or with a skin paddle. The skin paddle may be oriented transversely or ver-

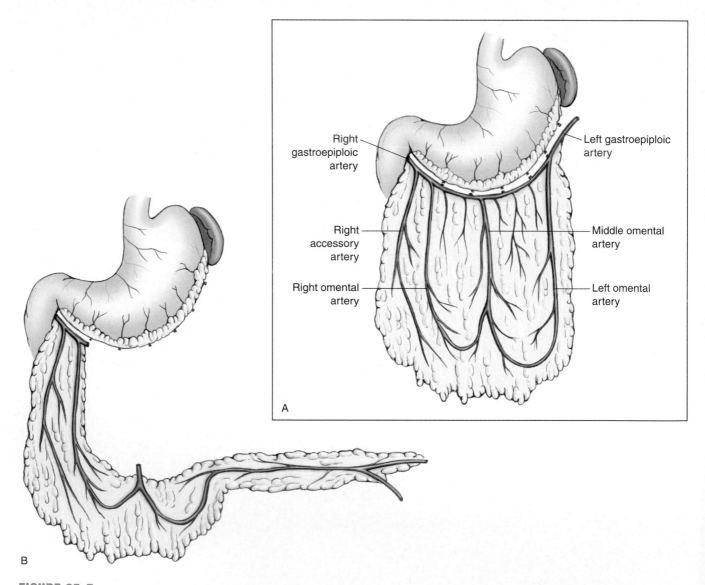

FIGURE 35-7

A: Omentum can be used for coverage in difficult situations following pelvic resection and soft tissue deficit. While the omentum lacks significant structural strength it provides a well vascularized bed which can support skin grafting. The division of the left gastroepiploic arch allows the omentum to be mobilized off the greater curvature of the stomach. The right gastroepiploic vessels are preserved to supply the flap. **B:** The omentum may be lengthened by dividing the omental arcade along the lines within the illustration, creating a long vascularized pedicle. *(Continued)*

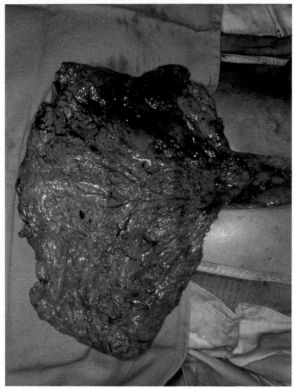

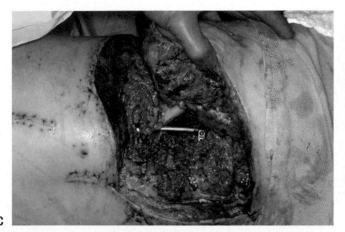

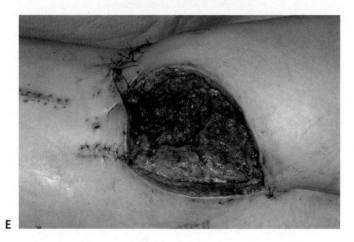

FIGURE 35-7

Continued **C–E:** Clinical example of a 16-year-old woman with exposed spinal hardware **(C)** following sacrectomy. The omentum was harvested through a midline anterior incision **(D)**, lengthened as shown in **(B)** and then passed through the back to provide coverage for the spinal hardware.

tically. The transverse rectus abdominis musculocutaneous (TRAM) or vertical rectus abdominis musculocutaneous (VRAM) flaps can be utilized as either pedicled or microvascular free flaps. The rectus abdominus muscle has a dual blood supply from the superior and inferior epigastric vessels. For the purposes of pelvic soft tissue reconstruction, the rectus abdominus muscle flaps are based on the inferior epigastric vessels when pedicled to cover the pelvis or sacrum.

Several key elements of preoperative planning are important in preparation for this procedure. A detailed history of previous intra-abdominal surgery needs to be obtained, because the inferior epigastric vessels may be divided during operations such as appendectomy, inguinal hernia repair, C-section, and colostomy creation (Fig. 35-8). The pedicle may also be damaged by radiation therapy. If there is any question about the integrity of the vascular pedicle, duplex evaluation should be performed.

Flap elevation is performed prior to abdominal exploration. We open the rectus sheath close to midline and dissect it off the rectus abdominis muscle (Fig. 35-8A–C). In this part of procedure, care should be taken to dissect inscriptions due to their proximity to the underlying vessels that run on the undersurface of the muscle. Once the flap has been dissected for coverage of the sacrum and posterior defects, the flap is placed in a plastic bag or wrapped with towels and placed over the anterior

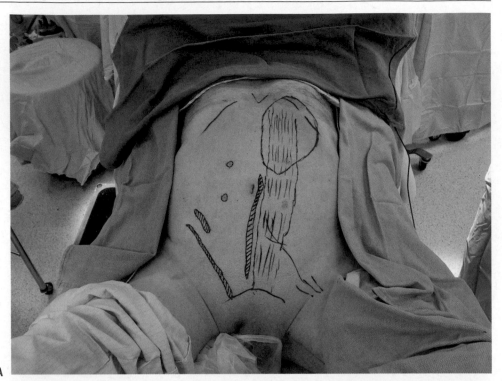

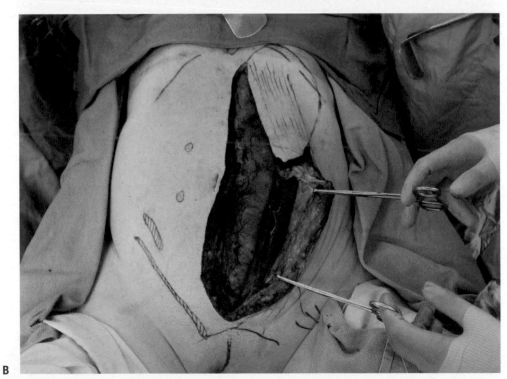

FIGURE 35-8

A: VRAM flap is planned for reconstruction of the defect from *en bloc* abdomino-perineal resection with sacrectomy. Skin paddle is designed to overlie rectus abdominus muscle. **B:** The rectus sheath is open and the rectus abdominis muscle is exposed. The anterior fascia is preserved with the skin paddle. *(Continued)*

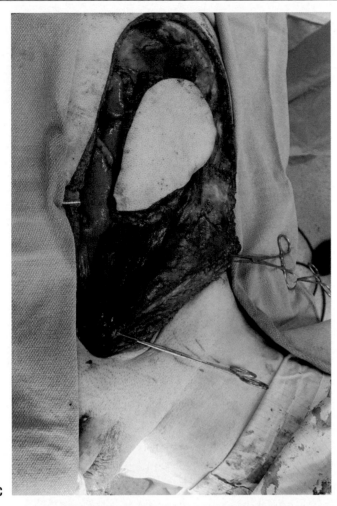

C

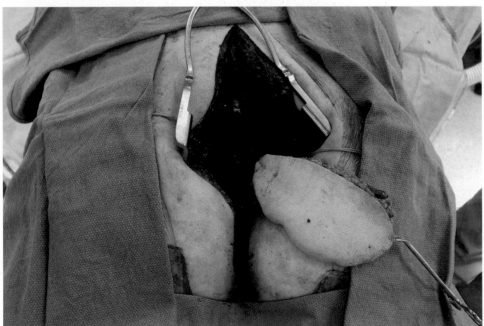

D

FIGURE 35-8

Continued **C:** The flap elevation is complete. The rectus abdominus muscle has been divided superiorly from its insertion into the ribs. The inferior epigastric vessels have been mobilized to prevent kinking as the flap is passed into the abdomen. **D:** The flap is placed into the abdomen and the anterior incision is then closed. The patient is then placed into the prone position and the sacrectomy is completed. At this point the VRAM flap is retrieved from the pelvis. *(Continued)*

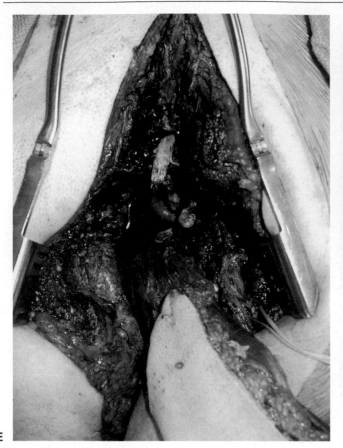

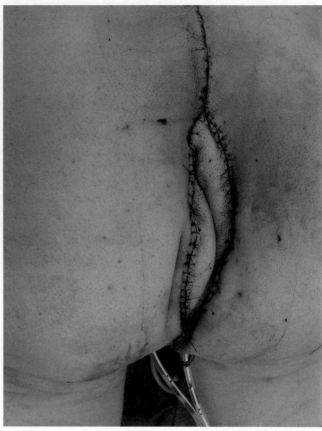

FIGURE 35-8

Continued **E:** Prior to its inset the muscle and vascular pedicle are examined to ensure there is no evidence of kinking or twisting. Note exposed dural sack. **F:** VRAM inset is complete with generous amount of skin remains to accommodate for sitting.

portion of the lumbar spine and sacrum. The abdominal portion of the procedure is then completed and the abdomen is closed. If a large fascial defect remains following VRAM harvest, this is reconstructed with synthetic mesh or allograft fascia. Following abdominal closure, the patient is placed in the prone jackknife position for the sacral portion of the operation, and the flap is easily visualized after removal of the specimen (Fig. 35-8D–F). Inset should ideally be performed with no tension to prevent sacral closure breakdown when the patients starts to sit.

Other Flap Options   In many instances, the safest approach to patients with pelvic sarcomas is a laparotomy and, when it is performed, omentum becomes a valuable reconstructive material. Omentum, if present, should always be interposed between hemipelvectomy flap and intra-abdominal viscera. This provides an additional protective layer in the event of hemipelvectomy wound problems. Omental flaps can be effectively used for dead space obliteration.

Although omentum and VRAM are truly the workhorses of pelvic reconstruction, several other flaps may become important as second line reconstructive options. Rectus femoris, tensor fascia lata, and anterolateral thigh flap can be used as pedicled flaps. Latissimus dorsi and anterolateral thigh flaps can be transferred as microvascular flaps depending on soft tissue requirements and availability of recipient vessels.

V-to-Y Advancement Gluteal Flaps   This versatile reconstructive technique can be performed in escalating complexity and is usually tried in the following sequence:

1. Unilateral fasciocutaneous
2. Bilateral fasciocutaneous
3. Unilateral musculocutaneous in conjunction with contralateral fasciocutaneous
4. Bilateral musculocutaneous
5. VRAM and bilateral fascio- or musculocutaneous advancement flaps (Fig. 35-9)

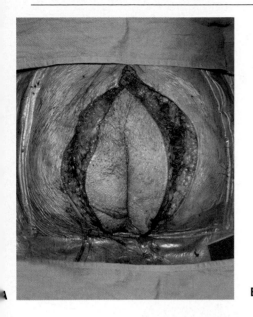
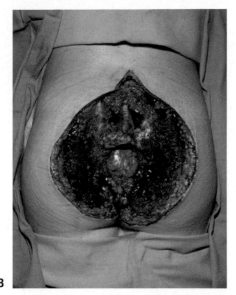
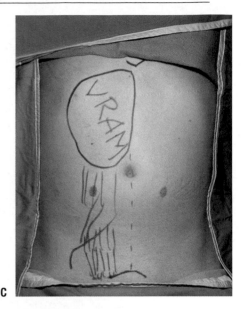

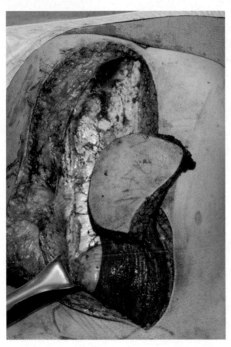
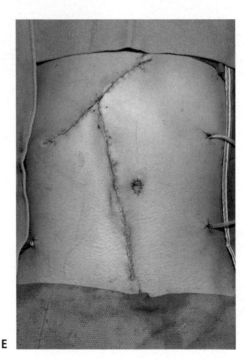

FIGURE 35-9

A,B: Combination of inferiorly based pedicled VRAM flap and bilateral fasciocutaneous V-to-Y advancement flaps for closure of a large sacral defect after wide local excision of the sacral sarcoma. **C–E:** Inferiorly based VRAM is elevated with large skin island based over superior portion of rectus abdominus muscle. The abdomen is closed with the aid of extensive undermining. The umbilicus is repositioned beneath the skin flaps to lie in the midline. *(Continued)*

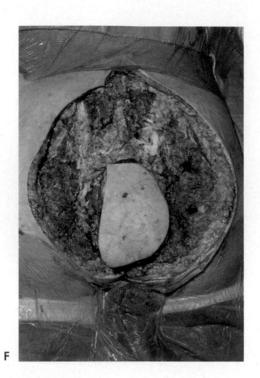
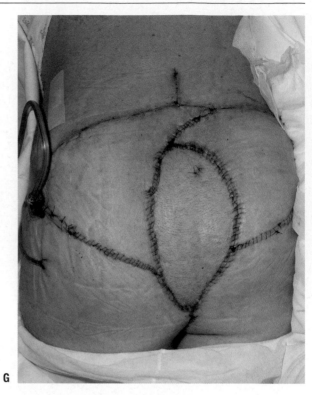

FIGURE 35-9

Continued **F:** VRAM flap allows for soft tissue coverage over sacrectomy defect and allows for reconstruction of pelvic floor; however large soft tissue defect remains at margins of sacrectomy incision. **G:** Remaining portion of sacral wound is closed with use of bilateral fasciocutaneous flaps. Flaps are elevated with fascia only to avoid injury to gluteus muscles to maximize post-operative ambulatory ability.

The surgeon must be careful in utilizing this flap in an ambulatory patient as it may affect functional performance. It is safer to reserve musculocutaneous gluteal flaps for paraplegic individuals. For large buttock defects, lateral donor sites of the V-to-Y advancement flaps sometimes may need to be temporarily covered with Vacuum-Assisted Closure (VAC®) dressings to be closed later when the edema subsides, skin is grafted, or allowed to heal by secondary intention.

In the face of insufficient amounts of local tissues, the donor part of the V-to-Y advancement flap can be skin grafted or covered with a wound VAC to allow healing by secondary intention.

Abdominal Wall Reconstruction in Pelvic Surgery   Integrity of the abdominal wall has to be maintained to prevent postoperative hernias. For a standard external hemipelvectomy defect without extensive resection of the abdominal wall, in the patients with musculocutaneous design of hemipelvectomy flap, no specific reconstruction of the abdominal wall is necessary other than meticulous layered closure of the hemipelvectomy wound. We did not observe postoperative hemipelvectomy hernias under these circumstances because sturdy fascia of the anterior compartment of the thigh or gluteus muscle along with muscular bulk of the flap effectively withstands pressure of the intra-abdominal viscera. Conversely, abdominal wall reconstruction becomes important for internal hemipelvectomy defects because frequently in these patients there is a very clear area of weakness in the lower abdominal wall. This situation is also aggravated by higher functional level of the internal hemipelvectomy patients.

Reconstructive efforts are guided by the extent of the abdominal wall deficit and degree of operative contamination. Time-tested surgery principles of ventral hernia repair apply. Hernia repair should be tension free with liberal use of prosthetic mesh materials. Well-incorporated prosthetic mesh is superior to nonneurotized autologous options because it secures the dimensions of the abdominal wall and prevents postoperative bulge and recurrent hernia formation. The downside of prosthetic mesh reconstruction is its propensity to infection in the presence of intraoperative contamination. Although prosthetic mesh can be used in clean-contaminated cases, most surgeons are reluctant to use nonabsorbable mesh in this setting and prefer either absorbable mesh such as Vicryl or a biologic substitute such as AlloDerm®, processed cadaveric human acellular dermis (Life Cell Corporation, Branchburg, NJ, USA) or Surgisis®, a product obtained by the processing of porcine small intestine sub-mucosa (Cook Surgical, Bloomington, IN, USA). Vicryl® mesh is a temporary abdominal reconstruction solution that permits a conversion of the contaminated situation into a clean one at the time of the second procedure. The latter aims for definitive reconstruction, but requires utilization of costly biologic materials and postoperative formation of abdominal wall hernia or bulge continues to be a problem.

POSTOPERATIVE MANAGEMENT

Postoperatively, patients usually require an ICU admission after major pelvic resections or hemipelvectomies. They are commonly kept on mechanical ventilation overnight until intravascular volumes are stabilized and gas exchange is adequate. To optimize postoperative recovery as well as systemic and flap perfusion the patient needs to be kept well hydrated. Adequate urine output needs to be maintained. The patient with pelvic or sacral flap is usually kept on a Clinitron bed® to avoid pressure injury to the flap. Recovery of bowel function, ostomy care, DVT prophylaxis, and wound care is similar to that for a general surgery patient undergoing abdominal procedures.

   Physical and occupational therapy services are involved early in the care of these patients. Even when the patients are on bed rest, range of motion exercises on nonoperated extremities and activities of daily living should be started. When it is safe, from a surgical perspective, to resume ambulation, the patients are evaluated for short-term rehabilitation placement.

RESULTS

Our experience shows that the outcome of external hemipelvectomy wounds was not dependent on hemipelvectomy flap selection. Reliability of its blood supply determines the success of the reconstruction. Historically, classic hemipelvectomy flaps that are based on the random circulation are exceedingly prone to necrosis. Preservation of the gluteal muscle as a part of the flap decreased, but did not solve, the problem of hemipelvectomy flap necrosis. We also observed that preservation of the branches of the internal iliac vessels providing direct blood supply to the gluteus maximus muscle further decreased hemipelvectomy flap necrosis rates. Hemipelvectomy wound outcomes therefore can be improved by increased utilization of microvascular fillet flap transfer that provides superb blood flow to the transferred tissue, not comparable with the periphery of a random hemipelvectomy following common iliac vessel ligation.

COMPLICATIONS

Wound complications such as surgical site infection and skin flap necrosis are the most common postoperative complications in musculoskeletal oncology. There are multiple reasons for the high rate of wound complications following major resections of musculoskeletal malignancies. Despite the fact that the vast majority of these procedures are clean cases with only occasional visceral resection that is applicable for pelvic tumors, wound complication rates are well beyond what one would expect. In modern musculoskeletal oncology practice, many sarcoma patients undergo neoadjuvant (preoperative) radiation and chemotherapy. Soft tissue complication rates approach 40% to 50 % in this group of patients. Moreover, even without neoadjuvant therapy, the duration and operative extent of the procedures significantly influence rates of postoperative wound complications. As noted earlier, wound complications that delay the administration of postoperative adjuvant therapies may have serious oncologic consequences. Rapid, uncomplicated wound healing is essential for patients who require postoperative adjuvant therapy, highlighting the need for early and close collaboration with plastic surgeons.

   A hematoma can occur after any oncologic surgery, ranging from incisional biopsy to extensive surgery. All tumor resections should utilize at least one suction drain, although larger resections may require several drains placed deep and in more superficial tissues. The pressure from the collection of blood products in a wound can compromise soft tissue reconstructions and may become infected. Drain sites and tracks are contaminated and usually are resected at the time of definitive tumor removal. For this reason, drains should exit the skin in line with the longitudinal incision used for biopsy. It is important to remember that drain placement can be as important as where one makes an incision. Drains should come out in line and close to an incision.

Hematomas are especially problematic following incisional biopsy, potentially compromising future resection and successful local control of a tumor. A hematoma can spread neoplastic cells beyond the immediate area and even into surrounding compartments if a transverse incision is used. Rigorous attention to hemostasis is therefore essential. Compressive dressings bolstered with plaster can also help minimize hematomas in the immediate postoperative period.

Seromas can occur following tumor resections, again potentially compromising soft tissue reconstructions and wound closures. Most surgeons therefore take a conservative approach to removing drains, allowing output to decrease (to less than 30 mL/day) and remain low before removal. Drains usually remain in place for a minimum of several days, but often are left in for much longer in large or irradiated wound beds. As with other facets of patient care, good communication with plastic surgery is important regarding the timing of drain removal. It is recommended that patients going home with suction drains remain on oral antibiotics.

Oncology patients often have a compromised nutritional status, making them prone to wound infections. Moreover, these patients are subject to the immunosuppressive actions of chemotherapy agents and the local wound effects from radiation. As many oncologic reconstructions rely on allografts, endoprostheses, or combinations of the two, surgeons should approach wound infections extremely aggressively. This approach entails a low threshold for surgical débridement. As with all surgical procedures, orthopedic oncology patients should receive pre- and perioperative intravenous antibiotics as well as postoperative coverage when appropriate.

Sacrectomy is prone to wound complications that are related to the extent of the procedure, intraoperative contamination, use of preoperative radiation therapy, local tissue ischemia, hematoma, positional pressure, dead space, and tight closure. In the setting of preoperative radiation, wound complication rates are as high as 50%. These factors can be minimized by meticulous surgical technique, obliteration of the dead space with a flap, and postoperative use of a Clinitron bed®.

Over the past 20 years, 160 external hemipelvectomies were performed in our institution. External hemipelvectomy has been associated with high morbidity but low mortality (5% to 7%). Overall, 54% of patients had at least one complication. Hemipelvectomy wound morbidity was the most common postoperative complication. Thirty-nine percent of patients experienced wound infection and 26% had hemipelvectomy flap necrosis. Wound complications were managed with serial débridement until control of the wound was achieved; however, this may result in a sizable defect.

In a delayed reconstruction setting, the amputated extremity is no longer available for tissue procurement and the contralateral pedicled VRAM flap becomes critical in closure of such defects. This flap provides a superb reconstruction and in fact is the flap of choice for postoperative hemipelvectomy wounds. In a very rare circumstance, when VRAM is unavailable and the hemipelvectomy wound is so large it cannot be closed by local tissue rearrangement or a skin graft, a free flap such as a contralateral anterolateral thigh flap or latissimus dorsi may be required. One has to consider a paucity of recipient vessels and the need for vein grafts or saphenous arteriovenous loop that significantly increase the risk of flap failure.

Oncologic outcomes of musculoskeletal tumors are largely dependent on tumor pathology. Limb salvage is possible in the vast majority of sarcoma patients. In those patients who still require proximal amputations such as external hemipelvectomy, stable soft tissue coverage is almost uniformly achieved. Despite postoperative wound complications related to the operative extent of the resection, intraoperative contamination, and preoperative radiation therapy, the vast majority of the patients heal the surgical wounds. Both successful wound healing and high rates of limb salvage became possible due to advances in reconstructive surgery over the past three decades. In our practice, we emphasize early involvement of a plastic and reconstructive surgeon in care of a sarcoma patient.

PEARLS AND PITFALLS

- Plastic surgery consultation early
- Early, durable reconstructions are important for functional recovery and also prevent delays in administration of postoperative chemotherapy and radiation therapy
- All surgeons should be present in the operating room at the start of a combined case

- Don't use an Esmarch—exsanguinate, if necessary, by elevating extremity and digital arterial compression
- Use compressive Robert Jones dressings when feasible, even after soft tissue resections

REFERENCES

1. Senchenkov A, Moran SL, Petty PM, et al. Predictors of complications and outcomes of external hemipelvectomy wound: account of 160 consecutive cases. *Am Surg Oncol.* 2008;15(1):355–363. Epub 2007, Oct 23.

RECOMMENDED READING

Abramson DL. Single-stage, multimodality treatment of soft-tissue sarcoma of the extremity. *Ann Plast Surg.* 1997;39:454–460.

Aflatoon K, Manoso MW, Deune EG, et al. Brachytherapy tubes and free tissue transfer after soft tissue sarcoma resection. *Clin Orthop and Rel Research.* 2003;415:248–253.

Apffelstaedt JP, Driscoll DL, Spellman JE, et al. Complications and outcome of external hemipelvectomy in the management of pelvic tumors. *Ann Surg Oncol.* 1996;3(3):304–309.

Bowden L, Booher RJ. Surgical considerations in the treatment of sarcoma of the buttock. *Cancer.* 1953;6(1):89–99.

Butler CE. Reconstruction of an extensive hemipelvectomy defect using a pedicled upper and lower leg in-continuity fillet flap. *Plast Reconstr Surg.* 2002;109:1060–1065.

Chang DW, Robb GL. Recent advances in reconstructive surgery for soft-tissue sarcomas. *Curr Onc Reports.* 2000;2:495–501.

Dickey ID, Mugate RR, Fuchs B, et al, Reconstruction after total sacrectomy: early experience with a new surgical technique. *Clin Orthop.* 2005;438:42–50.

Doi K, Hattori Y, Tan SH, et al. Basic science behind functioning free muscle transplantation. *Clin Plast Surg.* 2002;29:483–495.

Doi K, Kuwata N, Kawakami F, et al. Limb-sparing surgery with reinnervated free-muscle transfer following radical excision of soft-tissue sarcoma in the extremity. *Plast Reconstr Surg.* 1999;104:1679–1687.

Enneking WF, Dunham WK. Resection and reconstruction for primary neoplasms involving the innominate bone. *J Bone Joint Surg Am.* 1978;60(6):731–746.

Fuchs B, Dickcy ID, Yaszemski MJ, et al. Operative management of sacral chordoma. *J Bone Joint Surg Am.* 2005;87(10):2211–2216.

Frey C, Matthews LS, Benjamin H, et al. A new technique for hemipelvectomy. *Surg Gynecol Obstet.* 1976;143(5):753–756.

Georgiade N, Pickrell K, Maguire C. Total thigh flaps for extensive decubitus ulcers. *Plast Reconstr Surg.* 1956;17(3):220–225.

Ghert MA, Davis AM, Griffin AM, et al. The surgical and functional outcome of limb-salvage surgery with vascular reconstruction for soft tissue sarcoma of the extremity. *Ann Surg Oncol.* 2005;12:1102–1110.

Ihara K, Shigetomi M, Kawai S, et al. Functioning muscle transplantation after wide excision of sarcomas in the extremity. *Clin Orthop Rel Res.* 1999;358:140–148.

Ihara K. Pedicle or free musculocutaneous flaps for shoulder defects after oncological resection. *Ann Plast Surg.* 2003;50:361–366.

Kane JM, Gibbs JF, McGrath BE, et al. Large, deep high-grade extremity sarcomas: when is a myocutaneous flap reconstruction necessary? *Surg Oncol.* 1999;8:205–210.

Karakousis CP, Emrich LJ, Driscoll DL. Variants of hemipelvectomy and their complications. *Am J Surg.* 1989;158(5):404–408.

Kulaylat MN, Froix A, Karakousis CP. Blood supply of hemipelvectomy flaps: the anterior flap hemipelvectomy. *Arch Surg.* 2001;136(7):828–831.

Kunisada T, Ngan SY, Powell G, et al. Wound complications following pre-operative radiotherapy for soft tissue sarcoma. *Eur J Surg Oncol.* 2002;28:75–79.

Langstein HN, Chang DW, Miller MJ, et al. Limb salvage for soft-tissue malignancies of the foot: an evaluation of free-tissue transfer. *Plast Reconstr Surg.* 2002;109:152–159.

Langstein HN, Robb GL. Reconstructive approaches in soft tissue sarcoma. *Semin Surg Oncol.* 1999;17:52–65.

Lee HY, Cordeiro PG, Mehrara BJ, et al. Reconstruction after soft tissue sarcoma resection in the setting of brachytherapy. *Ann Plast Surg.* 2004;52:486–492.

Lohman RF, Nawabi AS, Reece GB, et al. Soft tissue sarcoma of the upper extremity. *Cancer.* 2002;94:2256–2264.

Lohman RF. Soft tissue sarcoma of the upper extremity. *Cancer.* 2002;94:2256–2264.

Lotze MT, Sugarbaker PH. Femoral artery based myocutaneous flap for hemipelvectomy closure: amputation after failed limb-sparing surgery and radiotherapy. *Am J Surg.* 1985;150(5):625–630.

Mastorakos DP, Disa JJ, Athanasian E, et al. Soft-tissue flap coverage maximizes limb salvage after allograft bone extremity reconstruction. *Plast Reconstr Surg.* 2002;109:1567–1573.

Meyers PA, Heller G, Healey J, et al. Chemotherapy for nonmetastatic osteogenic sarcoma: the Memorial Sloan-Kettering experience. *J Clin Oncol.* 1992;10:5.

Miller TR. 100 cases of hemipelvectomy: a personal experience. *Surg Clin North Am.* 1974;54(4):905–913.

Mugate RR Jr, Dickey ID, Phimolsarnti R, et al. Mechanical effects of partial sacrectomy: when is reconstuction necessary? *Clin Orthop*. 2006;450:82–88.

Mugate R Jr, Sim FM. Pelvic reconstuction techniques. *Orthop Clin North Am*. 2006;37(1):85–97.

Royer J, Pickrell K, Georgiade N, et al. Total thigh flaps for extensive decubitus ulcers. A 16 year review of 41 total thigh flaps. *Plast Reconstr Surg*. 1969;44(2):109–118.

Senchenkov A, Clay RP. Vacuum-assisted closure (VAC) dressing as a temporary coverage for brachytherapy afterloading catheters. *Ann Plast Surg*. 2006;57(3):355.

Spira M, Hardy SB. Our experiences with high thigh amputations in paraplegics. *Plast Reconstr Surg*. 1963;31:344–352.

Sugarbaker PH, Chretien PA. Hemipelvectomy for buttock tumors utilizing an anterior myocutaneous flap of quadriceps femoris muscle. *Ann Surg*. 1983;197(1):106–115.

Temple WJ, Mnaymneh W, Ketcham AS. The total thigh and rectus abdominis myocutaneous flap for closure of extensive hemipelvectomy defects. *Cancer*. 1982;50(11):2524–2528.

Wallace RD, Davoudi MM, Neel MD, et al. The role of the pediatric plastic surgeon in limb salvage surgery for osteosarcoma of the lower extremity. *J Craniofac Surg*. 2003;14:680–686.

Wei F, Jain F, Celik N, et al. Have we found an ideal soft-tissue flap? An experience with 672 anterolateral thigh flaps. *Plast Reconstr Surg*. 2002;109:2219–2226.

Wilcox TM, Comerota AJ, Mitra A, et al. Functional free latissimus dorsi muscle flap to the proximal lower extremity. *Clin Orthop Relat Res*. 2003;410:285–288.

Yamamoto Y, Minakawa H, Takeda N. Pelvic reconstruction with a free fillet lower leg flap. *Plast Reconstr Surg*. 1997;99:1439–1441.

PART VIII
REPLANTATION

36 Management of Major Upper Limb Amputation

Tsu-Min Tsai and Huey Y. Tien

INDICATIONS/CONTRAINDICATIONS

Replanting the upper limb above wrist level involves a large quantity of muscle and, consequently, is regarded as major replantation. Because muscle does not tolerate anoxia well, the success of arm replantation depends on the effects of ischemia, and warm ischemic time is much more detrimental than cold ischemic time. The tissue damage caused by 1 hour of warm ischemia is equal to that caused by 20 hours of cold ischemia. When warm ischemic time is more than 6 hours, the success rate is markedly decreased and the complication rate is significantly increased. When arm amputation is incomplete, there might be a venous blood regurgitation that causes capillary refill to be present. In this situation, health care personnel may be unaware that the injured limb is devascularized, and therefore fail to keep the injured limb in a cool environment. This oversight further lengthens warm ischemic time and jeopardizes the survival of the injured limb. Furthermore, one should remember that on-table time to revascularization is often warm ischemia time, as well. Daigle and Kleinert reported that the average warm/total ischemia times were 4.8/14.8 hours in failed replantation, which is significantly higher compared with the average of 1.1/7.5 hours in successful replantation.

As a rule, the more proximal the amputation, the poorer the prognosis. Although some debate its efficacy in cases of amputation proximal to the mid forearm, the upper limb should be replanted if at all possible, both for function and cosmesis. However, there are some conditions that contraindicate arm replantation, including:

- Significant associated injury
- Extensive injury to the affected limb or to the amputated part
- Severe medical illness

Significant associated injury to major organs prolongs the patient's time in surgery and, therefore, increases blood loss and the need for transfusion. Limb replantation is clearly contraindicated if it may jeopardize the life of the patient. Injury factors that require significant consideration are:

- Avulsion versus guillotine injury
- Ischemia time elapsed
- Quantity of tissue loss
- Presence of multiple levels of injury
- Degree of wound contamination

Chronic illness also may complicate, and even contraindicate, limb replantation. For example, vessel anastomosis may be more difficult among patients with diabetes, who have a higher prevalence of arteriosclerosis. Diabetes, autoimmune disorders, and prolonged steroid use increase patients' susceptibility to infection. Serious illnesses, including organ failure, preclude replantation surgery.

In addition to severity of injury to the limb and chronic medical illness, one also needs to take patient factors into consideration. Although there is no absolute cut-off age for replantation, the prognosis for a favorable functional outcome decreases with the increase of age. Children, as a rule, tend to be excellent candidates for major upper limb replantation. They have an advantage over adults in tissue regeneration generally, and especially in nerve regeneration. Patient factors in addition to age include the patient's occupation, hobbies, and wishes.

PREOPERATIVE PLANNING

Of course, always treat any life-threatening associated injury first. As soon as possible, control bleeding on the amputated stump with pressure dressings. Do not use any clamp instrument to try to stop bleeding because this increases the chance of damaging the vital structures (e.g., nerve) next to the bleeding vessels. The cut arterial end, however, can be tied to stop bleeding. Preserve the amputated part in a plastic bag, and cool it in ice slurry to just above freezing, usually 4°C. Then arrange rapid transportation to the replantation center.

In cases of incomplete amputation, wrap the limb snugly with gauze and elastic bandage so that bleeding stops, but not so tightly that blood flow is cut off to healthy tissue. Then, splint the injured area and place a regular ice pack on it. Special attention should be paid for any sign of hypovolemia.

While the patient is prepared for surgery or during transportation, the amputated part can be perfused with organ preservation solution, for example, Tsai's solution or UW solution, as shown in Table 36-1. Perfusion may have several benefits over simple immersion for large tissue parts, including the physical benefits of more rapidly cooling deep tissues and flushing stagnant blood. If the ischemic time is more than 6 hours, and especially if the amputation is incomplete, the amputated part also can be perfused with 1 unit of heparinized arterial blood obtained from the patient (Fig. 36-1). When the amputated part is brought to the operating room for cleaning and initial debridement, continue to keep it in a cool condition at all times.

SURGERY

The patient is taken to the operating room and placed on the operating table in the supine position. Because arm replantation surgery may take as long as 16 to 18 hours, general anesthesia is practi-

TABLE 36-1. **Solutions Used in Arm Replantation**			
Solution	**Content**	**Concentration**	**Preparation**
Tsai's solution	Injectable lactated Ringer's, heparin, preservative-free Lidocaine		Lactated Ringer's 150 mL + heparin 3,000 units + 1% Lidocaine 30 mL
Papaverine	Papaverine	1.5 mg/mL	Papaverine 1 mL (30 mg) + normal saline 19 mL
LMD/heparin drip	LMD, heparin	10 units/mL	LMD 500 mL + heparin 5,000 units

LMD, low-molecular-weight dextran.

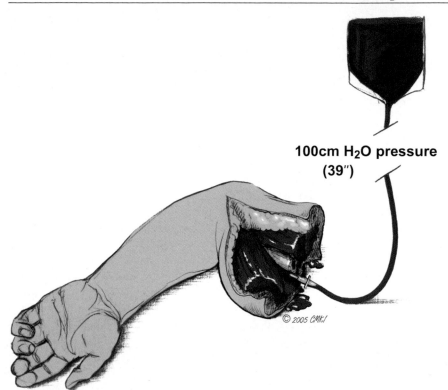

100cm H₂O pressure
(39″)

© 2005 CMKi

FIGURE 36-1

Perfusion of an amputated limb with heparinized blood. The blood bag is hung 100 cm above the amputated limb and the infusion flows by gravity.

cally always required. The patient is given a dose of intravenous antibiotics 30 minutes before surgery. The patient's injured limb is prepared and draped in standard sterile fashion. An upper-arm tourniquet is inflated to 100 mm IIg above the patient's systolic pressure to minimize bleeding. If necessary, the contralateral lower limb is also prepared and draped for possible skin, nerve, and/or vein grafting; it may even be used to provide a free flap.

The order for arm replantation is quite different from finger replantation. Before proceeding with replantation, lactated Ringer's solution or plasma is used to flush organ preservation solution from the limb. The recommended order of surgical procedures is as follows:

1. Arterial shunt or perfusion to shorten anoxia time
2. Thorough debridement
3. Bone fixation
4. Artery and vein repair, with or without vein graft
5. Repair of nerves
6. Repair of muscle and tendon
7. Skin grafting or flap for coverage
8. If indicated, fasciotomy

The artery from the amputated limb is cannulated with a standard vascular shunt to establish the connection between the proximal and distal artery and to intermittently perfuse the devascularized limb. A segment of regular intravenous infusion tube can also be used if no vascular shunt device is available. During perfusion, if the patient becomes hypotensive, temporarily clamp the perfusion. After 20 minutes, the venous shunt can be performed to minimize blood loss.

Thorough debridement is essential for a successful replantation. The injury may occur in an environment such as a farm, an automobile accident, or water sport in which the wound would be severely contaminated. Any crushed, grossly contaminated tissue must be removed. Muscles distal to the amputation level that have lost their contractility must be debrided. Effective debridement converts a dirty, crushed wound to a clean and guillotine-like wound. Residual dead tissue provides a substrate for bacterial growth after major limb replantation. The resulting gas gangrene or septicemia from postoperative infection may be life threatening. In addition, bone infection may result in non-union, delayed functional recovery, and secondary amputation.

Bone shortening is almost always the rule; usually a shortening of at least 2 to 3 cm is required. Bone shortening not only provides more healthy bony structure for an improved chance of bone healing, but also helps to release tension on the soft tissue and eliminates the need for vein grafting, nerve grafting, or tendon grafting.

Either internal or external bone fixation can be used, depending on the surgeon's preference. Internal fixation can be chosen for more definitive treatment, especially if there is minimal concern for infection. Plates and screws provide better stability and are most commonly used. Kirschner wires can be used when the amputation is around wrist level. Although intramedullary nailing is an option, it is rarely used. External fixation should be considered when there is a high risk of infection or when internal fixation is contraindicated. External fixation can be used for temporary fracture stabilization until soft tissue is healed. When the limb is viable, internal fixation can be implemented. Occasionally, however, external fixation can be a problem when free tissue transfer is required for soft tissue coverage. If this is the case, external fixation should be switched to internal fixation at the time of the free tissue transfer procedure or should be avoided from the beginning, if at all possible.

One should repair as many arteries and veins as possible, although there is no magic number for optimal results. In general, at least one artery and two vein anastomoses are required. The two-to-one ratio also holds when greater numbers of anastomoses are performed: Repair two veins for each arterial repair. The stump of the vessel on each end is gently debrided to remove crushed or severely contused vessel. Special attention is paid in cases of avulsion to make sure there is no hidden intima injury that might cause delayed thrombosis and, eventually, failure of replantation. The adventitia at the stump is then carefully trimmed to provide better exposure for anastomosis. A syringe with a small angiocath filled with Tsai's solution (150 mL lactated Ringer's + 3,000 units heparin + 30 mL 1% preservative-free Lidocaine) is used to flush the vessel lumen to remove any blood clot or debris (see Table 36-1). Vascular anastomosis is performed under a microscope with 8-0 or 9-0 nonabsorbable suture in interrupted fashion. For a more proximal amputation, for example, at the upper arm, anastomosis can be achieved with 6-0 or 7-0 suture. Clamps are removed after each anastomosis is completed, and the replanted part is observed for return of circulation. In the past, we would give a bolus dose of heparin (3,000 units) followed by a low-molecular-weight dextran (LMD)/heparin drip (500 mL LMD + 5,000 units heparin at 20 mL/hr) for anticoagulation. Nowadays, after the bolus of heparin, we use a low fractionated heparin (e.g., enoxaparin sodium injection or Lovenox 30 mg given subcutaneously) due to its efficacy and simplicity. If there is any sign of vessel spasm, the replanted part should be kept warm with warm normal-saline–moistened gauze or abdominal pads. Occasionally, papaverine (1.5 mg/mL) can be used to reverse vasospasm (see Table 36-1).

If the gap of the arterial defect is too big for primary anastomosis without increased tension, arterial reconstruction with a vein graft should be considered. The donor site of the graft can be a superficial vein from the contralateral arm or a saphenous vein from the lower extremity. The vein graft should be reversed routinely to prevent the valve effect. Venous anastomosis is performed in the same manner as arterial repair, but doesn't require reversal if a vein graft is used. As many veins as possible should be repaired.

Careful monitoring is necessary to avoid a systemic effect from revascularization (i.e., hyperkalemia, increased creatinine, and myoglobinuria). In complete amputation, the first 100 to 200 mL of venous blood, carrying with it toxic metabolites, is allowed to bleed out without going back to systemic circulation. For incomplete amputation, especially when part of the venous system is intact, the repaired artery is intermittently clamped to allow adjustment of systemic circulation.

All major nerves should be repaired, including the radial, median, and ulnar nerves and their branches. Epineurial repair with interrupted 8-0 or 9-0 nonabsorbable suture under a microscope is recommended. If a nerve graft is required, it can be obtained from the lateral or medial antebrachial cutaneous nerve or the sural nerve, depending on the length and size of the nerve graft desired.

Different techniques of tendon suturing can be chosen, according to the surgeon's preference. Strong tendon repair with early protective range of motion provides the best chance of functional recovery. If muscle and tendon are severely damaged, a tendon transfer is performed.

The authors recommend that fasciotomy be performed in anticipation of postischemic swelling. In the forearm, both the volar and dorsal compartments must be opened (Fig. 36-2). The incision on the volar distal forearm can be made along the ulnar side of the distal forearm to minimize tendon exposure. In the hand, all nine compartments (thenar, hypothenar, three volar, and four dorsal interosseous) are opened. This can be achieved with four incisions: one each on the side for the thenar and hypothenar eminences, and two dorsal incisions along second and fourth metacarpal bones in order to approach all interosseous compartments (Fig. 36-3).

Soft tissue coverage for exposed vital structures becomes easier after bone shortening and, in some cases, no extra skin is required. In most cases, primary wound closure can be accomplished with skin

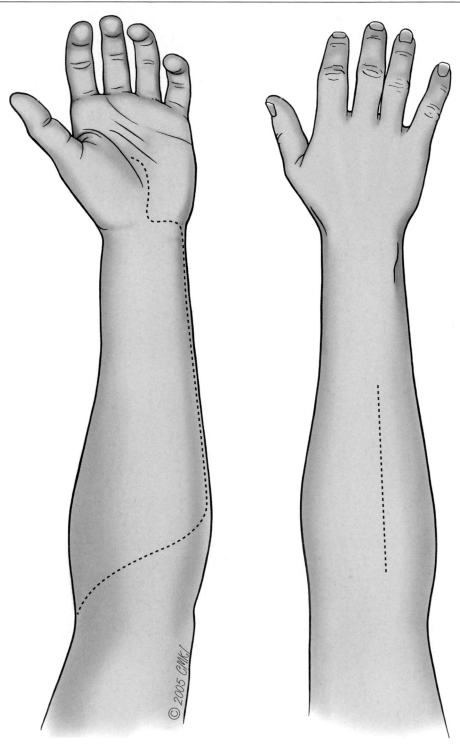

© 2005 CMK

FIGURE 36-2
Volar distal forearm incision along the dorsal side.

grafting only. Occasionally, especially in complicated amputations, additional soft tissue coverage is required. This can be achieved by forming a pedicled or free vascular flap. It can be done either in an immediate, emergent setting or in a semi-emergent setting (i.e., a few days after initial surgery).

POSTOPERATIVE MANAGEMENT

The patient is admitted and is given nothing by mouth for at least 12 hours in case it becomes necessary to return to the operating room. The replanted limb is elevated to heart level with an intravenous pole or pillows and is monitored at least every hour for color, temperature, blanching, and capillary refill. Among them, temperature is the most sensitive parameter. A temperature drop of

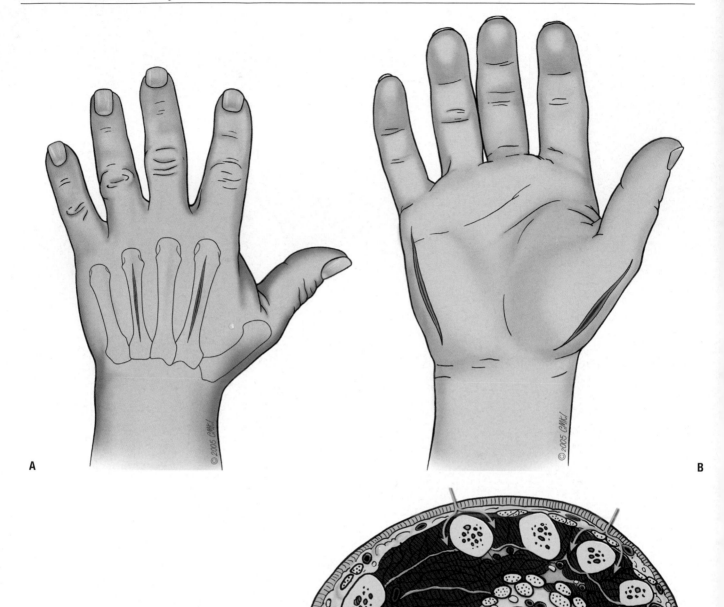

FIGURE 36-3

A: Dorsal incisions along the 2nd and 4th metacarpal bones. **B:** Incisions on the thenar and hypothenar eminences. **C:** Interosseous compartments.

more than 2°C represents an early sign of vascular compromise. It is also important to make sure that the capillary refill is the result of arterial flow, not venous congestion. The patient is instructed to refrain from smoking and caffeine products for 3 weeks after surgery because they may decrease circulation to revascularized tissue. Dressing change is avoided in the first 3 days to minimize the chance of vasospasm.

By tradition, heparin and LMD are routinely given intraoperatively and postoperatively. However, a new trend is to give one dose of heparin when revascularization is completed or, sometimes, not giving any heparin at all. In these cases, patients are given only aspirin postoperatively. Heparin and LMD are given only when there is any doubt about the efficacy of circulation. Prostaglandin E_1 is also reported to provide some benefit because of its effects of general vasodilation, leukocyte adhesion inhibition, and platelet aggregation inhibition. The dose given is 40 to 120 μg per day for 3 to 10 days.

Hyperbaric oxygen (HBO) treatment is very useful when the replanted limb shows marginal circulation. According to Nylander et al, HBO treatment significantly reduces phosphorylase activity, a sensitive marker for muscle damage, in the post-ischemia phase. Hyperbaric oxygen treatment is given at 2.5 atm of absolute pressure for 45 minutes, and usually three treatments are necessary.

In the weeks and months that follow replantation, additional surgeries may be required to improve the function of the replanted limb. These procedures may include debridement, tenolysis, and improvements in coverage.

COMPLICATIONS

Postoperative complications include persistent ischemia from the no-flow phenomenon, hyperkalemia/metabolic acidosis, myoglobinuria/renal failure, tissue necrosis, and wound infection. Any of these complications may either jeopardize the survivability of the replanted limb or endanger the life of the patient. The no-flow phenomenon is mainly due to long ischemic time and is often irreversible. Although free-radical scavengers (e.g., allopurinol) can be used to treat this condition, the result is often unsatisfactory.

During surgery, frequent test measurements should be used to monitor for the development of hyperkalemia and metabolic acidosis. High alertness and close monitoring of serum potassium during surgery, especially right after the vascular clamp is released, are key. The vessel should be intermittently clamped in the first couple of minutes of revascularization to allow time for adjustment. It's also important to maintain adequate hydration and avoid high potassium-content IV fluid. If it does develop, hyperkalemia/metabolic acidosis can be treated with alkalization and IV insulin. According to Waikakul et al, serum potassium concentration in the amputated segment was the best objective predictor of replantation success. When it is higher than 6.5 mmol/l 30 minutes after reperfusion, replantation should be avoided. A high systemic venous serum potassium concentration was also found before clinical signs of the reperfusion syndrome were seen.

Myoglobinuria and renal failure can be prevented with adequate hydration, alkalinization of urine, osmotic diuretics (mannitol), and free-radical scavengers. Frequent urine myoglobin monitoring is required until two consecutive results are within normal range. Tissue necrosis and infection are mainly due to inadequate debridement; therefore, adequate debridement is essential.

During the last 10 years, cases of myoglobinuria or renal failure are rarely seen following tissue perfusion or shunt anoxia time. Compared with minor replantation, patients with major replantation require longer hospital stays, more surgical procedures, and the functional results are not always satisfactory. The process also has a high psychiatric impact to both patient and family members.

Ultimately, the most important measure of outcome is the recovery of hand function. If there is no recovery of hand function, forearm amputation and a switch to below-elbow prosthesis can be considered. In one study from our institute, 8 of 34 patients with apparently successful major replantation underwent secondary amputation. Among them, four amputations were done because of poor function, one because of dysfunctional pain, and one because of poor cosmesis. The other two were part of planned staged procedures to preserve the length of the stump or joint. In general, a replanted limb tends to have a better functional outcome compared with a prosthesis. A replanted limb typically has better performance in gross prehensile activities and allows pronation and supination that prostheses do not offer.

In summary, arm replantation remains a major challenge to surgeons. The surgeon needs to consider the safety of the patient, to preserve limb viability, and to reconstruct the limb function. The final goal of a successful replantation is to achieve adequate function without pain. In addition, cosmesis must not be ignored, and secondary amputation sometimes is required. According to our experience, ideal conditions do not guarantee ideal results, although more distal amputation and shorter ischemic time predict a more favorable outcome.

CASE STUDIES

A 45-year-old man sustained a blast injury resulting in total amputation at proximal upper arm level. Total ischemic time was 11 hours before revascularization was accomplished (Fig. 36-4).

A 17-year-old boy was involved in a mining accident and sustained bilateral forearm amputations (Fig. 36-5).

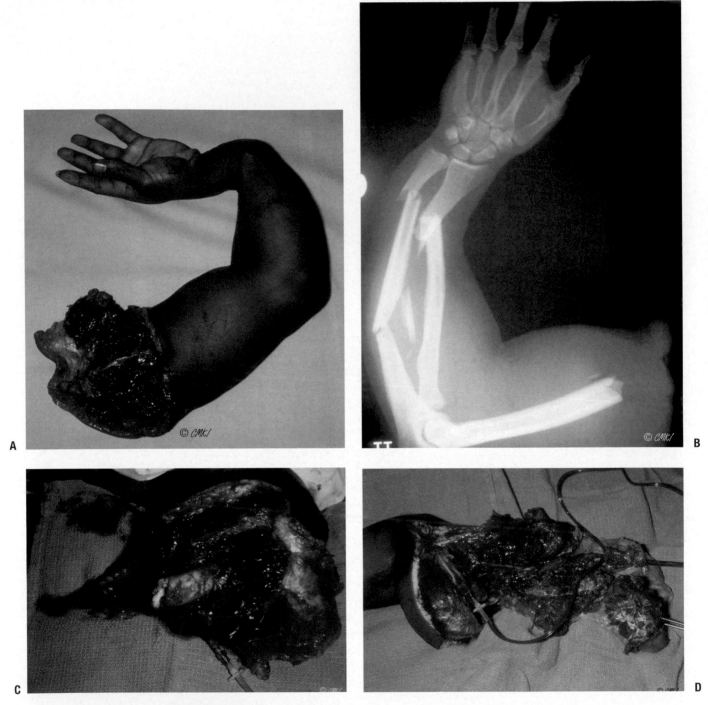

FIGURE 36-4

A: Amputated part demonstrated gross deformity at forearm level. **B:** Radiographic examination revealed amputation at proximal humerus level with segmental forearm fractures. **C:** Proximal part showed soft tissue defect with large area of bony exposure. **D:** Amputated part was perfused with 1 unit of heparinized arterial blood 2 hours before revascularization. *(Continued)*

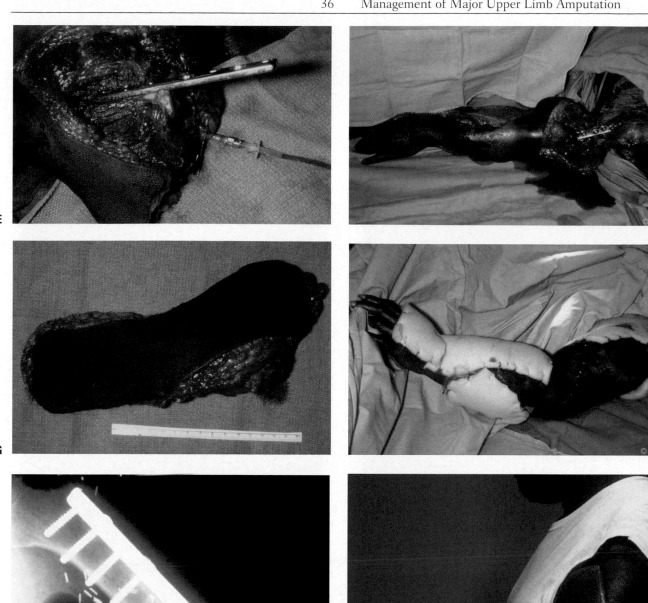

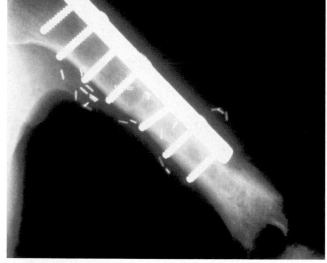

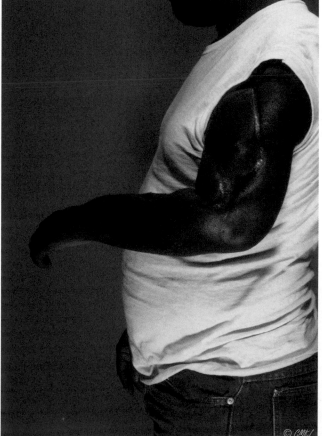

FIGURE 36-4

Continued **E:** While patient was getting ready for surgery, amputated limb was debrided and internal fixation partially readied for replantation. **F:** Completion of internal fixation, revascularization, and fasciotomy. **G:** Free tensor fascia lata flap for soft tissue coverage. **H:** Completion of initial surgery with free flap and skin grafting. **I:** Radiographic examination demonstrated healed humerus with plate in place. **J:** Final result after multiple surgical procedures including pectoralis major muscle transfer for elbow flexion. *(Continued)*

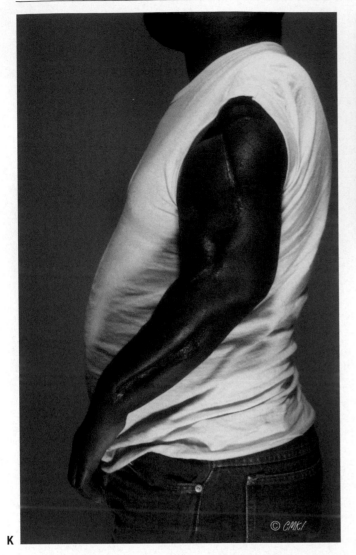

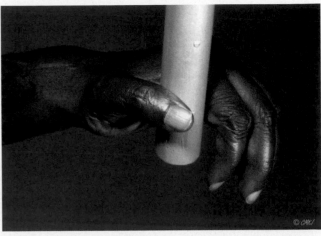

FIGURE 36-4

Continued **K:** Final result of elbow extension. **L:** Final result of hand gripping. The patient has some hand gripping function but has very little intrinsic muscle function. Sensory recovery is protective only.

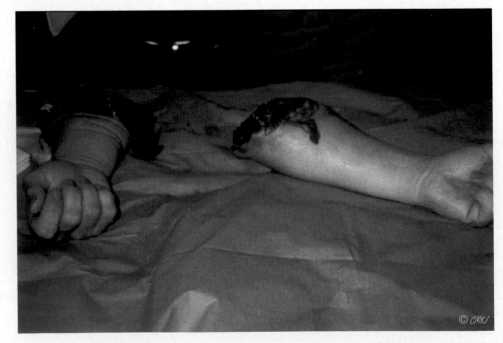

FIGURE 36-5

A: Right forearm amputated at mid-forearm level and left forearm amputated at proximal forearm level. *(Continued)*

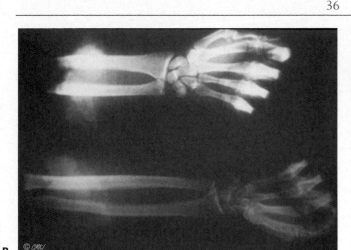

B

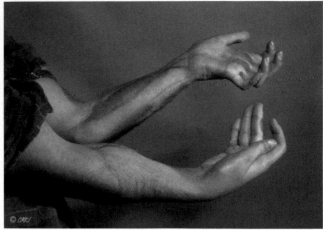

C

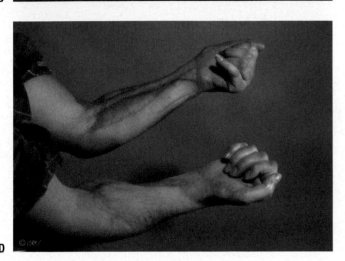

D

FIGURE 36-5

Continued **B:** Radiograph of amputated parts. **C:** Finger extension at final follow-up. **D:** Finger flexion at final follow-up.

RECOMMENDED READING

Bandyk DF. Vascular injury associated with extremity trauma. *Clin Orthop Relat Res.* 1995;318:117–124.

Chang J, Jones NF. Secondary soft-tissue reconstruction. In: Weinzweig N and Weinzweig J, eds. *The mutilated hand.* Philadelphia: Elsevier Mosby, 2005;355–370.

Chen Z, Huang Q. Principles of replantation and revascularization. In: Weinzweig N and Weinzweig J, eds. *The mutilated hand.* Philadelphia: Elsevier Mosby, 2005;193–216.

Chew WY, Tsai TM. Major upper limb replantation. *Hand Clin.* 2001;17:395–410.

Chitwood WR, Rankin JS, Bollinger RR, Moylan JA. Brachial artery reconstruction using the heparin-bonded Sundt shunt. *Surgery.* 1981;89:355–358.

Cooley BC, Tadych KL, Gould JS. Perfusion of free flaps with heparinized whole blood during ischemic storage. *J Reconstr Microsurg.* 1990;6:49–53.

Daigle JP, Kleinert JM. Major limb replantation in children. *Microsurgery.* 1991;12:221–231.

Edwards RJ, Im MJ, Hoopes JE. Effects of hyperbaric oxygen preservation on rat limb replantation: a preliminary report. *Ann Plast Surg.* 1991;27:31–35.

Fukui A, Tamai S. Present status of replantation in Japan. *Microsurgery.* 1994;15:842–847.

Goldner RD, Nunley JA. Replantation proximal to the wrist. *Hand Clin.* 1992;8:413–425.

Gordon L, Levinsohn DG, Borowsky CD, et al. Improved preservation of skeletal muscle in amputated limbs using pulsatile hypothermic perfusion with University of Wisconsin solution. A preliminary study. *J Bone Joint Surg Am.* 1992;74: 1358–1366.

Grunert BK, Weis JM, Anderson KJ. Psychological aspects of mutilating hand injuries. In: Weinzweig N and Weinzweig J, eds. *The mutilated hand.* Philadelphia: Elsevier Mosby, 2005;509–518.

Hicks TE, Boswick JA Jr, Solomons CC. The effects of perfusion on an amputated extremity. *J Trauma.* 1980;20:632–648.

Idler RS, Steichen JB. Complications of replantation surgery. *Hand Clin.* 1992;8:427–451.

Kocher MS. History of replantation: from miracle to microsurgery. *World J Surg.* 1995;19:462–467.

Leow ME, Pho RW, Pereira BP. Esthetic prostheses in minor and major upper limb amputations. *Hand Clin.* 2001;17:489–497.

Levin LS, Erdmann D. Primary and secondary microvascular reconstruction of the upper extremity. *Hand Clin.* 2001;17:447–455.

Mathieu D, Wattel F, Bouachour G, Billard V, Defoin JF. Post-traumatic limb ischemia: prediction of final outcome by transcutaneous oxygen measurements in hyperbaric oxygen. *J Trauma.* 1990;30:307–314.

Moneim M, Young SD, Mikola EA. The mutilated wrist. In: Weinzweig N and Weinzweig J, eds. *The mutilated hand.* Philadelphia: Elsevier Mosby, 2005;291–298.

Nichols JG, Svoboda JA, Parks SN. Use of temporary intraluminal shunts in selected peripheral arterial injuries. *J Trauma.* 1986;26:1094–1096.

Nichter LS, Morwood DT, Williams GS, Spence RJ. Expanding the limits of composite grafting: a case report of successful nose replantation assisted by hyperbaric oxygen therapy. *Plast Reconstr Surg.* 1991;87:337–340.

Norden MA, Rao VK, Southard JH. Improved preservation of rat hindlimbs with the University of Wisconsin solution and butanedione monoxime. *Plast Reconstr Surg.* 1997;100:957–965.

Nunley JA, Koman LA, Urbaniak JR. Arterial shunting as an adjunct to major limb revascularization. *Ann Surg.* 1981;193:271–273.

Nylander G, Nordstrom H, Frazen L, Henriksson KG, Larsson J. Effects of hyperbaric oxygen treatment in post-ischemic muscle. A quantitative morphological study. *Scand J Plast Reconstr Surg Hand Surg.* 1988;22:31–39.

Rosen HM, Slivjak MJ, McBrearty FX. The role of perfusion washout in limb revascularization procedures. *Plast Reconstr Surg.* 1987;80:595–605.

Scheker LR. Emergency free flaps. In: Weinzweig N Weinzweig J, eds. *The mutilated hand.* Philadelphia: Elsevier Mosby; 2005:339–354.

Shatford RA, King DH. The treatment of major devascularizing injuries of the upper extremity. *Hand Clin.* 2001;17:371–393.

Shimizu H, Tsai TM, Firrell JC. Effect of ischemia and three different perfusion solutions on the rabbit epiphyseal growth plate. *Microsurgery.* 1995;16:639–645.

Slodicka R, Lautenbach M, Eisenschenk A. Using prostaglandin E1 in microvascular reconstruction of the upper extremity after acute trauma [in German.] *Unfallchirurg.* 2002;105:14–18.

Strauch B, Greenstein B, Goldstein R, Liebling RW. Problems and complications encountered in replantation surgery. *Hand Clin.* 1986;2:389–399.

Tsai TM, Jupiter JB, Serratoni F, Seki T, Okubo K. The effect of hypothermia and tissue perfusion on extended myocutaneous flap viability. *Plast Reconstr Surg.* 1982;70:444–454.

VanGiesen PJ, Seaber AV, Urbaniak JR. Storage of amputated parts prior to replantation—an experimental study with rabbit ears. *J Hand Surg [Am].* 1983;8:60–65.

Waikakul S, Vanadurongwan V, Unnanuntana A. Prognostic factors for major limb re-implantation at both immediate and long-term follow-up. *J Bone Joint Surg Br.* 1998;80:1024–1030.

Wang WZ, Anderson GL. Intervention approaches against I/R-induced arterial insufficiency in reconstructive surgery. *Hand Clin.* 2001;17:357–369.

37 Replantation of Digits

Samir Mardini, Kuang-Te Chen, and Fu-Chan Wei

INDICATIONS/CONTRAINDICATIONS

Replantation is defined as reattachment and revascularization of a completely amputated part, whereas revascularization is defined as restoration of arterial inflow or venous outflow to or from a part that is incompletely amputated. In revascularization cases, it is of utmost importance that the true severity of the injury is not underestimated due to the grossly intact image of the injured finger. The introduction and improvements in microsurgical instrumentation and techniques have lead to successful revascularization and replantation of amputated parts as distal as the finger tip and pulp. Overall, the results of finger replantation are encouraging and have provided many amputation victims with extremely rewarding results.

Amputations of upper extremity digits are devastating for the patient who is initially stunned by the events of the trauma. Therefore, care is taken to discuss the situation in a gentle and thoughtful manner, considering that the patient has just lost a part of the upper extremity, and that this loss might be permanent if the reconstructive effort is not indicated or is unsuccessful. Generally accepted indications for finger replantation include amputations of the thumb in almost every situation, a single digit with the level of injury distal to the superficialis insertion, multiple digits, and any amputation in children (Table 37-1). The patient's desires have a strong influence on the approach.

Success in replantation is based on the functional outcomes as judged by objective parameters such as strength, range of motion, and sensory function, and not on the survival of the replanted or revascularized parts alone; therefore, the potential outcome must be considered for each individual patient. The potential for a long operative procedure, immediate or late failure, the potential requirement of regional or distant tissue flaps to complete the reconstruction, and the possible need for multiple procedures even after survival of the replants should be included in the formula for decision making and discussed with the patient and his or her family. The location, mechanism of injury, number digits involved, level of injury, condition of the amputated part, condition of the hand, length of ischemia time, the patient's general health, age, and associated injuries, and the patient's desires dictate the course of action. One advantage of replanting any digit is prevention of neuroma formation. A thorough knowledge of the anatomy and adequate exposure of structures aids in attaining optimal results (Figs. 37-1 and 37-2).

The thumb is the most important single digit, and its replantation is the most rewarding since provision of a post for opposition, even with lack of motion at the metacarpophalangeal and interphalangeal joints, is significant. In avulsion cases, the defects of the vessels and nerves may be segmental and the use of vein grafts for the arteries and veins, and nerve grafts or vein grafts for the nerves, may be required. The long nerve stumps of the amputated thumb can be anastomosed to the dorsal sensory nerves in the first web space, to a transposed nerve from the index finger, or to the more proximally located nerve stumps using nerve grafts. Despite the fact that sensory return may only be protective in nature, the replantation of thumb avulsion injuries usually results in significant improvement in function.

Patients presenting with multiple digit amputations are candidates for replantation, and efforts are made to replant all fingers with potential for good functional outcomes. The surgeon uses his or her judgment in deciding the location where an amputated part should be replanted. Replanting a digit onto the stump of the thumb is the first priority, and the other amputated digits should be replanted with the idea that a better grip is achieved when the long, ring, and small fingers are replanted with-

TABLE 37-1.	Indications and Contraindications for Finger Replantation

Indications	Controversial Indications
Amputations of the thumb at any level	Single-digit amputation at a level proximal to the insertion of
Amputation of multiple digits	the flexor digitorum superficialis tendon
Any amputation in children	Ring avulsion injuries
Single-digit injury in zone I	Severe contamination

Contraindications
Amputated parts that are severely crushed or damaged
Multiple-level amputations
Significant associated trauma and/or medical conditions

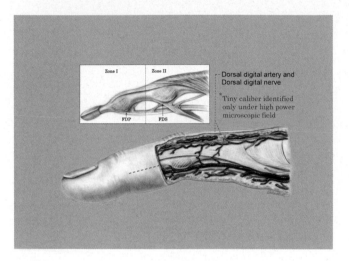

FIGURE 37-1

Lateral view of a finger demonstrating the location of arteries, veins, and nerves relevant to finger replantation. Also demonstrated are zones I and II as well as the level at which incisions are made for exploration of the neurovascular bundle.

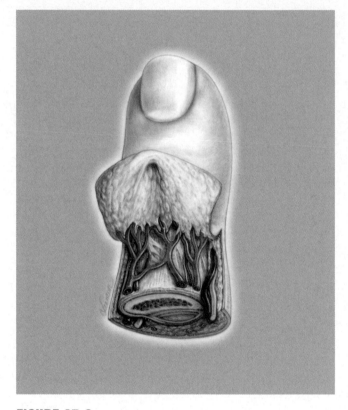

FIGURE 37-2

Mid-axial incisions and exposure of structures in the amputated part.

out gaps between the digits, and better fine pinch is achieved when the index and long finger are replanted. Efforts are made to replant each amputated digit to its natural position; however, less severely damaged amputated digits may be better placed onto a stump that is less damaged and is located in a more functionally significant position. For example, in a case of multiple digit amputations with involvement of both the thumb and index finger, in which the amputated thumb has sustained irreparable damage, the index finger is replanted to the stump of the thumb. After the thumb position has been filled, the replantation should begin with the one most appropriate for the patient's daily activities and functional needs at work.

Single-digit amputations distal to the insertion of the flexor digitorum superficialis (FDS) tendon (zone I) yield good outcomes following replantation, with little need for secondary surgery, even if the distal interphalangeal (DIP) joint requires fusion. In some instances, venous outflow cannot be reconstituted and postoperative leech therapy or heparinization and purposeful exsanguination can achieve digit survival. Four millimeters of dorsal skin proximal to the nail fold must be present for adequate vein size to be repaired. Tsai, McCabe, and Maki described their technique of finger tip replantation, which used leech therapy and other methods of decongesting the finger when venous congestion developed postoperatively. These authors noted a 69% survival rate, a 75% rate of return of some form of two-point discrimination, and an average range of motion of the DIP joint of 56 degrees. Replantation of a single digit amputation at a level proximal to the insertion of the flexor superficialis tendon and distal to the first annular pulley (zone II) often results in stiffness of the proximal and DIP joints and limited motion of the finger, with the replanted finger interfering with movement of the other fingers. Therefore, single-digit replantation may be only suitable for well-motivated individuals who are willing to undergo appropriate postoperative physical rehabilitation for a maximal functional recovery. Unless they are highly motivated, concerned about cosmetic outcome, or are children, patients are not usually replanted in this situation, as they often require secondary surgery and end up with disappointing outcomes.

Ring avulsion amputations present with segmental injuries of structures such as arteries, veins, and nerves; therefore, vein and nerve grafts are often necessary to bridge the gaps after debridement of unhealthy appearing neurovascular tissue. Otherwise, transposition of the neurovascular bundle from an adjacent digit (Fig. 37-3) or the use of arteriovenous shunting for inflow to the replanted digit can also yield successful outcomes. Most surgeons consider ring avulsion amputation patients to be poor candidates for replantation; however, replantation of an avulsed digit still can be attempted if the patient insists on replantation and he or she understands the likeliness of a suboptimal outcome.

The mechanism of injury plays an important role in decision making. Sharp, incisive injuries predict better functional outcomes than crush or avulsion injuries.

In elderly patients and patients with compromised medical conditions, the decision is based on the balance between the risk of undergoing the surgery, the functional outcome anticipated, and the significance of the replantation to the patient. Life-threatening injuries and significant medical conditions that preclude long anesthesia times are contraindications to digit replantation. Microsurgical replantation in children or infants is indicated and can yield good functional outcomes. In elderly patients, the surgeon should take into consideration the potential systemic insult from the anesthesia and operation, the arteriosclerosis of vessels, and the poorer potential of functional recovery.

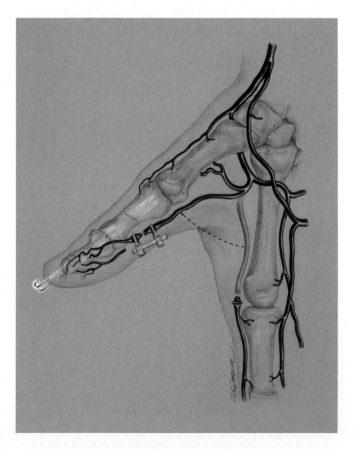

FIGURE 37-3

Transposition of an artery from an adjacent finger.

Warm ischemia times of less than 8 to 12 hours and cold ischemia times of less than 30 hours, measured from the time of amputation to the time of restoration of blood flow, are tolerated in digit replantation. Survival of replanted digits has been reported after as long as 42 hours of warm ischemia and 94 hours of cold ischemia. Immediate and proper cooling of the amputated part lengthens tissue survival.

A preoperative history of cigarette smoking does not seem to confer as negative an effect on the replantation as postoperative smoking. It has been shown to have significant negative effects on blood flow for up to 3 months. If the patient is unwilling to stop cigarette smoking, this could be considered a contraindication.

Amputated digits that are not commonly replanted are ones that are severely crushed or damaged, severely contaminated, have undergone multiple-level amputations, or are those of patients with multiple associated traumas or severe medical problems.

PREOPERATIVE PLANNING

A team approach is essential to the success of replantation. The transport team and the emergency room physicians should place the amputated part in appropriate dressings and arrange efficient transport to a center that has a replantation team. This team includes microvascular surgeons, anesthesiologists, operating room personnel and facilities, a microscope, and postoperative monitoring capabilities.

Minimal time should be wasted in obtaining unnecessary examinations. Many of the studies can be performed on the patient while the operating room is being prepared and, subsequently, the amputated finger is being prepared. If the operating room is ready and the patient is not, the finger can be taken to the operating room and prepared for replantation.

Obtaining a history and physical examination is necessary to aid in determining indications for surgery and avoiding postoperative complications and disappointing outcomes. Current events related to the injury are detailed, including the time and mechanism of injury, the location and conditions where the trauma took place, and the way the amputated digits or stumps were handled prior to admission. Information regarding the patient's general condition, including other injuries that occurred in relation to the current trauma and the patient's medical and surgical history, are obtained. The general examination of the patient is performed to exclude other major injuries. The amputated digit and the stump are examined in the emergency room. This examination is performed without digital blocks, which may cause injury to structures essential for successful replantation.

The amputated part is carefully preserved in a cool condition to minimize damage from ischemia. The amputated part is wrapped in gauze moistened with Ringer's lactate or saline solution, and placed in a plastic bag or specimen cup, which is then placed on ice. The amputated part is never placed directly on or immersed in ice or ice water, as this can cause freezing and permanent damage to the tissues.

Radiographs of the amputated digit and hand are taken to evaluate the condition of the bones and the presence of foreign bodies. The patient is kept in a warm environment, provided with adequate hydration, tetanus prophylaxis, and broad-spectrum antibiotics that are appropriate for the mechanism of injury and condition of the wound.

A discussion with the patient and the patient's family should include the risks of anesthesia, possibility of long operating times, potential need for blood transfusions, requirement for postoperative hospitalization, possibility of further surgery to salvage the finger in case of vascular compromise, the likely need for secondary procedures such as tenolysis, and the definite need for extensive physical rehabilitation postoperatively to achieve optimal outcomes. Patients are informed of the possibility that revision of the stump and closure of the wound might be performed; that vein grafts, nerve grafts, skin grafts, local flaps, regional flaps, or free flaps might be necessary to complete the reconstruction; and that bone shortening is often necessary in the primary reconstruction. The patient is made aware that there is a chance of immediate or late failure of the reconstructive effort and that other options for rehabilitation, such as prosthetic devices, might need to be resorted to in the future. Finally, if the patient is a smoker, he or she is told that smoking can affect the outcome and that postoperative smoking for up to 3 months can be detrimental to the final outcome of the surgery. The patient is given clear and realistic expectations regarding the expected outcomes.

Appropriate consultations with medical specialists are obtained. If a psychiatric disorder is suspected, a psychiatric consultation is obtained which in some circumstances might affect the decision as to whether to proceed with the replantation.

If an operating room is available, the amputated part is taken there first, examined under magnification, and set up for replantation while the patient is being prepared and anesthetized. Replantation is performed as soon as possible to shorten the ischemic time.

SURGERY

Patient Positioning

The patient is placed in a supine position with the arm abducted and placed over an arm table. A tourniquet is placed high up on the arm and on one of the lower extremities (in case vein, nerve, or skin grafts are required). Appropriate warming devices are placed to maintain normal body temperatures throughout the procedure.

General anesthesia is recommended, as replanting each digit requires between 2 to 4 hours to complete, and this usually becomes uncomfortable for the patient when an axillary block is performed. A brachial plexus block can be used to decrease the requirement for pain medication and decrease the incidence of vascular spasm in the operating room and postoperatively. Some authors use a brachial plexus block in addition to sedation in adults and older children with single-digit amputations in one extremity who are thought to be non-anxious and may tolerate 2 to 5 hours of immobility.

Preparation and cleansing of the stump and amputated part are performed using a povidone-iodine solution followed by copious irrigation with normal saline. A tourniquet is placed on the involved arm and one leg, and both are prepared and draped.

Technique

A two-team approach is used whenever possible, with one team working on the amputated part and the other working on the hand. The operative sequence for digit replantation varies slightly among surgeons and depends on the individual situation and ischemia time; however, our general routine is (1) identification of structures, (2) debridement, (3) bone shortening and fixation (Fig. 37-4), (4) repair of the extensor tendon, (5) repair of flexor tendons, (6) anastomosis of the artery, (7) coaptation of nerves, (8) anastomosis of veins, and (9) closure of the wounds.

Identification of Structures   During the dissection, the amputated part can be kept cool by placing it over a cooled apparatus. Bilateral mid-axial incisions are made, and the volar skin flap and dorsal skin flap are elevated, folded back, and sutured in position (see Fig. 37-2). If one team is performing the surgery, the exploration begins by identifying the neurovascular bundles and other structures in the amputated part using an operating microscope. High magnification minimizes inadvertent injury to important structures and decreases the chances of vasospasm. The digital arteries, one or two dorsal veins, and the digital nerves are identified and tagged with 6-0 sutures. The extensor and flexor tendons are located, trimmed, and tagged. If there is no artery available in the amputated part for anastomosis as is sometimes the case with ring avulsion amputations, the options for replantation become more limited. The use of an afferent arteriovenous shunt for the revascularization of unfavorable amputations of fingertips and distal phalanges may be an option (Fig. 37-5), or the replantation effort is halted and a revision and closure of the stump is performed (12,28–30).

Debridement   All non-viable tissue is excised while being careful not to cause inadvertent injury to important structures including the pulleys, particularly the A2 and A4 pulleys.

Bone Shortening and Fixation   Without excessive periosteal stripping, the bone is trimmed to provide surfaces that allow for good bone contact during fixation. Bone shortening also allows for direct vessel or nerve repair without tension, minimizes the need for using vein grafts and nerve grafts, and permits a more relaxed skin closure as postoperative edema can create compression of the vessels. Preservation of 5 to 10 mm of bone near a joint helps increase the range of motion that can be achieved. In traction avulsion amputations, the bone may require further shortening (19,36). Amputations through a joint are commonly treated with arthrodesis at the time of replantation. If this is not performed in the initial setting, eventual use of a silastic arthroplasty can solve some problems related to joint stiffness but is insufficient when the collateral ligaments are not present or do not provide adequate stability.

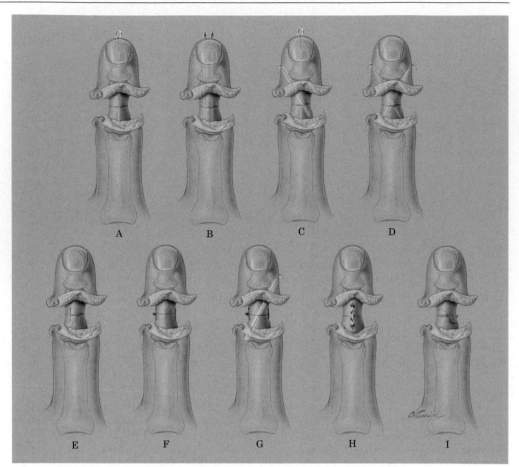

FIGURE 37-4

Different methods used for bone fixation. (*A*) One longitudinal Kirschner pin, (*B*) Two parallel Kirschner pins, (*C*) one longitudinal and one oblique Kirschner pins, (*D*) two oblique Kirschner pins, (*E*) two parallel interosseous wires, (*F*) two perpendicular interosseous wires, (*G*) one interosseous wire and one Kirschner pin, (*H*) plate fixation, (*I*) a screw for oblique fractures.

Bone fixation can be performed using crossed Kirschner wires (K-wires), two longitudinal K-wires, a single intramedullary K-wire, interosseous wiring, intramedullary screws, or external fixation devices (see Fig. 37-4). The type of fixation used depends on the stability of the fragments, the desire for early mobility, the compliance of the patient, and the preference of the surgeon. Plate fixation may be beneficial for fractures at the mid-shaft level as it allows for early mobility; however, plate fixation requires more extensive soft tissue dissection and periosteal stripping, and requires more time to perform. Longitudinally placed intramedullary or crossed K-wires that do not cross non-involved joints are the most commonly used methods. For replantations distal to the DIP, one K-wire may suffice. The authors prefer the use of interosseous wires when the replantation is performed at the level of the proximal part of the proximal or middle phalanx. Interosseous wiring provides adequate stabilization for early mobility and allows for adjustment of the alignment on an outpatient basis if malalignment is noted within the first week postoperatively.

Repair of the Extensor Tendon The extensor tendon is repaired using 4-0 medium-lasting sutures placed as horizontal mattresses or in a figure-of-eight fashion. Excessive and unnecessary manipulation, pinching, and grasping of tendons are avoided. In amputations at the proximal phalangeal level, the disrupted lateral band is repaired to achieve optimal extension function of the interphalangeal joints.

Repair of Flexor Tendons The flexor tendons are repaired by applying a modified Kessler technique using 4-0 nonabsorbable sutures followed by a running circumferential suture using a 6-0 monofilament nonabsorbable suture. Both the FDS and flexor digitorum profundus (FDP) are repaired meticulously. In zone II, only the FDP tendon is repaired to minimize subsequent tendon adhesion.

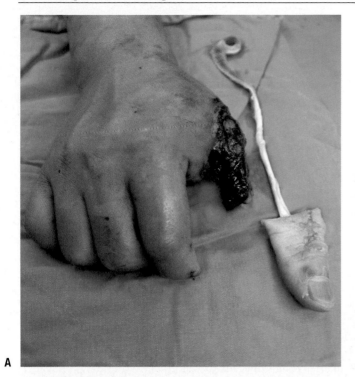

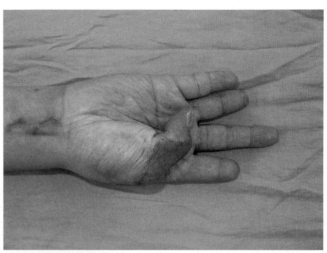

C

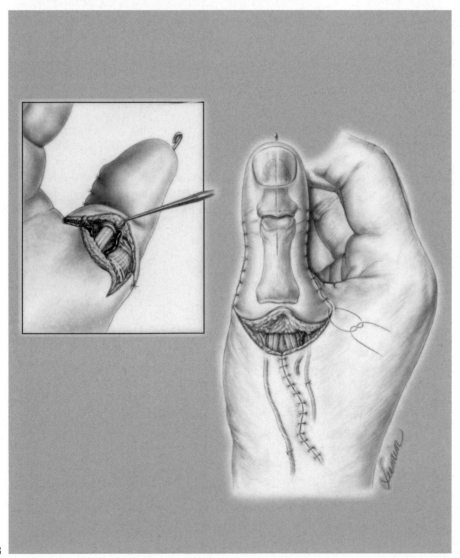

A

B

FIGURE 37-5

A: A 28-year-old man suffered from an avulsion amputation of his right thumb. The thumb was disarticulated at the interphalangeal joint and the skin envelope was avulsed proximally near the level of the metacarpophalangeal joint. Both digital arteries were avulsed from the distal amputee around the interphalangeal joint. The digital nerves were avulsed proximally near the level of wrist. The flexor pollicis longus tendon was avulsed at the level of the tenomuscular junction. **B:** Illustration demonstrating intraoperative details. The recipient artery in the hand was anastomosed to one of the volar veins to create an arteriovenous fistula. One dorsal vein was used as the outflow of the finger (a vein graft was necessary to bridge the gap). The bone was fixed using one longitudinal Kirschner pin through the interphalangeal joint. Both nerves were coapted to the superficial branches of the superficial radial nerve at the level of the anatomic snuffbox. **C:** Six months after replantation of the thumb using the arteriovenous technique.

Anastomosis of the Artery   The artery on both the amputated part and the proximal stump are examined under microscopic visualization and are cut at a level that causes no apparent damage to the vessel wall. The presence of bruising or thrombus, or the appearance of a coiled artery, indicates the need to trim the vessel further. The presence of thrombus within the lumen, or separation of the vessel wall layers, indicates damage and requires the vessel to be trimmed further. The outflow from the proximal stump of the artery is checked and should be spurting before it is considered adequate for revascularization. Hydration of the patient and maintenance of a systolic blood pressure over 100 mm Hg are important to achieving this purpose. Adventitia stripping often aids in relieving and preventing vessel spasm. Vein grafts from the volar aspect of the forearm or the dorsal foot are used as conduits whenever the gap is too large to complete the anastomoses without tension.

Revascularization can be provided by mobilizing a healthy undamaged artery from the adjacent digit (see Fig. 37-3). This technique provides inflow from a vessel that is unaffected by trauma, and obviates the need for vein grafting with its inherent risks. This can be performed in conjunction with transfer of the digital nerve in cases of thumb replantation. Vein grafts, nevertheless, are reliable, readily available, and avoid the need for incisions and scars in adjacent non-injured fingers.

When the digital artery is not available on the amputated part, afferent arteriovenous shunting can be used to perfuse the digit. Fukui and Yabe used this technique and found that a higher success rate was found when the inflow was from the artery of the stump to the volar veins rather than the dorsal veins. Anatomic studies by Moss and coworkers revealed that the direction of valves in the oblique communicating veins between the dorsal and volar veins favor flow from the volar veins to the dorsal veins. This technique can be successful in replantation of amputations as high as the interphalangeal joint (see Fig. 37-5).

If after release of the clamps the replant does not pink up, a waiting period up to 30 minutes is suggested. The vessels and the anastomosis are carefully inspected, adventitial stripping is performed, and the patency test is performed. Side branches, both proximal and distal to the anastomosis, can be tested to see if blood flow exists. Redo of the vascular anastomosis may become necessary because of either inadequate debridement of injured vessels or thrombosis at the anastomotic site due to inadequate microsurgical technique. Injection of high concentration heparin solution and/or thrombolytic agents is performed if all other factors are optimized and reperfusion seems to be inadequate.

Coaptation of Nerves   The nerve repair is performed by approximating the epineurium of both ends of the digital nerves using 10-0 or 11-0 sutures. Nerve grafts are used liberally to avoid any tension on the repair. Depending on the severity of the injury and outlook for wound coverage, secondary nerve grafting may be a better option to avoid exposure of this nonvascularized graft which may act as a source of infection and may result in poor function. The medial antebrachial cutaneous nerve and the sural nerve provide good sources of nerve fascicles for grafting purposes. In multiple-digit amputations, nerve grafts can be harvested from parts that are not planned for replantation. In avulsion cases of the thumb, sensory nerves from the avulsed finger can be attached to the dorsal sensory nerves of the first web space to restore protective sensibility.

Anastomosis of the Veins   The veins of the amputated part are inspected carefully after releasing the arterial clamps, and the ones with the most bleeding are anastomosed to the recipient veins in the hand. Dorsal veins are preferred for anastomosis. After separating the dorsal veins from the skin for a short distance and ligating a few branches, the length is usually adequate to complete the anastomoses primarily.

At least two veins are anastomosed whenever possible. Matsuda and coworkers evaluated the correlation between the number of anastomosed veins and survival rate in finger replantation. Their conclusions were that the essential amount of venous anastomoses is one in zone II (lunula to distal interphalangeal joint), two in zone III, and one in zone IV (proximal phalangeal region).

In situations where perfusion of the flap is good and there are no available dorsal veins for anastomosis, volar veins may be used. If there are no available veins or no outflow from any veins after a long waiting period, a last resort is to inspect the contralateral digital artery. If retrograde flow is present from the contralateral artery, that artery may be anastomosed to a recipient vein which can serve as an outflow vessel for the finger.

When replanting finger tip amputations and no sizable vein is present, other options include removal of the nail to keep continuous bleeding from the raw nail bed, postoperative periodic digital massage, and/or use of medical leeches. All these methods are performed with or without systemically heparinizing the patient.

Vein gaps can be bridged with vein grafts from the volar forearm or dorsal foot. If soft tissue is also lacking in the area where a vein graft is needed, a venous flap can be used which will provide a vein graft and a soft tissue cover.

Skin Closure   Meticulous hemostasis is obtained prior to closure of the wound. Under microscopic visualization, free ends of disrupted veins and arteries are carefully ligated. If only one artery is used for a finger, the contralateral digital artery is ligated to avoid postoperative bleeding. The skin is loosely approximated with a few interrupted sutures. The vessels are checked to make sure there is no compression or kinking with placement or manipulation of the hand and finger in different positions. Although a skin graft can be placed directly over the pedicle, rotation of a local skin flap is preferred and the defect from the rotation is skin grafted. Antibiotic ointment, non-adherent dressings, and wet gauze are placed over the incisions. No significant dressings are placed between the fingers to avoid potential compression of the digital vessels. Loosely placed circumferential dressings cover the hand.

Additional Procedures   Carpal tunnel release is performed for patients who have undergone avulsion amputations. The transverse metacarpal ligament is released, and the carpal tunnel is explored. In cases of severe avulsion amputations of the digits, forearm fasciotomies may be necessary.

RESULTS

Survival of replanted fingers ranges from 70% to 95% in both children and adults, with many patients achieving extremely satisfying results (Figs. 37-6 and 37-7). Survival rates are reported to be lower in avulsion and crush injury cases. Re-exploration due to vascular compromise is necessary in fewer than 20% of replantations and carries a salvage rate of approximately 70%.

Replantations of single or multiple digits when the amputation is distal to the sublimis insertion are highly satisfactory, both in terms of function and appearance, even without motion at the DIP. Secondary surgeries in these cases are rarely necessary.

A replanted thumb results in satisfactory outcomes in most patients, regardless of the type of injury or level of amputation (see Fig. 37-6). Even if a replanted thumb has a limited range of motion, it still plays an important role as a post for opposition. Schlenker et al reviewed their experience with 64 thumb replantations and found that 50% of the patients had two-point discrimination of less than 10 mm and an average active range of motion after replantation of 35% of normal for the interphalangeal joint and 29% of normal for the metacarpophalangeal joint. Most patients were able to return to work after approximately 7 months.

Sensory reinnervation is extremely important for the fingers to achieve optimal function. Glickman and Mackinnon reviewed the recovery of sensibility in 367 fingers and 87 thumbs that were replanted successfully. Average static two-point discrimination (S2PD) was 9.3 mm in clean thumbs versus 12.1 mm in crush/avulsion thumb replantations. Average S2PD was 8 mm in incisive injuries and 15 mm in crush/avulsion finger replantations. Mean S2PD was 11 mm in thumb replantations and 12 mm in finger replantations. Sixty-one percent of the thumbs and 54% of the fingers regained S2PD that was useful. They found that the factors that influenced sensibility were the age of the patient, the level and mechanism of injury, digital blood flow, cold intolerance, and postoperative sensory re-education. It was concluded that recovery of sensibility in the replanted digit is comparable to simple nerve repair and to nerve grafting techniques.

Cold intolerance is a significant problem following replantation. The exact mechanism of cold intolerance following digital nerve injury is not clear but may have a neurogenic or vascular origin. The more recovery of sensibility, the less cold intolerance seems to occur. Cold intolerance usually improves after approximately 2 years, but can persist for many more years.

POSTOPERATIVE MANAGEMENT

The patient is transported to a unit equipped with a warming device and highly trained nursing staff capable of performing hourly checks and recognizing signs of vascular compromise (Table 37-2). Every check includes an inspection of finger color, capillary refill, skin Turgor, and temperature. Pinprick testing and evaluation of vascular flow by hand-held Doppler ultrasonography are performed when the finger displays clinical signs of circulatory compromise. Temperature monitoring

FIGURE 37-6

A: A 57-year-old man sustained a crush injury of his right hand by a rolling machine. **B:** The thumb was completely amputated and the index and middle fingers were incompletely amputated at the level of the proximal phalanx and middle phalanx, respectively. **C:** The thumb was avulsed at the level of the proximal phalanx and the flexor pollicis longus tendon was torn from its tenomuscular junction. **D:** Nine months follow-up demonstrating adequate positioning of the replants and good strength. **E:** At 9 months follow-up the patient is able to grasp a pen.

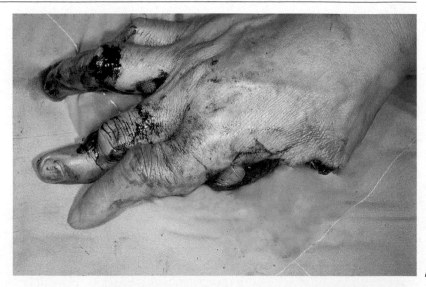

A

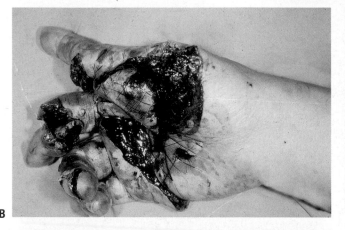

B

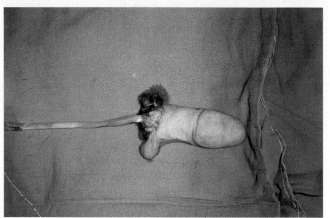

C

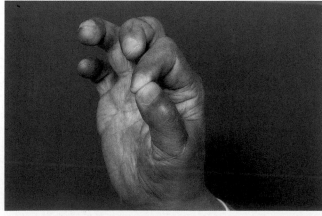

D

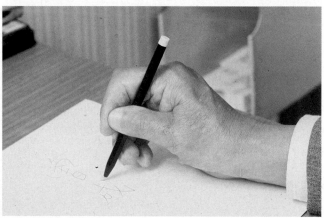

E

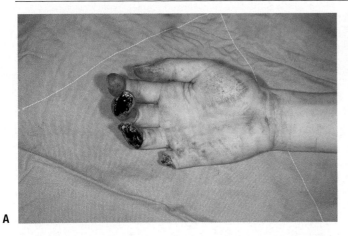

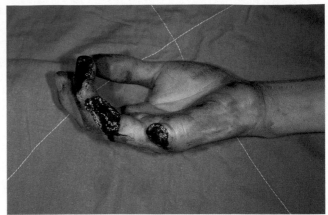

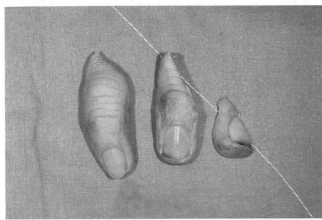

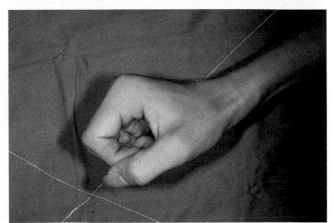

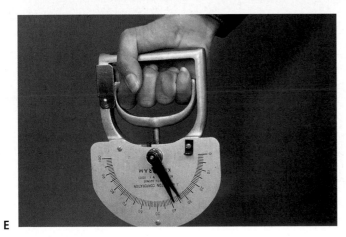

FIGURE 37-7

A: An 18 year-old man suffered from a sharp cutting injury by a machine saw. Volar view demonstrating the level of amputation of the three ulnar digits. **B:** This lateral view demonstrates the level of amputation of the long, ring, and little fingers. **C:** Dorsal view of the three amputated digits. **D:** At 9 months follow-up the patient has a good cascade and is able to make a fist. **E:** At 9 months follow-up, the patient is able to grip with good strength.

TABLE 37-2.   Signs of Arterial and Venous Compromise in Finger Replantation

	Arterial Compromise	Venous Compromise
Finger color	Mottled, bluish, or pale	Bluish, cyanotic, or dusky
Capillary refill	Sluggish (>2 sec)	Brisker than normal
Tissue turgor	Flat, decreased turgor	Tense, increased turgor
Temperature	Cool (>2° difference compared to control)	Cool (>2° difference compared to control)
Pinprick test	Scant amount of dark blood or serum	Rapid bleeding of dark blood
Doppler signals	Absence of pulsatile arterial signals	Absence of continuous or venous augment signals

of replanted digits has proved a reliable indicator of vascular status, as replanted digits are located in a terminal site with a terminal vascular loop that will not be influenced to a significant degree by heat exchange from the underlying bed. In general, a drop in temperature greater than 2°C from that of the control digit, or below 30°C, indicates the possibility of circulatory compromise.

A pulse oximeter placed distally on the replanted digit can be used to monitor changes in oxygenation. Laser Doppler flowmetry and photoplethysmography are used at some centers, but the cost of the instruments and the need for interpretation of the data have not proven its benefit over traditional methods such as clinical monitoring and temperature monitoring.

Intensive monitoring of replanted digits is undertaken for 3 to 5 days post replantation. Although thrombosis of vessels can occur up to 2 weeks following the replantation procedure, it is rare; and when it does occur, the chance of salvage is lower. This may be partly due to the delay in diagnosis in late thrombosis cases. In Betancourt's series of 71 replanted digits, the highest risk of critical thrombosis after replantation occurred in the first 3 days after surgery.

Patients' activities are monitored closely for the first 3 to 5 days to ensure that injury to the replanted part does not occur. The arm is elevated above heart level to decrease swelling, pain, and venous congestion. The level of arm elevation should not be excessive as to decrease arterial pressure in the hand and digits. Urine output and electrolytes are monitored to ensure adequate hydration to avoid vasoconstriction. Intraoperative placement of a continuous axillary brachial plexus block catheter can be a source of postoperative pain relief and can provide a chemical sympathectomy which may be applied for 3 to 5 days postoperatively.

The use of anticoagulants is controversial; however, heparin is often used in replantation cases. The authors favor the use of low-molecular-weight dextran starting in the operating room at the time of completion of the first vascular anastomosis. Systemic heparinization is used in replantation of crushed or avulsed digits or in cases where intraoperative vascular thrombosis occurs and requires revision of an anastomosis. Some authors recommend the use of aspirin at 325 mg per day, with the first dose administered prior to the replantation.

A warming lamp placed in the region of the replant and warming the patient's room may have some benefit. All patients are advised to avoid caffeine intake and cigarette smoking for at least 2 to 3 months following the surgery.

COMPLICATIONS

Immediate complications include partial or complete loss of the replanted digit due to circulatory compromise, infection, and bleeding. The presence of infection can lead to vascular thrombosis. This can be partially avoided by performing an adequate debridement and administering proper antibiotics based on the level and type of contamination. Skin necrosis can also be seen in the early phase due to inadequate debridement or compromise of blood supply to a part of the replanted digit. This scenario requires debridement and closure with local skin flaps, skin grafts, or transfer of more distant flaps.

Vascular Compromise Post Replantation

Following the detection of a change in one of the parameters used to assess finger or thumb perfusion, the decision is made on whether to proceed with exploration. It is our practice to have an aggressive approach to re-exploration and attempts at salvage. If arterial occlusion is suspected, the patient is immediately taken back to the operating room for re-exploration. If venous compromise is suspected, several maneuvers may be attempted prior to re-exploration: the dressing and some of the sutures are removed, the limb is elevated, and the patient is placed on a systemic heparin drip. If the digit does not show signs of improvement within 20 to 30 minutes, it is highly likely that the veins draining the replanted finger have undergone thrombosis. In this situation, the decision is made by the surgeon whether to take the patient back to the operating room or pursue a nonsurgical approach. For venous outflow obstruction in distal replantation, management by using medical leech therapy or continuous bleeding can be performed with high success rates. The nail plate is removed, a stab incision in the paraungual area is made, and a heparinized saline drip is placed over the incision site to maintain external bleeding. The smaller the replanted digit, the higher the salvage rate using these methods. In Han's series of 144 finger tip replantations with venous outflow through the use of this technique, the salvage rate was 70% (101 of 144 digits). The average period of the salvage procedure was 7.6 days. The duration of bleeding was different for different types of injuries: guillotine injuries required 5.9 days, crush injuries 8.2 days, and avulsion injuries 8.0 days.

Medical leeches, *Hirudo medicinalis*, have been reported to be effective for the treatment of venous outflow obstruction. The leech secretes hirudin, a potent anticoagulant, which acts locally without significant systemic effects. The therapeutic period required is approximately 3 to 5 days. Significant blood loss and the risk of infection (7%–20%) are the main disadvantages of this modality. The organism involved in infections from leeches is *Aeromonas hydrophilia*, and a third-generation cephalosporin is prescribed as a prophylactic method to prevent infections.

On exploration, the artery and vein are inspected. Occasionally, a hematoma is the cause of problem; however, a venous or arterial occlusion is often found. The thrombus is evacuated and arterial inflow or venous outflow are re-established. Vein grafts are used to reach healthy vessels when necessary. The steps are similar to the previously described procedure, including the occasional need to infuse high-concentration heparin solution and/or thrombolytic agents.

Late Complications and Secondary Procedures

The mechanism and level of injury, ischemia time, quality of the original repair, the postoperative rehabilitation program, and the effort put forth by the patient as well as the healing process all determine the final outcome. Depending on the combination of these factors, the resultant quality of finger function and the patient's lifestyle and motivation will determine whether the patient will seek secondary procedures to improve outcome. The majority of patients undergoing replantation (approximately 30% to 40% of patients who underwent finger replantation and up to 90% of patients with injuries in zone II) will require one or more secondary procedures. The physical therapist and surgeon follow the patient closely after the replantation and provide an aggressive and thorough physical rehabilitation program. Once the improvement has plateaued, usually at 6 months post-replantation, an evaluation of finger function and overall hand function will determine the need for secondary procedures. The patient's desires and level of function are of utmost importance in determining the need for surgery.

Frequent sequelae include tendon adhesions and joint stiffness. Avoiding transfixation of non-involved joints and performing a meticulous tendon repair decreases the incidence of these complications. Tenolysis as a secondary procedure is required in approximately 50% of finger replantations and up to 90% in patients with the level of amputation in zone II. Stiff proximal interphalangeal (PIP) and DIP joints are sometimes acceptable if the metacarpophalangeal (MCP) joint is mobile and allows for adequate grip. This is particularly true for the more ulnar digits. If the patient is able to use the thumb, index finger, and long finger to pinch objects adequately, he or she may be satisfied with the result and elect not to undergo further surgery. During the procedure of flexor tenolysis and/or tendon grafting, care is taken not to injure the repaired neurovascular bundle during the dissection. A detailed knowledge of the previous operative procedure can aid in avoiding injury to repaired structures. Pulleys are preserved, particularly the A2 and A4 pulleys. The tendon is exposed and inspected. If tendon rupture has occurred, tendon grafts with or without tendon rods are necessary in some patients. Ruptured or atrophied tendons are debrided. If the tendon is of poor quality, particularly in zone II injuries, reconstruction of the pulleys and insertion of a tendon rod followed later by tendon reconstruction may be the procedure of choice. Tendon grafts can be used to reconstruct the tendons if the quality of tendon appears good and the pulleys are intact. Pulley reconstruction and tenolysis are usually not performed in the same procedure. Extensor tenolysis is performed through dorsal longitudinal incisions and usually yields good results. Intrinsic reconstruction and dorsal arthrolysis are worthwhile when active and passive flexion are present. Arthroplasty can yield excellent results and is indicated for some MP and PIP joints. Arthroplasty can be performed along with other procedures such as tenolysis, capsulotomies, and capsulorrhaphies. Arthroplasty is performed through the same volar incisions that are used for the flexor tenolysis, or dorsal incisions are made. Vascularized joint transfers are indicated for replacing an MP or PIP joint, a flaccid thumb, or a fused MP or PIP of the index or other digits when the global hand function is good. The second or third toe metatarsophalangeal, PIP, or DIP joints are used from the toes.

Certain procedures are not performed simultaneously, such as tenolysis with procedures that require finger or hand immobilization (i.e., nerve repair, osteotomies, joint fusions, vessel repair and bone grafts). Some procedures can be performed together, such as tenolyses and arthroplasties. Malunion or nonunion can occur in up to 20% of replanted digits and seems to occur more commonly with replantations fixed with K-wires. Neurolysis, nerve repairs, and nerve grafts are indicated when the Tinel sign fails to cross the site of repair for 3 months. Early repair is advocated. Nerve grafts are used if the nerve injury is on the same side as the vascular repair to avoid injury to the vascular structures. It is important to find a healthy proximal stump for anastomosis. If not found, nerves from the dorsal radial sensory branches or the same or adjacent digits may be transferred.

Soft tissue coverage such as pulp transfers for thumb or opposable digits are sometimes necessary. Local flaps or free tissue transfer is sometimes necessary to cover open wounds or defects after contracture release of the flexor or dorsal side or the webspace. Perforator flaps and the lateral arm flap are good options for this.

Cold intolerance can be found in the majority of patients and most often resolves with time. Delayed circulatory compromise may occur up to 2 to 3 weeks post replantation, and often is caused by cigarette smoking or infection. Severe infections after digit replantation are rare and are usually related to inadequate debridement during the initial surgery or poor perfusion to the digit. Severe complications are unusual in digit replantation. Compression syndromes at the forearm or wrist level can occur and are usually associated with severe avulsion injuries. Fasciotomy and carpal tunnel release may be required in those cases. Web space contracture can occur as a result of thenar muscle contracture and/or soft tissue contracture in the web space. If the initial replantation is successful, late problems are usually related to suboptimal function due to poor motion and can be corrected with secondary procedures. Other secondary procedures that may be required are re-amputation, rotational osteotomies, and bone grafts.

RECOMMENDED READING

Axelrod TS, Buchler U. Severe complex injuries to the upper extremity: revascularization and replantation. *J Hand Surg Am.* 1991;16(4):574–584.

Baek SM, Kim SS. Successful digital replantation after 42 hours of warm ischemia. *J Reconstr Microsurg.* 1992;8(6):455–458.

Betancourt FM, Mah ET, McCabe SJ. Timing of critical thrombosis after replantation surgery of the digits. *J Reconstr Microsurg.* 1998;14(5):313–316.

Buncke GM, Buncke HJ, Kind GM, Buntic R. Replantation. In: Achauer BM, Eriksson E, Guyuron B, Coleman JJ, Russell RC, Vander Kolk CA, eds. *Plastic surgery indications, operations, and outcomes.* St. Louis: Mosby; 2000:2131–2147.

Buncke HJ, Alpert BS, Johnson-Giebink R. Digital replantation. *Surg Clin North Am.* 1981;61(2):383–394.

Buncke HJ, Whitney TM, Hill MK. Bony fixation in replantation. In: Buncke HJ, ed. *Microsurgery: transplantation-replantation. An atlas text.* Philadelphia: Lea & Febiger; 1991.

Buncke HJ, Whitney TM, Valauri FA, Alpert BS. Replantation surgery. In: Bncke HJ, ed. *Microsurgery: transplantation-replantation. An atlas text. Philadelphia:* Lea & Febiger; 1991.

Buncke HJ, Whitney TM. Secondary reconstruction after replantation. In: Buncke HJ, ed. *Microsurgery: transplantation-replantation. An atlas text.* Philadelphia: Lea & Febiger; 1991.

Cao X, Cai J, Liu W. Avulsive amputations of the thumb: comparison of replantation techniques. *Microsurgery.* 1996;17(1):17–20.

Chang LD, Buncke G, Slezak S, Buncke HJ. Cigarette smoking, plastic surgery, and microsurgery. *J Reconstr Microsurg.* 1996;12(7):467–474.

Zhong-Wei C, Meyer VE, Kleinert HE, Beasley RW. Present indications and contraindications for replantation as reflected by long-term functional results. *Orthop Clin North Am.* 1981;12:849–870.

Chen KT, Chen YC, Mardini S, Wei FC. Salvage of an avulsion amputated thumb at the interphalangeal joint level using afferent arteriovenous shunting. *Br J Plast Surg.* 2005;58(6):869–872.

Chen L, Gu J. Replantation of a completely detached degloved thumb. *Microsurgery.* 1996;17(1):48–50.

Chuang DC, Lai JB, Cheng SL, Jain V, Lin CH, Chen HC. Traction avulsion amputation of the major upper limb: a proposed new classification, guidelines for acute management, and strategies for secondary reconstruction. *Plast Reconstr Surg.* 2001;108(6):1624–1638.

Conrad MH, Adams WP Jr. Pharmacologic optimization of microsurgery in the new millennium. *Plast Reconstr Surg.* 2001;108(7):2088–2096.

de Chalain TM. Exploring the use of the medicinal leech: a clinical risk-benefit analysis. *J Reconstr Microsurg.* 1996;12(3):165–172.

Ekerot L, Holmberg J, Niechajev I. Thumb replantation or not? *Scand J Plast Reconstr Surg.* 1986;20(3):293–295.

Engkvist O, Wahren LK, Wallin G, Torebjrk E, Nystrom B. Effects of regional intravenous guanethidine block in posttraumatic cold intolerance in hand amputees. *J Hand Surg Br.* 1985;10(2):145–150.

Foucher G, Norris RW. Distal and very distal digital replantations. *Br J Plast Surg.* 1992;45(3):199–203.

Fukui A, Maeda M, Inada Y, Tamai S, Sempuku T. Arteriovenous shunt in digit replantation. *J Hand Surg (Am).* 1990;15(1):160–165.

Glickman LT, Mackinnon SE. Sensory recovery following digital replantation. *Microsurgery.* 1990;11(3):236–242.

Goldner RD, Urbaniak JR. Replantation. In: Green DP, Hotchkiss RN, Pederson WC, eds. *Green's operative hand surgery.* 4th ed. New York: Churchill Livingstone; 1999:1137–1157.

Gordon L, Monsanto EH. Skeletal stabilization for digital replantation surgery: use of intraosseous wiring. *Clin Orthop Relat Res.* 1987;214:72–77.

Graham B, Adkins P, Tsai TM, Firrell J, Breidenbach WC. Major replantation versus revision amputation and prosthetic fitting in the upper extremity: a late functional outcome study. *J Hand Surg Am.* 1998;23(5):783–791.

Green DP, Anderson JR. Closed reduction and percutaneous pin fixation of fractured phalanges. *J Bone Joint Surg Am.* 1973;55(8):1651–1654.

Han SK, Chung HS, Kim WK. The timing of neovascularization in fingertip replantation by external bleeding. *Plast Reconstr Surg.* 2002;110(4):1042–1046.

Ikeda K, Morikawa S, Hashimoto F, Tomita K. Fingertip replantation: pre-osteosynthesis vein graft technique. *Microsurgery.* 1994;15(6):430–432.

Jones NF. Replantation in the upper extremity. In: Aston SJ, Beasley RW, Thorne CH, eds. *Grabb and Smith's plastic surgery.* Philadelphia: Lippincott-Raven; 1997:981–998.

Khouri RK, Shaw WW. Monitoring of free flaps with surface-temperature recordings: is it reliable? *Plast Reconstr Surg.* 1992;89(3):495–499.

Kleinert HE, Jablon M, Tsai TM. An overview of replantation and results of 347 replants in 245 patients. *J Trauma.* 1980;20(5):390–398.

Kleinert HE, Juhala CA, Tsai TM, Van Beek A. Digital replantation: selection, technique and results. *Orthop Clin North Am.* 1977;8(2):309–318.

Koshima I, Soeda S, Moriguchi T, Higaki H, Miyakawa S, Yamasaki M. The use of arteriovenous anastomosis for replantation of the distal phalanx of the fingers. *Plast Reconstr Surg.* 1992;89(4):710–714.

Lendvay PG. Replacement of the amputated digit. *Br J Plast Surg.* 1973;26(4):398–405.

Matsuda M, Chikamatsu E, Shimizu Y. Correlation between number of anastomosed vessels and survival rate in finger replantation. *J Reconstr Microsurg.* 1993;9(1):1–4.

McC O'Brien B, Franklin JD, Morrison WA, MacLeod AM. Replantation and revascularization surgery in children. *Hand.* 1980;12(1):12–24.

Merle M, Dautel G. Advances in digital replantation. *Clin Plast Surg.* 1997;24(1):87–105.

Moss SH, Schwartz KS, von Drasek-Ascher G, Ogden LL II, Wheeler CS, Lister GD. Digital venous anatomy. *J Hand Surg Am.* 1985;10(4):473–482.

Nunley JA, Goldner RD, Urbaniak JR. Skeletal fixation in digital replantation: use of the "H" plate. *Clin Orthop Relat Res.* 1987;214:66–71.

Pederson WC. Replantation. *Plast Reconstr Surg.* 2001;107:823–841.

Reagan DS, Grundberg AB, George MJ. Clinical evaluation and temperature monitoring in predicting viability in replantations. *J Reconstr Microsurg.* 1994;10(1):1–6.

Schlenker JD, Kleinert HE, Tsai TM. Methods and results of replantation following traumatic amputation of the thumb in sixty-four patients. *J Hand Surg Am.* 1980;5(1):63–70.

Sherman R, Pederson WC, La Via AC. Replantation. In: Berger RA, Weiss AP, ed. *Hand surgery.* Vol 2. Philadelphia: Lippincott Williams & Wilkins; 2003:1543–1554.

Soucacos PN, Beris AE, Malizos KN, Vlastou C, Soucacos PK, Georgoulis AD. Transpositional microsurgery in multiple digital amputations. *Microsurgery.* 1994;15(7):469–473.

Stirrat CR, Seaber AV, Urbaniak JR, Bright DS. Temperature monitoring in digital replantation. *J Hand Surg (Am).* 1978;3(4):342–347.

Strauch B, Greenstein B, Goldstein R, Liebling RW. Problems and complications encountered in replantation surgery. *Hand Clin.* 1986;2(2):389–399.

Su HH, Lui PW, Yu CL, et al. The effects of continuous axillary brachial plexus block with ropivacaine infusion on skin temperature and survival of crushed fingers after microsurgical replantation. *Chang Gung Med J.* 2005;28(8):567–574.

Tamai S. Twenty years' experience of limb replantation: review of 293 upper extremity replants. *J Hand Surg (Am).* 1982;7(6):549–556.

Tark KC, Kim YW, Lee YH, Lew JD. Replantation and revascularization of hands: Clinical analysis and functional results of 261 cases. *J Hand Surg Am.* 1989;14(1):17–27.

Tsai TM, McCabe SJ, Maki Y. A technique for replantation of the finger tip. *Microsurgery.* 1989;10(1):1–4.

Tseng OF, Tsai YC, Wei FC, Staffenberg DA. Replantation of ring avulsion of index, long, and ring fingers. *Ann Plast Surg.* 1996;36(6):625–628.

Tupper JW. Techniques of bone fixation and clinical experience in replanted extremities. *Clin Orthop Relat Res.* 1978;133:165–168.

Urbaniak JR, Evans JP, Bright DS. Microvascular management of ring avulsion injuries. *J Hand Surg Am.* 1981;6(1):25–30.

Urbaniak JR, Hayes MG, Bright DS. Management of bone in digital replantation: free vascularized and composite bone grafts. *Clin Orthop Relat Res.* 1978;133:184–194.

Urbaniak JR, Roth JH, Nunley JA, Goldner RD, Koman LA. The results of replantation after amputation of a single finger. *J Bone Joint Surg Am.* 1985;67(4):611–619.

Weeks PM, Young VL. Revascularization of the skin envelope of a denuded finger. *Plast Reconstr Surg.* 1982;69(3): 527–531.

Wei FC, Chang YL, Chen HC, Chuang CC. Three successful digital replantations in a patient after 84, 86, and 94 hours of cold ischemia time. *Plast Reconstr Surg.* 1988;82(2):346–350.

Whitney TM, Lineaweaver WC, Buncke HJ, Nugent K. Clinical results of bony fixation methods in digital replantation. *J Hand Surg*

Index

Page numbers in *italics* indicate figures. Page numbers ending in *t* indicate tables.